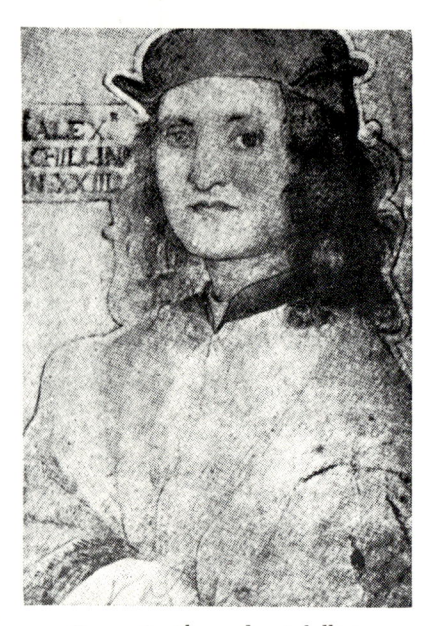

PLATE 1. Alessandro Achillini (1463-1512)

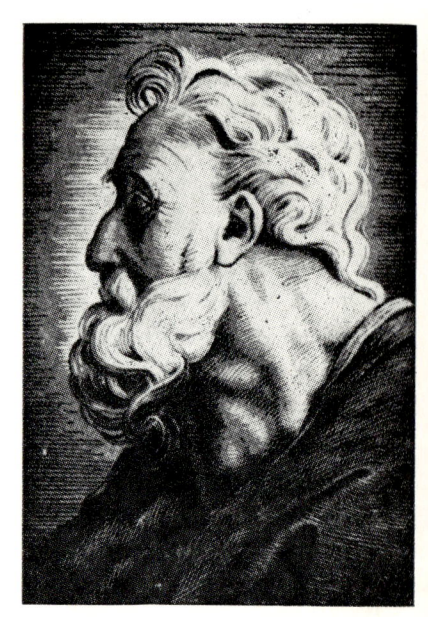

PLATE 2. Avenzoar (1113-1199)

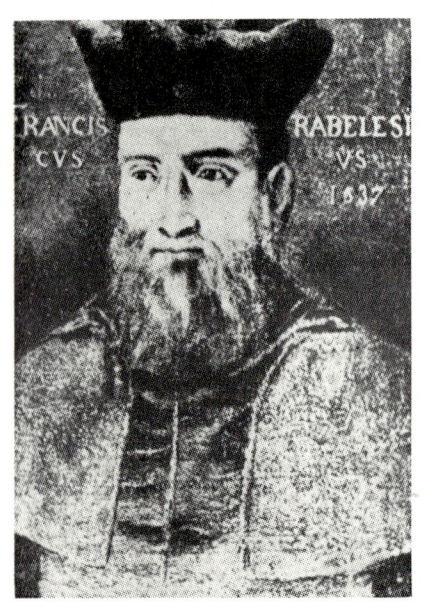

PLATE 3. Rabelais (1490-1553), wearing doctor's beret. One of the oldest pictures of the physician and writer. Medical faculty of Montpelier.

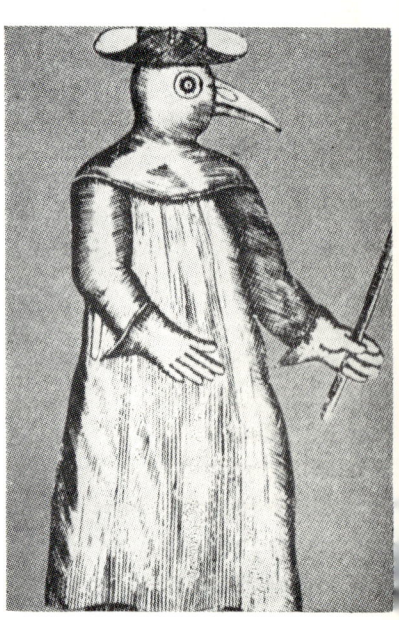

PLATE 4. Protective clothing of leather used by doctors, 1721. Frontispiece from Relation da la peste de Marseilles.

MEDIEVAL AND RENAISSANCE MEDICINE

by

BENJAMIN LEE GORDON, M.D., F.I.C.S.

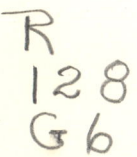

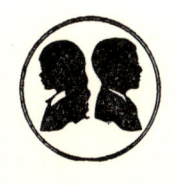

PHILOSOPHICAL LIBRARY
New York

Copyright, 1959, by Philosophical Library, Inc.
15 East 40th Street, New York 16, N. Y.

All rights reserved

Printed in the United States of America

DEDICATION

This book is affectionately dedicated to my eldest son
Cyrus H. Gordon, A.B., M.A., Ph.D.
Professor of Near Eastern Studies at Brandeis University,
a truly great scholar.

TABLE OF CONTENTS

		Page
	Preface	xi
Chapter		
I	Introduction	1
II	Early Medieval Medicine in the Western Empire	13
III	Byzantine Medicine	41
IV	Lay Medicine During the Early Middle Ages	69
V	Medicine in the Koran	86
VI	Post-Koranic Medicine	115
VII	The Arabian School of Translators	132
VIII	Famous Medical Authors of the Arabic Past	149
IX	Arabian Contributions to Chemistry and Pharmacology	183
X	The Arabo-Spanish Period	198
XI	Jewish Contributions to Medicine in the Middle Ages	237
XII	Scholasticism and Medicine	261
XIII	The Invention of Spectacles	288
XIV	The Rise of the Universities	299
XV	Medicine in Medieval Italy	313
XVI	Medieval French Medicine	338
XVII	Medieval Medicine in England	356
XVIII	Medicine in Medieval Germany	384
XIX	Medicine in Medieval Russia	399
XX	Anatomy in the Middle Ages	416
XXI	The Chirurgeon and the Barber Surgeon	427
XXII	Epidemic Diseases in the Middle Ages	456
XXIII	Tuberculosis and Other Infectious Diseases During the Middle Ages	474
XXIV	Smallpox During the Middle Ages	481

Chapter		
XXV	Leprosy in the Middle Ages	489
XXVI	Diphtheria During the Middle Ages	495
XXVII	Cholera, Dysentery and Trachoma in the Middle Ages	500
XXVIII	Malaria During the Middle Ages	514
XXIX	Syphilis and Other Diseases During the Middle Ages	524
XXX	Diabetes During the Middle Ages	539
XXXI	Epidemic Psychoses During the Middle Ages	545
XXXII	The Dancing Mania and Other Emotional Disorders	561
XXXIII	The Renaissance of Medicine	580
XXXIV	Medical Reformers	594
XXXV	The Revival of Anatomy	616
XXXVI	The Renaissance of Physiology	641
XXXVII	The New Birth of Pharmacology	657
XXXVIII	The Progress of Surgery	670
XXXIX	The Advance of Obstetrics	686
XL	The Growth of Ophthalmology	696
XLI	Theories and Studies of Contagion	702
XLII	Diseases Recognized During the Renaissance	724
XLIII	Sweating Sickness During the Renaissance	732
XLIV	The Liberation of Medicine	744
	Notes	765
	Index	825

LIST OF ILLUSTRATIONS

Plate 1. Alessandro Achillini.
Plate 2. Avenzoar.
Plate 3. Rabelais.
Plate 4. Protective clothing of leather used by doctors.
Plate 5. Hieronymus Fabricius.
Plate 6. Hieronymus Fracastorius.
Plate 7. Vesalius.
Plate 8. Portrait of Jewish physician.
Plate 9. Anatomical illustration from parchment roll.
Plate 10. The nervous system.
Plate 11. Theophrastus von Hohenheim.
Plate 12. Van Leeuwenhoek.
Plate 13. Vesalius.
Plate 14. Leonhard Fuchs.
Plate 15. Famous miracle of St. Cosmas and Damian.
Plate 16. Fabricius Hildanus.
Plate 17. Jean Baptista Von Helmont.
Plate 18. Luzzi de Mondino.
Plate 19. William Harvey.
Plate 20. Guy de Chauliac.
Plate 21. Guglielmo De Saliceto.
Plate 22. Fridericus Hoffmannus.
Plate 23. The Village Doctor.
Plate 24. The Medieval Physician.
Plate 25. Georg Bartisch.
Plate 26. St. Agatha.
Plate 27. Nicholas Culpepper.
Plate 28. The Physician, Joseph del Medigo.
Plate 29. Felix Platter.
Plate 30. John Caius.
Plate 31. Bernard De Cordon.
Plate 32. Thomas Sydenham.

Plate 33. Jean Pitard.
Plate 34. Conrad Gesner.
Plate 35. Averroes (Ibn Rushd).
Plate 36. Otto Brunfels.
Plate 37. Lanfranc.
Plate 38. Picture of a delivery.
Plate 39. Fransiscus De Le Boe Sylvius.
Plate 40. Nicolo Leoniceno.
Plate 41. Jesse Bennett.
Plate 42. Jerome Mercuriale.
Plate 43. Avicenna.
Plate 44. Vesalius.
Plate 45. Illustration of Caesarean section from Murcurio.
Plate 46. Rhazes.
Plate 47. Andres Laguna.
Plate 48. Arab physician preparing cough medicine.
Plate 49. Jean Astruc.
Plate 50. Jerome Cardan.
Plate 51. From Ketcham's Edition of *Mundinus*.
Plate 52. Silhouette of Jesse Bennett.
Plate 53. Facsimile of title page.
Plate 54. Traditional Portrait of Moses Ben Maimon.
Plate 55. Marcellus Malpighi.
Plate 56. João Rodrigues de Castelo Branco.
Plate 57. Ambroise Paré.
Plate 58. John Haryngton.
Plate 59. Arnold of Villa Nova.
Plate 60. Berengario de Carpi.
Plate 61. Ulrich von Hutten.
Plate 62. Frontispiece of the Hebrew text of Kitab-al Fusul fi-l-Tibb.
Plate 63. Amputation and Cauterization of Breast.
Plate 64. Jacobus Sylvius.
Plate 65. Athanasius Kircher.
Plate 66. Giovanni Alfonso Borelli.
Plate 67. Roger Bacon.
Plate 68. Thomas Linacre.

PREFACE

The favorable criticism received from members of the profession here and abroad by the book "Medicine Throughout Antiquity" and particularly from the two outstanding medical historians, Professors Max Neuberger and Arturo Castiglioni, has encouraged the author to present the present work, "Medieval and Renaissance Medicine."

It is the author's hope that the present work will at least partly fill the gap that lies between Claudius Galen and Thomas Sydenham.

Despite the dark shadows of superstition and barbarism which envelop medieval medicine, no one can study this period without becoming interested in it.

In preparing this work, the author has had to delve into widely diversified fields of literature to pick up salient facts, sift and classify them. The writer hopes that he has honestly striven not to be influenced either by polemics or by apologetics, but to serve the truth alone.

Many subjects in a work of this scope cannot be discussed as their importance might seem to warrant. A determined effort has been made to place emphasis on important facts.

Physicians who may read these pages may come across things that are well known to them. I cannot hope they will agree with all of my interpretations, but I trust they will get a sense of my pleasure in dealing with them.

The author is aware of the errors which in spite of every care taken to eliminate them must creep in when dealing with so many centuries of historical facts. He has attempted, wherever possible, to list all major sources at the end of each chapter.

The author is grateful to every writer from whom he has gleaned important knowledge. As much as he would have liked to mention everyone upon whose research he has drawn by name, some and doubtless even those who have furnished important information, have unintentionally been left unmentioned.

The author is greatly indebted to those who have supplied him with the interesting photographs and drawings, and to the editors of the various Medical Journals who have permitted him to use certain parts of his own articles previously printed in their publications. On this latter account I am especially indebted to Dr. H. A. Davidson, Editor of the Journal of the Medical Society of New Jersey, and to Dr. Wilfrid Haughey, Editor of the Journal of the Michigan State Medical Society.

The author wishes to acknowledge with thanks the advice and help received from his sons, Dr. Maurice B. Gordon and Dr. Cyrus H. Gordon. His son, Mr. Norman E. Gordon, assisted with the proofs.

BENJAMIN LEE GORDON, M. D.

MEDIEVAL AND
RENAISSANCE MEDICINE

CHAPTER I

INTRODUCTION

It is difficult to draw sharply defined lines in demarcating the beginning and ending of the Medieval Period. Old textbooks usually refer to the year 476 A.D. (the date of the final fall of Rome) as the start of this epoch and the year 1453 A. D. (the date of the fall of Constantinople) as the termination. This antiquated designation of a period of a thousand years is purely arbitrary.

The deposition of Romulus Augustulus, the last Roman Emperor in the West, in the year 476, was certainly not one of those events upon which the cultural history of the Western World depended. It did not even mark the final end of the Roman Empire for imperial unity was restored two years later for a short period. Likewise European culture did not suddenly regain ascendancy with the fall of Constantinople for the new conquerors of the Eastern Empire, the Turks, had little ambition for cultural advancement. To the contrary, their conquest of the Arabic countries extinguished the last vestige of Saracen civilization. The trend of historical investigations leads one to doubt the validity of any medieval period where the evolution of man became altogether stagnant. The advance of society has always continued. Of course, progress has not always been uniform. There was retrogression when barbarous races superimposed their substandard civilizations.

The period between modern and ancient times, however, does include a period of roughly a millennium. During most of these years, civilization was dragged down to a low level and mankind, hopelessly restricted by the authority of the Church, frittered away its existence with war and monastic dreams.

From the fifth to the eleventh century little progress was made in Europe. This epoch, often referred to as the Dark Ages, was a period in history when the higher ideals of European learning were relegated to a very base position. Only faint glimmerings of the great European civilization that had died continued to flicker in the dark cells of the monasteries where moth-eaten volumes of the works of the ancient Greeks were preserved but seldom referred to.

The power of the old civilization to absorb the new races had been exhausted by the fifth century and consequently the political history of Europe turned toward a different path. The fifth century witnessed the actual dismemberment of the Roman Empire. The peoples of Spain, Gaul, parts of Italy and Britain began forming the rude beginnings of what were to become the European national states of later centuries. This revolution was of sufficient magnitude to be regarded as the opening of a dark new era.

Both secular and independent learning deteriorated but the greatest stagnation took place in the fields of philosophy and medicine. A certain type of religious philosophy (known as Scholasticism) absorbed the attention of many thinkers from about the eleventh to the fifteenth centuries. Historians often refer to Scholasticism as the only intellectual interest of the Middle Ages. Most medieval intellectuals concerned themselves with petty and undeterminable problems as, for instance, how many angels can stand at one time on the point of a needle. There were a few medieval investigators who had true scientific eagerness—men like Roger Bacon, Duns Scotus and Occam were hopelessly outnumbered by those who were unscientific and uncritical in their learning.

FACTORS RESPONSIBLE FOR MEDIEVALISM

An important factor in creating the medieval intellectual vacuum was the continuous wars and the resulting famine and pestilence. Crops withered and vineyards rotted for lack of men to harvest the crops. Great epidemics that resulted from the general squalor and unsanitary conditions helped to destroy whatever cultural values remained from the days of the Old Roman Empire. It is known that a severe epidemic of bubonic plague ravaged Rome during Galen's time and that another one ravaged the city in the year 565 toward the end of the reign of Justinian.[1]

It is also known that many virulent epidemics prevailed in the year 543, which did much to weaken the domination of Italy over the Lombards. According to Gibbon,[2] 10,000 people died in Constantinople daily in the year 543. The venerable Bede (672-735) records pestilence in England in the years 664, 672 and 728.

Another major factor which must be considered when searching for the causes of the intellectual stagnation of the Middle Ages is the hierarchy of the Holy Roman Empire, although science was already on the verge of decay before Christianity was in a position to have any real effect on pagan thought. "Christianity," says Singer, "came to the ancient world as a protest and a revulsion against the prevailing and extremely pessimistic pagan outlook. Christianity brought men something for which to live. It was natural that it should oppose the philosophical basis of pagan thought. In this sense Christianity was certainly anti-scientific. Early Christian thought exhibits an aversion to the view which places the whole of man's fate under the dominion, the inescapable tyranny, of Natural Law. It is, however, essential to remember that the early Church, in developing this opposition, was not dealing with living observational Science. The conflict was simply with a philosophical tradition which contained dead, nonprogressive and misunderstood scientific elements." [3]

External factors, according to Plato, whether of nature or of human life and history, only become real when apprehended by the mind and the inconceivable is, in truth, impossible. According to the patristic doctrine, however, external facts can be considered as such only when they agree with theological dogmas. Under the disguise of neo-Platonism, the modes of thought inaugurated by Plato were circumvented to permit absorption of religious doctrines and, for that matter, all popular superstition. As a matter of fact, in the first few centuries of the present era, there coexisted a deep and prevailing undercurrent of primitive magic rites and beliefs, with the formal religious philosophies which were formulated by the early Fathers.

Natural knowledge was valued only in so far as it elucidated or exemplified the doctrines of the Church, or the passages of the Scriptures. Under such domination, critical power all but ceased to exist, and anything was believed if it was in accord with the Scriptures as interpreted by the Fathers.

One may appraise the contemporary knowledge of natural history in the second century from the compilation called *Physiologus* or *Bestiary,* in which the subjects originally were intended to be used as allegories taken from the animal world, but which, by doctrinal considerations, were later taken to be factual in nature. For example, it is seriously stated in this work that the cubs of the lioness are born dead, and on the third post-mortem day, are brought to life by the lion breathing between their eyes. This is used to illustrate "the resurrection of our Lord, the Lion of Judah."

Although a synod in 496 condemned *Physiologus* because it provoked scoffing in some and led others to heresy, this work continued to be widely read and even Gregory the Great did not disdain to allude to it on occasions. As a matter of fact, for an uncomfortably long period, *Physiologus* was considered *the* textbook of natural history. It illustrates the intellectual status of Europe when the last gleams of the sunset of ancient civilization were fading away into the dark night of the sixth and seventh centuries. Everything was accepted when endowed with supernatural sanction, and there was no critical insight.

In view of the fact that medicine was an art in which all men were personally interested, it was impossible for the Church to entirely control the art as was done with other branches of secular knowledge. It was, however, as much as possible removed from the secular field and confined to the monastery and cloister. Its practice was turned over to monks and priests. Henceforth, the tending of the sick remained a Christian duty.

In the sixth century the Benedictine monks began to study compendiums of the works of Hippocrates and Galen and this order gradually spread this knowledge throughout the West. The monks also had some knowledge of agriculture and were particularly interested in plants and herbs which were used as remedies.[4]

The belief however that monks and friars were the rational doctors of the Middle Ages is definitely unfounded. If the chroniclers, here and there, celebrate a monk's skill, the context itself nearly always shows that such skill was exceptional. The famed abbot Faricius was an excellent physician but he had mastered his profession outside the Church in his "worldly" days. A few early friars may be found tending lepers as an exercise of extreme Christian charity, but it would be difficult to find a single case, after the days of Francis and Dominic, of leper-hospitals regularly visited by them. Indeed, the distinguished ascetic, St. Bernard, addressed himself to a monk practicing medicine, as follows: "Thou art a monk, not a physician."

Medical books are often found in monastic libraries but the weight of evidence suggests that little was known or practiced in the monastic infirmaries beyond what was contained in the traditional leechdoms, or lists of old wives' remedies. The voluminous evidence of ecclesiastical prohibitions or restrictions of medicine is briefly and clearly summarized by the editors of *Johannes de Mirfeld*. Father Hilarin Felder quotes the text of two of the most important official prohibitions, and comments: "It is plainly signified by these that the study of medicine, since it is not directly connected with theology, is not adapted as a worldly occupation for the clergy. The Dominicans, in fact, expounded the relevant decisions in that sense, and considered the study of physic, in the sense of medicine, as forbidden by the Church."[5]

Until the latter part of the twelfth century medicine could hardly be considered a science, for it was not based on exact knowledge. Its practice was stereotyped, dogmatic, and devoid of any lofty outlook. The physician had no means of checking his conclusions by scientific measures nor did he care to devise means beyond those which were known to antiquity. He had no instruments to prove whether he was right or wrong in his diagnoses. He did not possess even so simple a device as a clinical thermometer without which modern physicians would be completely lost. The thermometer of course, is of comparatively recent design.[6]

The medieval physician did not seek to attain an understanding of the pathology of disease nor to investigate its etiology so that he might be enabled to prevent it or treat it intelligently. His only ambition was to collate ancient opinion about the particular case in question. This is practically what the Arabic medical writers, with the exception of Rhazes (850-950), Avenzoar (1113-1162) and Maimonides (1135-1204), have accomplished.

THE ARABIAN INFLUENCE

The Arabian mind was essentially concerned with compiling and remembering knowledge from all sources rather than initiating inquiry. In this direction great and useful work was carried out during the most happy days of the Saracen empire. The modern world is greatly indebted to these careful preservations of knowledge and to the additions of numerous copies of standard works on medicine before the period of printing, even though the science and art of medicine did not advance a single step through such efforts.[7]

Avicenna (950-1037), the greatest of Arabian scientists, followed the teachings of Galen and Hippocrates without questioning any of them. He was not an experimenter as much as a philosopher and his power over so many centuries in the field of medicine may be attributed to his masterly grasp of all contemporary science. His skill in dealing with fundamental mathematics is even now hardly surpassed. He is almost the sole instance of a great mind applying mathematical concepts to medicine.

It is not unfair to say that most of the writers of the Middle Ages were mere recorders, devoid of any spark of new thought, who preserved with reverence old traditions and knowledge. They lost themselves in subtle speculations. They found new meanings in old phrases. They were "diligent in dressing old words with new meanings" and their ingenuity in so doing became the standard of their scholarship.

In all this period, no new thought is found, no new methods, and no new experiments. To dissent from the authority of Hippocrates and Galen was not merely wrong but a heresy punishable by extreme penalties.

But even with such gross lack of initiative in the East, the physician of Europe was considerably behind his Islamic colleague. For a period of five hundred years the doctor of the West manifested no tendency to free himself from intellectual bondage.

The revival of medicine in the West may be traced to the translations of the Arabic versions of the Greek medical and more particularly philosophical authorities into Latin.

The new secular home of medicine was Salerno on the bay of Pacestume, and from this center appeared many works founded on the writings of Hippocrates and Galen. The physicians of Salerno were already known in the ninth century and in the eleventh century they began to read translations in the Latin language from the Arabic works. It is possible that there existed in Salerno an unbroken link between ancient learning and that of the modern world, for Salerno was a Greek colony and a Roman health resort and the tradition of Greek medicine appears to have never been interrupted.

The chief translator was Constantine Africanus (1020-1087) of Carthage who traveled extensively in Egypt and India in the pursuit of knowledge.[8] He was accused of sorcery when he returned to Carthage and was obliged to flee for his life. He fled to Salerno where he was appointed secretary to Robert Guiscard who had shortly before captured the town. He soon resigned his position and entered the monastery at Mount Cassino where he wrote the many medical works bearing his name. According to J. Freind's

History of Physics (1750), most of what he wrote was merely translations of the Greek and Arabian authors and in many instances he did not scruple to pass off other men's books as his own. In spite of the fact that he was guilty of gross plagiarism we owe Constantine the credit for the injection of Arabic medicine into the medical learning of Europe. This led to the advance of the first medical school in Salerno and to the publication of the *Regimen Sanitatis Salernitanum*.[9]

The twelfth and thirteenth centuries, which witnessed the great struggle between the secular and spiritual powers in the state, witnessed also the rise of a lay-inspired literature which helped medicine to emancipate itself from the slavery of the stereotyped ecclesiastical teachings.

The science of medicine made its way from the East by way of Spain. The names of Messua, Geber, Hunain ibn Ishak, Rhazes, Isaac Judeus and Avicenna gradually became familiar in European circles. In Spain, Arabian medicine made great headway. It brought forth physicians of the type of Abul Casim, Avenzoar and Maimonides.

To the Arabs we are indebted for the survival of science through the Middle Ages. Their conquests brought the Arabs into contact with the Greek literary tradition through the Syrian translations of the Greek writers.

Most of the physicians in the Caliph's dominions were Nestorians and there can be no doubt that many learned Nestorians professed Islam without any serious compunction or any great change in their work and thoughts. To these Nestorian teachers came the young, keen and curious Arab minds fresh from the desert. These students learned much and even improved upon the teachings of their professors.

The Nestorians were not the only teachers available to the Arabs. Throughout all the rich cities of the East the Jews were scattered with their own distinctive literature and traditions. It can safely be stated that the Arab and the Jewish minds reacted upon one another from common advancement. The scholarship of the Jews has never been tied down by linguistic barriers. A thousand years before Islam, they spoke Greek in

Alexandria, and now all over this new Moslem world they were speaking and writing Arabic. Some of the greatest Jewish literature of all time was written in Arabic, e.g. *Emunoth We-Deoth,* by Saadyah Gaon (882-942), *Fons Vitae* or *Mekor Hayyim* by Avencebral or ibn Gabriol and *The Guide of the Perplexed* by Maimonides.

It can be reiterated that while European learning was at its lowest ebb, a considerable amount of culture of mixed Greek, Roman and Jewish origin, survived in the countries which stretch from Syria to the Persian Gulf. One of the earliest centers of this culture was the Persian school of Jondisabur, which gave refuge to Nestorian Christians in 489, and to the Neo-Platonists who left Athens when Plato's Academy was closed in 529. Here translations, especially of Plato and Aristotle, brought Greek philosophy into touch with the philosophies of India, Syria and Persia, and led to the growth of a school of medicine, which survived until the tenth century.

One hundred and fifty years after the Arabian conquest, Harun-al-Rashid, the most famous of the Abbasside Caliphs, and his followers, helped to initiate the great period of Arab learning by encouraging translations of Greek authors. At first the advance was slow, for new terms and constructions suitable for the expression of philosophic and scientific medical thought had to be formed in the Arabic language, but gradually the hidden and forgotten stores of Greek knowledge were recovered and incorporated into Islamic culture. Finally, the Islamic scholars added their own contributions to the art and science of medicine.

Dr. Stanley Lane-Poole says: "No more astonishing movement in the history of civilization has occurred than the sudden passion of the whole Islamic world for culture . . . this was the supreme service of Islam to general culture. Bagdad was its great Hall of Science built by the son of Harun-al-Rashid. Cordova with its schools of renowned physicians, and Toledo (the center from which after its capture by Christian forces in 1085 a stream of translations issued) became bright glowing stars in the firmament of Arabic learning."

The Classical Period of Arabic medicine, during the ninth

and tenth centuries may be said to have its origin with the medical works of the Persian, Abu Bakr al Razi, known to Europe either as Rhazes or Bubacher, who practiced in Bagdad and compiled many encyclopedic textbooks, including a famous treatise on measles and smallpox. He is held to be not only the greatest physician of Islam but, indeed, of the whole world during the Middle Ages. He also applied chemistry to medicine and used the hydrostatic balance to measure specific gravities. Alexandrian alchemists of the first century were the first to attach chemical problems to medicine but little was done after them for six hundred years until the Arabians took up their work.

The most famous Arabian alchemist was Abu-Musa-Jabir-ibn Hayan, who flourished about 776. He is thought to be the original of many writers whose works appeared later in Latin and were designated as having been authored by the shadowy "Geber." [10]

While learning in Europe was at its lowest ebb, a considerable amount of culture of mixed Greek, Roman, and Jewish origin survived in the Byzantine imperial court of Constantinople and in the countries which stretch from Syria to the Persian Gulf. One of these schools was Jondisabur. The students of Jondisabur were basically philosophers, who desired to investigate the whole world—the visible as well as the invisible. Medicine in these days was considered a branch of philosophy. These philosophers none-the-less exercised great influence upon the development of the natural sciences.

THE BYZANTINES

The Byzantines were principally eclectics. They collected the writings of the best Greek authors and preserved them for posterity. Men of the type of Oribasius, Aetius, Paul of Aegina, Alexander of Tralles, Theophilus, Johannes Actuarius and Caelius Aurelianus considered themselves the pupils of ancient authority. They adhered strictly to their views and added only slight variation. They greatly increased their knowledge of Galen over other Greek writers. As Wittington has aptly remarked: "Had Galen's work been lost there can be little doubt that the dark age of medicine would have been darker, and more prolonged than it was."

The medieval physician preferred Galen's teaching of monotheism and his doctrine of teleology to that of Hippocrates' teaching "On the Secret of Disease," and he preferred the queer "Herbals" and the strange "Beastiaries" (the beast books) of Pliny to the "Materia Medica" of Dioscorides.

MEDIEVAL ENGLAND

In England literary and historical development culminated in the works of the Anglo-Saxon monk, Bede of Jarrow (673-735), author of *Historia Ecclesiastica Gentis Anglorum* who incorporated into his writing all the knowledge available in western Europe. His science was founded chiefly on the natural philosophy of Pliny. Bede stands between the Latin commentators Boethius, Cassiodorus, Gregory and Isidore of Seville who caught the last direct echoes of the classical or patristic learning, and the scholars of the schools of the abbey, founded by Charlemagne, chief among whom was Alcuin of York. Alcuin did much to overcome the prevalent idea that secular knowledge was opposed to religion and he carried the tradition of classical knowledge well into the middle ages.

Bede wrote his works in Latin, mainly for monks, but 150 years later culture had so advanced that Alfred the Great (849-901) translated or caused to be translated many Latin books into the Anglo-Saxon language.

From the *Medicinale Anglicume* known as the "Leech Book of Bald," the earliest Anglo-Saxon manuscript that exists, something may be gleaned concerning the leeches of the period. Bald himself, the owner of the book, was a man of learning. He refers to his library and tells us that he loves his precious volumes "more than fees or stored wealth."

Pagan medicine began, as we know, in faith, or rather in

theurgic superstition, and finally became a philosophical science. The same statement holds true with regard to the Christian medicine of the Middle Ages. Its philosophical phase extended through the scholastic period, and here too it represents a real advance, which must be regarded as one of the historical proofs that medieval medicine in general belongs to a progressive development. Medieval medicine was not, and did not remain, simply the medicine of the ancients, but began to combine with popular medicine. This was a new phase of development, with which of course, an important part of ancient medicine was combined. New and old, indeed, in every metamorphosis of civilization, join hands with each other.

When Michelangelo was asked how he had carved the Statue of Night on the Medici Tombs, he replied: "I had a block of marble in which was concealed that statue you see there. The only effort involved was to take away the tiny pieces which surrounded it and prevented it from being seen. Every piece of stone whether large or small, has a statue or effigy concealed within it, but of course one must know exactly how to carve away only that which hides it and this is very dangerous in that one may take away too much or too little." The medieval scholar did not carve away the pieces which concealed the effigy, but instead carved away the tiny pieces of the effigy itself. He discussed the nature of universals, and the relationship between ideas and matter and other such subtilities, but forgot that nature herself was not consulted for her secrets.

In conclusion one may say that medieval medicine was the growth of faith in authority which permitted no induction nor experimentation in contradistinction to ancient medicine which was a science of thoughtful observation and experimentation.

CHAPTER II

EARLY MEDIEVAL MEDICINE IN THE WESTERN EMPIRE

In order to get a clear idea of the circumstances that led to the decadence of medicine after the fall of the Western Roman Empire, it is pertinent to review briefly the political condition of Rome during its declining days.

A census of the Roman Empire taken when Julius Caesar (102-44 B.C.) held sway would have revealed perhaps more than a hundred million inhabitants, scattered throughout Europe, North Africa, and Asia Minor. At this period, the vast majority of the peoples of Europe were subject to Roman rule and the entire Empire was effectively governed by several thousand more or less worthy persons. In later years, however, the ruling power became concentrated in the hands of a score or more of unscrupulous individuals, who assumed dictatorial powers over the vast dominions.

The Roman colonial population consisted primarily of tribesmen of the plains and forests who were known among the Greeks and Romans as "barbarians." The main tribes of barbarians were, to the west: the Goths, the Vandals, the Angles, the Saxons, and the Jutes; and to the east: the Huns. The earliest Germanic settlers in the Roman Empire had been the Goths. They originally lived on the shore of the Baltic and wandered to the south. The Visigoths settled on the shores of the Black Sea and the Ostrogoths on the Danube.

Some of these barbarians found their way to the Roman capital and to the larger cities of the Empire as slaves. Others came as soldiers who were trained in the motherland either to help in further conquest or to guard the homeland against the machinations of its enemies.

In the course of time, the barbarians literally lived to pay tribute to the mother country so that a comparatively few native Roman citizens might live in luxury.

Wealthy Romans bought their way into high office and controlled the Empire with the wealth they had accumulated through slave labor. On the one hand, they built temples and erected magnificent public buildings, and on the other, they amused themselves with elaborate but sadistic gladiatorial shows and circuses. They constructed roads extending to their most distant possessions. To the *vulgus* or masses of common people at home, and to those barbarians who traveled the fine roads to find a better living condition in Rome, they handed out doles of grain and oil.

The barbarians, although primitive in their way of life as compared to their masters, loved freedom. They never gave up looking for a chance to become free. Naturally enough, none of the things that pleased the native Roman citizens brought contentment to the oppressed peoples of the conquered lands who outnumbered the native Roman citizens manyfold. The concentration of wealth and political power in the hands of a few carefree, pleasure-loving individuals merely hastened the moral decadence of the Roman Empire. This centralization of power by wealthy but unscrupulous individuals gave rise to well-nigh universal depravity and lawlessness, to betrayal of parents, husbands, and wives. Adultery degenerated into incest. Women became lascivious, depraved and dangerous and their depravity resulted in further wicked practices. The marriage institution was violated by general accord and concubinage became the order of the day. Promiscuous bathing and naked exhibitions were legalized. Even the very Vestal Virgins were guilty of inconceivable immoralities.

Rome, during the closing years of the Western Empire, thus sank deeper and deeper into an abyss of corruption, depravity, and moral decadence. True Roman culture vanished; education no longer was a standard of social distinction; wealth and political power became the only yardsticks by which one was esteemed.

Tacitus (55-120 A.D.) gives an eye-witness' description of the depravity of Rome:

"The holy ceremonies of religion were violated. Adultery reigned without control. The adjacent islands became filled with exiles. Rocks and desert places became stained with clandestine murders. Rome itself became a theater of horrors where nobility of descent and splendor of fortune marked men out for destruction; where the vigor of mind that aimed at civil dignities, and the modesty that declined them, were offenses without distinction; where virtue was a crime that led to certain ruin; where the guilt of informers and the wages of their iniquities were alike detestable; where the sacerdotal order, the consular dignity, the government of provinces, and even the cabinet of the prince, were seized by that execrable race as their lawful prey; where nothing was sacred, nothing safe from the hand of rapacity; where slaves were suborned, or by their own malevolence excited against their masters; where freemen betrayed their patrons, and he who had lived without an enemy died by the treachery of a friend." [1]

The corruption among high state officials soon reached a point where they did not shrink from murder to get rid of a political opponent.

Valentinus III was murdered by Petronius Maximus (455 A.D.) who succeeded him. Valentinus' widow, Eudoxia, in order to avenge her husband's death, invited Genseric from Africa to take possession of the capital, thus exposing the nation to bloodshed and pillage and to the rule of the barbarians.

With such conditions prevailing in the mother country, it is not surprising that many European provinces took this opportunity to throw off the Roman yoke and become independent. The Vandals who had settled in Spain, the Angles and Saxons who had migrated into Britain, and the Huns who had moved into France achieved varying measures of autonomy.

The captures of Rome by the Visigoths in 410 and again by the Vandals in 455 were not unexpected. Almost a century earlier (355 A.D.), Emperor Theodosius the Great, foresaw the fate that was already overtaking his great empire and divided his dominion between his two sons. The western division he bequeathed to Honorius and the eastern division, which consisted of Greece, Egypt, Macedonia, Asia Minor, East Africa and Thrace, to Arcadeus who established his capital at Byzantium (Constantinople).

The division of the great empire was primarily made because of the organic difficulties that had arisen in attempting to govern the eastern provinces from the western capital. The Romans, as is well known, were not a seafaring nation. They traveled largely by land for which purpose they constructed fine roads. The Italian peninsula, projecting as it does far out from the mainland, rendered traveling to the distant provinces more difficult. In order to enable soldiers and tax collectors to control the eastern provinces more substantially, it was deemed best to have a central headquarters located in the eastern division. This became particularly vital after some of the European colonies declared themselves independent of the mother country. The division was not one that was logical on a geographical basis only; there also was a linguistic reason for the more cultured element of the eastern states spoke the Greek language, while the population of the western division spoke Latin.

The cities of the western division, as the period of Roman sovereignty reached its termination, had a large population of barbarians who intermingled freely with the native Romans not as slaves but as equals. A large number of the barbarians had come to Rome even prior to this period as mercenaries or draftees from the colonies to be mustered into the Roman army. When Rome became politically weak these colonists formed a first-rate fifth column so that when Odoacer finally attacked Rome, King Romulus, the last reigning king of the once great Roman Empire, was easily defeated. (It was indeed a curious coincidence that the last Roman emperor bore the same name as the legendary founder of Rome.)

The dismemberment of the Western Roman Empire proved a great loss to science, art and literature. Great literary treasures were destroyed for the barbarian conquerors did not appreciate the value of the written word. Of course, the Church, as will be shown later, saved some of the wreckage of this ancient culture. Some medical treasures found asylum in the monasteries and other Graeco-Roman manuscripts were carefully guarded in the libraries of Alexandria and among the scholars in the Eastern Empire.

The fall of Rome (476 A.D.) left the empire with no central controlling power. Europe was in a chaotic state and law and order as such ceased to exist. Learning and culture in general became more and more a matter of the past. Medicine became a rich harvest for the quacks, the drug peddlers, the sorcerers, and the exorcists who flocked to the old capital from near and far in the hope of attaining quick riches.

Even nature seemed desirous of adding its own chaos to the political disruption. Earthquakes, inundations, epidemic diseases, and famines which helped stifle all scientific and cultural progress, were the order of the day, and succeeded in bringing down medical science to complete stagnation.

The severe epidemics in Italy, often following earthquakes or inundations, swept away entire communities. The poet Ovid (43 B. C.-17 A.D.) graphically described one of these pestilences that ravaged Rome during his time. It not only destroyed humans but even animals and fish.[2]

The epidemic of 79 A.D. followed the eruption of Vesuvius which destroyed Pompei and Herculaneum. This plague rapidly spread through Campagna where it is said that ten thousand people perished daily. There was hardly enough time to forget this terrible scourge when an even worse epidemic broke out in Orosius (125 A.D.). This latter plague was attributed to an invasion of the crops by hordes of grasshoppers which resulted in famine and later a severe form of bubonic plague broke loose. More than eight hundred thousand were recorded to have died in Numidia alone. Like wildfire, the holocaust spread to the African coast where more than two hundred thousand died in Carthage and Utica. In Utica alone, more than thirty thousand soldiers succumbed to this disease.

The Plague of Galen (166 A.D.; so called because Galen's enemies accused him of leaving Rome because of this epidemic) lasted for a period of six years. It was brought home to Rome by soldiers who returned from the East. According to contemporary writers, thousands of persons died daily in the capital. From the symptoms described by contemporaries this epidemic appears to have been a severe form of typhus. The most fearful plague of all is said to have been a smallpox epidemic which raged in the year 312 A.D. This resulted in an incalculable destruction of life.

These frequent catastrophes all did their share in enormously weakening the Roman nation politically, physically and spiritually. A people, harassed by bitter foes from without and facing death at every corner from within, have little inclination to pursue the studies of the arts and sciences.

On scientific medicine particularly, these periodic scourges had a most disastrous effect. People lost confidence in their physician when they observed that his efforts to help them were obviously so futile. At such times particularly, people take to spiritual and miraculous cures.

The fall of Rome left the empire no general controlling power. The mixed political authority was too weak to enforce any hygienic regulations when a calamity such as a severe epidemic broke out.

On the one hand, medicine became the happy hunting ground of the quack, the drug peddler, the sorcerer, and the exorcist who flocked to Rome in search of quick riches, and on the other hand, the new Christian religion drew to itself a large share of those who were not satisfied with the services of either the physician or the quacks. The members of the new religion attended to the sick on the highest ethical level and did not accept any pecuniary returns. They founded hospitals and free benevolent institutions in the larger cities. They admitted the sick to the religious shrines without question and the ecclesiastics assiduously watched over the patients to the peril of their own lives.[3]

The Apostles claimed that they had the faculty of curing dis-

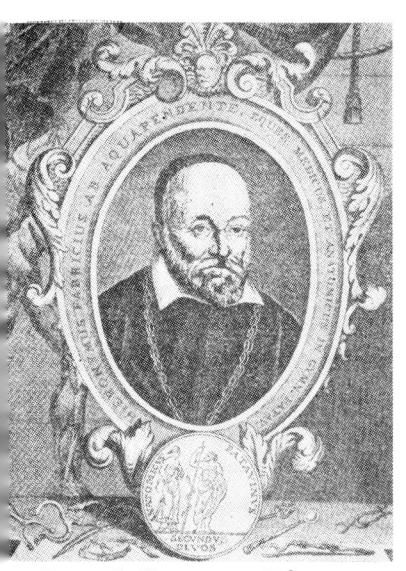

PLATE 5. Hieronymus Fabricius, eminent physician.

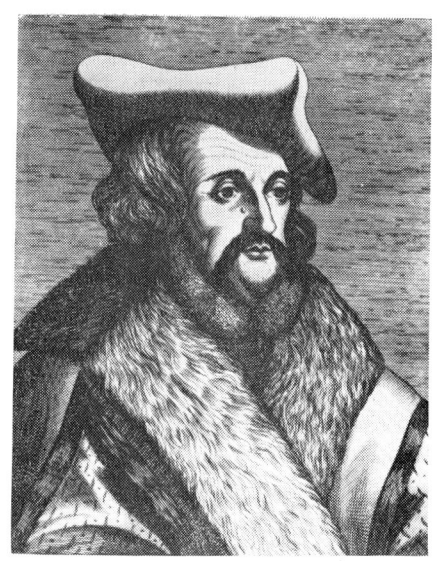

PLATE 6. Hieronymus Fracastorius (1494-1553). Famous for poem, *Syphilidis, sive Morbi Gallicii*. Published, Venice, 1530.
(Armed Forces Med. Lib. Wash.)

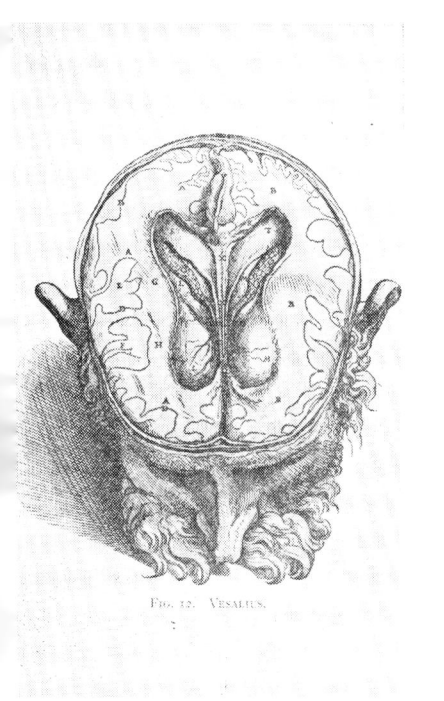

PLATE 7. Vesalius

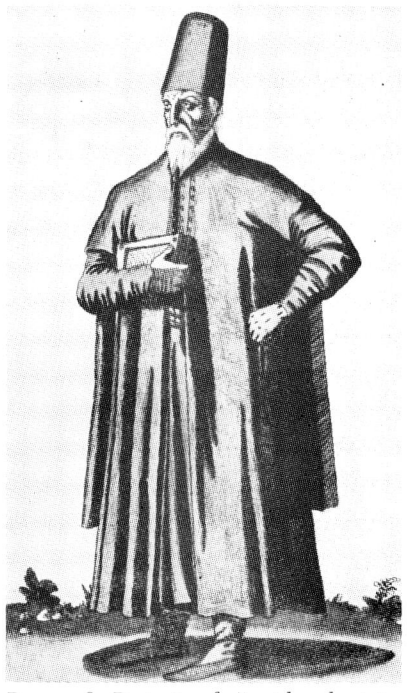

PLATE 8. Portrait of Jewish physician (from Nicolas de Nicolay, Les Navigations, 1576).

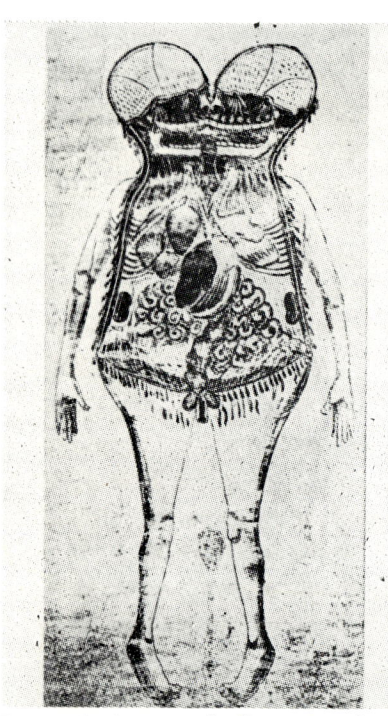

PLATE 9. Anatomical illustration from parchment roll of John Arderne (about 1370).

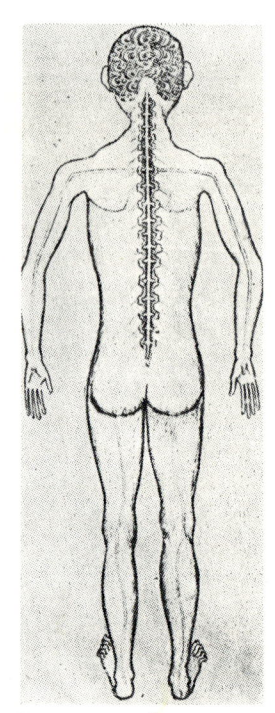

PLATE 10. The nervous system, from "Anatomy of Guido de Vingevano," ca. 1350.

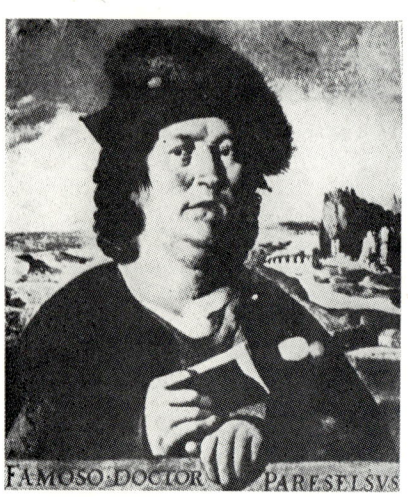

PLATE 11. Theophrastus von Hohenheim, called Paracelsus (1493-1541).

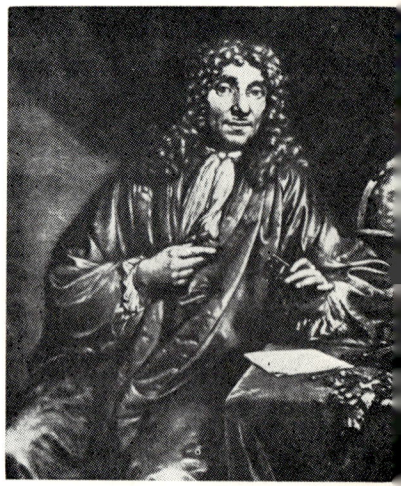

PLATE 12. Van Leeuwenhoek (1632-1723)
(From photographic reproduction in Collection of New York Academy of Medicine

eases by means of apposition of the hands or by inunction with holy oils and ointments. It was believed that the Apostles transmitted this miraculous therapeutic power which they had received from their Master, to the elders of each community.

The medicine of the Church Fathers closely followed Christian dogma.

This Christian compassion towards the sick and disabled led to a departure of medicine along lines practiced hundreds of years earlier in the temples of Aesculapius in Epidaurus and elsewhere. As early as the second century A.D., the pagan gods turned over their healing shrines to Christian saints. The sick were brought to the shrines or to the hospices to be cured under the supervision of priestly healers. There was a pagan shrine firmly established on Mount Cassino before St. Benedict took it over and established his great monastery.

Early Christians considered sickness to be a mark of divine displeasure. Before commanding a lame man to walk, Jesus first announced the forgiveness of the victim's sins. On another occasion, he admonished one whom he had healed to "sin no more, lest a worse thing befall thee." [4] Paul also saw in the sickness and death of certain members of the Corinthian community the chastening of the Lord for their improper observance of the Eucharist.[5]

Early Christians concerned themselves little if at all with medicine as a natural art. As a matter of fact, the Christian Church taught that the one concern of human existence was preparation for a future life. The faulty shell of the temporal body was of no importance; it was impious to devote any attention to, or care for, such a mundane thing. So widely was this doctrine accepted that several pious men and women were canonized solely on the basis of the fact that they did not wash.

Luke plainly indicated that, for Christians, the healing of disease was distinctly an affair of religion. Christian tradition represents Jesus himself in the role of a great physician during his earthly career. When a woman "who suffered many things of many physicians" barely touched the hem of Jesus' garment, she was immediately healed.[6] During his travels Jesus went about among the people curing all manner of sickness; and after his demise the same therapeutic energy, emanating from him to his disciples, was declared by Christians to be the only hope for the ills of humanity.[7] James said: "Is any sick among you? Let him call for the elders of the Church; and let them pray over him, anointing him with oil in the name of the Lord: And the prayer of faith shall save the sick, and the Lord shall raise him up; and if he have committed sins, they shall be forgiven him." [8]

Lay physicians were not trusted by the Church. There is an old maxim that "out of every three physicians two are atheists." Two frequently recommended therapies were placing the text of the Gospels upon the affected part of the patient and spreading the clothing of a pious man over him. The cloak reputed to have been worn by the apostle Paul was held to possess such healing power and was therefore frequently employed as a healing device.[9]

Gibbon, in his *Decline and Fall of the Roman Empire*, states that one of the most powerful causes for the spread of Christianity was the miraculous power believed to be inherent in the primitive Church; this included the power to cast out demons. Of course, Gibbon scoffs at exorcism as a practice of superstition, but he states that the great masses of people were sunken in a deep abyss of superstition.[10]

PATRISTIC MEDICINE

The Church Fathers frequently found an opportunity to touch upon medical subjects when discussing religio-philosophical problems, particularly when these discussions were in relation to the immortality of the soul. Clement of Alexandria (150 A.D.), in his "Pedagogue," dwells at length on how one ought to behave and what he should eat, drink and wear under various conditions. He considers milk to be modified blood and therefore naturally very nutritious. He goes into detail on social and sexual matters.

St. Jerome, also known as Hieronymus, has left an interesting summary concerning the diet of various nations. He warns against overeating and excessive drinking of alcoholic beverages. He particularly decries excessive consumption of meat. "Whosoever is ill," he states, "recovers health only through restricted expenditure and a rigid mode of life (i.e., through a meager diet). The food which serves to restore health will also preserve it. None need think that vegetables cause disease. If, however, they do not give rise to such strength as was possessed by Milo of Crotona which only results from flesh-eating, one may well question why it is necessary that a wise man and a Christian possess that which, in the case of soldiers and fighting men, only excite them to vice . . . I admire those who have chosen a life of moderation and desire only the drink of temperance—water; who shun wine as they would danger from fire. It suffices that boys and girls should in general be denied this drink . . . grown-up people cannot be prevented from consuming a more heated drink, but even for them there is a limit."

"In the use of baths," wrote St. Jerome, "there are four motives: cleanliness, warmth, health, and pleasure. For pleasure alone, one should not bathe. Women should bathe in the interest of health and cleanliness; men in the interest of health alone. The motive of warmth alone is superfluous, for limbs stiffened with cold can be warmed in other ways. Continuous use of baths induces weakness and saps the natural energy; it often leads to lassitude and faintness." [11]

St. Jerome's letter to Nepotian, reads: "It is a part of your (clerical) duty to visit the sick, to be acquainted with people's households, with matrons, and with their children, and to be entrusted with the secrets of the great. Let it therefore be your duty to keep your tongue chaste as well as your eyes. Never discuss a woman's looks, nor let one house know what is going on in another. Hippocrates, before he would instruct his (medical) pupils, made them take an oath and compelled them to swear obedience to him. That oath exacted silence from them and regulated their language, gait, dress, and manners. How much greater an obligation is laid on us (as clergymen)!"

St. Jerome also states that one ought not spurn earthly medicine since it is advantageous rather than harmful and since it has not been held in contempt by holy men (e.g. St. Luke, St. Cosmas, and St. Damian were physicians). "Wherefore let us honor the physicians so that they will help us when sick, remembering (the word of) that wise one: 'Honor the physician of necessity for the Most High created him.' [12] And do not hesitate to take what potions he gives you. That same wise one said 'The Most High created medicine from the earth, and the prudent man will not reject it.' [13] Therefore he who does not seek medicine in time of necessity deserves the name, 'stupid' and 'imprudent'. I say that it is wise to do well by the physician while you are well so that you will have his services in time of illness . . . God wishes to be honored by His miracles performed through man. According to Isaiah, whatever good is done by man is effected by God; he said 'The Lord does all of our works through us.' " [14] The exhortation ends on the following note of Christian idealism: "Aid the sick, your reward coming from Christ, for whatever gives you a cup of cold water in His name is assured of the eternal kingdom wherewith Father and Holy Spirit He lives and reigns for eternity. Amen." [15]

Gregory of Nyssa (c. 331-c. 396) was well posted on contemporary theories of medicine. He refuted the prevailing idea that the soul was created before the body. "There is one beginning for body and soul alike," he declared. "The power of the soul unfolds gradually with the growth of the body; just as the seed contains in germ all future developments, so does the principle of life in man." The closeness of intercommunion of body and soul is a characteristic teaching of Gregory of Nyssa. His concept that in Adam the whole of mankind was represented, sounds like a premonition of the modern science of genetics. According to Gregory, three organs are absolutely essential to life; the heart, the liver, and the brain.

Gregory of Nyssa wrote that flesh is capable of sensation and that movement results from force conveyed through the nerves, after the impulse originates in the meninges. Rupture of the meninges causes instant death. The entire body is permeated by canals, some of which spring from the heart and contain *pneuma* (arteries); others arise from the liver and contain blood (veins). The *pneuma* reaches the lungs by the process of respiration and is drawn from the heart. The respiratory process occurs involuntarily. The heart is attached to the lungs and by its contractions alternately expands and compresses them. By this method inspiration and expiration take place.

Three forces maintain life: the first permeates the whole body with warmth; the second provides moisture to that which is warmed; and the third holds the limbs together and endows everyone with the power of independent and voluntary movement.

Gregory of Nyssa explains the process whereby food is digested by the alimentary tract, as follows: "The stomach, the heat of which is maintained by the heart, yearns after food; the more it does so, the greater the amount of heat it absorbs. Digestion is a process of coction of matter, which is divided into coarser and more refined portions. The residuum passes through the intestines and for a time provides them with nourishment. The many convolutions of the intestines serve the purpose of retarding evacuation so that appetite may not recur too rapidly."[16] This Christian author goes on to explain how food is assimilated and changed into blood.

Gregory of Nyssa further states: "The liver, to which the *pneuma* is brought by means of an artery whereby the blood acquires its red color, lies at so great a distance from the heart in order that the two sources of vital force should not be brought together in too confined a space. The vapors originating from the admixture of moisture and warmth nourish the brain, the coverings of which are prolonged in a tube-like fashion through the spinal column."

According to Gregory of Nyssa, all the different constituents of the body are fashioned in a most marvelous manner from the same primary nutriment: Hairs for example, are formed by the escape of vapors through the pores; long and straight ones when the emanations take a direct path and wavy or curly ones when they are expelled through tortuous channels.[17]

Gregory of Nyssa's namesake, Gregory of Nazianzus, marveled at the structure of man. "Consider O man," he said, "how thou art made and shaped and how greatly God's wisdom showed itself in thy creation." In this statement Gregory of Nazianzus appears to have emulated Galen in his teleological concepts.

One of the most learned and keen-witted Church Fathers was St. Tertullian of Carthage (c.155–c.220 A.D.). He was a frequent medical critic. He denounced the barbarity of the obstetricians who "in order to save the life of the mother dismember the embryo" and he bitterly condemned Herophilus, the medical sage of Alexandria, whom he accused of practicing venesection on prisoners. Yet he nevertheless made frequent use of medical terms and similes. Among other things, he said: The highest faculty of the soul is in the heart. Growth of soul goes on parallel with bodily development. The only natural impulse is that towards nourishment.

St. Tertullian, with great emphasis, advanced the view that the soul is not first united with the body at the moment of birth, but rather is begotten with it. He makes note of the fetal movements which are felt by pregnant women as proof of this.

St. Tertullian states that the function of the bile is to assist digestion and to hasten evacuation of the bowels. He differentiates nerve tissue from tendons by their sensitivity.

A study of Greek philosophy directed St. Tertullian to the Greek medical writers whose treatises occupied an important place in his working library.[18]

One of the patristic philosophers who followed the science of medicine with great interest was Nemesius (c. 400) Bishop of Emesa, Syria, the author of "Human Nature." John of Damascus (d. 754) and the Schoolmen including Albertus Magnus (1193-1280) and Thomas Aquinas (1225-1274) held him in the highest esteem as a scholar. He was ranked by his admirers as greater than Aristotle and Galen. He is credited by some as having anticipated Harvey in the discovery of the circulation of the blood.

The unbiased reader of Nemesius' works, however, cannot

find evidence to substantiate such claims, especially with reference to the latter subject: "The movement of the pulse originates from the heart, particularly from the left chamber, the so-called *pneumatic*, which distributes the *vital warmth* through the arteries to all parts of the body, just as the liver distributes nutriment by means of the arteries. . . . When the pulsating vessel expands it draws into itself blood from the nearest vein, which serves as nourishment to the *vital spirit*; when it contracts it expels all impurities from the body through the invisible pores."

His contributions to physiology do not appear to have been original for he largely follows the medical views of antiquity. For example, he adheres to the ancient Pythagorean teaching that the male germ (*semen*) originates in the brain and reaches the testicles through vessels contained behind the ear. He places the faculty of human imagination in the anterior ventricle of the brain, that of reason in the lateral ventricles, and that of memory in the posterior ventricle. In this he follows the teaching of Posidonius (b. 360).

Another eminent patristic philosopher who was greatly interested in medicine was Lactanius Philomenus (born circum 220). Because of the beauty of his writings he has been referred to as "the Christian Cicero." Lactanius, who was an African of heathen parentage, is considered one of the most eminent scholars of his period. In his work *"De Opificio Dei,"* he treats the subjects of anatomy, physiology, and psychology with more than passing interest. He believes with Aristotle, Galen, and Varo in the principle of teleology which postulates that the bodily structures and functions were all created according to a purposeful pattern in every detail and that the wisdom of the Creator is reflected in the formation of each and every organ and tissue of the body.

His teachings included the following: Perception of taste is situated in the tongue, not in the gums. Ocular convergence is brought about by tension only. Embryonic developments begin with the head, not with the heart. Determination of sex depends upon the predominance of male and female seed. Male embryos are developed in the right side of the uterus and females in the left (an Aristotelian concept).

In his description of the internal organs of reproduction, Lactanius gives two theories concerning the origin of semen: *ex medullus*, and *ex amni corpore*. Since his sex theories had been repeatedly maintained by various ancient writers, however, few if any of them have any claim to originality.[19]

The early theologians, with great zeal and thoroughness, prepared themselves in the technical language of Aristotle, Galen and others, not so much to acquire knowledge of the ancient learning as to place their theological studies upon a firm foundation.

Generally speaking, the early ecclesiastics were highly cultured men and if they had devoted themselves to the arts and sciences they probably would have reflected scientific credit upon their age. Since, however, science with them was subordinate to religion, when science ran counter to religious dogma, science had to give way.

To the credit of the Church it must be admitted that, during the early centuries of Medievalism when all worthwhile knowledge was threatened with decay, the Church, unshaken by the catastrophic changes, preserved a link with the more enlightened past. Passively, at least, it rescued the works of art and what was left of the sciences, from complete destruction.

It would be a mistake, however, to conclude that the Church made a direct contribution to the science of medicine. It strictly prohibited the dissection of human bodies and looked upon surgery as a sinful shedding of blood. In ecclesiastical hands, prayer, exorcism, charms, votive offerings, blessings and relics of the saints, eclipsed rational therapeutics.

In the year 529, the same year that Justinian closed the School of Philosophy at Athens for all time, St. Benedict of Nursia (c. 480-c. 550) came from Subiaco to Mount Cassino, and established a monastery there where monastic life was deprived of its Oriental character and made to be more in keeping with Occidental conditions.

Mount Cassino is an isolated hill overhanging the town of

Casinium, midway between Rome and Naples. It is related that an ancient Roman temple had been situated on Mount Cassino before it was taken over by St. Benedict. The latter overthrew the pagan altar, destroyed the grove and set up a temple to St. Martin where all ailments were treated.

The influence exercised by the Benedictine Order in the West may be compared to that of St. Basil in the East. St. Benedict, having dwelt for a time as a hermit in the Sabine mountains, later gathered disciples around him, founded monasteries first at Subiaco and then at Mount Cassino, and wrote a "Rule," which after the lapse of two centuries, was to become the one monastic Rule of the West. It may, in fact, be said that the history of Western monasticism is practically identical, for the greater part of the Middle Ages, with that of the Benedictines.

The "Rule of St. Benedict" teaches the virtues of humility, obedience, and poverty, and enjoins the practice of silence, hospitality, and manual work. It regulates the hours of prayer and lays down the order of the Psalmody. His monastery developed into a little city where a complete society provided all necessary functions. A monastery, according to St. Benedict, had to possess a garden, a mill, and all essential offices and workshops. He insisted that monasteries offer facilities for the sick and that all guests be received with honor.

The monastery of Mount Cassino was the very first in Western Europe where the teaching of medicine was fostered. The Benedictines were the most scientific of the monks and they cultivated medicine to a considerable extent. The monastic infirmary at Mount Cassino had a pronounced influence upon medieval medicine. Many manuscripts dealing with medicine were collected there and members of the Order of St. Benedict became famous as copyists of Greek and Arabian medical documents. The medical works of Hippocrates, Galen and Avicenna were translated there.

Often, however, the translations were made to harmonize with the religious doctrines of the day. For example, the Galenic theory of *pneuma* was associated with the Christian doctrine of the soul. While, in theory, medical classics were read in the original, in practice the healing of disease was attributed to Providence. Later, when an amalgamation took place of the monasteries founded by St. Benedict and Cassiodorus, scientific material came to be included in the Benedictine Rules or rather in their practices. The Benedictines in the West came to be the counterpart of the liberal Nestorians in the East.

Archius Cassiodorus (480-575), like Nestor in the East, helped bring about this change among the inmates of the monastery. Cassiodorus after many years of political activity as private secretary to Theodoric (reigned 493-326) and his successors, turned monk in order to dedicate himself to God and science for the rest of his life. He made the monastery not only a house of contemplation and prayer but also an institution for education and learning. Cassiodorus, who later joined the Benedictine Order recommended that the monks take up the study of medicine and he went so far as to name the writers of antiquity whose works were to be studied as a foundation for a knowledge of medical science.[20]

It should be borne in mind that although the statutes of the Benedictine Order made the cultivation of the sciences a part of the Rule, the cure of disease by prayer and conjuration alone was permitted. Cassiodorus particularly recommended certain writings of Hippocrates and the works of Galen and Dioscorides. His recommendation helped to preserve the names of many ancient physicians.

One of the greatest educators of the Middle Ages was Bishop Isidorus of Seville (626-750), sometimes referred to as Isidorus Hispalensis. In his twenty volume "Etymologiae," he collated all that he considered of value in ancient medical literature. This encyclopedic work exercised a considerable influence upon the art of healing particularly among the clergy. The fourth book of this work, which largely follows the text of Caelius Aurelianus, presents a survey of the entire range of medicine. Bishop Isidorus emphasizes that a wide and many-sided education is necessary for the practitioner of medicine and he classifies medicine on a level with philosophy. He gives the therapeutic action of the various drugs which he lists and the methods by which they are administered. He discusses the use of various medical instruments and other professional equipment.

In contradistinction to the more enlightened elements of medieval Europe, Gregory of Tours (538-593) in his "History of the Franks" and his books on the miracles of the Saints, illustrates how the Franks in Merovingian times were deeply permeated with superstition. Among the forms of healing which the Franks preferred were healing by prayer and exorcism; treatment by contact of the involved parts with sacred relics such as pieces of tombstones and dust of saints; therapy by dropping wax from votive candles or ashes from their wicks on the affected parts; and cure by employing oil from church lamps either internally or externally. However, one can infer from isolated pages in the writings of Gregory some experience in surgical matters. The people, however, even in such matters, placed their confidence in surgeons who professed belief in the miraculous power of the saints.

Medicine in medieval Italy originated from both clerical and secular sources and these subsequently tended to approach one another. In the original Benedictine monastery, like in other monasteries, the sick were first tended in accordance with the usual ecclesiastic principles of medical practice. Later, copying the non-clerical physicians, monks and even non-monastic clergy began to employ healing herbs and medicaments in addition to their spiritual therapeutics. It can honestly be said that monks and clerical healers filled the gap which had been created by the decline and fall of the lay educational institutions. They also undertook that part of the state care of the poor and sick which at one time had fallen to the *"archiatri popularis."* In this respect Italy, in contrast with other countries, at no time lacked at least some form of medical facilities. The medical prowess of the monks may be inferred from the following medical works of the abbot of Mount Cassino, Bertharius (857-884): "De Innumeris Remedorium Utilitabius," and "De Innumeris Morbis."

In Spain, under the tyranny of the Visigoths, the medical status sank to a very low ebb. The profession declined to the level of a trade. If the patient died the physician had no claim to remuneration. For technical errors such as an unskilful venesection, the physicians had to pay a fine of 150 *solidi*. If the death of a freeman was brought about by the treatment of the physician the latter laid himself open to arbitrary punishment from the relatives of the deceased. Even in urgent cases, venesection could only be performed on a freewoman in the presence of relatives. Failure to abide by this statute was punishable by a fine of 10 *solidi*. Such regulations hindered medical practice to the utmost for none but quacks would take a chance in facing criminal charges following the administration of therapy.

In France, the establishment at Tours was the most famous center of monastic learning. This school was founded by the Anglo-Saxon Alcuin (735-804), the teacher of Charlemagne. Tours also has the distinction of having conserved and transcribed many manuscripts that would otherwise have been lost.

Lay "doctors" were considered, in England and France, inferior to the cloister healers. Germany, because of the undeveloped state of the monastic schools, was in a far inferior position with regard to the knowledge of medicine, law and theology. In the early Middle Ages, clerics were throroughly learned men, not only in theology, but also in medicine and law. Lay healers were unlettered individuals who gained practical experience by serving as apprentices to other healers of the same caliber.

The services rendered by monks to civilization during the transition from ancient times to the Middle Ages were exceedingly important. Among these ecclesiastics were first-rate agriculturists and skilled artisans in the various handicrafts. Every monastery was surrounded by gardens which were taken care of by the monks of the monastery. Many modern botanical terms may be traced to these monks or through them to Greek and Latin sources. For instance, the plant *atropa belladonna,* from which are derived various important medicinal derivatives still in use, was cultivated by monks and first introduced as a pharmaceutical herb from the convent gardens. Since antiquity, monks have always been deeply interested in botany. The reader will recall that it was a monk, Gregory Mendel (1822-1884) who, in the middle of the nineteenth century, by his experimentation in the cultivation of peas, arrived at the Mendelian Doctrine which has revolutionized biological science and laid the groundwork for the modern science of genetics.

Bound by the strict confines of the rules of their respective orders with regard to bodily labors and mental pursuits, the monks performed various tasks of priceless value. It is through them that many classical works of antiquity have come to us. Gerbert (d. 1003), an abbot who held sway at the close of the tenth century speaks of his large collection of books and of the ecclesiastic scholars who were interested in them. The order of Carthusians (founded in 1087) and that of Cistercians (an offshoot of the Benedictine stock) had an unusual craving for luxurious books, beautifully written, illuminated and bound. The members of these orders constantly strived to build up their libraries.

At first the monks attended only to their own brethren in the infirmaries in the vicinity of the cloisters, whence the arts of medicine and pharmacy were taught to the young clerics. Later they practiced medicine and dispensed drugs to the public in general. Still later, owing to certain abuses which will be mentioned later, the Church forbade the practice of medicine on patients from outside of the monasteries.

In monastic writings, the terms *"medicus"* and *"infirmarius"* are often met with. According to Wickersscheimer *"medicus"* applies to the head of an infirmary and *"infirmarius"* applies to an assistant.

The teachings of monastic medicine were largely theoretical for dissection was forbidden by the Church and surgery was a violation of the second Commandment. Even when drugs were used they were prepared with religious ceremonies and prayers. Generally speaking, monk therapeutics were of a spiritual nature. Miracles like those alleged to have occurred in the shrines of Aesculapius were also said to have transpired in some monasteries.

It should be pointed out that monasticism cannot be regarded as an institution belonging exclusively to Christianity, although it received its full development in this religion. In the second and third centuries the Alexandrian school of philosophy taught a kind of mysticism in which moral ideas and ascetic practices occupied an important place. An attempt has been made by some Christian philosophers to find in the Alexandrian mystic philosophy the source of Christian asceticism. While Alexandrian asceticism might have influenced early Christian monasticism, the origin of monasticism is much older.

A life of poverty, chastity, humility, and obedience came to be essential to the monastic life, in carrying out the evangelic counsels and necessary fundamentals in the attempt to imitate as closely as possible the life led by Christ Himself, and after Him, by the Apostles and first disciples.

The first monks, like the ascetics before them, took the words of the Gospels literally and abandoned all their worldly possessions in order to live in poverty and by the labor of their hands. They considered chastity to include complete celibacy and perfect continence.

The intellectual work of the monks consisted chiefly in the *lectio divina:* the reading and study of the sacred Scriptures and other holy writings. In the West, this part of the monastic curriculum underwent great development and more and more time was given to intellectual work. Gradually the endeavors of the scholarly monks were extended to more or less non-religious tasks. The copying of ancient manuscripts in the scriptorium of the monastery became one of the principal occupations of the monk, and it is to this fact that medicine as other sciences owe the preservation of the greater part of the works of classical antiquity. The arts of calligraphy, drawing, painting, and the illumination of manuscripts, soon followed as a natural consequence. Some monasteries produced masterpieces of manuscript and bookmaking which are now among the most precious possessions of the libraries of Europe.

THE USE OF SHRINES IN CHRISTIAN MEDICINE

Investigations of the catacombs of Rome have shed light upon the early use of shrines and relics for healing purposes. The catacombs were official burial places protected by Roman law with entrances open to the public. Their chapels and altars were used for memorial and communion purposes. People who prayed at these tombs took with them relics from the revered dead and oil from the lamps which burned in the tombs. Such oil was considered of great therapeutic value. If the body of a saint reposed beneath the altar, the oil was known as "oil of the saint" and was particularly precious and much sought after by the sick and disabled.[21]

Gregory of Tours related a number of cures effected at the shrine of St. Martin (316-396). He himself claims to have been relieved of a severe headache by merely pressing his head on the rail of the sepulcher. Pellets of wax burned at the sepulchers or altar, or a pinch of dust scraped from the tomb of St. Martin and dissolved in water, were believed to cure severe attacks of dysentery. Licking the railing that enclosed the tomb of St. Martin is said to have cured a severe attack of glossitis. The incantations, chanted at the bedside of a patient who was in possession of a relic of St. Martin, read as follows: "Oh ineffable theriac! Ineffable pigment! Honorable antidote! Celestial purge! Superior to all drugs of the faculty! Sweeter than aromatics! Stronger than unguents together! Thou cleansest the stomach like scammony, the lungs like hyysop, thou purgest the head like presthrig!"

To illustrate how deeply the belief in the therapeutic value of the relics of St. Martin was rooted among the masses, the following story is mentioned by White. Two lazy beggars, one blind, the other lame, tried to avoid contact with the relics of St. Martin, which were carried about in a procession, so that they would not be cured and lose their claim to alms. The blind man took the lame man on his shoulders to guide him and escape the procession, but they were caught in the crowd and cured against their will.[22]

33

The relics of saints gradually came to be the favorite substitute for the previously employed charms, and curing by relics gradually grew in importance and became firmly established. Toward the end of the fourth century miraculous curing powers were ascribed to the very images of saints which adorned the walls of the churches. Saintly intercession became more and more frequently evoked and saintly relics were believed to work wonderful therapeutic miracles.[23]

In deep antiquity the cure of disease was directly governed by the gods. In the "Book of the Dead" of the Egyptians the human body is divided into thirty-six parts. The function of each organ or part was thought to be controlled by a deity.[24] The eye, for example, was governed by the god Hathor, the ears by Assud, the lips by Anibis, the growth of the hair by Nei and the face by Ra. All these individual powers were governed and coordinated by Thoth, who supervised the functioning of the entire body. The individual god concerned with the affected part was appealed to in time of illness.

When spirits and demons displaced the gods as the etiological agents of disease, the whole subject became much more complicated. Attempts were actually made to explain the difference in disease by advancing the theory that there were separate demons not only for every disease but even for every symptom of every disease.

The names of pathogenic demons originated in Babylonia and Persia and such spirits were designated according to the diseases they produced, the organs they attacked or the symptoms they presented. Frequently they were named after the localities in which they were said to be most numerous.[25]

In medieval times gods and demons yielded to saints. These were believed to possess the power of inflicting as well as of curing disease. Kerler names no less than 130 saints who were invoked in various diseases. Some of the saints associated with various diseases are as follows:[26]

Ague was called St. Pernel's Disease. Hookworm became known as St. Gothard's disease. Chorea had five patron saints and was variously termed St. Anthony's Dance, St. Vitus' Dance, St. Guy's

Dance, St. Modestus' Disease and St. John's Disease. Stammering was called St. Vitus' Dance of the voice and St. Vitus was also the patron saint of this affliction. Delirium tremens assumed the name of St. Martin's Evil. Dental disease and toothache were referred to as St. Apollonia's Disease. Epilepsy was known as St. Avertin's Disease, St. Valentine's Disease, St. John's Evil and St. Mathurin's Disease. Erysipelas was known as St. Francis' Fire, gout as St. Maur's Disease and hydrophobia as St. Herbert's Disease. Hemorrhoids was referred to as St. Fiacre's Disease. Intestinal colic was termed St. Erasmus's Disease.

Diseases of the legs and feet were under the supervision of St. Bechus and St. John. Leprosy and cancer were known as St. Gete's Disease. Cancer was also known as St. Gile's disease. All diseases of childbirth as well as those of children, regardless of their nature, became known as St. Margaret's Disease. Diseases of the lungs and throat were named after St. Blasius (Blaise) and quinsy was termed St. Blaise's Disease. Mania, regardless of its variety, was termed St. Dymphna's Disease. Measles became known as St. Lazarus' Disease. Ophthalmia was governed by two saints: St. Lucy and St. Clair. Plague was called St. Sebastian's Disease. Pellagra was identified as St. Aman's Disease. Pruritus was known as St. Main's Evil.

Rheumatism was designated as St. Gervasius' Sickness. Ringworm became identified with St. Aignan. Syphilis had a saint for every stage of this malady. An established case was often referred to as St. John's Disease. Primary syphilis, or the manifestation of a bubo, became familiar as St. Roch's Disease. Secondary syphilis was know as St. Sement's Disease. Yellow fever was called St. Anthony's Fire. St. Zachary was connected with dumbness.

The relation of saints to disease was usually determined by the manner in which the saint died. For example, Saint Agatha was cruelly tortured before she was put to death, her breast being cut off. Hence, disease of the female breasts was placed in her charge, and she became the patron saint of nursing women. Saint Apollonia had her teeth knocked out and her jaw broken. Hence prayers were directed to her to relieve toothache.

Saint Lucy became the patron saint of ocular pathologies by virtue of the fact that she sacrificed her own eyes for the sake of her faith. St. Cyriacus, who cured a princess possessed by a demon, is the patron saint of mental diseases. St. Blasius rescued a boy from suffocation and is called upon to help people with diseases of the neck.

The elevation of members of the Church to sainthood may be traced to the old Greek and Roman practice of raising humans to the position of godhood.

Until the end of the sixteenth century the only recourse for the sufferers of certain ailments was to make a pilgrimage to the shrines of saints where holy men were present and furnished the sufferers with certain prayers appropriate to every disease. As late as the eighteenth century the hospital of the Order of Saint Anthony of Vienna had a collection of relics of the afflicted who had received relief there.[27]

Even where drugs were administered to reenforce the spiritual healing, these therapeutic agencies were connected with saints. In modern pharmacopoeias, there are still drugs known as St. Bartholomew's fever liniment (a preparation of oil of turpentine, tincture of opium, and camphor), St. Bartholomew's tea (Paraguay), St. Jacob's oil (a liniment containing aconite), St. Lucas' bark (Caribbean bark), St. Thomas' Balsom of Tolu, St. German's tea (known as *spices laxantis*; a mixture of senna elder flowers, fennel, anise and potassium bitartrate) and Jesuit bark (cinchona).[28]

Miracles formed part of the evidence which led to the canonization of saints. A large number of healing miracles were usually included in the list of attributes of particular saints.[29]

St. Benedict was the patron saint of all diseases. Great faith was placed in the medal of Saint Benedict. It consisted of a round, coin-like piece of metal, on one side of which is the figure of the saint holding a cross in his right hand and the Holy Rule in his left hand. On the other side is a cross and around it the letters "C.S.P.B.," which stands for "Crux Sancti Patris Benedicti" (The Cross of the Holy Father Benedict). Saint Benedict was considered by the Church to be the most potent *efugator daemonu.* His name was evoked in cases of spiritual peril and deadly attacks.

The custom of carrying the sick to the monasteries is reminiscent of the ancient practice of taking them to the temples. This was first practiced among the Egyptians in the temples of Isis and Serapis. "Temple sleep," before the deities, was conducive to recovery and health. The soul, which was believed to depart from the body during sleep, was in a better position to communicate with the divine power and ask forgiveness in the temple than when imprisoned in the body.

In ancient Greece maimed and disabled persons were brought to the temple of the priestly physician Aesculapius and were placed before his deified figure to be cured. Aesculapius is accepted as the patron saint of medicine. Epidaurus, the reputed birthplace of Aesculapius, grew into the most popular health resort of ancient Greece. It became a medical center. The students were trained for the dual calling of priest-physician. One of the essential methods of treatment was the "temple dream," during which the gods manifested themselves in the form of serpents who visited the patient and licked the diseased portion of the body. The two daughters of Aesculapius, Hygeia and Panacea, were also deified. The former became the patron saint of preventive medicine, and the latter, of drugs that cure all diseases.[30]

During the outbreak of an epidemic, dozens of possessed persons were carried to the temples. They were left on the floor of the holy places until they died or the demon was expelled.

In early medieval times, the exorcist, when called on to exercise his calling, always appeared in a dignified form. He was, as a rule, attired for the occasion in a bright-colored mantle ornamented with shiny decorations. He never failed to impress the patient with his authority and power. The spell often began as follows: "With the wand of Moses and the plate of Aaron and the seal of Solomon and the shield of David and the miter of the high priest, I perform this spell." This was followed by conjuration of the evil spirit to leave the body of so and so, the son of so and so. In one of Montgomery's collection,[31] the spell began, "I, Paback, come clad in iron and fire vested with garments of Hermes the Logos and my strength is in Him who created heaven and earth."

Celsus censured the exorcists of his day in no mistaken terms. "There are," he said, "often seen every day on the public square men taught among Egyptians who for a copper perform wonderful miracles, drive out spirits by their breath from those who are ill, evoke the souls of heroes." Then he asked: "Is it reasonable to conclude that they are the sons of God or should we not rather think them wretched and wicked men?"

Among the earliest healing saints were Cosmas and Damian (third century). The physician and surgeon guilds later chose these saints as their patrons. In the sixteenth century a coin was designed by Benvenuto Cellini on which were inscribed the figures of Cosmas and Damian. Pope Felix IV erected a church devoted to these saints on the Forum in Rome. Cosmas and Dameon were martyred in 303 by Emperor Diocletian, while they were engaging in the practice of medicine in Cilicia. According to legend, these saints are credited with having amputated the legs of a dead Negro and successfully grafted them on a living white person whose legs had been removed.

St. Gall (556-640) is said to have employed fervent prayer to cure the daughter of a nobleman who was at death's door. He exorcised the demon of the sickness and forced it to depart instantly.

The outstanding female *medicus* of the cloister was St. Hildegard of Bingen (1098-1180). Her book, "Physics," written partly in Latin and partly in German, contains a description of medical plants, minerals and various biological products. It contains prescriptions for suppressing sexual desire and for relieving pain in pregnant and parturient women. She quotes freely from the writings of Pliny, Isidorus, Constantine Africanus, Walafried and others.

Faith cure was sometimes costly. When the remains of St. Sebastian (about the third century) and St. Gregory were brought to the cloister of Soisson, patients flocked to this sanctuary from far and wide. "The net revenue brought in by those that sought medical help was eighty measures of money and one hundred pounds of coin."

The shrine at the Cathedral of Cologne claimed to have obtained the skulls of "The Three Wise Men of the East," and sufferers from all over Europe came there to be treated. The Church of St. Ursula, which was filled with relics of her eleven thousand virgin martyrs, drew to its shrine thousands of troubled persons searching for cures.

The mortal remains of St. Margaret, the virgin, martyred at Antioch in 303 A.D., were handed down from one queen to another much in the fashion of crown jewels. The body of Margaret was brought into the lying-in chamber during the queen's labor, so that an heir to the throne might safely, speedily, and painlessly arrive.

During the time of the Crusades, wealthy knights carried on their persons or kept hidden in holy shrines, relics made from pieces of wood claimed to have come from the original cross. Receptacles alleged to be filled with the tears of Virgin Mary were also sold at a premium, for curative purposes. A grove of a hundred acres could not have furnished all the wood sold in little morsels as remnants of the true cross; and the tears of Mary sold drop by drop for large sums would have formed a veritable rivulet.[32] The Venetians for many centuries boasted that they possessed a fragment of the original cross, a part of the head of St. John, the entire skeleton of St. Luke, and an arm of St. George.

Athens, the Greek capital, was a great center in this traffic of sacred relics. Athens claimed to possess a fragment of the stone on which Jacob slept, the very staff which was transformed into a serpent by Moses, the cradle in which Jesus had lain, the Virgin's garments and her spindle, a morsel of the bread used in the last supper, and many other holy relics.

While it is true that under the direction of the Church many institutions and orders for the purpose of helping the maimed and the diseased came into existence, the medical practices in such institutions were theurgic to an extreme degree. Prayers, amulets and exorcism were employed even for the cure of everyday diseases. Sickness was regarded purely as a punishment from God, or a visitation from the devil (ideas which are by no means foreign to this very day).

While it should be stated that the sick were not compelled to employ Church healers, there was actually little choice. Few laymen who practiced medicine were held in high esteem. The lay physician was not a learned man as was his competitor the Church healer. The latter had been duly instructed in a monastic school, where the curriculum included the study of medicine, and he dispensed his services gratis. On the other hand, the lay physician who charged for his services, was considered an artisan or tradesman. Moreover, regulatory laws were enacted to restrain and govern lay healers. They were made legally responsible for any want of skill or malpractice, and their fees for surgery or medical advice were strictly stipulated. They were generally of very low caliber.

In summation then, it may be stated that a process of disintegration took place during the course of the chaotic sixth century when, from the Alps to the southernmost point of Italy, havoc and devastation, famine and misery, savagery and brutality, were spread far and wide by the long-drawn-out fights between the Ostrogoths and Byzantines, by the invasions and occupations of the Lombards and Vandals, and most of all, by the pestilences which, accompanied by terrifying natural phenomena, followed upon the murderous wars. Deprived of almost every other aid, medicine, like other branches of science was forced to seek refuge in the monastic seclusion of the Church to maintain its very existence in an unsympathetic world.

CHAPTER III

BYZANTINE MEDICINE

The transference of the Roman capital to Constantinople did not improve the intellectual status of Europe to any great extent. Historians invariably note the profligacy of the Byzantines. They are described as an idle, depraved people who spent their time for the most part in loitering about the harbor or carousing over their wine. It has been said that in war they trembled in terror at the sound of a trumpet and that in peace they quaked before the wickedness of their demagogues. It is reported that during the assault of Philip II, the Byzantines could only be prevailed upon to man the fortifications on the city walls by the aroma emanating from temporary kitchens distributed along the ramparts.

To be sure a wise monarch could have found a sufficient number of honest intellectuals in the Byzantine dominions for the development of learning. Alexandria still retained some of its ancient splendor and Pergamos still maintained its great schools of learning. The Greek classics were still read in their original language in Old Greece and in many sections of Asia Minor. The cultural traditions of the East, which were even older than those of Rome, were still revered in many lands under Byzantine rule. There was a mingling of Greek culture, Roman law, Egyptian mysticism and the Jewish and Christian religions. Yet Constantine the Great found no interest in cultural matters beyond the development of architecture and the art of painting.

Dazzled by the splendor of his birthright, Constantine lacked both the inclination and the capacity for original achievements.

He and his court in the palaces of Constantinople carried on the traditional practices of the Roman monarchs. Lecky gives this characteristic description of the Byzantine rule of this period:

"Of that Byzantine Empire the universal verdict of history is that it constitutes, without a single exception, the most thoroughly base and despicable form that civilization has yet assumed . . . There has been no other enduring civilization so absolutely destitute of all the forms and elements of greatness, and none to which the epithet, mean, may be so emphatically applied . . . Its vices were the vices of men who had ceased to be brave without learning to be virtuous. Without patriotism, without the fruition or desire of liberty . . . slaves, and willing slaves, in both their actions and in their thoughts, immersed in sensuality and in the most frivolous pleasures; the people only emerged from their listlessness when some theological subtlety, or some chivalry in the chariot races, stimulated them to frantic riots . . . . The history of the Empire is a monotonous story of the intrigues of priests, eunuchs and women, of poisonings, of conspiracies, of uniform ingratitude, of perpetual fratricides." [1]

The coalition of the government with the Church brought about an intellectual depression. Many secular schools were closed, and those that for some reason could not be closed, were under the supervision of the clergy. Bona fide medical schools were closed. Priests usurped the office of the physician. Magic and quackery prospered. To be sure there were some learned physicians who would not submit to priestly rule but they were a small minority and were not able to form an organized resistance.

Constantine the Great (288-337) left the cultivation of the sciences in the hands of the Christian ecclesiastics to whose religion he had become converted. Constantine was satisfied that his duties toward learning were fulfilled by the theologic speculations of the Church Fathers. He sought to divert the attention of the peoples from nature and the real facts of life, and to establish a universal canonical authority on matters of education.

The study of anatomy on the human cadaver was forbidden as

being definitely prohibited by Christian dogma. It was well-nigh impossible to obtain a dead human body for the purpose of study because of the belief in resurrection and because of the prevalent notion that the body is too base to deserve intimate study and that only the soul is worthy of consideration. Religious dogma influenced even anatomic terminology. For example, the coccyx became known as the "resurrection bone" because of the belief that this bone served as a nucleus from which the body would be restored and resurrected.

The Church however could not entirely crush ancient medical learning because the few non-clerical learned individuals of the Eastern Empire would not accept such a doctrine. Such persons were willing to compromise with the Church on the use of prayer or even charms in addition to rational remedies, but they would not agree to abandon rational medicine altogether.

The more broad-minded ecclesiastics who supervised the education of the youth allowed certain traces of secular learning to filter through to their pupils although they were most cautious in dealing with subjects that were in direct conflict with Christian dogma.

The subjects that were more or less adequately taught without much interference from the Church were theology, jurisprudence, astrology, history, military science, and, to a lesser degree, mathematics and astronomy. However those subjects which required unbiased observation and independent rational criticism, such as the sciences of medicine and philosophy, were discouraged. Under such conditions it was well-nigh impossible to make any open original contributions to the sciences of medicine and philosophy. As a matter of fact, even poetry, apart from the religious hymns, came under Church ban. Under such an environment, stagnation and retrogression needs must ensue for no true progress can be made in such a stifling atmosphere.

It is always the case, in time of intellectual depression, that certain basic impulses find refuge in the obscurity of mysticism. Astrology flourished and superstition reared its ugly head. Advances in learning cannot be made where there is neither infusion of experimentation nor true scientific spirit and where boundless respect for ancient authority squelches independent criticism and discourages original research.

Great stress, almost to the point of worship, was laid on ancient tradition. The medicine of Galen and other ancient physicians (as interpreted by the Church of course) was considered the last word on the subject of medicine. Independent thought was considered a heresy even by physicians themselves. Galen enjoyed the admiration of the profession at large. His word was law. The greatest ambition of a physician was to be able to collect and comment on ancient authorities.

It is natural for a people who have no opportunity for education to preserve the memory of their ancestors and follow folklore blindly. This is precisely what happened with the few Byzantine medical writers. They looked upon the doctrine of the ancients as an unassailable canon in which no important changes could be made.

Byzantine medicine thus became the art of copying and repeating what ancient physicians had said. The works of Galen and Dioscorides were especially open to opprobrium but even the writings of the credulous Pliny, who compiled his history from fairytales told to him by the barbarians during his travels, were revered without any personal critical judgment. Byzantine medicine, to be exact, is a mechanical preservation of ancient thought or an anthology of the classical medical writings.

CLASSIFICATION OF MEDIEVAL MEDICINE

Medieval medicine may be divided into three periods: the Byzantine, the Saracenic and the Western. Inasmuch as this classification is made on a geographic basis, the different periods necessarily overlap each other chronologically and, in order to facilitate the study of each period, it seems advisable to discuss the leading physicians and compilers involved with the period with which they are connected.

The most prominent physicians of the Byzantine period who

were responsible for the preservation of classical medicine were Oribasius (325-403), Aurelianus Caelius of Numidia (5th century) a Roman colony of North Africa, Aetius of Amida (510-574), Alexander of Tralles (525-608), Theophilus Protospatharius (b. 540), Paul of Aegina (625-696) and Johannes Actuarius (c. 1275).

ORIBASIUS (325-403 A.D.)

Among the medical compilers and commentators of this period none is more prominent that Oribasius. His compilations were greatly admired by students of medicine for many centuries after his death. His superiority over other compilers rests on the fact that he quotes his authorities accurately. Medical science is especially indebted to him for rescuing from oblivion the surgical works of Archigenes of Afanna (48-117), Heliodorus (c. 100), Antyllus (3rd century) and others who have contributed so much to the progress of surgery. Were it not for the painstaking researches of Oribasius the aforementioned works would have been completely lost. Like his master authority Galen, Oribasius wrote about manifold subjects in his remarkable anthology, and unlike other compilers, he carefully eliminated superstition from his therapeutics. What courage it took to ignore mysticism when everyone expected the physician to practice it!

Oribasius was born in Pergamos, Asia Minor, a city famous for its great schools and eminent scholars. He studied in the medical schools of Alexandria under the tutorship of Zeno of Cyprus (A.D. 330). At the request of Julianus Apostata (331-390), Oribasius came to Constantinople in the year 355. His great talents and exceptional qualities were soon recognized by Julianus, and, when the latter became governor of Gaul, he took Oribasius along with him. When Julianus became Emperor he appointed Oribasius Court Physician, and bestowed upon him the rank of *Quaestor* of Constantinople. To show his appreciation, Oribasius dedicated the 70 volumes of his Greek encyclopedia to Julianus, his friend and benefactor.

In his "Synagoguae Medicae," he preserved the more important medical texts. Unfortunately only about one-third of the 70 volumes of his "Collecta Medicinelia" have escaped the ravages of the ages.[2] Later in life he completed an abridgement, in his work "Euporista" (A.D. 390) for the benefit of his son, Eustathius, which work is still extant.[3] This epitome, which was intended as a physician's quick reference book and first aid manual for educated laymen, contains sections on simple drugs which were later quoted by various Arabic authors. Oribasius does not consider surgery in the epitome because this branch of medicine was only intended for specialists.

After Julianus' untimely death, jealous colleagues of Oribasius falsely misrepresented his fidelity to his demised benefactor. He was publicly disgraced, deprived of his honors and property, and banished among the barbarians. His exile, however, did not in any way discourage him. His reputation followed him wherever he went. He was venerated even by the uncivilized tribesmen among whom he sojourned and many of these considered him to be divine. He effected such extraordinary cures that his fame soon reached the ears of Valens and Valentinian, the new emperors. They recalled him to Constantinople, restored his honors, and reimbursed him for his losses. In Constantinople he continued to enjoy the highest reputation as a scholar and physician to the end of his days.

As has been intimated Oribasius excerpted huge amounts of worthwhile ancient medical literature. He carefully included almost all important passages from ancient medical authorities. Oribasius reproduced the ideas of others with such clarity, order, and precision that his summaries are frequently preferable to the originals. The only liberties he permitted himself were to arrange and systematize his material and, at certain times, to comment on the works of his authorities. He hesitated to express his own opinions on debatable subjects and instead cited the opinions of his authorities. His own opinions and achievements are conspicuously relegated to the background. He sometimes cites two different authorities, holding opposite opinions. In one place he gives a description of Galen's opinion on a certain anatomical question, and in another place he cites Soranus' varying view on the same subject. He does not intimate with whom he agrees.

Oribasius was particularly careful not to refute the opinions of Galen whom he greatly revered, even when he was in a position to amplify upon or revise his teachings. In one place, while discussing venesection, he reports that, while dissecting apes, he discovered a nerve which was located beneath and close to the median vein of the arm, but he would not amplify on this finding lest somehow he might contradict the opinion of his revered master. On the whole it may be said of him that he was against putting his own ideas permanently on the record because of his great reverence for his predecessors. In debatable questions his modesty seldom permitted him to weigh his own valuable judgments on the scale.

His works deal with anatomy, physiology, pathology, symptomatology, obstetrics, surgery, embryology, climatology, hygiene, dietetics, baths, massage, plasters, poultices, bandages, and other external remedies.

His genius as a compiler and commentator is particularly shown in the chapters dealing with hygiene, diet, pregnancy, parturition, lactation, and the early education of children. Under the heading of surgery he describes fractures, dislocations, urinary and sexual diseases, hernia, tumors, and many operations. He lists therapies for inflammations, wounds, and ulcers.[4]

Oribasius' works were copied verbatim by writers for twelve centuries after his death. They were translated into Syrian and Arabic by Hunain ibn Ishaq and his pupil Isa ibn Yahya, but no fragments of these translations are left. Many fragments of Ruphus of Ephesus are preserved in Oribasius' books.

CAELIUS AURELIANUS (5th century?)

Caelius Aurelianus was another compiler and he may be regarded as the last celebrated writer of the Eastern Empire. He was born at Sicca in Numidia but the date of his birth has not been definitely established.

His writings indicate, however, that he flourished in the fifth century. It is not certain whether he was a student in Alexandria or not but it is well known that he displayed a wide literary activity while still young. His works, which are written in Latin, embrace all branches of the medical art. Medicine is greatly indebted to him for presenting an exposition of the entire theoretical and practical contents of the Methodist School. Extracts from his writings give a glimpse of rational medicine during a period of history when superstitious practice was the order of the day.[5]

The chief achievement of Caelius Aurelianus is his more or less free translation of the Greek works of Soranus into Latin. "De Morbis Acutis et Chronicis" is a compendium of the entire subject of medicine which is designed in uniformity with modern requirements. More than in other writings of antiquity, this work clearly describes diseases in accordance with their etiology, symptomatology, pathology, diagnosis and therapy. Not infrequently Caelius Aurelianus enlarges upon the anatomy of a particular case and he often enters into the subject of differential diagnosis and presents reviews of medical literature from Hippocrates down to Soranus.

Caelius Aurelianus' therapeutics excludes all mystic and supernatural methods of treatment. Methods of physical examination receive his careful attention. He puts himself on the record against many doubtful operations and he was definitely averse to venesection when performed to the point where the patient fainted. In his treatment he pays attention to hygiene, dietetics and physical therapy. Whereas he does not hesitate to point out divergences of opinion, he seldom, if ever, oversteps the bonds of decorum. His attitude thus fits in with the actual character of the Methodic School of Soranus, rather than the passionate school of Galen. Soranus was Aurelianus' fountainhead of medicine.

Caelius Aurelianus' writings on neurology and psychiatry are particularly important. He classifies two forms of paralysis:

spastic and flaccid. He describes, in addition to paralysis of the extremities, paralysis of the eyes, lids, pupils, tongue, larynx, lips, gums, esophagus, other portions of the gastrointestinal tract and bladder. In treatment of paralysis, he lays particular emphasis upon physical therapy and exercise. He states that the chief difference between paralysis and apoplexy is that the former is chronic and the latter is acute. He distinguishes between clonic and tonic forms of convulsion. Epilepsy is distinguished from hysteria by its more profound disturbances of consciousness. He considers incubo or nightmare in children a precursor of epilepsy.

The first symptoms of phthisis are hemorrhage of the lungs and constant coughing; gradually a characteristic clinical picture develops. Caelius Aurelianus, in the diagnosis of consumption, lays stress upon the breath sounds and the nature of the sputum. In treating phthisis he recommends fresh air, appropriate diet, sea voyage, inhalation of steam, and frequent baths. Cough in general is a symptom of the disease but may arise independently from other ailments. He distinguishes "atrophy" of the lungs from phthisis and empyema. He refers to differences of opinion among authorities on the subject of pleurisy. He gives Soranus' definition of pleurisy as "pain in the side of the chest associated with fever and cough." This disease comes mostly in the winter and attacks men and old persons rather than women and children. Caelius Aurelianus lists the symptoms of pleurisy as follows: pain radiating upward, fever, dyspnea, cough (sometimes dry, other times associated with expectoration), coated tongue, insomnia, and relief by lying on the affected side. He recommends venesection on the sound side.

Aurelianus gives the following symptoms of pneumonia: labored breathing, pain in the chest, cough, expectoration, air-hunger, and copious sweats.

He attributes habitual diarrhea to protracted disorders of the digestive tract and abdominal inflammation. He prescribes enemata and suitable diet for this condition.

The differential diagnosis between tympanites and edema rests on the fact that the former condition leaves no pitted mark after digital pressure and the latter does. Percussion on a tympanitic area sounds like tapping on a drum but on an edematous area elicits a flat note.

Gout, according to Caelius Aurelianus, is prevalent in certain neighborhoods and is more common among men than women. The symptoms are formication in the limbs, disturbances of digestion and respiration and a choleric predisposition. A certain type of spring water is the best remedy for gout.

Caelius Aurelianus divides dropsy into a generalized form (anasarca), a localized form in the limbs, and a type confined to the abdomen (ascites).

Passio renalis or nephritis runs a course with fever, constipation, abdominal pain, and vomiting and leads eventually to weakness and emaciation. The urine in this condition appears at times to be fatty or ichorous. The ureters are often implicated and become inflamed. The causes of nephritis are listed as chills, injuries, digestive disturbances, spiced food, and improper diet. Vesical calculi are associated with severe pain radiating to the pubis, navel region and testes. The diagnosis of vesical calculi is made by examination of the urinary sediment and subjective symptoms.

Caelius Aurelianus, like all ancient physicians, favors complete segregation of lepers in order to avoid the danger of contagion. His books on chronic diseases were published first by Aldus in 1547 in a collection entitled *"Medici Antiqui Omnes."* His works were regarded as standard textbooks on medicine by Cassiodorus who recommended them enthusiastically to the monks.

AETIUS OF AMIDA (510-574)

One of the most prominent of the Byzantine medical writers was Aëtius of Amida who occupied in Byzantium almost the same position that Oribasius held in Rome. Aëtius was born at the beginning of the sixth century (c. A.D. 510) in Amida, a city located on the banks of the Tigris in Mesopotamia. He studied in Alexandria following which he settled in Byzantium

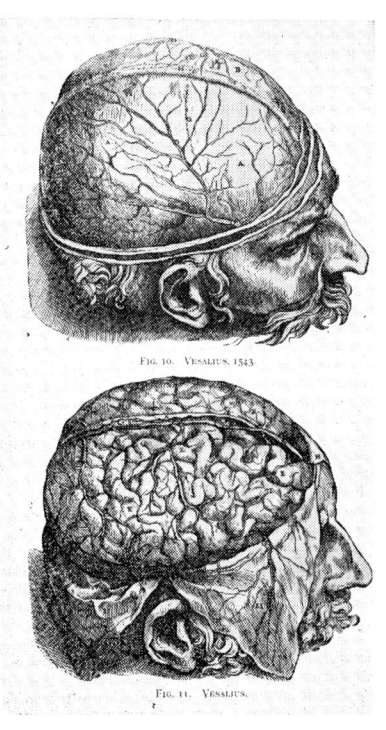

PLATE 13. Vesalius

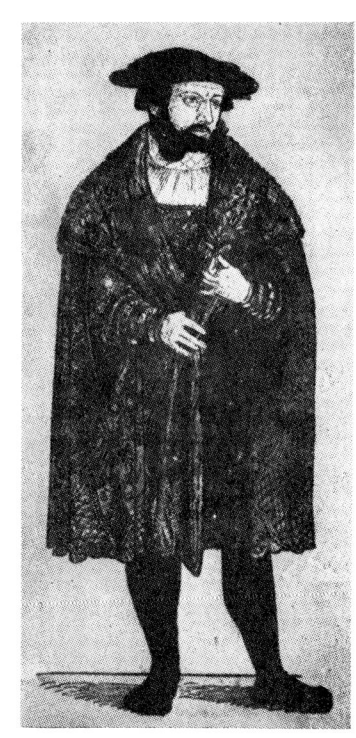

PLATE 14. Leonhard Fuchs, author of De Historia Stirpium (Basel 1542)

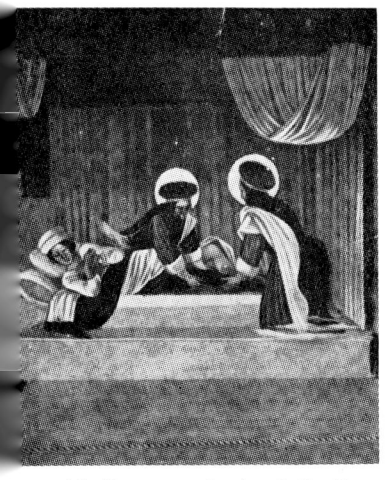

\TE 15. Famous miracle of St. Cos-
s and Damian. An amputated leg is
replaced by that of a dead Moor.

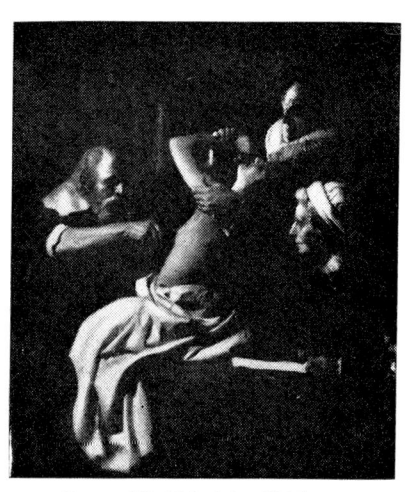

PLATE 16. Fabricius Hildanus (1560-1634)

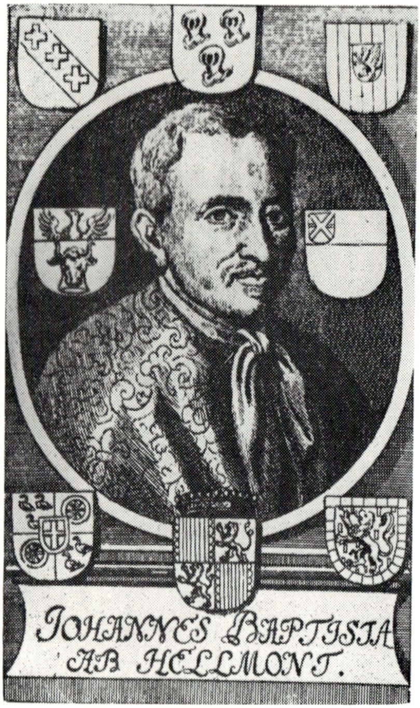

PLATE 17. Jean Baptista Von Helmont
(1577-1644)
(Armed Forces Medical Library, Washington, D.C.)

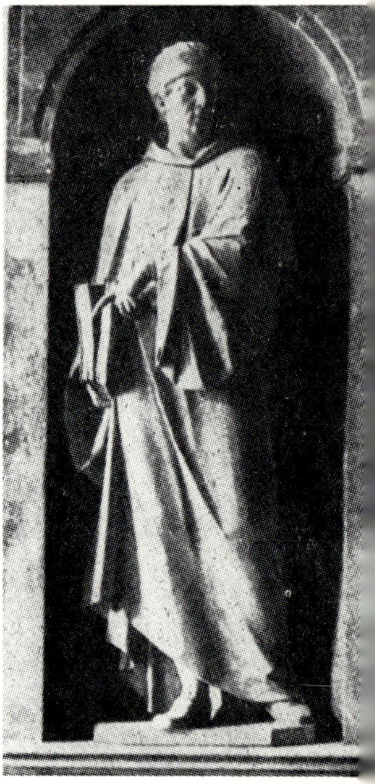

PLATE 18. Luzzi de Mondino
(Courtesy Armed Forces Medical Library, Washington, D.C.)

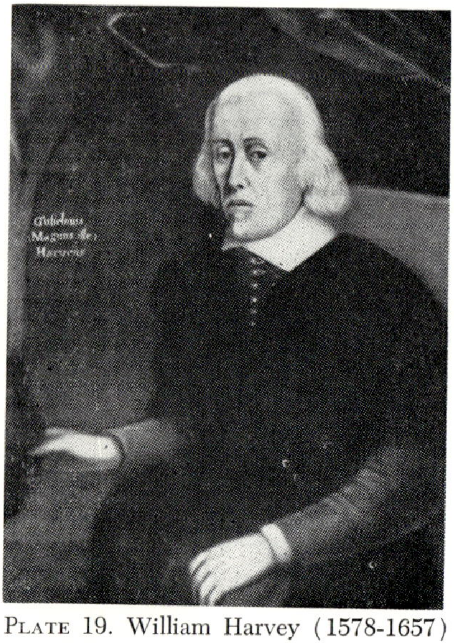

PLATE 19. William Harvey (1578-1657)

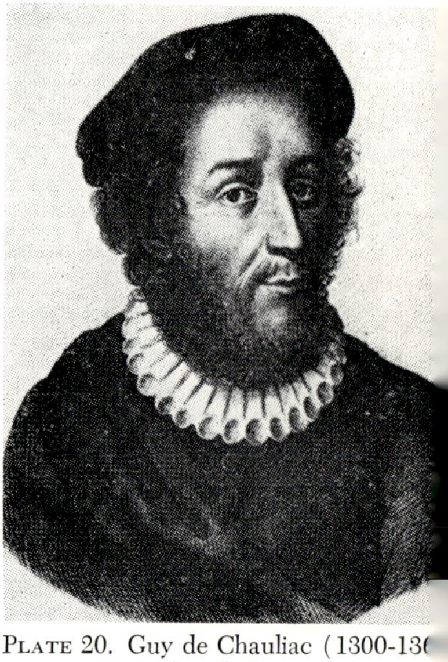

PLATE 20. Guy de Chauliac (1300-13..)
French Surgeon

during the reign of Justinian. He became court physician to the Byzantine ruler and finally was appointed *Comes Abseqii*—one of the chief officers of the imperial household. He was a prolific writer and his largest medical work is the "Tetrabiblos" written in Greek and so named because in some manuscripts it is subdivided into four parts, each consisting of four books (a total of 16 books). This work was based on Oribasius' writings and, like the latter, it is a compilation of the writings of Greek and Roman physicians.

Aëtius embraced Christianity and this religion played an important part in his treatment of disease. There is no complete edition in the original Greek language. A complete Latin translation was published in Venice in 1534 and a more reliable one, made by Carnarius, was published in Basel in the year 1542.

Aëtius was regarded by some of the Renaissance physicians as one of the greatest medical writers. He was praised by Boerhave (1668-1738) and severely criticised by Puschmann and Walmann. His lasting fame as a medical writer, however, is based on the fact that he was a careful compiler rather than an original thinker. In his "Tetrabiblos," Aëtius quotes Galen on general medicine, Soranus and Philomenus (80) on obstetrics and gynecology, Rufus (c. 50 A.D.) and Leonides (c. 200) on surgery and many other prominent medical writers. He defended the Hippocratic maxim of *vis medicatrix naturae*—a precept concerning which very different explanations have been given from the day of the "Father of Medicine" down to the present time.

Aëtius' anatomical descriptions were based largely, although not exclusively, upon Soranus and he also largely followed Soranus in his obstetrical teachings. According to Aëtius, the process of birth is determined by the condition of the membranes and the blood supply. If the membranes are small and the blood supply insufficient the movement of the child will tear the membranes and precipitate labor. Approaching labor is recognized by the size of the upper abdomen, frequent micturition and increased vaginal mucous secretions. The causes of dystocia are ossification of the symphysis pubis and excessive concavity of the sacrum which forces the uterus over to one side.

Aëtius employed the method recommended by Philomenus for extracting the fetus in case of dystocia. This method included (1) embryotomy, (2) embryulcia (the instrumental removal of the fetus from the uterus) and (3) removal of the placenta. If the head of the child became wedged during labor, resort was had to podalic version. Aëtius also described the indications and technique for induction of labor, cephalotripsy (crushing of the fetal head in order to facilitate delivery), decapitation and dismemberment.

In adherent placenta, direct traction downward is to be avoided so as to avoid prolapse of the uterus. Dilation of the closed *os uteri* is to be performed by injecting oil into it, by gradually stretching it with the hand or by the administration of emmenagogues and sitz baths. Artificial abortion is indicated in those cases where labor at the normal time would be dangerous to the mother; the most favorable time for this is during the third month. The main indication of approaching abortion is the discharge of watery or blood-stained fluid from the vagina. Among the means of procuring the expulsion of a dead embryo from the uterus is the introduction of dry sponges or papyri into the vaginal vault.

The heart is the seat of fever; fever results chiefly from diseases of the stomach and the intestinal canal. The general vitality suffers in diseases of the various organs only in so far as it functions through these organs.

In inflammation of the stomach, according to Aëtius, the internal portion becomes scorched with heat and the external portion freezes. If the starting point of inflammation is in the liver, typhus fever arises; if in the lungs, ague results.

Aëtius gives an excellent description of diphtheria in children: "It develops almost always from previously existing aphthae. The ulcers are at times white and run in patches; at other times they are of an ashy-grey color; they resemble the scabs caused by the use of the cautery. The patient is seized with dryness of the throat and this is complicated by great difficulty in breathing, particularly when redness is seen under the chin and paralysis of the soft palate develops . . . After the acute stage is over, noma and gangrene may ensue . . . Care should be taken of the fever which usually sets in with great severity . . . In many cases the uvula is destroyed and if after a long time the ulceration stops and cicatrization begins, children speak indistinctly and swallowed fluid returns through the nose . . . I have seen a girl die after forty days who was already in convalescence. Most cases, however, are in danger until the seventh day." [6]

Aëtius makes some clever observations on mania and other diseases of the mind and his methods of diagnosis are interesting.

He employs digital pressure in detecting anasarca and gross palpation in diagnosing enlargement of the spleen. Aëtius recommends inspection of the urinary sediment in ascertaining the existence of kidney disease. He discusses the value of a form of percussion in diagnosing ascites and pleurisy.[7] In cerebral congestion he advises probing the nose of the patient with a stick until bleeding ensues so that the resulting hemorrhage may render the cure more certain.

Aëtius' pharmacology includes the use of pimpernel plant (a species of the primrose family) for hydrophobia and pomegranate bark for worms. He employs a novel method to detect poison in a wound: first a poultice of walnuts is placed on the wound and later this is thrown to a fowl. If the fowl eats the poultice, the wound is considered free of any poison. If the poultice is rejected by the fowl and not eaten, the wound is surely poisoned.

While he admonished his colleagues not to be dazzled by the glare of "the authorities," Aëtius himself follows the teachings of Galen, Rufus, Leonides, Soranus, and others almost blindly. The few instances where he shows independence of thought are the exceptions rather than the rule. For example, in the case of venesection, he advocates the bleeding of both sides of the body—the diseased side as well as the sound side. He held the opinion that since "all the veins of the body communicate," it is immaterial whether the venesection is performed in the vicinity of the diseased part as was taught by Hippocrates, or on the opposite side of the body as was taught by the leading Methodists.

While in medicine Aëtius employed religious charms, in surgery he used rational methods. Aëtius gives the following methods of stopping hemorrhage: the application of digital pressure, bandage pressure, cold compresses, astringents, and corrosives, the use of ligatures and section of the bleeding vessels. His treatments of bone pathologies and of ulcers are Galenic. His treatments for coxalgia, and sciatica are those of Archigenes which consist of actual cautery and the moxa. He follows Leonides in recommending incision and drainage of abscessed tonsils and employs Leonides' pathology and treatment for glandular tumor of the neck, and cystic tumors. He advocates actual cautery in the treatment of prolapse of the rectum. He describes operations for fistula, fissures, diseases of the prepuce, hydrocele and hernia.

Aëtius was opposed to operating upon aneurysms except where this condition resulted from injury. He suggests a treatment for malignant ulceration of the rectum. His remarks concerning the differential diagnosis of malignant ulcers are most interesting. His recognition of lung-stones gives evidence that he made dissections on the human body.

His operation for carcinoma of the breast is that of Archigenes and Leonides. He suggests surgical methods of treatment for atresia of the uterus and vagina, calculus of the bladder, and inguinal hernia, and he describes amputation of the clitoris.

Aëtius' best and most exhaustive descriptions are those which he presents on diseases of the eye in which he depends upon many leading ophthalmologists that preceded him. He appears to have been familiar with the common external affections of the eye which he classifies on an anatomical basis. Internal diseases of the eye, of course, were *terra incognita* until Helmholtz invented the ophthalmoscope in 1851.[8]

Among diseases of the lids, Aëtius mentions swelling, ecchymosis, chemosis, and cancer. Among diseases of the conjunctiva, he notes inflammation, dry catarrh, blepharitis, blisters, sebaceous cysts, roughness (probably trachoma), styes, blepharoncus, ptosis, and staphyloma. He also lists pupillary pathologies including myosis, mydriasis and irregularity of the pupils.

The causes of visual disturbances include opacity of the

aqueous humor, shrinking of the lens and "amaurosis." The last is a condition where the patient is unable to see anything but the pupils appear clear. Aëtius does not describe a method of extracting cataract. He refers to nyctalopia (night blindness).

He describes a treatment for purulent conjunctivitis in the new-born (ophthalmia neonatorum), which includes the instillation of oil into the eyes soon after the birth—a treatment which had been recommended by Soranus. Other diseases of the eye listed by Aëtius are abscess of the lids, ectropion (he refers to Antyllus' operation for ectropion), entropion, foreign bodies, carbuncle of the lid, and trichiasis. He frequently quotes Demosthenes and Severus, the most famous ophthalmologists of their day.

All in all the ophthalmology of Aëtius consists of 90 chapters which, for the first time in history, takes in the entire field of ophthalmology.[9]

In striking contrast with the numerous sound principles promulgated by Aëtius are the unscientific nostrums and superstitions of which he frequently approves. For example, in gout, he recommends a very complicated remedy, the use of which is to be begun in January. It is to be taken for 100 days and then its use suspended for 30 days. Following this it is to be again employed for another 100 days and stopped for 15 days. When this is completed it is prescribed again every second day for 260 days. Aëtius treats the agony of a renal colic with a stone upon which is engraved the figure of Hercules strangling the serpent, or by an iron ring, upon one side of which is exhibited an incantation and on the other side a mystic diagram.

The preparation of salves and plasters must take place with certain ceremonies and employing certain religious charms. Thus, while triturating such preparations, until the required consistency is obtained, one must continually repeat in a loud but solemn tone the following charm: "The God of Abraham, the God of Isaac, the God of Jacob, give virtue to this medicament."

For a bone stuck in a patient's throat, Aëtius orders the patient to swallow a sponge moistened with turpentine and fastened to a strong thread in order to catch the foreign body so that it can be withdrawn. If this manipulation fails, he advises the physician to grasp the patient by the throat and repeat the following charm in a loud voice: "As Lazarus was drawn from the grave, and Jonah out of the whale, thus Blasius, the martyr, commands, 'Bone, come up or go down!' " [10]

ALEXANDER OF TRALLES (A.D. 525-608)

One of the most illustrious physicians of the Byzantine period was Alexander of Tralles, frequently referred to as Alexander the Physician. Alexander was born at Tralles, a celebrated city of Lydia. The inhabitants of this city, perhaps because of their proximity to the city of Ionia, famous for the Ionic School of Philosophy, were distinguished for the linguistic purity of their Greek. Alexander was the son of Stephanus, a famous physician of that city, under whom he was instructed in the first rudiments of medicine. It is uncertain whether he was a Christian or a Jew,[11] but from some formulae subjoined to the eleventh book of his works, Dr. Freind concludes that he was not a pagan since the pagans rarely employed incantations formed out of texts of Scripture—a practice which appears to have originated with the earlier Christians.[12]

Alexander's writings show him to have been directly opposed to the Methodist sect. He never once named the grand division of diseases established by the Methodists or the rule of fasting for three days preparatory to beginning a course of medicine. His constant use of purgatives in almost every complaint, and especially in gout, is utterly repugnant both to the Methodist precepts and practice. He was the youngest of five brothers all of whom became distinguished in their chosen fields. His oldest brother Anthemius acquired fame as the builder of Hagia Sofia; he also was one of the foremost mathematicians and physicists of his time. Metrodorus was distinguished as a grammarian. Olympus became renowned as a jurist and Diocorus as a physician.

Alexander of Tralles traveled extensively to obtain practical experience, and finally settled in Rome where he practiced and taught medicine to a number of students.

Alexander flourished during the time of Justinian during the middle of the sixth century. He was a writer of far more originality than either Aëtius or Oribasius, drawing much upon his own personal professional experience, instead of being, like his predecessors, a mere servile compiler.

Alexander of Tralles exhibits a personal style of his own and his methods of arrangement of material are unique. His style is clear, concise, and orderly and he employs chiefly the most common and intelligible expressions. While other writers adopted no methodical arrangement of diseases, he classified them according to a definite and reasonable plan. He is the only Greek writer who can be compared, in this respect, with Aretaeus (30-90).[13] Alexander describes and arranges medical subjects according to the part of the body affected, beginning with the head and proceeding downwards. He distinguishes the true etiology of disease from the exciting and predisposing causes. He offers the opinion that the composition of the morbid humor determines the character of the disease. He divides disease into primary and secondary types and states whether the involvement is local or general. Symptoms, he states, are of two kinds: essential and accidental. Treatment depends upon the diagnosis. "The first purpose of the physician is to eliminate the causes of the disease."

His guiding principle in therapeutics is *contraria contrariis curentur*. "The duty of a physician is to cool the warm, to warm the cool, to dry the moist, and to moisten the dry." "Overinterference with nature and drastic cures must be avoided." "Unfortunately," he states, "there are many who consider those physicians who take pleasure in burning and cutting more competent than those who attempt to cure by the rational system of diet." The choice of drug must be guided by reason and still more by experience. He cautions the physician against adopting a plan for treatment of disease without first having studied the specific and individual causes. Especially in acute conditions, he urges the physician not to follow any routine but to always consider the patient's strength, his constitution, and his mode of life as well as the season of the year and atmospheric variations.[14]

After Alexander retired from his extensive practice he decided to write his medical observations in book form. His clarity of expression, style and keen knowledge of Hippocrates and Aretaeus show good background and independence of thought and practice. He does not hesitate to express his own personal opinions on medical questions although in matters of theory he claims to be a close follower of Galen.

One passage in which Alexander criticizes Galen's therapeutics is noteworthy. He excuses himself in the following manner: "Here may be applied the saying of Galen concerning Archigenes: 'He was a man, and it is therefore difficult to assume that he never made mistakes, since he must have been ignorant of many things, have misinterpreted others and described them superficially.' Yet would I not have dared to say this of a man who stood so high in science, if truth had not inspired me with confidence and if I had not held silence to be a sin. For if a physician form an opinion and fail to express it he does a great wrong, behaves wantonly, and by his silence is much to blame. Herein one should follow the principle which, as he tells us, Aristotle has laid down: 'I love Plato, but I also love truth, and so, if choice must be made between them, I give preference to truth.' " [15]

Considering Alexander's remarkable powers of observation and his great store of common sense, one is surprised to find in his prescriptions the current Byzantine superstitions including spells and charms. Perhaps he had to give at least lip service to the practices of the epoch in which he lived. Particularly when rational treatment failed, he could hardly oppose such superstitious measures as amulets, charms, and incantations, which, after all, appeased the public and did the patient no harm. Perhaps he ordered these much as physicians of the present day prescribe a placebo—for psychological reasons, and particularly to satisfy the rich and fastidious Byzantine patients who could not be persuaded to adopt more rational treatment. For many centuries the teachings of Alexander were universally accepted as authoritative, not only among the Byzantine physicians, but among all physicians, for translations of his works penetrated both the East and West.

Alexander left a medical treatise of 12 books, some of which he dedicated to his father, from whom, as has already been mentioned, he received a considerable part of his education.[16] In this, his *"Libri Duodecim de re Medica,"* he presents the results of his medical labors and he includes his treatises on pathology and the therapeutics of internal diseases. He wrote his "Twelve Books on Medicine" before his death when no longer able to practice and dedicated this work to his friend Cosmas.

Alexander of Tralles was a contemporary of Aëtius. Their works, which are all based on ancient authors, give excellent examples of how Graeco-Roman medicine had degenerated, and that even men of great ability and medical skill resorted at times to superstition. Alexander recommends a mixture of green lizards, live dung beetles and henbane as the best cure of gout and states that these ingredients are only effective if dug up with the thumb and third finger of the left hand when the moon is in Pisces or Aquarius, and when a suitable incantation is recited. This superstitious reliance upon the efficacy of charms and incantations (which may or may not have been sincere), Alexander attempts to vindicate by even appealing to the authority of Galen. Although an admirer of the ancients, he was not afraid to express his dissent with them on occasion, and he even had the courage to question the opinions of Galen on some points.

THEOPHILUS PROTOSPATHARIUS (603-649)

Theophilus Protospatharius, physician and captain of the guard of the Emperor Heraclius (603-641), was one of the most popular physicians and medical authors of the early Middle Ages. Very little is known of his early history. Like so many of the learned physicians of his day, he probably had studied in Alexandria. His treatise, "On the Structure of the Body," contains extracts from Galen's *"De Usu Partum."* He was more physiologist than anatomist, but the basis of his physiology was inspired by piety and teleology. In his physiological writings he refers to the wisdom and goodness of the Divine Being which has ordered everything to be infinitely perfect and which has given to the hand of man precisely five fingers and to the skull a spherical form. The doctrine of teleology had been elaborated by Galen who endeavored to explain physiological processes on the basis of teleology.

The writings of Theophilus, which, like those of the other Byzantine writers, were accepted as authoritative for many centuries, were based primarily on the works of Galen. However Theophilus occasionally made comments on, additions to, and alterations of the concepts of the master. He modified the theory of Galen to the effect that urine arises from the inferior vena cava, by his own hypothesis which states that the fluid part of the urine is already present in the portal vein and reaches the vena cava via very fine capillaries.

The nature of the urine, he states, indicates the condition of the blood and the entire body. He was thus a great believer in uroscopy.

In anatomy, he mentions for the first recorded time, that the olfactory nerves are a special pair of cranial nerves. He gives an original description of the palmaris brevis muscle. He directs attention in his work to the dependence of the development of the skull and vertebral column upon that of the brain and spinal cord. When examining a patient, Theophilus put much stress on the nature of the pulse. His work, "On the Structure of the Body," was used as a textbook in medical schools for many centuries.

PAUL OF AEGINA (PAULUS AEGINETA—625?-690?)

One of the most celebrated of the Byzantine physicians was Paul of Aegina, who received his name because of his birthplace on the island of Aegina. He was among the last of the Greek compilers. Very little is known of his personal life history, and even the period of his birth is disputed. According to Le Clerc's (1652-1728) calculations, he lived in the fourth century. Vander Linden places his birth in the fifth century. Francis Adams in his English translation of the "Epitome," produces documentary evidence that Paul flourished at the end of the sixth or beginning of the seventh century.[17] Garrison records his life span as 625-690 A.D.[18]

Paul was the last great physician of Byzantine culture and background to practice and teach in Alexandria just prior to the destruction of the great medical and cultural center by Omar, whose armies captured the city in the name of the Prophet Mohammed.

Almost all distinguished writers of his own generation and for centuries later quote his opinions frequently in their medical works. Many consider him to be the most eminent of the Byzantine masters.

In the preface of his "Epitome," which consists of seven books, Paul tells why he compiled the "Epitome":

"On this account I have compiled this brief collection from the works of the ancients, and have set down little of my own, except a few things which I have seen and tried in the practice of the art. For being conversant with the most distinguished writers in the profession, and in particular with Oribasius, who, in one work, has given a select view of everything relating to health (he being posterior to Galen, and one of the still more recent authors), I have collected what was best in them, and have endeavored, if possible, not to pass by any one distemper. For the work of Oribasius, comprehending seventy books, contains indeed an exposition of the whole art, but it is not easily to be procured by people at large on account of its bulk, whilst the epitome of it, inscribed to his son Eustathius, is deficient in some diseases altogether, and gives but an imperfect description of others, sometimes the causes and diagnosis being omitted, and sometimes the proper plan of treatment being forgotten, as well as other things which have occurred to my recollection. Wherefore the present work will contain the description, causes, and cure of all diseases, whether situated in parts of uniform texture, in particular organs, or consisting of solutions of continuity, and that not merely in a summary way, but at as great length as possible."[19]

In the first of the seven books of his "Epitome," Paul concerns himself with hygiene, prophylaxis, dietetics (including the nourishing power and uses of the different articles of food), and therapeutics in their connection with the various ages, seasons and temperatures.

The second book is devoted to the various kinds of fever and the symptoms they produce. The third book, covering topical affections, begins at the top of the head and descends down to the toenails. The fourth book concerns itself with complaints that are exposed to view on any part of the body, and this volume also covers intestinal worms. The fifth book describes wounds and bites of venomous animals. The sixth book is a treatise on general surgery. The seventh book is devoted to materia medica. The entire work consists of 242 sections containing everything that was known about the medical arts in his time.

As Paul states himself, his work is based on the seventy books compiled by Oribasius, although throughout his work he quotes a large number of Greek medical masters. The material which he collected is systematically arranged. His style is fluent and easily adapted to the needs of medical students.

Medicine is indebted to Paul for preserving in the seventh book of his "Epitome" one of the best descriptions of the Plague which had been described by Rufus of Ephesus (98 B.C.- 17 A.D.).[20] Because of its classical importance, it will be presented here in full:

"In the plague there is everything which is dreadful, and nothing of this kind is wanting as in other diseases. For there are delirium, vomitings of bile, distension of the hypochondrium, pains, much sweatings, cold of the extremities, bilious diarrheas, which are thin and flatulent; the urine watery, thin, bilious, black, having bad sediments, and the substances floating on it most unfavorable; trickling of blood from the nose, heat in the chest, tongue parched, thirst, restlessness, insomnolency, strong convulsions, and many other things which are unfavorable. Should a person foresee that the plague is coming, by attending to the badness of the season, and the unhealthy occupations of the inhabitants, and from observing other animals perishing; when one observes these things, let him also observe this—what is the character of the present season, and what that of the whole year, for you will be able thereby to find out the best regimen; such, for example, as if the temperature of the season ought to have been dry, but has become humid; in that case, it will be necessary, by a drying diet, to consume the superabundant moisture. Care also must be had to the belly, and when there is phlegm in the stomach it must be evacuated by emetics. And when a fulness of blood prevails, a vein should be opened. Purgings also by urine, and otherwise by the whole body, are proper. But, if the patient is affected with ardent fever, and has a fiery heat about the breast, it will not be improper to apply cold things to the breast, and to give cold drink, not in small quantities, for it only makes the flame burn more; but in full draughts, so as to extinguish it. But if an ardent fever prevails within, and the extremities are cold, and the skin cold, the hypochondrium distended, and the stomach sends the matters which have been melted, some upwards, and others downwards; if watchfulness, delirium, and roughness of the tongue, are present; in these cases, calefacient remedies are wanted to diffuse the heat all over the body, and every other means ought to be tried, in order to determine the heat from the internal to the external parts. The following proportions may be used: of aloes, two parts; of ammoniac perfume, two parts; of myrrh, one part; pound these in fragrant wine, and give every day to the quantity of half a cyathus. I never knew a person, says Rufus, who did not recover from the plague after this draught. So says Rufus: but Galen says, concerning pestilential putrefactions, that to drink Armenian bole, and, in like manner, the theriac from vipers, is of great service; and that in the plague which prevailed in Rome, all died who were not benefited by either of these things." [21]

The following translation from the Latin version of Paul of Aegina's works by Johannes Guinterius von Andernach is here appended:

"I consider moreover a colicy affection, which still becomes violent from a kind of collection of humors, which took its origin from regions in Italy, moreover in many other places in Roman territory whence it spread like the contagion of a pestilential plague. Wherefore in many cases it passed into epilepsy, to some there came a loss of motion, with sensation unhurt, to many both, and of those who fell victim to the epilepsy, very many died. Of those indeed who were paralyzed, not a few recovered; for the cause which attacked them ended by crisis." [22]

The sixth book of Paul's "Epitome" shows that he was a surgeon of note. His military surgery is complete, clear and suited for the kind of warfare of his period. It is based on rich personal experience. This book contains the oldest complete system of operative surgery which has come down to us.

In the treatment of fractures, Paul followed many of the methods of Hippocrates and Soranus with extraordinary thoroughness but here again he alters their teachings when he deems it necessary. He recommends application of splints immediately after the injury, not waiting a week until the swelling is reduced as taught by ancient authorities. In compound fractures he favors the immediate reposition of the protruding fragment despite Hippocrates' teachings that such practice is dangerous. He also advocates immediate reduction of dislocations, which procedure also contradicts the teachings of the ancient authorities.

The ophthalmologic section of the "Epitome" ranks second in prominence to that of Aëtius in his "Tetrabiblos." It was considered the most important treatise on diseases of the eye. His doctrine of trachoma was far advanced of his age.

Regarding the history of the "Epitome," this was published in Greek by the Aldine Press in Venice in 1528. A manuscript in Latin dating from the ninth century was discovered concealed in Mount Cassino. An Arabian translation became the standard textbook in Arabian countries during the fifteenth and sixteenth centuries. Abulcasim has drawn upon Paul for most of his information. An excellent translation of his work in English has been published by Dr. F. Adams.[23]

JOHANNIS ACTUARIUS (13th century)

From the eighth to the fourteenth century there was only one celebrated Byzantine medical writer and this was Johannis Actuarius, the son of Zacharias. The name "Actuarius" was a title applied to court physicians of the Eastern Empire and Johannis occupied the post of imperial court physician of Constantinople during the latter part of the thirteenth century and the beginning of the fourteenth century.

His best known work, *"De Urinis,"* gives evidence of his adherence to the spirit of Hippocrates. He treats each case on its own merits. His remedies are simple and mild and nature is always permitted to do its part; this is in contrast to the "double barrel shotgun" prescriptions with ten or fifteen ingredients dispensed by his medical colleagues.

Johannis made many valuable contributions to clinical medicine. His teachings on the pulse show that he does not always see eye to eye with Galen whom he tries to follow. He often tries to overcome the confusion found in the teachings of the "Pergament."

He wrote a compendium in seven volumes upon the subject of uroscopy which was accepted as authoritative, but he does not depend on the character of the urine alone in reaching a diagnosis. He also believes strongly in the value of the pulse in reaching a diagnosis. "De Urinis," according to Sprengel (Kurt, 1766-1833), is the best treatise on the subject up to his time.

Vierordt considers Johannis to be the first physician to describe paroxysmal hemoglobinuria. His knowledge of the urine was phenomenal. Perhaps even modern physicians have something to learn from him with regard to inspection of the urine. It might be best to let Johannis speak for himself concerning the significance of azure, livid and black urine:[24]

"The urine may be tinged with the same color, azure and livid as well as black, which in thickness as well as in thinness of the surrounding humors, are found in different varieties as well as with different names; so that we should study their significance in various different diseases. Therefore, it is earlier an azure blue in malignancy, but later the same appears blackish blue. Black is by no means allowed to be a bad color itself, since the door of the rich is distinguished by the gloominess of this color. Besides there are colors which can occur concerning which we have just spoken, and which will be discussed a little later. An azure color appears when one suffers a moderate mixing of the melancholy humor, or a more severe chilling, or when some mortification is encountered. Indeed a livid color is seen in the urine, produced in the same manner; moreover it surely suggests injuries or blows inflicted upon a man. On the other hand an azure urine which seems very thin, is generated on the surface of a thin, melancholic humor, which indeed inclines to thickness; this happens because of much coldness. However this azure color may appear from loss of strength, although there was no sign of mixing earlier, but it was changed from bad colors to worse ones. Thou mayest judge by the same reasons the significance of livid urine by saying the same: which indeed appears livid on account of injuries and blows, the bruises and marks of the body will point this out to the eye as well as other signs which thou mayest be able to obtain.

"Yea, indeed, an extremely black urine, moreover, is a sign of heat advanced to an extreme degree, especially where the urine shall have been green, or something approaching this. Moreover it signifies extreme chilliness. And thus thou shalt know this to be due to this cause. Moreover if the livid and azure urine was present before, it signifies chilliness . . . Nevertheless not in all or in part may we see the bad black colors of the urine demonstrated; this is to be understood by the same reason. Since indeed it is found that black urine in men is salutary in preceding diseases, which betray their origin from black humors; now also kinds of melancholia, when a quartan fever terminates, produce a black urine which appears very rapidly."

Johannis declares that urine is filtered from the blood derived from the inferior vena cava. Because of its origin, it may be assumed that changes in the blood have a marked effect on the urine. Therefore he advises the physician to examine the urine carefully using a graduated glass vessel divided into seven sections. Johannis declares that his studies conclusively prove that urine furnishes reliable information as to the humoral pathology of the individual.[25] He explains the occurrence of tetanus by the determination of the humor in the spinal column. He writes upon colic and lead poisoning. He was one of the first to detect and describe the pin worm. He is a great believer in venesection, not only in cases of plethora but also in other morbid conditions. He indicates the best areas for bloodletting in the various morbid conditions. For example, in headache, venesection is to be performed on the upper arms; in diseases of the chest, at the bends of the elbow; and in pleurisy, on the affected side.

His ideas of the workings of the human mechanism are based on the theory that the soul is unembodied and amorphous. The origin of the soul is in the *pneuma* which is formed in the liver. The *pneuma* reaches the heart through the inferior vena cava where it becomes united with the vital spirit, whence it is distributed throughout the body. The greatest transformation occurs when it reaches the brain where the soul spirit takes its origin. "Just as in plants the sap undergoes changes in all parts so does the *pneuma* undergo transformation in every part of the body and the different functions are conditioned by the varying structures of the organs, as light takes the color of the particular glass it shines through."

The mental functions which distinguish man are: (1) perception (2) imagination (3) judgment (4) understanding and (5) reason. He assigns to reason the highest mental function and reason is least bound up with the *pneuma*. The power of imagination is subordinated to all other mental faculties.

The works of Johannis show that he possessed a classical background and an exhaustive knowledge of literature. These facts, coupled with his independent criticisms and evaluations, set him apart from his times.

Johannis evidently belonged to the school of Pneumatics. He

explains all bodily and psychic processes in man by the action of the *pneuma*. His discussion of *pneuma* occupies two volumes of his work. Of course this subject was not new and had been much discussed by almost all ancient writers from Hippocrates and Galen down to Magnus and Theophilus. However, Johannis developed the concept to contain many of his own ideas.

Byzantine medicine comes to an end with the works of Johannis Actuarius, who was a well grounded writer in classical literature and a physician endowed with keen powers of observation and sound judgment. He was not only ahead of his predecessors and contemporaries but also far in advance of his age.

CHAPTER IV

LAY MEDICINE DURING THE EARLY MIDDLE AGES

Apart from a small number of Byzantine lay physicians, few lay doctors are mentioned in the history of the early Middle Ages. That such physicians existed can be inferred from the famous schools that existed during the fourth and fifth centuries in the East at Alexandria, Constantinople, Berytus, Caesarea, Laodicea, Pergamos, Antioch and Athens, and in the West at Rome, Athenaeum, Ravenna, Marseilles, Autun, Bordeaux, Treves, Toulouse, Poitiers, Lyons, Narbonne, Arles, Vienna and Besancon. These schools were mostly under the direction of pagan teachers, and their curriculum included philosophy, medicine, law, literature, grammar and astrology.

The physicians of pagan origin who were educated in these schools could not have suddenly passed off the face of the earth and turned their profession abruptly into the hands of the monks. As a matter fact, Italy at no time entirely lacked lay practitioners of good repute who gave private instructions to students in medicine. It is related that, in the second half of the sixth century, Alexander of Tralles practiced in Rome and, as it was the practice in those days for physicians to train aspirants for the profession, he most likely taught the art of medicine to disciples there. It is further reported that Pope Gregory invited the Archbishop of Ravenna, Marianus, to Rome in order to undergo medical treatment for a malady of the chest. This further bears out the supposition that, in the midst of the ruins of the past, glowing embers of the old Greek tradition never became completely extinguished, but continued to glow under the ashes and were from time to time—even with Church opposition—fanned into fresh flame.

As has been intimated, it woud be a mistake to conclude that the preponderance of clericism and monasticism brought about the complete disappearance of the lay practitioner. A survey of the entire period emphasizes the fact that the decay of medicine and culture in general did not keep pace with the decline of Roman domination. Rome continued her individual existence and many schools of learning kept their doors open although their brilliance faded. In the East we read of the Nestorians of the Bactishua family, of the Schools of Translators and of others.

In Italy there were some lay schools kept open in defiance of the Church. These schools were attended not simply by youths desiring to obtain an education, but also by grown men. The subjects taught were grammar, rhetoric, philosophy, jurisprudence, and medicine. The teachers were appointed by the municipal council and enjoyed certain privileges such as exemption from the duty of quartering soldiers and from other public burdens. Many students went to Italy for their general education, and some went to Constantinople, the capital of the Eastern Empire, where a few secular schools were still in existence. Generally speaking, physicians of pagan origin who practiced medicine outside of the Church, were not respected as their background was poor and their training only superficial. They had no formal school education.

Lay physicians were largely employed to give expert testimony in legal matters dealing with gynecology such as when the virginity of a litigant had to be established. Such cases, naturally, could not be openly handled by the clergy. Expert testimony, in cases of bodily injury and poisoning, also was given by lay physicians.

There existed hospitals under lay administration at Lyons in 542, and at Merida in 580. Besides the hospital physician, there was also the physician-in-ordinary with the title of "Archiater" who performed definite functions. Lay physicians were employed as personal physicians at the palaces of the rulers and even to care for the Popes.

Under Theodoric the Great (454-526), Italy, which in the fifth century had undergone such severe trials, passed through a period of peace and enjoyed material prosperity. The most jealous consideration was given for Roman tradition in the administration of government and the promotion of art and science. In the latter respect, it suffices to mention the names of Cassiodorus, Boethius and Ennodius (474-521). Theodoric, one of the noblest rulers who ever held sway over Italy, wished to be a protector of the Romans rather than a conqueror, and it is for this reason that he left them in possession of their laws and institutions. He established liberal laws and institutions for both the Romans and the Goths, and these people lived in proximity following their respective native customs without any marked antagonism.

Theodoric was the first king in Europe to recognize different nations living within their own clearly marked boundaries as equals. He was not only a patron of the arts and sciences but it is known that his own talented daughter Amalaswintha, spoke Greek with the Greeks, and Latin with the Romans. She saw to it that her son, Atalaric, was instructed in the Roman arts. The Goths possessed a comparatively high development of language and many of them evinced inclination toward scientific studies.

King Theodoric formulated wise regulations governing the practice of physicians (*archiatri*). His concern for medicine and his noble advice to the *archiatri* are well expressed in the famous "Eulogy and Counsel of Theodoric":

THE EULOGY AND COUNSEL OF THEODORIC

"Among the most useful arts that contribute to sustain frail humanity, none may be regarded as superior—or even equal—to medicine, which aids the sick with its maternal benevolence, puts our pains to flight, and gives us that which riches and honour are unable to give. . . . Leave aside, O men of the medical arts, those controversies that are prejudicial to the sick; and if you are not able to come to an agreement consult someone whom you can question without dislike, for every wise man is willing to seek counsel and he is regarded as the most zealous whose frequent questions prove that he is most wise. At the very beginning of your career in this art you are consecrated by oaths like those of the priests: you promise solemnly to your instructors to hate iniquity and love honesty. . . . Remember that to sin against the health of a person constitutes homicide. When I honour you with the title of *Comes Archiatrorum* so that you will be esteemed among the masters of the art of healing and everyone will ask your opinion, I warn you to demonstrate that you are a just arbiter in this notable art. . . . To the expert archiater may the pulse reveal our internal disorders, may the urine reveal them to his eyes. Enter freely into our palace, with full confidence, and may it be permitted to you to prescribe diets, to say things that one would not dare to hear said, and to prescribe even painful treatment in the interest of our health." [1]

The era of the Ostrogoths has bequeathed to us at least one work possessing a trace of originality:—"The Dietetics of Anthimus." Anthimus (5th century) was a Greek physician, and the last lay author who flourished before medicine passed over into the hands of the clergy. Anthimus was expelled from Byzantium and he journeyed to Italy with Theodoric the Great, where he lived for a while as an emissary of the Ostrogoths to the court of the Frankish King Theodoric. His work on dietetics is mainly based on ancient works although this includes his personal experience as a practitioner among the Goths. It is written in the form of an epistle.

He asserts in the introduction that rational dietetics is the foundation of health and the primary factor in preventing disease. He advises moderation in eating and drinking and states that personal preparation of food should not be neglected even on journeys. He states that food should be easily digestible.

Anthimus lists one hundred different articles of food and drink which are digestible and nourishing and discusses the preparation of each. He points out the nutritional value of each of the individual parts of the ox and swine. He warns against the use of pickled meat, bacon-rind and pigeons "because they feed on helebore" and he also cautions against the use of hard boiled eggs, old cheese, most mushrooms, old fish and oysters.

Anthimus, oddly enough, believes in the therapeutic efficacy of bacon in treating intestinal parasites and of partridge flesh and rice cooked in goat's milk in combating dysentery. He employs barley-meal porridge diluted with tepid water in treating fever and almond or fig emulsion in cases of catarrh and angina.[2]

Other lay physicians were the *archiater* Peter, who was court physician to a later Frankish king named Theodoric (about 605), and the *archiater* Reovalis (about 590). The latter mentions that he was called in to see a small boy who had a disease of his thigh; the little patient's case had been given up as hopeless. He writes: "I, having made an incision into the testicles (strangulated inguinal hernia?), as I had once seen done in the city of Constantinople, restored the boy sound to his sorrowing mother." This narrative indicates the existence at this time of a higher class of lay physician who possessed some surgical knowledge and skill. This was doubly important at a time when surgery was forbidden to monkish physicians.

Among the Alemanni,[3] lay physicians were employed for medico-legal duties. In the Germanic codes, mention is made of the fee to be granted the physician in the determination of the penalty for bodily injuries. The Langobard Code, promulgated in the year 650, contains this stipulation: "Whosoever has inflicted wounds upon anyone, he shall supply him with attendance and likewise pay the fee of the physicians, at a rate to be estimated by learned men."

Among the Visigoths, the lay physician, having undertaken the treatment of a case, was obliged to conclude an agreement concerning proper remuneration and also to post security for malpractice. For the cure of various diseases there were distinct fees: for example, a fee of 5 *solidi* was charged for a cataract extraction. If the patient died but the physician had performed his duties satisfactorily, the physician received no fee but he could withdraw without hindrance. If the physician committed any technical error, he had to pay a fine. If, however the death of the patient was brought about by the treatment of the physician, the physician was subject to fine or worse. If the patient were a servant, the physician had to provide another servant of similar value; if, on the other hand he were a freeman, the physician laid himself open to arbitrary punishment from the relatives. The physician could only perform venesection on free women in the presence of a relative—even if the procedure were deemed urgent. Any infraction of this regulation led to a fine of 10 *solidi*.

Such stringent enactments naturally hindered medical action —and particularly reputable medical action—for none but itinerant quacks could hope to escape criminal prosecution.

What ecclesiastic domination failed to accomplish in the process of disintegration of medical practice was completed in the sixth century by famine, by savage wars that raged between the Ostrogoths and the Byzantines and, most of all, by the pestilences which followed in the wake of the wars. This terrible devastation which continued to the eighth century strangulated all pursuit of science and undermined all confidence in lay medicine. In the face of the epidemics, the lay physicians became helpless and the people abandoned themselves entirely to faith. To be sure the clerical physicians could not avert an epidemic or cure those who were stricken by it but their methods were harmless and appealed to the religious sense and the patient at least was inspired by the hope of entering a new and brighter existence in the hereafter.

On the other hand the lay physician at that period had nothing to inspire confidence. His chief methods of diagnosis were based on uroscopy and palpation of the various pulses and even if he reached some conclusion as to the disease, his treatment was revolting and cruel and not devoid of superstition. To attempt to catalogue all remedies and cures that have passed through the alimentary tract of man throughout the ages is to undertake to compile a work on human folly. In the name of the healing art man has resorted to wild nostrums, loathsome and nauseating excreta of cats, dogs, goats and even bats and mice, and disgusting remedies such as snakes, toads, lizards and mice.

Hanging the victim by the feet or gouging out one of his eyes so that the poison might run out, were regarded as proper methods of curing poisoned patients. The last is said to afford the explanation as to how Emperor Albrecht lost one of his eyes. Even so eminent a naturalist as Conrad von Megenberg, as late as the year 1342, went from Vienna to Regensburg to the grave of St. Erhard for the sole purpose of creeping over his grave while a hymn of his own composition was sung.

The time of taking the various abominable mixtures prescribed by the physician was often determined by the position of the sun, moon and stars. At times the relative wealth of the patient guided the practitioner in compounding his prescription.

In addition to the lay doctors, there were old wives, eccentric individuals, shepherds, minstrels, jugglers, executioners and similar gentry who dabbled in medical practice.

"There is nothing men will not do," said Oliver Wendell Holmes (1809-1904), "there is nothing they have not done to recover their health and save lives. They have submitted to be half-drowned in water, and half-choked with gases, to be buried up to their chins in earth, to be scarred with hot irons like galley slaves, to be crimped with knives like codfish, to have needles thrust into their flesh, and bonfires kindled on their skins, to swallow all sorts of abominations, and to pay for all this, as if to be singed and scalded were a costly privilege, as if blistering were a blessing and leeches a luxury."

In the seventh century, the embryonic lay-physician studied in the traditional manner under the tutelage of an older physician.

All physicians were subject to certain rules and regulations. The "Fuero Juzgo," a Spanish translation of the original code of the Visigoths entitled "Forum Judicium,"[4] reads as follows:

1. "No physician may undertake to bleed a woman in the absence of her relatives; if he has done so, he shall pay 10 *solidi*[5] to the relatives or to the husband, since it is not impossible that occasionally some advantage may be associated with such an opportunity." In all Germanic legal codes (Salic, Ripuarian, Bavarian) carnal offenses were very severely punished. Whoever touched the hand, arm or breast of a maiden was fined 15,

30 or 35 *solidi,* in the order mentioned. A manservant who impregnated a maid of another, who died during pregnancy or labor was castrated. Hence it follows that this unchristian operation was still in vogue and was performed as a punitive measure. Castration was likewise performed from motives of pure revenge, as the case of Abelard (who was castrated by the friends of Heloise in consequence of his love for her) proves. The same vengeance too was commonly taken among the southern Slavs, Arabs, Abyssinians, Negroes, Turks, and Indians.

2. "No physician shall visit any person confined in prison without the presence of the jailer, lest the prisoner, through fear of his punishment, may seek the means of death at his hands."

3. "When anyone has called a physician to see a sick person, or to heal a wound, the physician, when he has seen the wound or recognized the pains, shall at once take charge of the patient under definite security."

4. "When a physician has assumed charge of a patient under security, he must cure him. If death ensues, he shall not demand the stipulated fee, nor shall a suit be instituted for it by either party." Some physicians, however, in serious cases, guarded themselves from prosecution by having the patients declared legally dead in advance of treatment, so that if death actually ensued it could not be ascribed to their treatment.

5. "If a physician has removed a cataract from the eye and restored the patient to his former health, he shall receive a fee of five *solidi.*"

6. "If a physician injures a nobleman in bleeding him, he shall pay 150 *solidi.* If, however, the patient dies, the physician (how equitable!) shall be delivered up at once to his relatives, to be dealt with as they may see fit. When however, the physician has killed or injured a slave, he must return a slave of the same kind."

7. "When a physician has accepted a student, he shall receive a fee of twelve *solidi.*"

8. "No one shall cast a physician into prison without hearing, except in case of murder." [6]

It should be noted that there was a distinction made between a visit to the sick, and a visit for treating a wound. In Sweden[7] the educated physician was expected to understand not only illness, but also treatment of fractures, incised wounds, wounds of the skin, stabs through the body and amputations. The unerudite lay physician was regarded as a mere mechanic and tradesman.

It does not follow, however, from the ordinance cited, that the physicians of the Visigoths were necessarily regarded with special disrespect. These ordinances, like all similar laws from the beginning of time to the present day, were instituted chiefly to provide against transgressions and to meet exceptional cases.

In spite of the fact that lay physicians were considered members of the so-called lower class, their high remuneration and severe penalties indicate their relatively high social position.

Toward the midpoint of the Middle Ages, monkish or clerical medicine had about entirely superseded all higher lay practice and for all practical purposes only herniotomists, lithotomists, oculists and lower medical itinerants survived. The position of the lay physician at this time particularly was considered disreputable as may be inferred from the action of King Gram, who, in order to remain unrecognized during a festival, put on the dress of a physician and took the lowest seat at the dining table.

The so-called *volksarzte* of the Germans were probably the uninterrupted successors of the lower itinerant physicians. The higher class lay physicians, who still existed among the Goths in the beginning of the Middle Ages, disappeared, or at least took a position of inferiority until the foundation of the school at Salerno and the European universities.

Anthimus, (5th century) to whom we have hitherto referred, is the last lay author of the West for a period of 400 years. Following him the conduct of literary affairs remained in the hands of the clergy and monks.

It is related that Cassiodorus, "the last Roman," amidst the chaotic confusion erupting in the West, undertook the responsibility of preserving the heritage of literature through monkish influence—without, however, taking measures to combat the superstition which flourished so universally in his unenlightened era.

Cassiodorus recommended the study of medicine to the monks giving them detailed advice as to which writers of antiquity should be studied as a foundation for learning the healing art. Addressing the monks, he declared: "Learn to know the properties of herbs and the blending of drugs, but set all your hopes upon the Lord, who preserves life without end. If the language of the Greeks is unknown to you, you have the herb-book of Dioscorides, who has described and depicted the herbs of the field with astonishing accuracy. Afterwards read Hippocrates and Galen in Latin translation especially the 'Therapeutics' of the latter, which he has dedicated to the philosopher Glaucon and the work of an unknown author, which, as would appear from investigation, is compiled from several writers. Study further the Medicine of Caelius Aurelianus, the Hippocratic book upon herbs and healing methods, as well as a variety of other treatises upon the healing art which I have brought together in my library and have bequeathed to you."

He stressed that the healing art was a worthy calling in that it concerns both the present and future well being of patients and aids them when other (i.e. spiritual) means fail. He warned physicians to avoid quarrels, jealousy, all forms of wickedness, and all methods of disreputable therapy. He exhorted physicians to ever seek knowledge, to read the works of the Ancients, to manifest zeal and cheerfulness in treating the sick, and to seek purity in their personal lives. For an effective bedside manner, the following advice was given: "Let your visits bring healing to the sick, new strength to the weak, certain hope to the weary. Leave it to clumsy (practitioners) to ask the patients they are visiting whether the pain has ceased and if they have slept well. Let the patient ask you about his ailment and hear from you the truth about it. Use the surest possible informant. To a skillful physician palpation of the pulsing of the veins reveals the patient's ailment while the appearance of the urine indicates the prognosis. To make things easier, do not tell the clamoring inquirer what these symptoms signify."

The seeds of Cassiodorus did not fall on barren soil. The works or translations recommended by him are still in part extant in numerous manuscripts.

One of the most liberal monarchs, Emperor Charlemagne (742-814), King of the Francs, was a patron of the classics. He organized schools at every cathedral modelled after the schools of the Egyptian temples and Arabian mosques, and from the year 806 onward, it was expected that medicine should be included in the curriculum. These institutions were important not only in the development of general education but also in the revitalization of medical knowledge. Such schools were developed in Paris, Fulda, Wurzburg, Hershaw, Metz, Lyons, Cremona, Parma and Florence. The personal physicians of Charlemagne were Wintraw and a Jew named Abul Faradsh; the latter must not be confused with the Arabian historian of the same name who is also known as Bar-Hebraeus (1226-1286).[8]

To the curriculum of the Cathedral Schools which originally embraced the seven sciences (the trivium: grammar, logic and rhetoric; plus the quadrivium: arithmetic, music, geometry and astronomy), he ordered that medicine should also be taught under the name of *physic*.

In England, King Alfred (849-901) is known not only as a warrior but also as a proponent of higher education. He is, without question, one of the greatest men England has ever produced. Under his sovereignty, good laws were enacted and his was a golden age of peace and happiness for his subjects. He always stood ready to improve the lot of his subjects. He founded schools for rich and poor in England. One of his schools was founded in the city of Oxford (*not* the famous university of the same name).

Like Charlemagne, Alfred, in his educational work, received assistance from monk scholars. He was also aided by the learned Jews who came to live at his court by invitation. He divided his time wisely between study, prayer and business of state. His

79

great tolerance is shown by a letter to his son in which he says, "For God's love my son and for the advantage of thy soul, let they (the slaves) be masters of their freedom and their own will; and in the name of the living God I entreat that no man disturb them; that they shall be as free as their thoughts to serve what Lord they please." [9]

Monks and clerical physicians appear to have filled the gaps which existed from the time the lay educational institutions declined until the universities made their appearance. They particularly undertook the state care of the poor which formerly had been performed by the *archiatri popularis* or municipal physicians.

By the close of the sixth century most secular schools had disappeared and had been replaced by cathedral or monastic schools. In England, monastic schools were founded at Iona (565), at Oxford, at Cambridge (c. 670), at Whitby (675) and at Jarrow (678), and later at York, Winchester and Canterbury. In Ireland monastic schools were introduced by St. Patrick (c. 440). Among the famous European schools were those of Fulda, Hershaw, Prum, St. Gall, Chartres, Tours, Weisenburg and Reichenau. It is not known whether medicine was included in the curriculum of any of these schools.

Clerical physicians belonged to the lower as well as the higher clergy. The Church at times declared the professional successes of the lower clergy to be miracles and canonized the parties concerned. In case of the death of one of these clerical physicians— indeed with other physicians too— it was customary to place manuscripts of the writings of Galen, Hippocrates, etc., in his coffin. In later years the rank and file of the higher clergy often produced well educated physicians, such as for example, John of St. Amand (c. 1200), Peter of Spain (died 1277) and Simon de Cordo (died 1330). When the practice of medicine was forbidden to the clergy, the decrees of councils were often ignored—even with regard to surgical operations which were strictly forbidden.

Various clerical physicians enjoyed Church benefits in return for which they were expected to instruct pupils gratis and to treat the sick without charge—a consideration, however, that was not always carried out. Hence Emperor Sigismund in 1406 enforced these regulations and declared: "The high Magistrati in Physica treat no one gratuitously, and hence they are going to hell." Clerical physicians, in many cities, gave free advice on appointed days, chiefly in the vestibules of the churches where the sick were brought. That some of the priests did not perform their duties very zealously is evidenced by the decree of the Council of Vienna.[10]

The earliest hint of clerical participation in surgery is found in the alleged performance of a Caesarean section by Bishop Paul of Merida. It is related that Bishop Masona built a large hospital at Merida in 580. According to Neuburger, it is extremely probable that in this institution the influence of the Nestorians' skill in medicine made itself felt.

Following the conversion of the Aryan Visigoths to Catholicism (586), monastical and ecclesiastical instruction received a considerable impetus. We may assume definitely that institutions and monasteries were provided with several physicians. From the ecclesiastical schools came Isidorus Hispalensis (Bishop Isidore of Seville 570-636), one of the most educated men of the Middle Ages.[11]

It will be recalled that the Church had prohibited the monks from exercising their activities beyond the walls of the monasteries. The practice of medicine beyond the cloister introduced an element of commercialism in the priests' lives and kept them away from their religious duties. Frequently monks were called away to distant places to give medical attention to dignitaries of the Church and princes of state. Monks engaged in medical procedure traveled about more and more and returned to the monastery only for important holy days. Some of the ecclesiastical healers actually forgot their traditional opposition to the shedding of blood and engaged in surgery and some even substituted drugs for prayer. Such practices finally culminated in the promulgation by the council of Rheims which prohibited monks and ecclesiastics from practicing medicine outside their orders altogether; after the year 1219, no member of a religious order was permitted to go outside of the monastery to practice medicine.

Ecclesiastic medicine began to decline in the tenth century due to a number of factors, chief of which was the fact that the people lost faith in the monks on account of the behavior of some of their number. While monks generally observed the "Benedictine Rule" with regard to virtue, humility, obedience and hospitality and engaged in manual labor and intellectual work, there were some whose capacity for evil counterbalanced their desire to do good. Exempt from all civil authorities, some monks took advantage of their privileged status and became unruly. At times the monasteries became actual hotbeds of insubordination to the state and even to the Church. Part of this temptation to evil arose out of Church celibacy. On rare occasions, the conduct of certain monks actually occasioned public scandals.

Another great influence which led to the decline of monkish medicine was the rising belief in the medical efficacy of the invocation of saints and relics. Every country had its saints and each saint had control over a certain disease or diseased organ. The healing power of saints was frequently exercised through relics in the shrines consecrated to them. These forms of healing were very costly and patients had to travel long distances and pay large sums for the privilege of employing them.

The Crusades, especially, brought an extended field of activity in the lay medical field. Innumerable hospitals were founded as a result of these military expeditions, and lay physicians ran these institutions. The great Hohenstaufer, Fredrick II, enlightened by the wisdom of the Orient was active in the promotion of education and especially in the elevation of the position of physicians. By his high regard for medical studies and educational institutions, he became a benefactor of mankind—especially in Italy. Through his medical ordinance, published in 1242, which paid no heed to the triple ban of Pope Gregory IX (1227-1241), he secured for himself an honorable place in the history of medical culture.

Roger, King of Sicily, and grandfather of Fredrick II, had

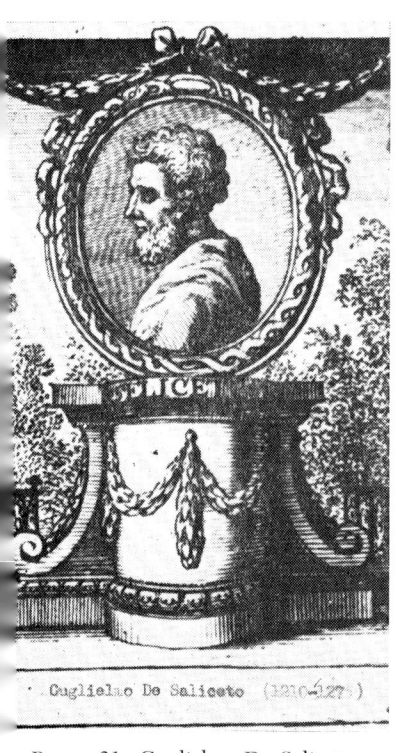

PLATE 21. Guglielmo De Saliceto
(1210-1275)
(Courtesy New York Acad. of Med.)

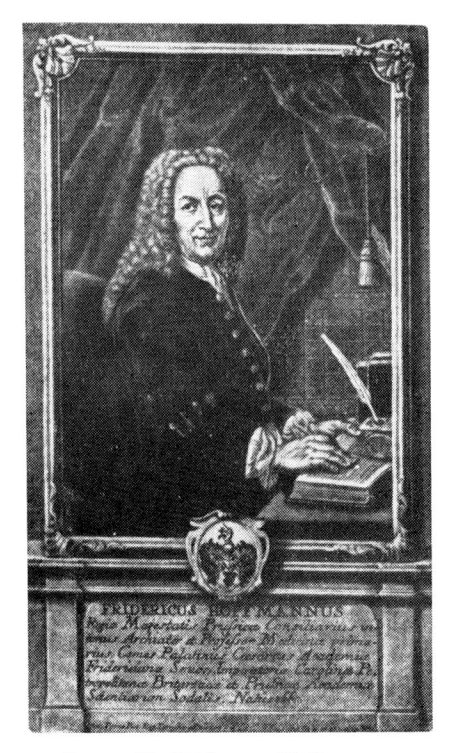

PLATE 22. Fridericus Hoffmannus

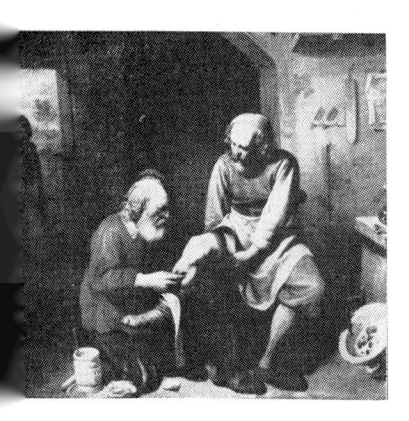

PLATE 23. The Village Doctor. This painting by Ryckeart (Flemish School, 1612-61) shows a village practitioner treating a leg injury. It is now hanging in the Kaiser Friedrich Museum in Berlin.

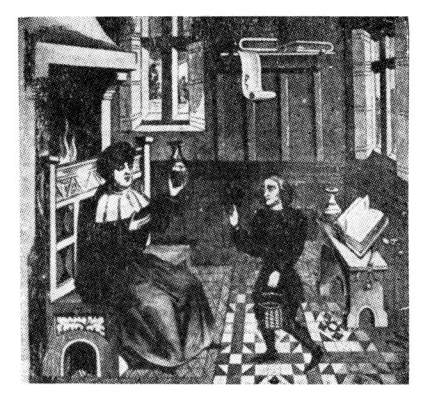

PLATE 24. The Medieval Physician in his office.

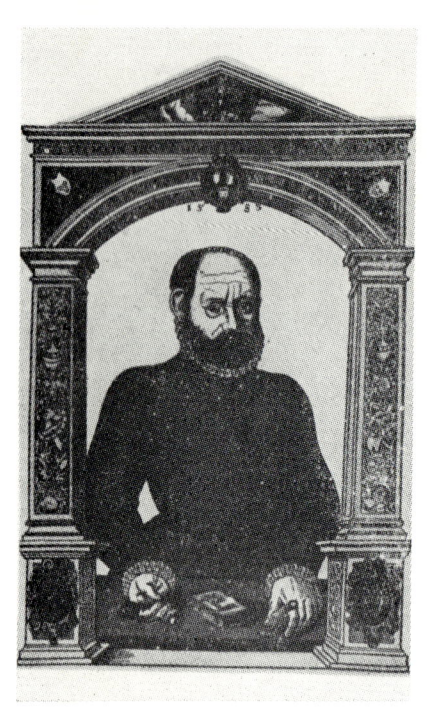

PLATE 25. Georg Bartisch, author of *Ophthalmoduleia* (1583), a book on the care of the eyes. In it he inveighs against quack oculists.

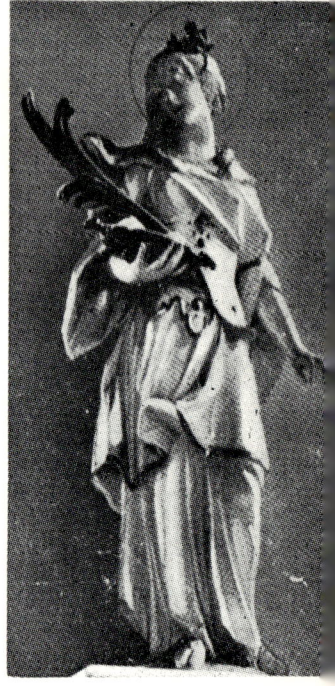

PLATE 26. St. Agatha, patron breast diseases.

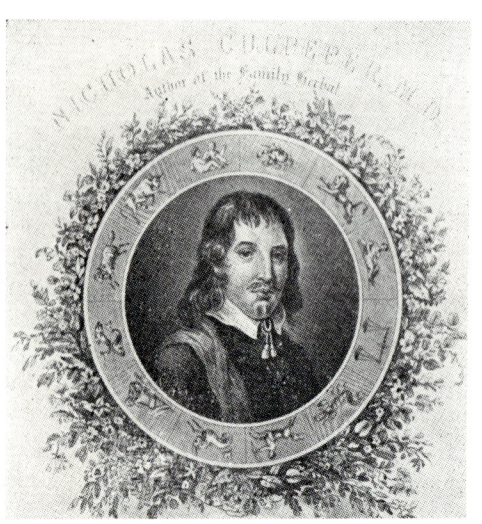

PLATE 27. Nicholas Culpepper, student in Physics and Astronomy.

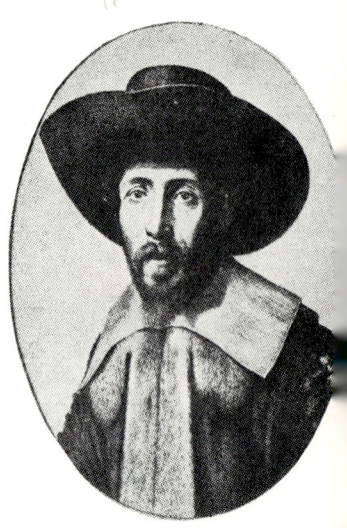

PLATE 28. The Physician, Joseph Medigo (1591-1655), engraved Willem J. Delff after painting W. C. Duvster.

already published an ordinance providing that the physician, before entering practice, must present himself to the civil magistrates and procure their permission, "in order that my subjects may not incur danger through the inexperience of the physicians." For violation of this ordinance the penalty of imprisonment and confiscation of all worldly goods was established. His grandson, Fredrick II, enlarged upon the important regulations of Roger's ordinance and came up with the following:

Code of Physicians and Surgeons

A. To practice in all branches of medicine (and surgery also), and to bear the title of physician, is permitted only to him who has passed an examination at Salerno, and received the state-license from the Emperor or his viceroy. Violators of the law are to be punished by fines of money and goods, and receive one year's imprisonment.

B. Before a physician is admitted to an examination, he must have attended lectures in logic for 3 years, and on medicine and surgery for 5 years, and must have practiced under the direction of an experienced physician for 1 year.

C. Physicians are to be examined on the books of Hippocrates, Galen, and Avicenna.

D. To be approved, the surgeon is to bring evidence that he has attended the lectures of professors, and pursued for one year the curriculum which surgeons hold necessary, including a satisfactory course in human anatomy. Surgeons of the first class are to be examined by three professors, of whom one teacher of surgery is to conduct the examination in the Latin language, and in the presence of recognized authorities of the nation of the candidate. The diploma is to be signed by all these persons, accompanied by the attestation of a notary, and must bear the seal of the Faculty. Surgeons of the second class are to be examined in Italian and by two teachers only, and the diploma is then to be subscribed by the two examiners alone.

Surgical candidates must take an oath never to treat internal disease, and they may never receive the title of doctor.

E. The physician must swear to give information of such fact if an apothecary sells adulterated drugs.

F. The physician must not be guilty of collusion with the apothecary as regards the price of drugs; still less might he keep a drug-store.

Fees of the Physician According to the Code

A. The poor must be treated without charge.

B. The physician must visit his patients at least twice each day, and, if requested, once also at night. For this he receives for each day's treatment:

    (1) In the city, or at his residence, half a *tarenus*.

    (2) Away from his residence, when:
        The patient paid his traveling expenses, 3 *tareni*
        The doctor paid his traveling expenses, 4 *tareni*

Of Apothecaries, Druggists and Their Tariff

A. The druggists (confectionari) must compound and keep their drugs properly and in the prescribed method, which fact must be certified by physicians, and even confirmed by an oath. Contravention of this regulation was punished by seizure of goods and even by death.

B. The apothecaries (stationarii) must keep all regular drugs and samples for no longer than one year from the day of purchase; they can charge 3 *tareni* per ounce; for medicines requiring aging for more than one year, they were permitted to charge 6 *tareni* per ounce.

Apothecary-shops could be kept only at places designated throughout the kingdom.[12]

Theodoric's famous *Chirurgia* was originally published in the year 1267. Divided into four parts, this work deals with wounds, dislocations, fractures and hemorrhage. He suggests control of venous bleeding by pressure and arterial bleeding by ligature above and below the point of severance of the artery. He treats skull fracture by elevation and removal of the loose pieces. His handling of lacerations with stitching and dry dressings left unchanged for four or five days is suggestive of modern surgery.[13]

CHAPTER V

MEDICINE IN THE KORAN

Very little is known of Arabian learning prior to the sixth century, beyond the fact that under Emperor Trajan (A.D. 53-117) there existed a Roman province in Arabia which included the fertile land of Haraun extending as far as Petra. Through this province, a certain amount of western learning must have filtered through to the Arabian people. During the fourth century there was a migration of the Nestorians from Syria to Edessa and of Jews to the suburbs of Mecca and to other of the larger cities of Arabia. Among the migrants, there were skilled physicians respected for their scholarship in the medical arts and science whose tenets were based on Greek learning. Nonetheless the fact that prior to the end of the seventh century Arabia had not produced a single personality of scholarly attainment shows that the foreign scholars did not make much impression on the native Arabians. In other words, although the aforementioned scholars were treated with hospitality by the Arabian tribes, their knowledge did not permeate the shell of Arabian ignorance and indifference.

A change of sentiment among the native Arabians was put into motion at the beginning of the sixth century when the pagan religion was assailed from many directions by the Zoroastrians, Christians, and Jews. To these attacks the native nomadic tribes could no longer be indifferent. Widespread discussion and public disputation ensued which led to tribal blood feuds. Yet until 569 the people of Arabia failed to produce a single individual wise enough to stand up against these external religious attacks.

In the year 569 A.D., two years after the death of Justinian, there was born at Mecca, in Arabia, the man who, of all men, has exercised the greatest personal influence upon the human race. He elevated his own nation from a religion of fetishism which involved the adoration of a meteoric stone and the basest idol-worship, to a monotheism which quickly and irrevocably wrenched from Christianity more than half its possessions. Reference is made to Mohammed and his code of laws, the "Koran."

In order to properly evaluate the medicine of the Koran one has to analyze the cultural status of the Arabs. Prior to the advent of Mohammed, Arabia was peopled by various nomadic races of pure Arab blood which roamed about the land in the never ending search to find pasture for their flocks. There were a relatively few individuals who occupied themselves with either tilling the soil of small farms or trading. When Mohammed came on the scene, the inhabitants of Arabia were far from independent; they were variously subjected to the governments of Abyssinia, Persia and the Byzantine Empire. Parts of the people were governed by members of leading families. The primitive Bedouins did not recognize any government. They considered their rights to the fields and prairies of the country for pasture of their flocks inalienable.

As has been intimated, prior to the appearance of the prophet, the people of Arabia were pagans. There were deities for every natural occurrence. The healing of the sick was the province of the holyman who claimed to know the way of the gods. Folklore and magic played an important role in curing disease. It is true that Christianity was penetrating from Syria to some degree and had made headway in the larger towns such as in Bagdad, Medina, and Mecca. Several prosperous Jewish settlements had also been established through the influence of the Byzantine government north of Mecca. The monotheistic principle of the Jewish and Christian elements of the city populations had just about begun to filter through to the native pagan populations.

Mohammed possessed that combination of qualities and attributes which more than once has decided the fate of empires.

A preaching soldier, he was eloquent on the pulpit and valiant on the field. His theology was simple and plain spoken: "There is but one God." He did not engage in vain metaphysics, but applied himself to improving the social condition of his people by regulations concerning personal cleanliness, sobriety, fasting and prayer. Above all other munificent acts, he esteemed almsgiving and charity. He was generous to other religions and admitted the salvation of men of any form of faith provided they were virtuous. To the declaration that there is but one God, he added, "and Mohammed is his Prophet."

The first monotheistic school to take definite form was the Hanifite School which had been founded by Abu Hanifa in Baghdad (767). This school vigorously opposed paganism. Its doctrine, known as Hanifism, to which Mohammed was converted, rejected all polytheistic beliefs with their superstitious practices and accepted the belief in one God. The Hanifites originally included only a small group but quickly grew into a large religious cult. They adopted the teachings of the Old and New Testament. Under the Hanifite influence, the deities which were appealed to by the pagans in disease and misfortune lost their prestige. Having lost faith in their gods, they turned to their wisemen for help in sickness. Thus trained lay healers from the Byzantine Empire, Persia and India came to Arabia and were consulted in case of sickness.

Naturally enough, superstitious medical practices were not abandoned altogether. Doctors and medical writers, as is their wont, yielded to the spirit of the times and did not hesitate to recommend charms and amulets in connection with their natural remedies.

At this period, a prominent Arabian physician, Al Harith ben Kalada, from el-Taif near Mecca, who was a contemporary of Mohammed, appeared on the medical scene. Al Harith was a student of the Academy of Jondisabur, Persia. Before he returned to Mecca he traveled through India in search of medical knowledge. Upon his return he spread the teachings of the Hippocratic lore among the more intellectual of his countrymen.

Some medical ideas in the Koran have been traced to Al Harith.

The preservation and restoration of health is one of the most important objects of all religious codes. Both Babylonian and Egyptian religious codes were associated with medicine. The priest also attended to the sick. Manu (in the holy books of the Brahman, Buddha and reformed Brahman religions), Confucius (in China), Zoroaster (in the Zend Avesta), Moses (in the Old Testament) and Jesus (in the New Testament) all concerned themselves with the health of their people.

Of course, the Koran is primarily a religious and ethical code and by no stretch of the imagination can it be considered a medical work. It touches upon medical subjects only indirectly and then only from the viewpoint of a layman.

The hygiene and the prophylaxis found in the Koran are not nearly so scientifically contrived and deeply rooted as those contained in the Old Testament and the medical subjects treated in the Koran are certainly not on a par with those of the Talmud (which system was written about 100 years before the appearance of the Koran).[1] However considering the cultural difference between the Jews and Arabs of that period, there is no question that the Koran served as an instrument for improving the health of the people.

The medical subjects dealt with in the Koran include dietary regulations, rules of cleanliness, problems of social hygiene, marriage regulations, sexual matters and laws of circumcision. While the medical phenomena of the Koran are generally of a supernatural nature, the hygiene of the Koran is essentially rational and is of no negligible worth.

Mohammed ordered that the sick be kept separate from the rest of the population. The Koran follows the Old Testament in dealing with leprosy: "They should cry out at him, 'Unclean! Unclean!'"[2]

The very touch of a dead body contaminates one. Such a doctrine is also found in the religious codes of Manu, Zoroaster and Moses.

The Koran states that Abraham was deserted by his people

because of his contact with the dead: "And he said, 'I am sick, then they turned back from him'." The Israelites left their houses by the thousands in fear of death.

Under the subject of hygiene may be included the methods of disposal of the dead. In tropical and subtropical climates, dead bodies have to be disposed of promptly in order to render them harmless to the living. Prompt burial was the most frequent method used. Cremation was at times employed and in some cases the dead were disposed of by throwing them in a box into deep water. Criminals were left for the vultures to consume: "Then the birds will eat from his head."[3] The Koran here refers to the "baker" of Pharaoh whose dreams were interpreted by Joseph.[4]

Hygienic directions are given with reference to clothing, dwelling-places, sleep, cleanliness of the skin, selection of food and drink, bodily care and attention to the sick. The Koran enumerates the objects Allah has created for the benefit of the faithful: "And God makes for you places of rest in your house and makes for you camps out of the skins of animals . . . and from their wool and their furs and their hair, there are household goods and things to use for a time."[5] "And he makes for you coats which shelter you against heat."[6]

ETIOLOGY[7]

The etiological doctrine manifested all through the Koran is that there is one cause for all diseases and misfortunes—sin. "Whatever good befalleth you, our men, is from God. Whatever evil befalleth you is from yourself." "And he against whom my wrath becomes due, he surely perishes, and most surely I am exceedingly forgiving to him who turns to me and believes and does good."[8] "If Allah were to take away your hearing and your eyes and put a seal upon your heart what deity other than Allah would bring it back to you?"[9]

It is clear if all diseases arise from one cause, there can be only one remedy and this is to obtain forgiveness from Allah.

With such a thought pattern there are naturally very few physical remedies mentioned in the Koran. A more complete discussion of Koranic Etiology is contained in this chapter later.

ANATOMY

Anatomy was a defunct science to the Arabs in the days of Mohammed. The Koran mentions very little of the bodily structure, and when it does refer to it, Mohammed's grave ignorance of anatomy is manifest. He apparently gave credence in the Koran to the idea that the trachea terminates in the heart. Evidently the Koran was influenced by the ancient concept that the *pneuma* supplies the body with life, and reaches the heart, "the organ of life," via the nostrils and the trachea. The heart was thought to be the seat of the soul and at death the soul was thought to return to Allah by the reverse route: i.e., from the heart to the trachea to the nostrils.[10]

The prophet seems to have had some knowledge of the large blood vessels (aorta or vena cava) near the heart. "And then we would have certainly cut his vein" near the heart.[11]

PHYSIOLOGY

What has been said of Koranic etiology and anatomy applies even more to physiology. Every human motion and sensation is controlled by Allah. The Koran discusses physiologic functions only to extol the wonders of Allah. When discussing the origin of milk, the Koran states, "We give a drink out of what is in their insides from betwixt the contents of the blood." To this the commentators add: "The coarse elements of food pass out through the kidneys and rectum and the more delicate ones turn into milk and the finest into blood."

EMBRYOLOGY

Only second to the creation of heaven and earth does the Koran marvel over the process of procreation. References to procreation are frequently made in the Koran. Two different versions of the mechanism of fecundation are presented: One is to the effect that "We have created man of the mingling seeds of both sexes."[12] The other harks back to a theory popular in the days of Aristotle: "We formerly created man of a finer sort of clay (referring to Adam); afterwards we placed him in the form of seed in a sure receptacle (the womb); afterwards we made the seed coagulated blood and we formed the coagulated blood into a piece of flesh (clot); then we formed the piece of flesh into bones (skeleton) and we clothed these bones with flesh (muscles); then we produced the same by another creation."[13]

From this rude description of the formation of the human body, one may assume that the male alone furnishes the seminal fluid and that woman's share in the process of fecundation is merely that of an incubator. The male germ mixes with the blood of the female in the uterus where it forms a clot which gradually changes into flesh, which in turn ossifies to form a skeleton, and finally the bones are covered with muscles to complete the formation of the new body. "And after birth God perfected him and breathed into him of his spirit and gave him hearing, sight and heart."[14] The only organs mentioned in the Koran are the ears, eyes, and heart. The last was considered the seat of the soul and the organ of understanding.[15]

As to the source of the seminal fluid, the Koran repeats the ancient idea that it arises from the head, reaching the testicles after transit through the spinal column. "He made man out of liquid poured forth coming out between the back bone and the breast bone."[16] This idea is also found in the Talmud.[17] The Koran repeats several times the observation that man originates from a "repulsive drop." "Have we not created you of a repulsive drop of seed which we placed in a sure depository until the fixed time of delivery?"[18] An expression used in the "Dicta of the Fathers" reads: "Reflect upon these things and thou wilt not fall a prey to sin: Know whence thou comest—from a repulsive drop; and whither thou goest—to a place of decay."[19]

The safety of the seed and the growth of the child are secured by three different layers of tissue: "He formed you in the womb of your mother by several gradual formations within three veils (the abdominal wall, the womb, and the membranes) of darkness in which the fetus is developed."[20] The description in the Koran of the *"conception immacula,"* while supernatural, is still within the range of natural laws. It tells the story not in the sense of Catholic dogma but in a natural sense; thus the angel appeared to Mary in the form of a man: "And he sent our spirit Gabriel into her and he appeared unto her in the shape of a perfect man."[21]

With reference to the newly born child the Koran directs mothers to nurse their babies on their breasts for a period of two years: "And the mothers suckle their children for two complete years.[22] In the case of those who wish to complete their period of suckling, it is the duty of the father of the child to feed them (i.e., the mothers) and clothe them with fairness."[23] This ruling makes it compulsory on the part of the father to provide the mother with special food and clothes. On the other hand, if both parents ". . . desire to wean the child by mutual consent or counsel there is no blame on them."[24]

Instead of the mother suckling her own child, Mohammed permitted the employment of a wet nurse: "But if you desire to provide a wet nurse for your children there is no blame on you."[25]

There has been a belief among Eastern races that the character and traits which a child develops are highly affected by the woman whose milk it sucks; thus parents were unwilling to nurse their babies on animal milk and were very careful in selecting a wet nurse. A wet nurse's character was closely investigated before she was permitted to nurse the baby. If her qualifications were found to be satisfactory she was provided with good food, clothing and shelter.

The Koran, referring to the child Moses, whom Pharaoh's daughter found in a box floating in the Nile, presents the following version: "And we had already forbidden the (Egyptian) wet nurse to him (Moses); then she (his sister, Miriam) said,

'I shall point out to you the people of a family who will take charge of him.'"[26] Thus, Moses, lest his purity be polluted, was not permitted to suck from an Egyptian wet nurse. The same version of this legend is also found in the Talmud.[27]

Because of the strong belief that milk has a physical and moral influence on the child, Mohammed prohibited one to marry his wet nurse or "milk sister" (the term employed for one who was nursed by the same wet nurse). To marry one's wet nurse was equivalent to marrying a blood relation. The Koran warns that one must not marry ". . . the mother who gives you to suck and your foster sister."[28] In this connection it is interesting to note that the Koran places the most stringent prohibitions upon incestuous marriages and the preservation of family purity: "Forbidden to you are your mothers, and your daughters, and your sisters, and your paternal aunts, and your maternal aunts, and the daughters of a brother, and the daughters of a sister, and the mothers who have given you suck, and your foster-sisters, and the mothers of your wives, and your step-daughters, who are being brought up under your care, from wives with whom you had intercourse; but if you have not had intercourse with them, then there is no harm for you, and the wives of your sons who are from your own loins; and it is forbidden to you to have two sisters as wives together but what is past is past; surely, God is forgiving, merciful."[29]

"And forbidden also are married women excepting those which your right hand possesses. This is God's prescribing for you; and allowed to you are all beyond those mentioned, that you seek them in exchange for what is your own, intending to marry them, not for lust. Therefore as to those with whom you wish to benefit yourselves, give them, then their stated dowries; and there is no harm on you in what you mutually agree after the dowry has been fixed. Surely, God is knowing, wise."[30]

The marriage of a free, believing woman was easy enough for the wealthier classes, but not for the poor who had to purchase their wives from the fathers of the girls whom they wanted to marry. To these Mohammed decreed: "And he amongst you who has not sufficient means to marry a free, believing woman, then he might marry one of those whom your right hands possess from amongst believing maids, and God knows best your faiths; you are one from the other (i.e., you are all one.) Therefore marry them with the permission of their masters, and give them their dowries with fairness, these women being duly brought into marriage, not acting for lust, and not being kept as mistresses; so that when they have been brought into marriage, if they then commit an act of indecency, then for them is half of the penalty prescribed for free women. This permission to marry a maid is for him who is afraid of falling into difficulties. And if you wait, it is better for you; and God is forgiving, merciful."

In order to preserve racial purity, Mohammed instituted strict prohibition against marrying prostitutes or others who are morally degenerated. "An adulteress shall not marry except an adulterer or a pagan. An adulterer shall not marry except an adulteress or a pagan woman."[31]

In pre-Islamic times, prostitutes were stoned to death for infidelity. In later times they were buried alive. The Brahmans threw their unfaithful wives to the dogs to be devoured and unfaithful men were buried alive. Mohammed abolished capital punishment except for murder.[32] Free women were punished for infidelity with one hundred lashes with a leather whip and slave women with a mere fifty lashes together with imprisonment in their own houses until death.

Nothing was easier in pre-Islamic days than to divorce a wife. All one had to do was to say "Be to me like the back of my mother."[33] Mohammed insisted that wives be treated with at least some semblance of fairness. He instituted strict divorce laws: "And when you divorce your wives so that they complete their term; then keep them with fairness or leave them with fairness. And detain them not to cause injury."

In order to understand the social regulations in the Koran one must bear in mind that women in pre-Islamic days had no rights at all. It was alleged that Allah had made men over-lords over them. Mohammed said, "Men are protectors over women."[34] In the same chapter Mohammed said, "And there are women of whose disobedience you may be afraid; then teach them and next punish them lightly; if then they obey you, then do not seek a way against them." [35]

While in this world women are not such a happy lot, those who believe in Allah are promised entrance into Paradise with their husbands, there to recline on raised and shaded couches. "They shall have therein fruit and whatever they call for." [36]

Particularly beautiful believing women are promised unlimited joy in Paradise. "In the garden of bliss seated upon a throne facing each other; a cup with a fine drink is made to pass around them . . . and with them are large eyed beauties with a modest glance." [37]

Notwithstanding Mohammed's reforms, the marriage laws in the Koran are very partial to men. Men have all the rights and women are always at the mercy of the men.

The sultan was permitted as many as 60 wives. Other believers were allowed only four wives although this number did not include concubines and plain slaves. "Marry whom you like two at a time from among other women, two at a time or three or four but if you are afraid over them that you will not be able to keep equally (among your wives) then marry only one." [38] Mohammed himself possessed 21 wives.[39]

Mohammed at least modified the practice of easy divorce. The Koran requires four months after a divorce decision is made for complete separation to be permitted. "Those who swear off their wives have to wait four months; then if they go back, surely God is forgiving, merciful. And if they have resolved on divorce . . . then the divorced woman must wait three courses, and it is not lawful for them to conceal what God has formed in their wombs . . . and their husbands have a right to take them back during this period if they desire to make peace, and, they (the wives) have a right against their husbands." [40]

The period of four months delay only applies in ordinary cases but if a man wants to separate from a pregnant or suckling woman he is obliged to wait two years after childbirth until the provided time of lactation is consummated and during this period it is the duty of the father to house, feed and clothe the mother. When a divorced wife has intentions of remarrying, it is provided that she has to wait an additional three months (besides the four month period). According to the Koran: "If the four monthly periods passed and they are divorced, the divorced woman still waits three monthly periods."[41] In other words it must be certain that she is not pregnant when she marries again. "The woman whose husband did not come close to her may be divorced at once."[42]

The following regulations apply to women who for one reason or another have amenorrhea (cessation of all menses without pregnancy): "And as to those of your women who have stopped their monthly courses (or) if you are in doubt (thereto) then their period is three months and the same with those who have not started their courses, and as to the pregnant women their term is up to the time of their giving birth . . . House them where you house yourself according to your means and do not harm them with a view to straighten their circumstances . . . Therefore if they suck for you then pay their due . . . and if you mutually disagree then let another woman do the suckling."[43]

"Widows must wait three months and ten days before they can wed."[44] The ten days longer wait for widows is evidently out of respect for their deceased husbands. The purpose of these regulations from a medical point of view can be explained on the theory that after an additional three months, pregnancy will be noted and there will be no doubt as to the paternity of the child. According to Jhel-al-Eddin, pregnant women were anxious to deny their pregnancy to their future husband in order that they could rear their own children with those of their second husband as full sisters and brothers.[45]

Another reason for compelling a woman to wait an additional three months before she remarries might have been to protect the new husband from diseases she might have contracted from her former husband. In this case the risk of contracting disease would be minimized. Pregnancy at seven months is easily recognized and all doubts as to paternity are removed with those wives who do not menstruate regularly.

The Koran's reference to the fact that those who have never menstruated need not wait three months to rewed, alludes to the marriage of young children which is not a rare phenomenon in the East where fathers commonly marry off their daughters at a tender age to rich men for pecuniary gain.

Cohabitation with menstruating women is forbidden in the Koran: "Avoid women during the menses and approach them not till they are in a state of purity."[46]

The following *sura* of the Koran shows that cohabitation was considered a religious act: "Your wives are a tilth for you; then come to your tilth as you please and send forward good for your souls and reverence for Allah and know you are going to meet him."[47] Prohibition of intercourse during menstruation undoubtedly was based on the medical opinion that at such a time cohabitation was injurious to both sexes. The pilgrims to Mecca were prohibited from cohabitation on purely religious grounds.[48] However such was permitted during the fast days.[49] The Koran does not go as far as the Old Testament which prohibits even touching women during their monthly period.[50]

The Levitical regulations regarding menstruating and lying-in women, while in accordance with hygienic principles, are traceable to earlier primitive practices. Indeed, the fear of menstrual blood among Semitic races appears to have been deeply rooted, as is seen in Genesis. Laban, searching for his missing *teraphim*, feared to approach Rachael's camel in the saddle of which they were concealed, when he was told by his daughter that "the manner of women is upon me."

To the primitive philosopher the menstrual discharge consisted of defiled spirits or unclean demons which had entered the body and whose escape through the monthly flow might injure those who were in contact with the woman; hence, in the interest of the community, all kinds of precautions were taken against close proximity with a menstruating woman. She was secluded from society until the imaginary danger was thought to have passed. The very touch of her eating vessels and garments was taboo; and not until she submitted to certain rites of purification was she free to mingle with her family and neighbors.

The precautions against contacting the lying-in woman were even more strict. She was, in certain instances, removed to an isolated place and forbidden to see any persons until her presence was no longer considered dangerous to the community. This custom was not confined to uncivilized or barbaric peoples. The ancient Greek religion prohibited persons who had been in contact with menstruating and particularly lying-in women to enter a temple or to approach an altar for a prescribed interval.[51]

According to Pliny, the belief that a woman is defiled during her monthly sickness was widespread among all peoples of antiquity. The most serious results were ascribed to proximity with such women. Pliny's statements with reference to menstruating women are amusing for their absurdity: "On the approach of a woman in this state," he writes, "must will become sour, seeds become sterile, grafts wither away, garden plants become parched and fruit will fall from the tree beneath which she sits. Her very look even dims the brightness of mirrors, blunts the edge of steel, and removes the polish from ivory; dogs licking the discharge are seized with madness and their bite is venomous and fatal."

"If the menstrual discharge coincides with the eclipse of the moon and sun," continues the gullible Pliny, "the evils resulting from it are irremediable and no less so when it happens when the moon is in conjunction with the sun; the congress with a woman at such a period is noxious and attended with fatal effects to man."

The story that the death of Lucretius (98-55 B.C.), one of the most illustrious men of antiquity, was caused by his jealous wife, who made him drink menstrual blood, while undoubtedly fabulous, shows how this belief was widespread all through the ages.

In modern times the mystic iconoclast, Paracelsus, asserted that the devil constructed spiders, fleas, caterpillars, and all other insects that infest the air and earth, from menstrual blood. At the present time this superstition is largely confined to primitive peoples. Bushmen of South Africa think if a man glances in a girl's eye during her menstruation, he will become stupefied and change into a talking tree. Cattle-raising tribes of South Africa hold that their cattle die if the milk is drunk by menstruating women. Among many tribes of the North American Indians, women retire from the camp or village during the time of their uncleanliness and live in special huts which are provided for that purpose, and where they strictly abstain from all intercourse with men, who fear them just as if they were stricken with the plague. Native Australian women at this time are forbidden under pain of death to touch anything that men use and even to walk on paths that are frequented by men. In Uganda, utensils which a woman touches in this condition are destroyed. The Bribri Indian women of Costa Rica use banana leaves instead of plates for food when they have their monthly flow, and these they bury in the ground when they are done lest animals eat them and waste away or perish.[52]

Sexual perversion as in the case of Sodom who practiced pederasty was considered a grave religious violation. "And Lot said to his people, Do you commit an indecency which no one of the people of the world has done before you? You are surely running to males with lust rather than to females."[53]

Changing wives was a widespread custom among the pre-Islamic Arabs but this was forbidden in the Koran. "And if you should desire to change one wife for another, and you have given one of them a heap, then take not anything thereof; will you take it unjustly and with open sinfulness?"[54]

Mohammed frequently expressed his opposition to the heathen Arabs who killed their newborn girls by burying them alive because they were ashamed to be known as fathers of girls: "And when any one of them is given the tidings of (the birth) of a female, his face becomes black and he is full of grief, he conceals himself from his people on account of the evil of what he has been informed . . . accepting the disgrace and shame, he buries her alive."[55] At times, because of poverty, pre-Islamic Arabs even slaughtered their new-born sons.[56] With reference to infanticide Mohammed followed the precepts of the Hanifites who condemned the murder of children of tender age.[57] The Koran also prohibits suicide.[58]

According to the Koran, killing is only allowed under two conditions: Firstly, in holy war, to enemies of the country and non-believers;[59] and secondly, when avenging the death of relatives.[60] In the latter case, killing is restricted to the class of society of the murdered person. A free man may be avenged by a free man, a slave by a slave[61] and a woman by a woman.[62] There is an alternate plan, however, whereby punishment may be redeemed by a pecuniary settlement.[63]

ETIOLOGY OF DISEASE

The chief cause of all infections, according to the Koran, is theurgic. Allah is the cause of all causes. There are, however, secondary causes such as malignant spirits. The idea that malignant spirits are the cause of disease and ill luck was general among peoples of the East as in the case of Job where Satan became the messenger of Allah: "And remember our servant Job, when he called to his Lord, 'Surely the evil one (devil) has touched me with weariness and agony.'"[64]

Possession by disease-demons (*"madschunun"* in Arabic) was another cause of disease. "Most surely your messenger who has been sent to you is a possessed man."[65] "Either he dared to be against God or he is possessed."[66] "He is but a possessed man; therefore bear with him for a time."[67]

The evil eye also could produce sickness. All that was needed was a look "from the evil one when he envies."[68] It must be remembered that the superstitious belief in the evil eye has been persistent throughout the ages. Epidemics such as black death, smallpox, cholera and other contagious diseases were thought to be transmitted by a glance of the envious eye.

Astrology was another subject which was related to disease: "And they find evidence by means of the stars."[69] "And he (Abraham) looked and observed the stars and said, 'Verily I shall be sick.'"[70] Curiously, the Talmud presents a similar legend with relation to Abraham.[71]

The dependence of Mohammed upon his teachers and upon what he heard of the Jewish Haggadah and Jewish practice is now generally conceded. This subject was first treated from a general point of view by David Mill in his "Oratio Inauguralis de Mohammedanismo e Veterum Hebraerum Scriptus Magna ex Parta Composita" (Utrecht, 1718).

J. Gastfreud has attempted in his "Mohammed Nach Talmud und Midrasch" to demonstrate similar parallels in later Mohammedan literature (Berlin, 1875; Vienna, 1877; Leipzig, 1882). The subject of the Jewish elements in the Koran has received an extensive treatment by H. Hirschfeld in his "Beiträge zur Erklärung des Koran" (Leipzig, 1880).

Witchcraft is mentioned in the Koran as a cause of disease: "But they are lost and made to get hold of the paths." [72] The Arabic word *"marhur"* is used for "they are lost" and indicates that the persons referred to have been bewitched.

Disease is also ascribed to magic. It could arise ". . . from the evil of those who blow on knots in things made firm." [73] It was a common practice to make knots in cords and blow on them to cause injury to enemies. One had to utter certain magical formulas at such a time.

Other causes of disease mentioned in the Koran are of a rational nature. Some are ascribed to emotional conditions such as anxiety, fright, and worry. "Jacob's eyes became dim from worry." [74] The Book of Psalms gives a similar cause for dimness of vision: "My eyes are dimmed because of vexation." [75] "Allow not your life to pass by with sighs and worry." "Therefore let not thy lives run off their account with regrets." [76] "Sarah cried out and stroke her hand on her face when she was told that she would have a manchild." [77] The Koran comments that fear caused her heart to palpitate and her skin to wrinkle. According to the Koran, her heart was in her larynx and "she could not look." [78]

Physical causes of disease include inflicted wounds: "We will soon brand him on his beastly nose." [79] Self inflicted injuries are referred to as in the case of Potiphar's wife in Egypt: "She provided each one of them with a knife and said, 'Joseph come out, and in their presence'; therefore, when they saw him, they made much of him and cut their hands." [80] "And their foreheads and their sides and their backs shall be branded therewith." [81] "Boiling water will dissolve their skins." [82]

There are many catastrophes mentioned in the Koran that

wiped out entire nations. Mohammed attributes them to the wrath of Allah, as a punishment for evils committed against Him, but some of the punishments can, of course, be explained rationally. These might have been caused by various forms of food poisoning, and severe epidemics of smallpox, typhus, dysentery, malaria, and other infectious diseases. The Koran states that the Thamudites were punished by a thunderbolt [83] for killing a holy camel and eating its flesh. For this crime the entire population was punished with a dire sickness: "They then hamstrung the she-camel and rebelled against the command of their Lord . . . Shaking cut them then so that they became dead corpses thrown down in their house."[84] The commentaries note on this verse, that ". . . the next day after eating of the camel's flesh their faces turned yellow, the second day red and on the third day black and finally all were lying prostrated on the floor dead." Looking upon this legend from a medical point of view one may come to the conclusion that the death of the Thamudites was caused by ptomaine poisoning, originating in the flesh of the dead camel that had been exposed for too long a period to the heat of the tropical sun.

A rational explanation may also be given for the destruction of the forest-dwellers who died in great numbers for their evil deeds against Allah. As the Koran expresses it: "So they belied Him and the agony of a dark day seized them."[85] The agony was preceded by seven days of terrible heat followed by the appearance of a cloud which was brought by a hot wind. Following this, death ensued. It is evident that their death was not a direct punishment from Allah, but came indirectly as it often does in tropical climates after a period of drought and protracted heat exhaustion.

The story of the "masters of elephants" in the Koran is also interesting for it affords an inside view as to how Mohammed attributed natural events to miracles. The Koran states: "Hast thou not seen how the Lord did with the companions of the elephants? Did he not cause the stratagem to be lost? . . . flocks of birds threw stones of clay on them and He made them stubble eaten away."[86] The destruction of the elephant boys apparently was not produced by the flocks of birds that passed over them. It is claimed that a smallpox epidemic broke out which annihilated the masters of the elephants.[87] Incidentally, this was the first smallpox epidemic observed in the Arabic countries. Smallpox spread to Egypt in the year 640 A.D. and from Egypt it reached the European countries.[88] The legend of falling stones from Heaven to punish the wicked is an old one. It reminds one of the method by which the people of Sodom were destroyed, as noted in the Old Testament.[89] "Then the Lord caused to rain upon Sodom and upon Gomorrah brimstone and fire from the Lord out of heaven; and He overthrew those cities, and all the plain, and all the inhabitants of the cities, and that which grew upon the ground."[90]

The destruction of Add was by cyclone which phenomenon is not unusual in the Arabian countries.[91] According to the Koran: "And as to the Addites they were then destroyed by means of a furious wind blowing with extraordinary force which Allah ordered against them for seven nights and eight days of great vigour." The Koran thus describes how the people of Add were destroyed: "The people were thrown down as if they were hollow trunks of palm trees; then doest thou see any remnants of theirs?"[92] "It was a wind containing painful agony. It destroyed all things by the command of the Lord so that they became such that nothing was seen of them except their dwellings."[93] It should be noted here that in the East the observation has been made that strong winds frequently precede epidemics —especially dysentery.[94] The Bible story of the destruction of Sodom referred to above may also be explained on rational grounds. It could have resulted from a volcanic eruption, which hurled "brimstone and fire" upon the city.

Death after the imbibing of water is frequently mentioned in the Koran as well as in the Old Testament. Such instances were not and still are not particularly supernatural. Many of the streams in the East have been and are contaminated. Concerning the case of Saul (David, in the Old Testament), the Koran states, "When Saul marched out with his forces, he said, 'Surely God is going to test you by means of a stream; then whoever drinks of it is not of me and whoever does not partake of it he is of me, but if he takes with his hand a handful (it matters not)'; then they drink of it except a few of them." Those that did not drink the water felt confident that they could overcome Goliath and his house.[95] Of course the effect of the water may be explained on a rational basis: Perhaps the clearer water on the surface which was more exposed to the air was relatively safe but the water drawn from the depths was badly contaminated and not potable. It should also be noted that a handful of water contains only a small volume. On this basis those who did not drink or drank only water scooped up from the surface were not affected but those who drank from the depths soon became gravely ill.

The only diseases mentioned by name in the Koran are leprosy and blindness: "And thou curest the blind and the lepers with My authority." [96]

The meaning of the Arabic word *"baida"* (white) which applies to certain skin eruptions is not clear and may refer to one or a number of diseases. The Koran refers to Moses whose healthy hand became "white" when he removed it from his bosom (during his miraculous performance before Pharaoh) and on one occasion mention is made that Jesus healed certain skin eruptions. In the case of Moses the text reads "And he put out his hand; then lo! it became as if white to the onlookers." [97] "And press thy hand under the armpit, it will come out shining white without any disease." [98] It appears that the Arabs looked upon the transformance of the color of the hand to white as a miracle.

PSYCHOSIS

Other pathologic conditions which the Arabs were well acquainted with were epilepsy, hysteria and psychosis. According to some of Mohammed's biographers, the Prophet himself was afflicted with such maladies and he suffered from attacks which lasted from hours to several months at a time. His symptoms included twitching of the muscles, movements of the lips and tongue as if he wanted to taste something, rotating of the eyeballs, shaking of the head sideways, a drunken stuporous expression, facial pallor, copious perspiration, violent headache, but no unconsciousness. These symptoms perhaps point to *petit mal* epilepsy.[99]

The fact that Mohammed was not unconscious during his attacks, however, effectively rules out *grand mal* epilepsy.[100] During or immediately after Mohammed's attacks he is reported to have dictated portions of the Koran.

Psychosis was not a rare condition among prophets, poets and holymen. Balaam [101] saw "a vision of the Almighty, fallen down, yet with open eyes." There have been many historic personalities afflicted with epilepsy.[102] The Persian king, Cambyses (521-611), is reported to have had epileptic attacks. Other alleged epileptics were Julius Caesar (102-144), Dante (1265-1321), Moliere (1622-1673) and Napoleon (1768-1821). In more recent times Swinburne and Swift were among the literary men said to have been epileptics.

Priest-physicians among the ancient Greeks regarded epileptic seizures as divine manifestations. Epilepsy was generally known as "the sacred disease" but some referred to it as "morbus Herculi" (Hercules' disease). Tradition has it that Hercules had epileptic attacks when he was communicating with the gods.

THERAPY

The therapy of the Koran, as must be expected, is of a theurgic character. God is the healer: "Then when I am sick He heals me." [103] "God created for every disease a remedy." Honey was considered a remedy for many ailments. It is produced "from the inside of a bee in which there is healing for mankind." Honey was widely used as a dietary supplement and as a remedy. "Diet was regulated to cure disease among the Arabs."[104] Water also was employed to cure many diseases and the efficacy of watercure is first noted by Job: "Here is a cool bathing place and drink." [105]

According to the Koran, when Jacob's eyes became blurred his son Joseph sent him a sherd (perhaps to be used as a compress about the eye) . . . "and he was cured." [106] In the Bible no such story as this is found. When Jonah was thrown on the land by the whale: "He cast him out on a desert land where he was sick and He caused a gourd plant to grow upon him." [107] The large leaves of this plant perhaps were intended to protect him from the sun.

The most important health measure of the Koran is rest. The Koran made it mandatory to utilize the night only for rest. "He also made a night for you that you may rest therein, and . . . for no other purpose." "Honor God for the long rest."

Frequent cleansing of the (entire) body has been the custom among the Arabs from early times. Aside from the regular cleansing of the skin which is ordered after touching unclean things, after urination and defecation, after sexual intercourse, and after sickness, the Moslem washes his hands, feet and head very often because these parts of the body are exposed to the elements. He also washes his hands before and after meals.

The believer is promised that in Paradise he ". . . will be dressed in green silks and velvets." Mohammed enjoined his followers to keep their clothes clean: "Purify thy raiment." Loyal Mohammedans were not permitted to sleep in their clothes: "Take off your garment at noon and after your night prayers." The Koran mentions taking off of clothes at noon because it is customary in warm climates to rest when the sun is high. Another purpose of clothing, according to the Koran, is to avoid the sight of a nude body—a disgrace to men as well as to women.[108]

WATER

Water has always figured as a spiritual and physical cleanser. In the Old Testament water was used as a prophylactic and cure. It was employed to cleanse the menstruating and lying-in woman, to purify those that had been defiled by touching unclean bodies,[109] to clean lepers[110] and to treat gonorrhea ("*zab*").[111] Sprinkling the body with water symbolized moral purity. Thus Ezekiel declares: "And I will sprinkle clean water upon you and ye shall be clean from all your uncleanliness, and from all your idols will I cleanse you." [112]

The New Testament speaks of the "water of life." [113] Holy water for actual purification of persons is still being used by the Church to drive away evil forces.

Among the Arabs, water was used as a purifier before prayer and was employed to cleanse persons who were contaminated by coming in contact with menstruating women, leprous persons, or bodies of the deceased. Water is still recognized as the most vital element in maintaining life. Pure, fresh water was and still is difficult to obtain in tropical climates, and was naturally considered a life-sustaining substance possessing marvelous powers to revive the lives of animals and plants.

Among the attributes of the Paradise which Mohammed promises the believers is the presence of an abundance of fresh water: "There are rivers of water which does not become noxious." [114] The Koran describes the Paradise as ". . . a garden beneath which flow rivers." [115] Mohammed promises to the believers water that does not get spoiled [116] but the unbelievers get a ". . . drink of boiling water and a painful agony." [117]

Camphor water appears to have been relished in Mohammed's time: "Surely the virtuous shall drink a cup tempered with camphor."[118] Although the Koran forbids alcoholic drinks,[119] wines are frequently extolled as sparkling fluids only second to water: "And out of the fruits of palms and grapes there are those which you use for making intoxicants." [120] Possibly grape and date brandy were the products referred to. Wine was commonly mixed with plain water or gingiber water to circumvent the prohibition of wine in the Koran.[121]

Alcoholic drinks are so polluting as to necessitate a bath before prayer to Allah is again permitted: "Come not nigh to prayer while you are intoxicated, nor when you are polluted until you have bathed yourself." [122]

Uncleanliness in a physical sense is a condition by which one may transmit disease to another, or subject one to contagion.

That which at the present time is ascribed to pathogenic microorganisms was in the time of Mohammed blamed on pollution by pathogenic demons—so to speak—which attack the person and contaminate him with disease.

MOHAMMED'S TOLERANCE OF THE SICK

Mohammed was tolerant of the sick and freed them from the observance of otherwise mandatory religious laws: "And carry out the pilgrimage and the visit to Kaaba for the sake of Allah . . . but if one of you be sick or suffering from injury in the head, he should compensate by fasting or alms-giving." [123]

According to the Koran: "There is no bar on the blind, no bar one lame, nor is there any bar on the sick, nor upon yourself whether you eat in your own house or the houses of your fathers, etc. Nor is there any blame on you if you eat together or separately." [124] With reference to eating with the blind it must be remembered that the blind in the East generally are a disgusting sight. Most of them have lost their sight as a result of chronic inflammatory diseases of the eye—especially trachoma. People customarily shunned the blind, but Mohammed encouraged believers even to eat with them. This leniency towards the sick is also extended to the ordinances concerning fasting: "For those who cannot fast . . . for anyone of you who is sick or on journey, there is then the same as on other days, and for those who find it hard to bear, there is redemption by giving alms to the poor." [125] The same tolerance is extended to prayer itself: "He knows that there will be among you who are sick and others among you moving on (about) the earth seeking God's grace; therefore recite whatever is easy thereof." [126]

FOOD

Vegetable and animal foods were used by the Arabs during the time of Mohammed. Mohammed said: "Eat of the good things we have provided you with."[127] "And He sent down upon you the manna and the quail, and He provides you with pure food."[128] "Allah promised to the believers a mixed kind of food in Paradise."[129] "And will increase them of fruits and flesh and what they wish."[130] It is not clear whether the Arab heathen, before Mohammed, indulged in cannibalism, but there is an injunction against this practice in the Koran.[131] The Koran specifies the kind of animals which may be eaten by believers. Sheep, goats, cows and camels were permitted as foods.[132] "Swine is forbidden."[133] "Food gained by hunt is permitted" provided one is not on a pilgrimage.[134] It was and still is customary to eat slaughtered young animals and even unborn embryos.[135] "Blood as an article of food is prohibited."[136] "Fat (from certain parts of the animal's body) may be eaten."[137] Nothing is mentioned about the eating of fowl. Birds were promised to believers in Paradise.[138] Wine as a drink is strictly prohibited. Fish played a great part in the Arab dietary regime. Both sweet water and salt water fish were eaten.[139]

The fruits of the palm tree and vineyards were highly recommended: "And out of the fruits of palms and grapes . . . there is healing for mankind."[140] Peas and lentils were highly prized articles of food. Dates, figs, olives, berries, olive oil, radishes, cucumbers and onions are listed as healthy fruits and vegetables.

The Koran mentions the "fruit of *Zakkum*" (the identity of which is not known) as a food for the sinful: "Like dregs of oil it shall boil in their bellies."[141]

BREAD

Strange as it may seem bread is mentioned only one time in the Koran and then only in connection with the dream of the "baker."[142] Of course, it is certain that at the time of Mohammed the Arabs baked bread from wheat. From deep antiquity, the Arabs always displayed an actual reverence for bread. They have been careful not to throw bread away and if perchance a piece fell on the ground, it was always picked up immediately and kissed. It is related that in 1942 when the American soldiers landed in Morocco they were instructed by their officers not to cut bread into slices but to break it in pieces so as to avoid offense to the natives who are averse to using a knife on such a revered substance.

MILK

Milk is frequently mentioned in the Koran as a drink.[143] The kind of animal whose milk was employed is not mentioned, but presumably sheep, goats, cows and camels were all used.

Mohammed appears to have considered milk as a fluid, the characteristics of which were midway between the chyle (the milky emulsion into which the fat of food is transformed by the intestinal juices) and the blood—an idea which he might have learned from El Harith ben Kalada, his contemporary: "And most certainly there is a lesson for you in the cattle who give you a drink of what is in the inside from betwixt the contents of the bowels and the blood—pure milk delicious to those who drink." [144] Elsewhere the Koran asserts: "It is a substance midway between the food and the blood." [145] The commentators add this: "The coarse part of the food passes out through defecation and urination. The finer part of the food turns into milk. The finest turns into blood." This comparison of milk with blood and the origin of both liquids occupied the attention of early physiologists. According to Avicenna (who probably quotes a still older theory), both blood and milk are derived from the chyle. Blood is manufactured from the chyle in the liver, and milk is made from the chyle in the mammary glands. In the liver the chyle which has a milky hue, turns red, and this in turn is restored to white in the breast.[146]

The food that God prepared for the helpless newborn infant after its separation from the womb was naturally looked upon with great admiration. Mothers felt religiously bound to suckle their babies for at least two years, partly out of reverence for this marvelous substance in their breasts.

Milk thus was accorded a special place in the Koran: "It is a fluid reserved for the believers in Paradise." "It will be imbibed in Paradise like water." [147]

SURGERY

No reference to surgery is found in the Koran. Even circumcision, which is an old religious ceremony practiced among the Arabs, is not mentioned. Perhaps Mohammed took this rite so much for granted that he felt there was no need to mention it. The laws the prophet laid down in the Koran were largely intended to prevent abuses. Apparently the Arabs never violated the circumcision rite and considered it just as important and commonplace as cutting the umbilical cord. The practice of circumcision is the oldest religious surgery known. Its original purpose, however, is still veiled in mystery.

Arabs practiced circumcision long before the time of Mohammed. According to the Old Testament, Ishmael, the progenitor of the Arab race, was circumcised at the age of 13. Mohammed himself believed in this religious practice. Pococke refers to a tradition which attributes to the Prophet the saying: "Circumcision is an ordinance for men and honorable for women." Arabs, like the Abyssinians, appear to have practiced female circumcision. It is not clear whether the operation was performed on the labia or over the clitoris. M. Murat is certain, however, that the operation was performed over the clitoris. In Arabia the profession of female circumcision expert (*resectricis nymphrum*) was as popular an occupation as that of engaging in cock castration or caponization. It is related by Abufelda that when Islam came close to a crushing defeat in the Battle of Ohod, Hamza, the uncle of the Prophet, cried out to the Koreish chief of the enemy: "Come on, thou son of a she-circumcisor."

Among African races circumcision is looked upon as a rite commemorating the advent of manhood. According to Livingstone, among the Bassoutus, the performance of *boyuera* (circumcision) is of purely civil significance and not connected with religion. Young girls have an ordeal similar to that of circumcision which they must pass when nearing the age of 13. In other words, the female rite bears a relationship to that of male circumcision, denoting entrance into womanhood. At a certain appointed time the girls are assembled at the bank of a neighboring river, where they are placed under the care of matrons. There they are schooled in the art of household duties, and after having undergone a rigid initiation, they are admitted into womanhood. In Sierra Leone, in addition to the aforementioned ceremonies, the skin over the clitoris of the young maids is excised at midnight in the full moon, and they receive new names by which they are to be known throughout the rest of their lives.

Lafargue states that circumcision among the native Australians is associated with elaborate ceremonies. Even when they are at war, the hostilities are stopped in order to perform the rites properly. Boys of about 13 or 14 years of age are rounded up and carried away amidst the cries and lamentations of their mothers and other female relatives, who, in their grief, mutilate themselves by cutting into their thighs so that they bleed profusely. The operation is performed in an isolated place where an old man suddenly appears from behind the trees announcing that the rite is about to be performed.

But whatever the origin of circumcision among the Egyptians and other races might have been, the purpose of the operation among the Hebrews is set forth in unmistakable terms: It was intended to serve as a blood covenant, as is seen in the Book of Genesis: "This is My covenant, which ye shall keep between Me and thee, and thy seed after thee; every man-child among you shall be circumcised. And ye shall circumcise the flesh of your foreskin; and it shall be a token of the covenant betwixt Me and thee." [148]

Circumcision was practiced among the Egyptians from an early period. Pythagoras had to submit to the operation before he was permitted the privilege of studying in the Egyptian temples. Herodotus relates that Psammetich, who reigned over Egypt towards the end of the sixth century B.C., almost brought down upon his head the wrath of his subjects by admitting uncircumcised strangers into Egypt. A bas-relief discovered in the temple of Khons at Karnak shows that the operation was extensively practiced in Egypt at that period. According to M. Chabas, the sculpture refers to the sons of Rameses II, who were circumcised by the Pharaoh himself. The knife appears to be a stone implement; his sons appear about 10 or 12 years of age.

Despite the fact that Christianity has abolished the practice of circumcision, some Christian Churches went out of their way to celebrate this practice to an extent never dreamed of by Jews and Mohammedans. Early Christians celebrated the Feast of Circumcision without resorting to the operation and the detached prepuce was greatly venerated.

Interesting from a surgical point of view is the legend of the seven sleepers who, according to the Koran,[149] slept in a cave for a period of 309 years. It is stated that God had them change their positions from one side to the other.[150] This seems to imply that it was known that individuals who reclined too long in one position are subject to sickness such as pneumonia and decubitus or pressure (bed) sores.

Tried by modern standards, Mohammed cannot be rated as a great religious leader and codifier, but neither can he be dismissed lightly as some of his critics have done. Even though he could neither read nor write, he was humble enough to admit that he had no education. He tried to emphasize the truth of the Koran: "And no one denies our signs except the disbelievers."

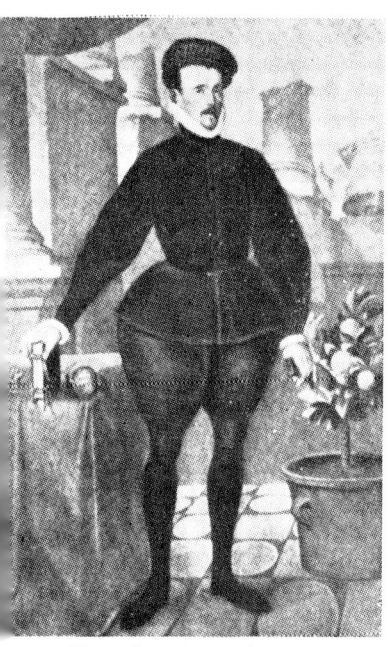

PLATE 29. Felix Platter (1536-1614), Professor of Medicine of Basel. After oil painting of Hans Bock the Elder.
(Public Art Collection of Basel)

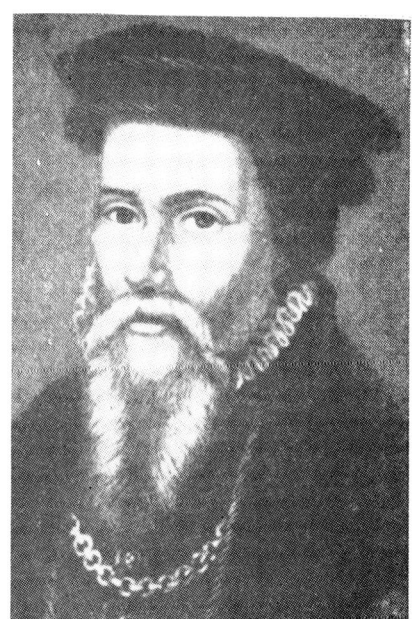

PLATE 30. John Caius: Physician and Educator.

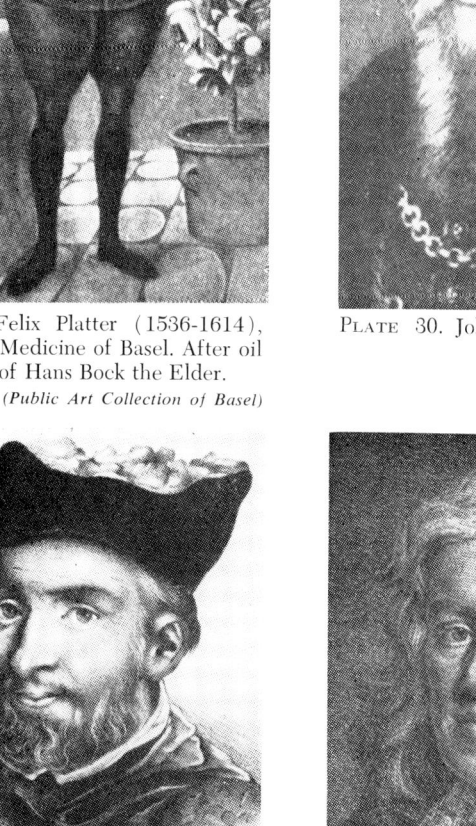

PLATE 31. Bernard De Cordon, 13th Century.
(Armed Forces Medical Library, Washington, D.C.)

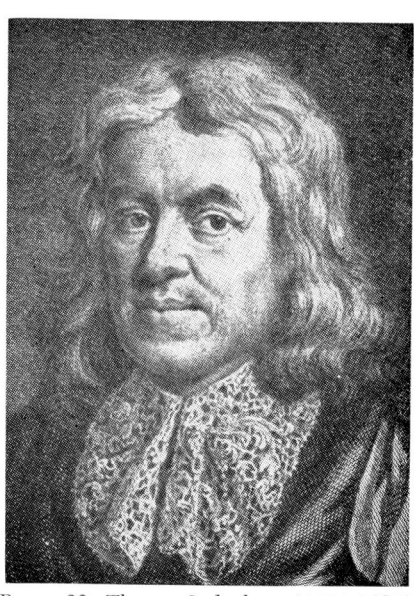

PLATE 32. Thomas Sydenham (1624-1689)

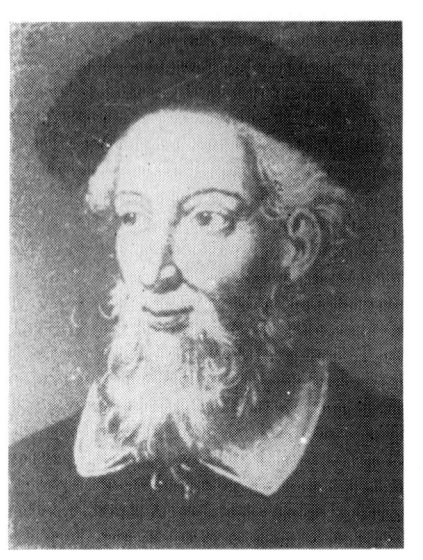

PLATE 33. Jean Pitard (1228-1305)
(Courtesy Armed Forces Medical Library, Washington, D.C.)

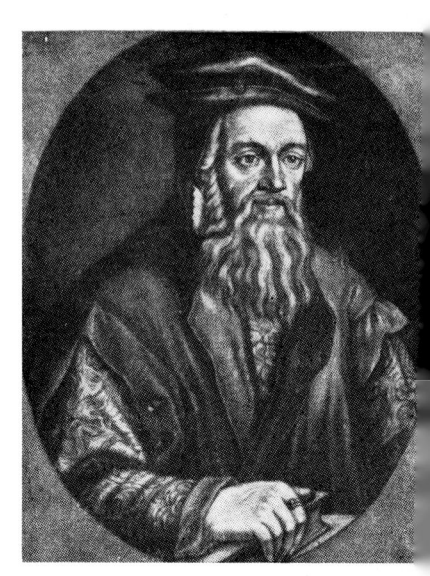

PLATE 34. Conrad Gesner (1516-1565

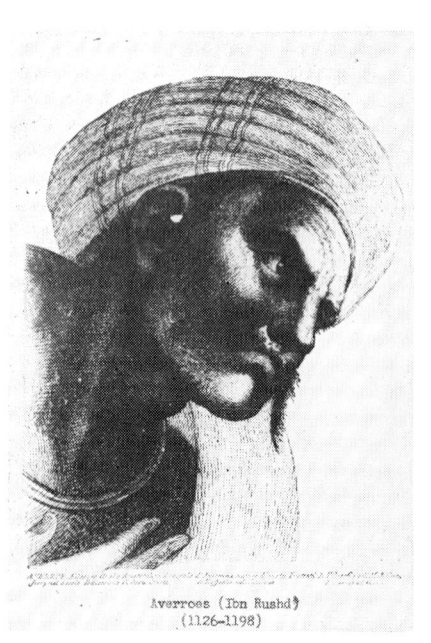

PLATE 35. Averroes (Ibn Rushd) (1126-1198)
(Courtesy Armed Forces Medical Library, Washington, D.C.)

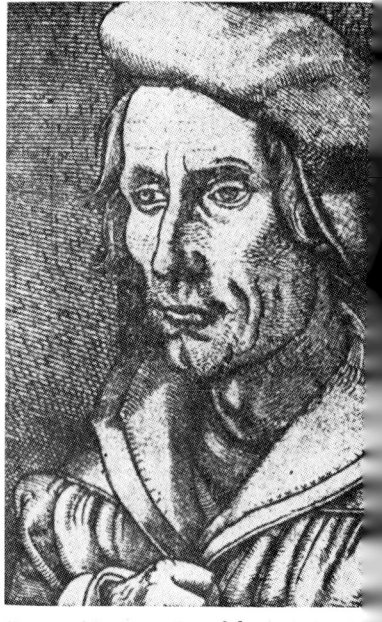

PLATE 36. Otto Brunfels (1464-153
Author of a catalogue of famous p
sicians published 1530.

CHAPTER VI

POST-KORANIC MEDICINE

The primitive medical concepts manifested throughout the pages of the Koran are surely no gauge of the secular medical knowledge which developed among the Arabian peoples during the Middle Ages. Ninth century records indicate that higher standards of universal knowledge existed among these Arabians than among any other contemporary people and that there were Arabian physcians who were not only trained in Greek and especially Galenic medicine but also in philosophy, mathematics, astronomy, law and theology. A mass of erudition was conveyed orally by *"rawies"* (reciters) from generation to generation. There were medical schools in Mesopotamia and Persia which taught systems based upon the plan of the Alexandrian schools.[1]

Arabic medicine is an outgrowth of the Arabic world outside of Arabia. It owed neither seed nor soil to the Arabian peninsula. It was written in the Arabic language which the physicians of the age employed irrespective of their nationality. The seed of the new learning was the legacy of Hellenism. The soil was Syria, where the Greek civilization was still in existence, and Persia, where the University of Jondisabur flourished. Yet the stimulus that quickened the intellectual life and induced the first vigorous growth of scholarly advance came from the religion of the Arabs.

Of course, there were in Arabia, as elsewhere, medical healers who disregarded medical standards and resorted to magic and similar deceptions. According to no less an authority than Rhazes, there were many doctors who employed a great deal of trickery in their practice. Many customarily hired confederates who claimed to be patients and spread the good word that their employer had wrought miraculous recoveries on them.²

The status of Arabian medicine in the early medieval period may best be derived by perusing the secular literature that developed after the completion of the Koran. One of the most celebrated of these texts is the "Arabian Nights," termed in Arabic, "Alf-Lailat wa Laila"—"The One Thousand and One Nights." This Arabic work includes material taken from the Indian and Persian languages reinforced with many Arabic elements. Some of these stories go back to the period of Koran. The entire work, in its present form, seems to have been collected into one large opus in about the thirteenth century A.D.³

The story which throws light upon the medicine of that period goes back to the reign of Caliph Harun al Rashid (786-802) at the end of the eighth century. It deals with one named Abu al Husn ("Father of Beauty")—an heir who squandered all his wealth recklessly and was left with one beautiful slave girl named Tawaddud who possessed an extraordinary amount of intellect and varied learning.

This slave girl realized her master's plight and urged him to sell her to the Caliph Harun al Rashid in order to raise sufficient money to get him out of his financial difficulties. The Caliph was much impressed with her beauty, but before he consented to purchase her for the stipulated price, he wanted to be convinced of the magnitude of her scholarship. He therefore summoned specialists in all branches of science to test the extent of her knowledge. These scholars put her through a severe examination in law, theology, philosophy, astronomy, astrology, music, chess playing, and medicine. The answers given by the slave girl Tawaddud to her medical examiners furnishes a fair idea not only of the sources and aspects of the Arabian medicine of that period but also of the current knowledge of Galenic as well as Talmudic medicine.⁴ Her replies to the queries are of great medical interest.

After she was questioned by the Islamic theologian and came out victorious, there ". . . came forward the skilled physician and said to her, 'We are free of theology and now to physiology. Tell me, therefore, how is man made? How many veins, bones and vertebrae are there in his body? Which is the first and chief vein and why was Adam named Adam?'"[5]

She replies, "Adam was called Adam, because of his *udmah*, that is, the wheaten color of his complexion and also (it is said) because he was created of the *adim* (the earth)[6] . . . There were created for him seven doors in his head, viz., the eyes, the ears, the nostrils and the mouth, and two passages, before and behind. The eyes were made the seat of the sight-sense, the mouth the seat of the taste-sense and the tongue to utter what is in the heart of man."[7]

After describing the biblical story of the composition of man she proceeds to the chemical and physical basis of the structure of man.[8] She then continues with the humoral physiology of Hippocrates and finally discusses the mechanism of man.

According to Tawaddud, Adam was made of a compound of the humor of fire, being hot-dry; the black bile that of earth, the four elements: water, earth, fire and air. The yellow bile is cold-dry; the phlegm that of water, being cold-moist, and the blood that of air, being hot-moist. There were made in man three hundred and sixty veins[9] and two hundred and forty-nine bones.[10]

There are three souls or spirits: the animal, the rational and the natural, to each of which is allotted its proper function. This is the Platonic idea of the division of the soul into three parts.

Tawaddud then goes on to speak of the wisdom of the Creator in the formation of each and every organ of the body. Here she gives voice to Galen's concept of teleology.

She continues: "Moreover, Allah made him (i.e. Adam) a heart and spleen and lungs and six intestines[11] and a liver and two kidneys and buttocks and brain and bones and skin and five senses: hearing, seeing, smell, taste, touch. The heart He set on the left side of the breast and made the stomach the guide and governor thereof. He appointed the lungs for a fan to the heart[12] and established the liver on the right side, opposite thereto. Moreover, He made, besides this, the diaphragm and the viscera and set up the bones of the breast and latticed them with the ribs."

Tawaddud was next interrogated as to how many ventricles are contained in a man's head.[13] She replies: "Three which contain five faculties, styled the intrinsic senses, to wit: common sense, imagination, the thinking faculty, perception and memory."[14]

The following is the slave girl's description of the osteology of the human body which is most remarkable for its time, for it includes some additions to Galenic anatomy:

Q. "Describe to me the configuration of the bones."

A. "Man's frame consists of two hundred and forty bones,[15] which are divided into three parts; the head, the trunk and the extremities. The head is divided into calvarium and face. The skull is constructed of eight bones, and to it are attached the four osselets of the ear. The face is furnished with an upper jaw of eleven bones and a lower jaw of one; and to these are added the teeth: two and thirty in number, and the os hyoides (the fork bone; Arabic "al-lami").The trunk is divided into spinal column, breast and basin. The spinal column is made up of four and twenty bones, called *fikar* or vertebrae; the breast, of the breastbone and the ribs, which are four and twenty in number, twelve on each side; and the basin of the hips, the sacrum (or 'holy bone')[16] and the os coccygis. The extremities are divided into upper and lower, arms and legs. The arms are again divided firstly into shoulder, comprising shoulder blades and collar bone; secondly into the upper arm which is one bone; thirdly into fore-arm, composed of two bones, the radius and the ulna; and fourthly into the hand, consisting of the wrist, the metacarpus of five, and the fingers, which number five, of three bones each, called the phalanges, except the thumb, which hath but two. The lower extremities are divided, firstly into thigh, which hath one bone; secondly into leg, composed of three bones: the tibia, the fibula and the patella; and thirdly into the foot, divided, like the hand, into tarsus, metatarsus and toes; and is composed of seven bones, ranged in two rows, two in one and five in the other; and the metatarsus is composed of five bones and the toes number five, each of three phalanges except the big toe which hath only two."[17]

No description is given of the muscles or ligaments, but the angiology of the human system and the function of the internal and external organs are discussed.

Q. "Which is the root of the veins?"

A. "The aorta, from which they ramify, and they are many, none knoweth the tale of them save He who created them; but I repeat, it is said that they number three hundred and sixty. Moreover, Allah hath appointed the tongue as interpreter for the thought, the eyes to serve as lanterns, the nostrils to smell with, and the hands for prehensors. The liver is the seat of pity, the spleen of laughter and the kidneys of craft; the lungs are ventilators, the stomach the storehouse and the heart the prop and pillar of the body. When the heart is sound, the whole body is sound,[18] and when the heart is corrupt, the whole body is corrupt."

The following concerns itself with diagnosis:

Q. "What are the outward signs and symptoms evidencing disease in the members of the body, both external and internal?"

A. "A physician, who is a man of understanding, looketh into the state of the body and is guided by the feel of the hands, according as they be firm or flabby, hot or cool, moist or dry. Internal disorders are also indicated by external symptoms, such as yellowness of the white of the eyes, which denoteth jaundice, and the bending back, which denoteth disease of the lungs."

Q. "Now what are the internal symptoms of disease?"

A. "The science of the diagnosis of disease by internal symptoms is founded upon six canons: (1) the patient's actions; (2) what is evacuated from his body; (3) the nature of the pain; (4) the site thereof; (5) swelling and (6) effluvia given off his person."

Q. "How cometh hurt to the head?"

A. "By the ingestion of food upon food, before the first be digested, and by fullness upon fullness; this it is that wasteth people. He who would live long, let him be early with the morning-meal and not late with the evening-meal; let him be sparing of commerce with women and wary of such depletory measures as cupping and blood-letting; and let him make of his belly three parts, one for food, one for drink and the third for air; for a man's intestines are eighteen spans in length and it befitteth that he appoint six for meat, six for drink and six for breath. If he walk, let him go gently; it will be wholesomer for him and better for his body and more in accordance with the saying of the Almighty, 'Walk not proudly on the earth.'" [19]

Q. "What are the symptoms of yellow bile and what is to be feared therefrom?"

A. "The symptoms are sallow complexion and bitter taste in the mouth with dryness; failure of the appetite, venereal and other, and rapid pulse; and the patient hath to fear high fever and delirium and eruptions and jaundice and tumor and ulcers of the bowels and excessive thirst."

Q. "What are the symptoms of black bile and what hath the patient to fear from it, if it get the mastery of the body?"

A. "The symptoms are false appetite and great mental disquiet and care; and it behooveth that it be evacuated, else it will generate melancholia and leprosy and cancer and disease of the spleen and ulceration of the bowels."

Q. "Into how many branches is the art of medicine divided?"

A. "Into two: the art of diagnosing diseases and that of restoring the diseased body to health."

Q. "When is the drinking of medicine more efficacious than otherwise?"

A. "When the sap runs in the wood and the grape thickens in the cluster and the two auspicious planets, Jupiter and Venus, are in the ascendant; then setteth in the proper season for drinking of drugs and doing away with disease."

Q. "What time is it, when, if a man drink water from a new vessel, the drink is sweeter and lighter or more digestible to him than at another time, and there ascendeth to him a pleasant fragrance and a penetrating one?"

A. "When he waiteth awhile after eating, as quoth the poet:—

'Drink not upon thy food in haste but wait awhile;
Else thou with halter shalt thy frame to sickness lead:
And patient bear a little thirst from food, then drink;
And thus, O brother, haply thou shalt wine thy need.'" [20]

Q. "What food is it that giveth not rise to ailments?"

A. "That which is not eaten but after hunger, and when it is eaten, the ribs are not filled with it, even as saith Jalinus or Galen the physician, 'Whoso will take in food, let him go slowly and he shall not go wrongly.' And to conclude with his saying (on whom be blessing and peace!), 'The stomach is the house of disease, and diet is the basis of healing; for the origin of all sickness is indigestion, that is to say, corruption of the meat in the stomach.'"

Q. "What sayest thou of the *hamman* (bath)?"

A. "Let not the full man enter it. Quoth the Prophet, 'The bath is the blessing of the house, for that it cleanseth the body and calleth to mind the fire.'"

Q. "What baths are best for bathing?"

A. "Those whose waters are sweet and whose space is ample and which are well aired; their atmosphere representing the four seasons—autumn and summer and winter and spring." [21]

Q. "What kind of food is the most profitable?"

A. "That which women make and which hath not cost overmuch trouble and which is readily digested. The most excellent of food is *brewis*[22] or bread sopped in broth. According to the saying of the Prophet, '*Brewis* excelleth other food, even as Ayishah excelleth other women.'"

Q. "What kind of kitchen, or seasoning, is most profitable?"

A. "Flesh meat" (quoth the Prophet) "is the most excellent of kitchen; for that it is the delight of this world and the next world."

Q. "What of fruits?"

A. "Eat them in their prime and quit them when their season is past."

Q. "What are the most excellent fruits?"

A. "Pomegranate and citron."

Q. "What sayest thou of drinking water?"

A. "Drink it not in large quantities nor swallow it by gulps, or it will give thee headache and cause divers kinds of harm; neither drink it immediately after leaving the *hamman* (bath) nor after carnal copulation or eating (except it be after the lapse of fifteen minutes for a young man and forty for an old man), nor after waking from sleep."

Q. "What of drinking fermented liquors?"

A. "Doth not the prohibition suffice thee in the Book of almighty Allah, where He saith, 'Verily wine and lots and images, and the divining arrows are an abomination, of Satan's work; therefore avoid them, that ye may prosper'? And again, 'They will ask thee concerning wine and lots: Answer, "In both there is great sin and also some things of use unto men but their sinfulness is greater than their use."'[23] As for the advantages that be therein, it disperseth stone and gravel from the kidneys and strengtheneth the viscera and banisheth care, and moveth to generosity and preserveth health and digestion; it conserveth the body, expelleth disease from the joints, purifieth the frame of corrupt humors, engendereth cheerfulness, gladdeneth the heart of man and keepeth up the natural heat: it contracteth the bladder, enforceth the liver and removeth obstructions, reddeneth the cheeks, cleareth away maggots from the brain and deferreth grey hairs. In short, had not Allah (to whom be honor and glory!) forbidden it,[24] there were not on the face of the earth aught fit to stand in its stead. As for gambling by lots, it is a game of hazard such as diceing, not of skill."

Q. "What wine is best?"

A. "That which is pressed from white grapes and kept eighty days or more after fermentation: it resembleth not water and indeed there is nothing on the surface of the earth like unto it."

Q. "Which is the most excellent of vegetables?"

A. "Endive."

Q. "Which is the most excellent of sweet-scented flowers?"

A. "Rose and Violet."

Q. "What sayest thou of cupping?"

A. "It is for him who is over-full of blood and who hath no

defect therein; and whoso would be cupped, let it be during the wane of the moon, on a day without cloud, wind or rain and on the seventeenth of the month. If it fall on a Tuesday, it will be the more efficacious, and nothing is more salutary for the brain and eyes and for clearing the intellect than cupping."

Q. "What is the best time for cupping?"

A. "One should be cupped 'on the spittle,' that is, in the morning before eating, for this fortifieth the wit and the memory. It is reported of the Prophet that, when anyone complained to him of a pain in the head or legs, he would bid him be cupped and, after cupping, not to eat salt food after fasting, for it engendereth scurvy; neither eat sour things as curdled milk immediately after cupping."

Q. "When is cupping to be avoided?"

A. "On Sabbaths or Saturdays and Wednesdays, and let him who is cupped on these days blame none but himself. Moreover, one should not be cupped in very hot weather nor in very cold weather; and the best season for cupping is springtide."[25]

Q. "Now tell me of carnal copulation."[26]

A. "Copulation hath in it many and exceeding virtues and praiseworthy qualities, amongst which are, that it lighteneth a body full of black bile and calmeth the heat of love and induceth affection and dilateth the heart and dispelleth the sadness of solitude; and the excess of it is more harmful in summer and autumn than in spring and winter."

Q. "At what time is copulation good?"

A. "If by night, after food is digested and, if by day, after the morning meal."

Q. "What are its good effects?"

A. "It banisheth trouble and disquiet, calmeth love and wrath and is good for ulcers, especially in a cold and dry humor; on the other hand, excess of it weakeneth the sight and engendereth pains in the legs and head and back: and beware, beware of carnal connection with old women, for they are deadly. Quoth the Imam Ali (whose face Allah honor!), 'Four things kill and ruin the body: entering the *hamman* (bath) on a full stomach; eating salt food; copulation on a plethora of blood and lying with an ailing woman; for she will weaken thy strength and infect thy frame with sickness; and an old woman is deadly poison.'[27] And quoth one of them, 'Beware of taking an old woman to wife, though she be richer in hoards than Karun.'"[28]

Q. "What is the best copulation?"

A. "If the woman be tender of years, comely of shape, fair of face, swollen of breast and of noble race, she will add to thee strength and health of body; and let her be even as saith a certain poet describing her."

Q. "How is the seed of man secreted?"

A. "There is in man a vein which feedeth all the other veins. Now water is collected from the three hundred and sixty veins and, in the form of red blood, entereth the left testicle, where it is decocted, by the heat of temperament inherent in the son of Adam, into a thick, white liquid, whose odor is as that of the palm-spathe."[29]

Regardless of the nature of the "Arabian Nights"—whether all fiction or part fact—the writer of the story of Abu al Husn and his slave girl must have been acquainted with many rational medical concepts including the humoral theory, the theory of the four elements, and considerable human anatomy, physiology and hygiene.

That the Arabian physician was held in high esteem is shown by the following tale from the "Arabian Nights":

"The most wonderful of the events that happened to me in my younger days (said the physician) was this: I was residing in Damascus, where I learnt and practiced my art; and while I was thus occupied, one day there came to me a Mameluke from the house of the governor of the city; so I went forth with him, and accompanied him to the governor's residence. I entered, and beheld at the upper end of the saloon, a sofa of alabaster overlaid with plates of gold, upon which was reclining a sick man. He was young; and a person more comely had not been seen at his age. Seating myself at his head I ejaculated a prayer for his restoration and he made a sign to me with his eye. I then said to him, 'O master, stretch forth to me thy hand': whereupon he put forth his left hand. I was surprised at that, and said within myself, 'What self-conceit!' I felt his pulse, however, and wrote a prescription for him. I continued visiting him for a period of ten days, until he recovered his strength. He entered the bath and washed himself and came forth. Then the governor conferred upon me a handsome dress of honor and appointed me superintendent of the hospital of Damascus."

This story indicates the ability of the doctors of the age to cure their patients, and is illustrative of the high standing of certain members of the medical profession.

There is another story in a lighter vein told by a doctor which contains a useful lesson for the sick. It tells how a man was afflicted with severe pains in the stomach. He sent for a doctor. The doctor inquired what the sick man had eaten. The patient said he had made a meal of a quantity of burnt bread. The doctor prescribed an eye lotion. This greatly astonished the patient who complained that this was certainly no occasion for horseplay.

The doctor assured him that he had prescribed advisedly. "I consider," he said, "that it is necessary to cure your eyes in order that you might see the folly of again eating burnt bread."[30]

It appears that even the legitimate Arabian physicians did not at all times refrain from devious and publicity-gathering conduct. Thus, on one occasion, a man fainted in the street close to a physician of undoubted reputation. The physician, using his cane as a cudgel and summoning the bystanders to follow his example, beat the sick man upon the soles of his feet and upon his body, until he aroused somewhat. Thereupon the others were encouraged and followed the physician's example. When the sick man, miraculously, finally came to, everyone among the assembled Arabians praised the cleverness of the doctor.

The following story is interesting because it contrasts the duly qualified physician and the quack: In a certain town there were two doctors: one of supreme merit and the other, although of not inconsiderable repute, little if anything more than a charlatan and quack. It chanced that the king's daughter became seriously ill. The two doctors were summoned to the palace and the king asked the first physician what he recommended. The good physician expressed his honest and capable opinion concerning the case and stated that a certain medicine contained in the imperial stores would restore the princess to health. "But," said the good doctor, "I am old and weak in sight, and I fear I could scarcely be able to find it, even were I permitted to make a search for the medicine."

Then the other doctor volunteered to make the necessary search. This was permitted, with the result that, not knowing anything about the matter, he selected a drug which was a deadly poison. No sooner had the princess swallowed the draught than she dropped dead on the spot.

In consequence of this terrible result, and in full accord with the usual Eastern custom, the careless quack was compelled to drink the remainder of the drug with the inevitable sequel that he just as rapidly passed out of the picture: Thus did the storyteller contrast the work of the qualified medical man with that of the disreputable medical man.

At times the Arabian physicians had recourse to mysterious procedures. They wrote with a purgative ink (perhaps prepared from the juice of colocynth, scammony, etc.) various charms in cups, to purge the faithful patient. They also employed uroscopy and astrology in treating their patients. Such unscientific methods as these were also transmitted by the Arabian physicians to the West.

From a woman's urine, pregnancy was allegedly diagnosed, and even the sex of the child foretold. Our modern pregnancy tests do not attempt to perform this latter task.

The kind of diagnoses frequently made may be inferred from the following case: Thabet ibn Corra (836-901) diagnosed a disease between the ribs and the pericardium, not from any local phenomena, but in the following manner (according to the patient): "I showed him my urine glass, and he saw in it what was hidden between my ribs and my pericardium. The concealed disease appeared to him as a stain on a polished sword looks to the eye."

As intimated previously, there are instances of quacks who impressed the sick by performing miraculous cures. They hired men to pose as patients and sent them around the neighborhood of their operations to tell the populace of the wonderful cures the doctor had performed upon them. Sometimes a doctor sent his confederate to find out as much as possible about the patient so that when he attended him for the first time, he appeared to have a profound knowledge of the sick person and his family. Such charlatans, of course, were not the monopoly of the Arabs. The European healing profession was by no means free of such impostors. The use of the magic cap (*Tarnkappe*) in Germany which rendered one invisible and therefore invulnerable to the attack of the "angel of death" may be regarded as a similar deception. Siegfried's baptism in dragon's blood by which he became vulnerable only in a place about the size of a leaf in the interscapular region, and Achilles' sole vulnerability at the heel, are famous mythological examples of the sort of thing that gullible patients believed possible.

The fee of such doctors seems to have always been stipulated in advance. As little chance as possible was taken that the death of the patient might terminate the fee. When a patient appeared to be getting worse, the physician demanded at least half the stipulated fee at once.

Physicians-in-ordinary and court-physicians enjoyed high salaries, and often attained great wealth. In case their treatment failed, however, or their masters turned on them for other causes, they were subject to imprisonment, whipping and even death.

We must remember, of course, that Arabian conditions and customs are not to be compared with our modern society. The relations of medical colleagues with each other among the Arabians were usually on a low level. Detraction of and calumny against one's colleagues was the customary procedure. There are instances where physicians actually poisoned their professional competitors in order to get rid of them.

The native medicine of the early Middle Ages in Arabia was for the most part practiced by unlettered and primitive barbarians who were on a lower level than the physicians of the peoples they conquered (i.e. Syria, Egypt, Mesopotamia and Persia). Holding no professional advantage over the physicians of the countries they occupied, they were none the less willing to learn from the more educated physicians of the conquered countries. The conquering Arabs did not impose a new civilization on their defeated enemies for the fact is that they had nothing to impose. But soon after their conquests were completed they became desirous of absorbing what was best from their vanquished foes. They certainly succeeded in invigorating the scattered civilizations then in decline and breathed into them a breath of new life.

During the early days of the Islamic Conquest, powerful Arab armies, aflame with religious exultation and aroused with the fruits of victory in one country after another—in the name of Allah and his prophet Mohammed—had not time nor inclination for cultural activities. The conquerors at first had only one desire—to establish their religious domination firmly over the new territories. As a matter of fact, they at first found many of the practices and customs of their new possessions incompatible with their own and whatever appreciation the invading Arab hordes might have had for the arts and crafts of the peoples of their newly conquered countries was more than offset by a basic antagonism and fear of foreign culture.

Even in these early days of conquest, however, the Arabians had some taste for religious poetry and particularly for Arabic grammar. The latter they felt was very necessary to facilitate the teaching of the Arabic tongue to the peoples of the conquered nations. The conquerors proudly boasted that Arabic was the most perfect tongue ever spoken by mankind.

The attention paid to the study of language produced many grammarians of distinction. A number of dictionaries were compiled, one of which consisted of 60 volumes and had each word illustrated by quotations from the Koran and other classic works. Later encyclopedias were also produced, the most noted one being that which was compiled by Muhammed ibn Abdulah of Granada.

A great change in the cultural activities of the Islamic peoples at large began to take place after the aggressive wars subsided and particularly after some of the Caliphates transferred their capitals from Arabia to Damascus-Syria, where a vestige of the Graeco-Syrian culture still survived. In their new possessions, the conquerors gradually dropped their native customs and practices when their own interests were not at stake and began to emulate the Graeco-Syrian savants. From alchemy, which originally attracted them because of its alluring character, they became interested in chemistry and medicine, and offered hospitality to foreign physicians, scholars, philosophers, and artists.

According to Marmaduke, in the entire history of mankind, the Arabians, after their conquests were completed, give the only large scale instance where conquerors voluntarily respected and emulated the conquered. Once Mohammedanism was firmly established, complete religious freedom was permitted. The only tribute exacted from the conquered lands was for the cost of protecting their liberty.[31] The Arabs freely allowed their subjects to continue their own legal usages and religious practices and employed no force in their proselytizing as was customary in Christian countries.

After the accession of Abu Bakr, father-in-law of Mohammed's favorite wife, to the Caliphate, Islam spread into Syria among the monotheistic Nestorians and came in contact with the Hellenism of the Nestorian monasteries—a fact which had an important bearing on the cultural fusion of the Hellenistic and Oriental elements. The Nestorians were the intermediaries between the ancient masters and the victorious Moslems.

It was this Christian sect, the members of which had been exiled to Persia, that first translated Aristotle into Arabic. Once their translations had been begun, they did not cease working on them for a century and a half, during which time nearly all of the Greek literature in the natural sciences passed into the Arabic language. The Nestorian culture thrived best in Persia during the tolerant rule of the Sassaman dynasty, where the heretical Nestorians found welcome refuge. The Academy of Jondisabur was greatly influenced by the scholarly Nestorians. This Academy became the greatest center of learning and attracted students from all the Eastern countries. This University was the first in the East where the system of medicine taught to the students was based on Greek medical science.

The founder of the Nestorian sect was Nestorius who was born at Germanicia, near Mount Taurus, where he studied theology. The Syriac subjects of Seleucis had been Christianized early. However, their views had been leavened by powerful Greek influences and they were unwilling to abandon the wisdom of Hippocrates and Aristotle at the behest of the bigoted, orthodox Patriarchs of the Eastern Christian Church. A major schism arose, and this heretic sect of Christians—at the head of which was Nestorius—established what is known as the Nestorian Church. The members of this schismatic subdivision acknowledged Christ but clung fiercely to the philosophy of Greece.

Most of their cities were originally Greek colonies in which institutions had been set up modeled on those of Athens. Richly endowed with the spirit of speculative science, they remained at heart true to the old traditions. Nestorius' fame as a scholar and teacher of the Christian religion became so widely spread that he was consecrated as a Patriarch of Constantinople. After a few years in office he became the victim of jealousies and intrigues and was deposed from his patriarchal position in 431 by the Council of Ephesus. The heretical doctrine imputed to him consisted in the allegation that he denied the complete mergence of the divine and human natures into one person, in Christ, and in claiming that Mary, the mother of Christ, ought not to be called the mother of God. He was retired into the monastery of Antioch in 435, and from this institution, he was banished to Petra, Arabia, and later to the Great Oasis in Upper Egypt.

His followers fled eastward. Many of them went to Edessa, where a school of medicine had been flourishing for centuries. The school was the center of Nestorian activities until 489, when it was closed by order of the Emperor Zeno, thus causing a further dispersion of the Nestorians. These zealous Nestorians then proceeded to carry the doctrines of Nestorius throughout the whole length of Asia. The Nestorians for many centuries formed the main links between East and West. In 762 considerable of their number came to Bagdad.

The Nestorians had a large share in the translation of many Greek works on mathematics and medicine into Syriac. Their activity continued until the ninth century. The translations of classic Greek works into Arabic were generally made with the help of Syriac versions. The Nestorians and Jews were especially well fitted for this task because of their knowledge of languages. Members of these groups had a first class knowledge of Greek, Syriac, Arabic and Persian.

CHAPTER VII

THE ARABIAN SCHOOL OF TRANSLATORS

The rise of the Mohammedan Empire, which influenced Europe so much both politically and intellectually, made its mark also on the history of medicine. As had been the case after the Roman conquest of Greece, the conqueror benefited intellectually from the victims of his conquest. After the military operations of the Mohammedans had become consolidated, schools of medicine and of general learning arose in all capitals of the Moslem Empire. The medical schools were often connected with hospitals and schools of pharmacy. At Damascus, Syria, Greek medicine was zealously cultivated under the guidance of Jewish and Nestorian teachers. Other schools were founded in Bagdad and in Sura, Mesopotamia. In Bagdad, the first translation of Greek medical works were made by ibn Masawaih and his pupil Hunain. Years earlier, the Arabs had become acquainted through commerce with Indian medicine, and Indian physicians lived in the royal courts of Bagdad.

It may be of interest here to explain in detail how this Arabian revival of culture came about. For centuries the University of Jondisabur,[1] which had been founded in the fourth century near Kazerun, between Susa and Ecbatanta Persia, was the primary means of spreading higher education all through the Near East. This University became a refuge for the Nestorians driven from Edessa in 489, for the Jews who fled from Syria at about the same time, and also for the Neoplatonists who were banished from Athens in 529.

The Nestorians and the Jews brought with them Greek medical works translated into Syriac, and the Neoplatonists conveyed to Jondisabur their philosophical ideas based on those of Plato. The works of all these groups were later translated into Arabic. Baas ascribes the frequent corruption of texts in the Arabic translations to the fact that the Greek works passed through the narrow cloisters of the Nestorian monasteries.[2]

Jondisabur became the greatest intellectual center of the time. There Greek, Jewish, Christian, Syrian, Hindu and Persian ideas were exchanged and synthesized. By royal decree Persian translations of Aristotle and Plato were made at this institution. Jondisabur reached the peak of its importance during the reign of Nushirwan the Just (he was called "Chosroes" by the Greeks, and "Kisra" by the Arabs), who ruled over Sassania from 531 to 579. Jondisabur became especially important as a medical center. The medical teachings were essentially Greek tinctured with Hindu, Syrian and Persian doctrines. The medical school flourished until the end of the tenth century. Its influence upon Islamic medicine was tremendous in the latter half of the eighth century.[3]

Among the first Arabian physicians of the sixth century was Al Harith ben Kalada al Thakefi of Taif, near Mecca, who studied medicine in Jondisabur and, for a time, practiced in Persia, where he accumulated quite a fortune. When he returned to Mecca he became a friend of Mohammed and a confidant of the first Caliph, Abu Bekr. It is known that some of Al Harith's ideas pertaining to medicine are found in the Koran even though it is not known whether or not Al Harith accepted Mohammedanism. He was fatally poisoned under obscure circumstances in the year 634. Perhaps it was because he was skeptical of the teachings of Mohammed that he met with his untimely end.

His son, Al Nader ben Harith ben Kalad, also a physician, was violently opposed to the teachings of Mohammed and he was with the opposing army at the Battle of Bedr which occurred on February 24, 624. He was captured and brought back to Medina where he was executed by Ali ibn Talif on the personal order of Mohammed.

One of the most distinguished physicians to influence Arabian medicine was Jordshis (Georgeus) of the medical faculty of the Academy of Jondisabur. In 769 he was invited by Caliph al Mansur to Bagdad to translate medical works from the Persian language into Arabic. He turned over the hospital duties of Jondisabur to his son, Bakhtishua, and traveled to Bagdad, taking along with him one of his students named Ifa ibn Shalahtha. He was received in Bagdad with great honor. While he was in this metropolis, occupied with the task of translating the medical works, the monarch took sick with some gastric disturbance. When all efforts on the part of his court physicians to relieve him were to no avail, he turned to Jordshis for relief. The latter, in the course of a few days, succeeded in curing him of his serious malady. As a reward Jordshis was appointed the Caliph's personal physician. The doctor, however, did not remain long with the Caliph for he contracted a severe illness and requested to be relieved of his duties so that he could return home. The Caliph presented him with many precious gifts before his departure. It is related that the interest in medicine of Caliph al Mansur and his princely sons was due to this famous physician. It is not definitely known which medical works he translated from the Persian to the Arabic language, but it has been assumed that the works of Hippocrates and Dioscorides were included.[4]

THE BAKHTISHUA FAMILY

The Bakhtishua family produced a number of famous physicians and scientists whose fame extended for several centuries. They occupied prominent positions in the courts of the Caliphates of Persia, Iraq, Syria and Arabia.

Perhaps the most distinguished physician of the Bakhtishua family was Jabril (Gabriel) ben Bakhtishua, who was appointed body physician at the court of Caliph Harun al Rashid (805)— an office previously occupied by his father and grandfather. Jabril successfully treated the Caliph after a cerebral accident, employing venesection. It is related that he employed a rather novel plan in treating the Caliph's favorite wife, who was afflicted with (hysterical) paralysis of an arm. He subjected her to a sudden mental shock that necessitated the use of the arm—a stratagem which enabled her to immediately regain the use of the arm. These two cures placed the doctor in high esteem with the Caliph. He became the most influential person in the court of Harun al Rashid. Anyone who desired promotion in rank or other favors sought the influence of Jabril. He, however, soon aroused the jealousy of many ranking officers. The death of Harun al Rashid at the beginning of the ninth century abruptly changed his fortunes. The succession of Rashid's son, Al Amin, to the Caliphate, gave Jabril's enemies the opportunity to revenge themselves against him. They trumped up serious charges against him, and he was deposed and imprisoned.

The new Caliph appointed a Bishop of Persia as his body physician. The latter, fearing that the famous Jabril might yet get out of prison and be called back to his former position, caused a rehearing of the charges. The tribunal thereupon sentenced Jabril to death. It was indeed fortunate for Dr. Jabril that al Amin's reign was short lived. After two years of rule, his brother, al Mamun, wrested the Caliphate from him with the aid of his friend, General Tahir ben Hasin (known as "the man with two hands"). Amin was promptly executed and Jabril was freed before his death sentence could be carried out.

The new Caliph, Mamun, brother of Amin, recalled Jabril to the position he had occupied under his father, Harun; but for some reason he later lost grace with the Caliph who appointed Jabril's son-in-law, Michael, as his physician. Michael, however, did not occupy the position long. Caliph Mamun took very sick and Michael proved hopelessly inept in handling the case. Jabril was summoned and he was successful in restoring the Caliph's health in three days. As a reward the Caliph ordered the return of Jabril's confiscated belongings and reinstated him in his former position. Jabril died in 828 and was buried with great honor and pomp in the Church of St. Sergius, in Medina. Jabril was the author of five books, the most important of which was "An Introduction into the Medical Art." [5]

One of Jabril's sons, Jahja (Johannes) ben Bakhtishua, became body physician to Caliph al Moctader. He died in the year 940. Another son, Obeidalla ben Jabril ben Bakhtishua, was the physician of Caliph al Motaki. He was the author of a work entitled "Hortus Medicinae," which was a medical compendium consisting of 50 chapters. His son, Jabril ben Obeidalla, a famous physician at the court of Sultan Adhad ed-Dalla ben Buweih, was professor of medicine and physics at the Hospital of Bagdad. He died in 1006 at the age of eighty-five. He is the author of "Pandecta Medicinae" in five volumes, and a book on the eye, "De Morbus Ocularum."

Fifty years after the death of Mohammed, the advancement of learning had became a settled policy under the Caliphs of Bagdad. The studies of medicine, mathematics and astronomy, as well as general literature, were encouraged.

The rise of Arabian civilization came to pass with the accession of the Abbasids to power (A.D. 750). Thanks to the enlightenment of the early Abbasid Caliphs of Bagdad, notably al Mansur and al Mamun, official Islam cast off from the moorings of narrow and intolerant orthodoxies and sailed out to the wide stream of learning. With the establishment of the Abbasid dynasty a new epoch in Arabian medicine began. The former pagan practice rapidly became antiquated and out of place. The Omayyads (with one exception) were not religious men and, while preserving the outward forms of Islam, allowed full liberty of belief and practices to the Christians and Jews.

The celebrated Abbasid family introduced Persian culture among the Islamic peoples through the Arabianized Persians. The growth of liberal tendencies among the Arabians reached its climax when their capital was tranferred to Bagdad. In a few years Bagdad became a great center of commerce, industry, and agriculture and a metropolis of secular learning. Its culture embodied both the traditions of the ancient Oriental world and the Western world. Bagdad, in its luxurious way of life, its glamour and its splendor, exceeded even the capitals of the Byzantine and Persian Empires. It grew to be the greatest and most influential city, not only of the Near East, but also of the world. It became the center of learning and the domain of the intellectuals. Foreign culture was greatly encouraged by the Abbasids. At the end of the eighth and beginning of the ninth centuries the Caliphates were at their height of power. Islam became the greatest spiritual and physical force in the world, and in a comparatively short time it exercised great intellectual influence upon the world's history.

Caliph al Mansur (reigned 754-775 A.D.) invited learned men, regardless of their religious views, to Bagdad and offered them hospitality and protection. He appointed the famous Nestorian ibn Masawaih to head the School of Bagdad.

The Academy of Bagdad was the most flourishing school of its time. The medical school had a hospital in its vicinity where bedside instruction was given to students and where examinations were conducted at the end of the period of instruction. Among the professors were Joshua ben Nun (c. 800 A.D.), a philosopher of high repute, and Yakub ibn Ishaq (c. 800 A.D.).

Al Mansur's son, Harun al Rashid (786-809 A. D.), founded a special institution for transcribing precious manuscripts. Under his direction a large collection of books were brought together. He issued an edict that no mosque should be built unless there was a school attached to it.

Caliph al Rashid gratified his curiosity by causing Homer to be translated into Syriac, but he did not venture to have the great epics rendered in Arabic. The translation of Homer into Arabic was not realized until deep in the tenth century.

Caliph al Mansur (754-775 A.D.) and his son Harun al Rashid (786-809 A.D.) deserve a prominent place in the history of medicine. The beginning of a new era of Arabian learning was unfolded during their reign. At first the advance was impeded by linguistic grounds, for new terms and constructions suitable for the expression of medical, philosophic and scientific thought had to be formed in the Arabic languages.

CALIPH ABDALLAH AL-MAMUN (786-833 A.D.)

The growth of Arabian medicine was particularly manifested during the reign of Caliph al-Mamun (813-833 A.D.), who was a great patronizer of the arts and sciences. He brought together a tremendous collection of the writings of great authors and founded a special institution for translation which was placed under the direction of distinguished scholars. It is related that one of the terms of peace which he forced on all whom he fought and conquered was absolute surrender of all literary treasures.

Abdallah al Mamun was born in Bagdad in 786 A.D. He was the seventh and greatest caliph of the Abbasid dynasty and reigned from 813 to 833 A.D. His mother and his wife were Persians, which explains his Persian proclivities. He himself pursued studies in languages and philosophy in Persia. He was an ardent Mutazilite or Secessionist, who held that God could not predestine man's actions because He was a moral being who was bound to do what was righteous. Al Mamun therefore demanded that theology should be subjected to investigation by the mind.

Caliph al-Mamun founded universities at Basra, Kufah and Samarac and medical schools in Bagdad. He equipped them well and furnished them with the best of teachers. He transferred many scientists and physicians from Jondisabur to Bagdad. He wrote four long letters to explain that the Koran was not divine but conceived by men, and he cruelly punished those who dared entertain different views (e.g., ibn Hanbal). He thus combined in a most remarkable way democratic thought and dictatorial intolerance.

Incidentally Caliph al Mamun was the first Caliph ever officially to admit that the Koran had been created by man during the course of recorded history. This doctrine was in serious opposition to the orthodox teaching that the Koran was eternal and had been created prior to the world, having coexisted previously with God. The Caliph, then, took a long stride forward in permitting reason to outweigh blind faith. Under al Mamun, the intellectuals did not hesitate to devote themselves to Greek science. With such a lack of bigotry, it is not surprising that the truth was pursued for its own sake, and traditional beliefs modified when they were irreconcilable with scientific facts.

A great library in Bagdad called "The House of Wisdom" was founded by al Mamun. The Grandees of the Court vied with each other in collecting books. A school devoted to translation was founded in Bagdad, where Hunain ibn Ishaaq (809-873 A.D.), a great physician and brilliant translator, was appointed director.

Jews and Christians were very welcome at al Mamun's court. He was even a greater patron of letters and science than his father Harun al Rashid. He went to considerable difficulty to obtain Greek manuscripts and he obtained a number of valuable holographs by purchase. He even sent a mission to the Byzantine Emperor Leon the Armenian (812-820) for this purpose.

The Caliphs al Mutassim, al Mutawakkil and al Mustamin continued the work of translation from the tenth century onward. They also provided commentaries on the works of the ancient Greeks. The remaining scholars and physicians of Jondisabur were transferred to the courts of Bagdad and Samara under Caliph al Mutawakkil.

The earliest translations into Arabic were the works of Euclid, the Almagest of Ptolemy and the physics of Aristotle. The translators were Syrians, Persians, Jews, and Greek scholars.

The Arabs based their scientific knowledge, not on original investigations, but upon the works of the Greek and other authorities which they so zealously translated. The first translations were not from the original Greek, but from Persian and Syrian versions. Later the bulk of the translations were made from original Greek sources. The Arabs never translated the Greek poets into their own tongue, although they assiduously collected and translated into Arabic the works of the Greek physicians and philosophers. Their strict religious sentiments and sedate character caused the Arabs to hate the lewdness of classical mythology. The Arabs went so far as to denounce indignantly any effort to connect the licentious, impure, Olympian Jove and the Most High God, as an insufferable and unpardonable blasphemy.

Since the translators did not add anything materially to ancient Greek medicine, the so-called "Arabian medicine" is only Arabian in the linguistic sense. The Arabic writers, as a rule, were not natives of Arabia. The only medical writer of importance who was of Arabian stock was al-Kindi. The other Arabian writers and translators were of different nationalities and included Syrians, Persians, Jews, Egyptians and Spaniards who made use of the Arabian language but were not racially Arabians.

The real Arabians, of course, excepting the Caliphs and a relatively few others, were indifferent to higher culture for a long period of time. They were interested more in religious speculations, such as for example, whether the Koran was created by God or produced by the hands of man, or whether man, philosophically speaking, possessed a free will, or was bound down by divine predestination. Nevertheless, medicine is greatly indebted to the Arabians both for stimulating a revival of the scientific spirit of ancient Greece and for preserving a substantial part of our knowledge of the art of healing. Thanks to the patronage of the Abbasids, Bagdad maintained for centuries great fame as the center of intellectual life.

The division of the realm into principalities had a beneficial cultural effect because the competition of the provinces with one another encouraged technical and scientific endeavors.

Gradually a large medical literature came into existence. Various works were produced which remained in use by physicians for many centuries, such as, for example, the medical works of Rhazes, ibn al Haitham, Holy Abbas, and Avicenna.

The works of Hippocrates, Dioscorides, Archigenes, Ruphus, Galen, Oribasius, Alexander of Tralles and Paulus of Aegina were all rendered in Arabic, as were the important medical works of Persia and India. Some of the Arabian translations of ancient Greek texts were more correctly transmitted than those which had been done by Latin translators. For example, Galen's anatomy was far more accurately described in Arabic than in any previous translation.[6]

The works of the Arabian writers that appeared in print form only a small fraction of the literature that was never published. Three hundred medical writers who wrote in Arabic are enumerated by Ferdinand Wustenfeld (1808-1899) and other historians have enlarged the list. Only three original printed Arabic translations have been preserved. A number more are known through Latin translations. The great majority still exist in manuscript form. There can be no doubt that these works were, in the main Greek medicine modified to suit the climate, habit and native lore with the addition of various Oriental sources.

Even though as has been mentioned, very few of the so-called Arabian medical authors were Arabian except with respect to language, the Arab historians, understandably enough, like to appropriate all that is written in their language as their own. Thus even the works of Maimonides are claimed by many Arab historians as their own.

It is obviously impossible to dwell upon all Arabic medical writers in the present work. Only those individuals who exerted an influence upon Western medicine will be considered here.

The following is a more or less chronological list of some of the more important medical authors and translators who flourished under the Eastern Caliphate:[7]

Name	Date
Aharun al Quis	c. 600 A.D.
Masarjawaihi	c. 622 A.D.
Burzwei ibn Adesher	c. 683 A.D.
Khalid ibn Yazid	d. 704 or 708 A.D.
Jordshis (Georgeus)	c. 720 A.D.
Abu Zakariya Yuhanna ibn Masawaih (Latin: Mesue Major)	777-857 A.D.
Al Kindi	d. 873 A.D.
Hunain ibn Ishaq	809-877 A.D.
Thabit ibn Qurra	826-901 A.D.
Isa ben Ali	c. 925 A.D.
Hubaish ibn al-Hasan	d. 912 A.D.
Isa ibn Yahya	c. 987 A.D.
Abu Yakub Ishaq	c. 910 A.D.
Kosta ibn Luka	864-923 A. D.

The first celebrated physician of the early Islamic period was Aharun al-Quis (Aaron the Priest or the Presbyter), who is often referred to as the last of the Alexandrian physicians. He appears to have been a contemporary of Paulus of Aegina (6th century). His work "Kunnash,"[8] also known as "The Medical Pandect of Aaron," consists of thirty books. He wrote in Greek and this was translated into Syriac. The Syriac version was translated into Arabic (c. 683 A.D.) by Masarjawaihi, a Persian Jew of Basra, Iraq.[9] This latter version is the oldest medical work in the Arabic language and for a time was literally the fountain head of Arabic medicine. Aharun al-Quis was the first writer to make mention of smallpox.

Masarjawaihi himself left an important medical work, "On Ailments and Simple Drugs," which is referred to by the celebrated Arabic physicians Rhazes and Ibn al Bathor. These famous doctors referred to him as "the Jew." Masarjawaihi was a pharmacologist of note. He recommended the juice located at the end of the branches of Persian lilac mixed with honey and boiled in grape juice as an effective antidote for certain poisons. He stated that the leaves of the Persian lilac when applied to bald spots make hair grow (no doubt this latter remedy was as effective as those presently employed for alopecia!). Masarjawaihi is the first to translate texts from Syriac into Arabic.

Another translator and writer of the pre-Islamic period was Burzwei ibn Adesher, a Persian physician who showed a great inclination toward medicine since his childhood. He absorbed the medical knowledge of the Persian and Indian schools while still a very young man. He probably attended the medical school at the University of Jondisabur. He became court physician to Nushirwan ben Cobad ben Firuz, King of Persia (reigned 531-571), at whose request he traveled to secure a copy of the famous work, "The fables of Bidpai." He copied this work and translated it into the Pelwih language. Later it was translated into Arabic under the title of "Calila and Dimna" and was eventually rendered in German under the title of "Die Fabeln Bidpai aus dem Arabischen."[10]

KHALID IBN YAZID (d. 704 or 708 A.D.)

The Caliphates produced one of their greatest translators in the person of Khalid ibn Yazid ibn Muswiya, called "the *Hakim*" (philosopher). He was a member of the Marwan family which flourished in Egypt. He was an Omayyad prince who, according to Muslim tradition, was supposed to have encouraged Greek philosophers in Egypt to translate Greek scientific works into Arabic. He was himself deeply interested in medicine, astrology and alchemy. He is said to have studied under an Alexandrian scholar named Marianos.

IBN MASAWAIH (777-857 A.D.)

Among the early translators was Abu Zakariya Yuhanna ibn Masawaih (Latin: "Mesue," or, more specifically, "Mesue Major" —Mesue the Elder; at times referred to as Johannis Damascenti). He was the son of a pharmacist in Jondisabur and was perhaps the first Arabic ophthalmologist. He came to Bagdad and studied under Jabril ben Bakhtishua in the Beit al Hikma. Jabril appointed him as director of the infirmary of Bagdad (at the Academy). He was a Christian physician who wrote in Syriac and Arabic. He later became physician to the Caliph Harun al Rashid, who appointed him head of the Medical School of Bagdad. He translated various Greek medical works into Arabic. Caliph al-Mutasim (c. 836) is said to have supplied him with apes for dissection. A number of medical writings are credited to him, notably the "Disorders of the Eye" (*"Daghal al ain"*), which is the earliest systematic treatise on ophthalmology extant in Arabic. Ibn Masawaih was also the author of a number of medical books on anatomy and dietetics. The Latin translation of his Aphorisms, *"Aphorisma Johannis Damascenti"* is ascribed to him and was very popular in the Middle Ages. His works are frequently quoted by later writers. He is referred to by Rhazes as the author of various medical works in the Arabic language on pharmacy and therapeutics. These works have not been recovered. He held that smallpox is caused by fermentation of the blood.[11]

AL-KINDI (d. 873 A.D.)

The only famous Arabic writer of Arabian stock was Abu Yusuf Yakub ibn Ishaq al-Sabbah al-Kindi (Latin, Alkindus). He was born in Basra at the beginning of the ninth century and flourished in Bagdad under al-Mamun and al-Mutasim (813-842). He was persecuted during the orthodox revolt led by al-Matawakkil (847-861). He was known as "the philosopher of the Arabs" because he was the first and only great philosopher of the Arabic East. His knowledge of Greek science and philosophy was considerable. He made a deep study of Aristotle from the Neoplatonic point of view.

Al-Kindi's theories of the soul, with some modifications, formed the basis of later Arabic philosophical thought. His conception of the universe was similar to that of Aristotle. Divine intelligence is the cause of all worldly existence. Its activity is disseminated from the heavenly sphere to the terrestrial world. The world soul is intermediate between God and the world of bodies. This world soul created the heavenly bodies. The human soul is an emanation from the world soul. It is tied to the human body, but insofar as it is true to its spiritual origin, it is free and independent. But true freedom is only attainable in the world of intelligence so that if man would attain this he must develop his intellectual powers by acquiring a true knowledge of God and the universe.[12]

Relatively few of al-Kindi's numerous works (207?) are extant. These deal with mathematics, astrology, physics, music, medicine, pharmacy, and geography. Many translations from the Greek into Arabic were made or revised by him or under his direction. He considered alchemy as an imposture. Two of his works are especially important to the study of vision: "De Espectibus," a treatise on geometrical and physiological optics (largely based on Euclid, Heron and Ptolemy), and "De Medicinarum Compositarum Gradibus Investigandis Libellus," which deals with the dosage and preparation of medicines and represents an extraordinary attempt to establish posology on a mathematical basis. Most of his works were translated by Gerald of Cremona.[13] Al-Kindi is still referred to by the Arabs as "Abu Yusuf, the philosopher."

HUNAIN IBN ISHAQ (809-877 A.D.)

The greatest of all Arabic translators was Hunain ibn Ishaq (Johannitius), or more fully, Abu Zeid ibn Ishaq al Ibadi. He was born at Alhira in Iraq and, like his master, Ibn Masawaih, under whom he studied medicine, he also was a Nestorian. He traveled in Greece and studied Arabic at Basra. He collected Greek medical manuscripts, translated many of them, supervised the activities of other scholars, and revised their translations. His role with regard to medical literature is analogous to that of Thabit ibn Qurra with regard to mathematical and astronomical texts. The school of Nestorian translators headed by Hunain must have been quite large, for its members managed to translate the greatest part of the Hippocratic and Galenic writings into Syriac and Arabic.

Hunain also wrote original works: notably, a history of Mohammed, a treatise on ophthalmology and an introduction to Galen's *"Ars Parva."* The last was immensely popular during the Middle Ages. Although Hunain was unquestionably a very great scholar, he was more of an encyclopedist than a scientist. He produced more than 150 translations and wrote more than 100 original books. Unfortunately, the bulk of this enormous output is now lost. Such important documents as his translations of Dioscorides' "Materia Medica" and Galen's "Simple Drugs" have not survived the ravages of time.

Hunain was not only a translator and author but a great linguist. He coined many of the Arabic scientific terms and identified the Greek names of drugs with the Arabic, Persian and Syriac equivalents. These names passed immediately into the medical works of his contemporaries. Moreover, Hunain made extracts of, and commentaries on, the pharmacological treatises which he had translated. Ibn Abi Usabia (1203-1269 A.D.), the historian of Arabian physicians, enumerates seven such tracts. None of them are extant. The "Isagoga" ("Introductiones in Medicinam") is an original work in which Hunain gives a systematic review of the Galenic system of medicine. It also contains the names and theories of medieval medical authorities. Hunain's name is frequently mentioned in al-Ghafiqui's pharmacology.[14]

Besides his translations of the medical and philosophical works of Galen, Aristotle and Plato, Hunain left several books, among them a treatise on simple drugs, which is now lost, but known by the quotations in Rhazes' and al-Ghafiqui's writings.

THABIT IBN QURRA (826-901 A.D.)

Another famous translator was Abu al Hasan Thabit ibn Qurra ibn Marwan al-Harran who was a native of Harran, Mesopotamia. He was a physician, mathematician and astronomer. One of the greatest translators from Greek and Syriac into Arabic, he actually founded a school of translators of which many of his own family were members. The works of Apollonius (Books 5 to 7), Archimedes, Euclid, Theodosius, Ptolemy (on geography), Galen and Eutocius were translated by him. Many anatomical, medical, mathematical and astronomical writings are ascribed to him. Most of these were in Arabic but some were in Syriac. He also translated Hippocrates' treatise "On Air and Water" and Galen's "De Chyle" and "Compendium Libris de Alimentis et Libris de Diebus Criticus."[15] He was the author of many original works on a number of medical subjects.

ISA BEN ALI (c. 925 A.D.)

Isa ben Ali (commonly known as Jesu Haly) was a pupil of Hunain ibn Ishaq. He practiced ophthalmology in Bagdad. He

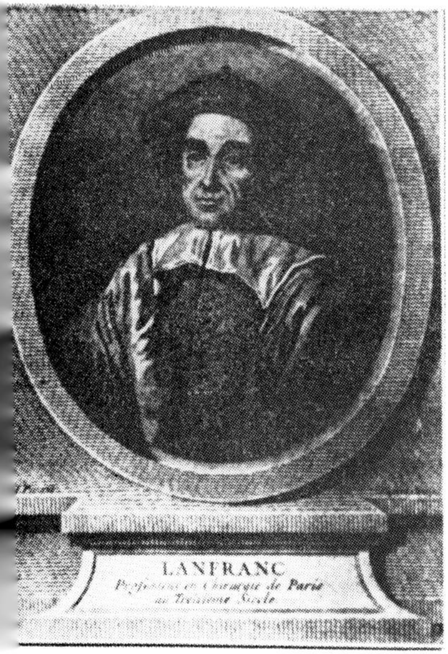

PLATE 37. Lanfranc
(Armed Forces Medical Library, Washington, D.C.)

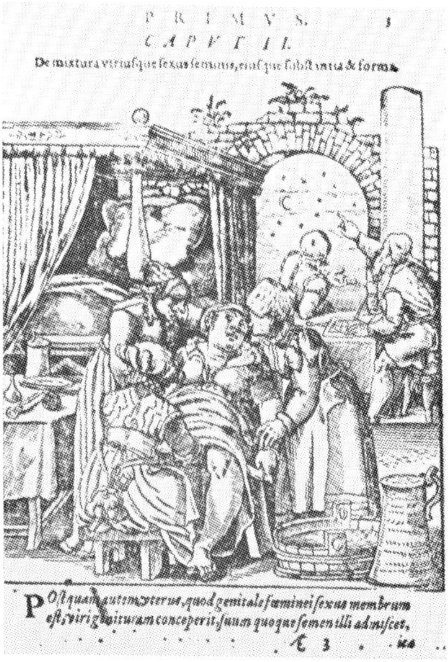

PLATE 38. Picture of a delivery. Jacob Reuff (1580).

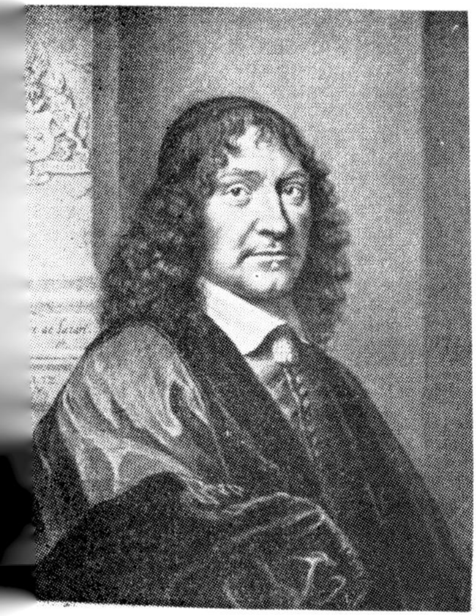

PLATE 39. Franciscus De Le Boe Sylvius (1614-1672)

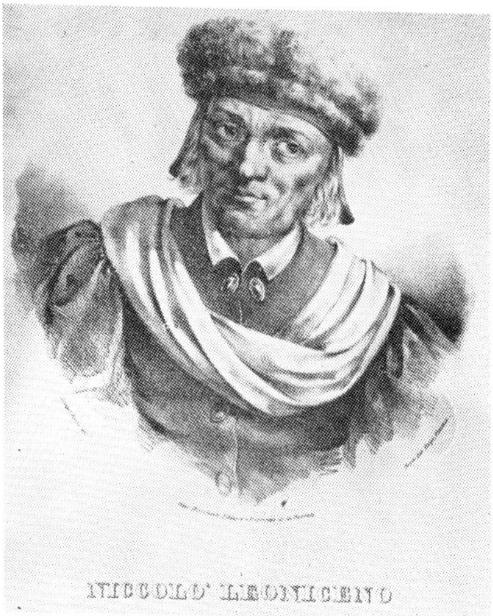

PLATE 40. Nicolo Leoniceno
(Courtesy Armed Forces Medical Library, Washington, D.C.)

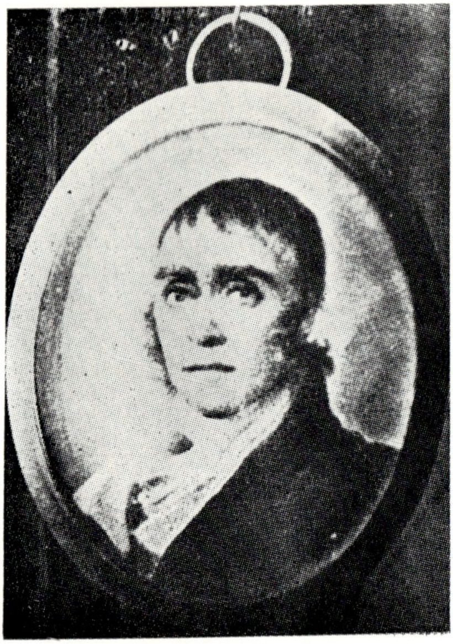

PLATE 41. Jesse Bennett. From Dr. Joseph L. Miller's article describing first Caesarean operation in this country.

(*Courtesy Virginia Medical Quart.*)

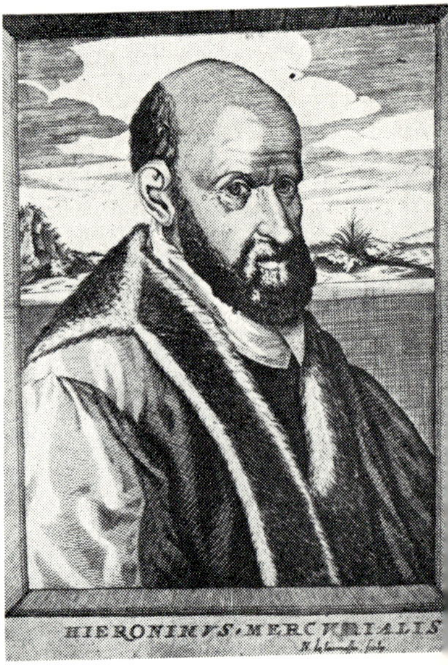

PLATE 42. Jerome Mercuriale (1530-1606)

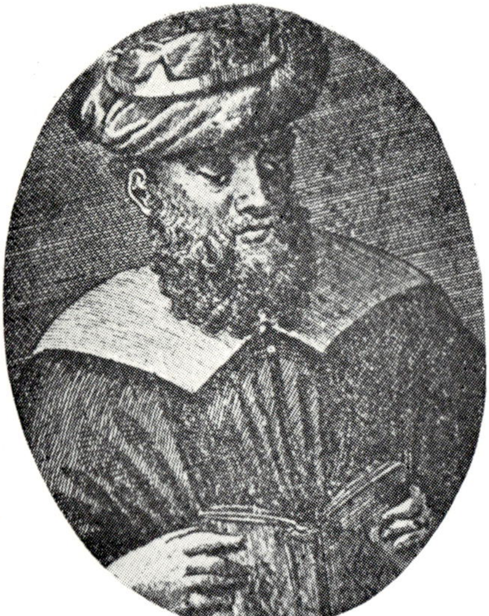

PLATE 43. Avicenna

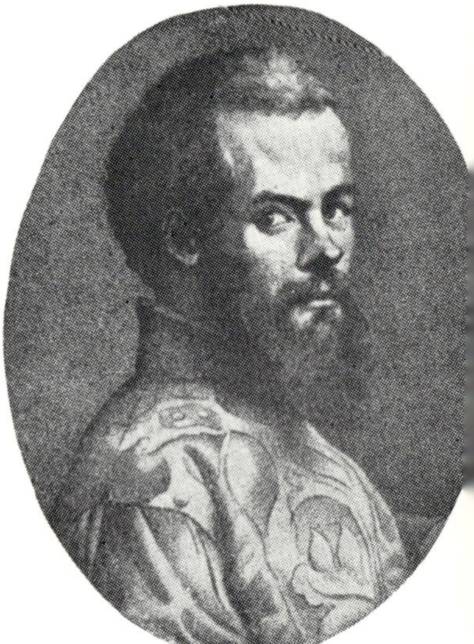

PLATE 44. Vesalius

wrote a manual on eye diseases entitled in the Latin translation, "Libra Memorialis Opthalmicorum," which consists of three parts: part one is devoted to the anatomy and physiology of the eye; part two concerns itself with the external diseases of the eye; and part three includes non-visible eye affections. This is the oldest book on ophthalmology which is still extant.[16]

There is also a manuscript at Dresden attributed to Isa ben Ali which, in the Latin version, is entitled: "De Cognitione Infirmitatem Ocularum et Curatione Eorum." Isa ben Ali left a pharmacological treatise which is only known by quotations from it in other works.

HUBAISH IBN AL-HASAN (d. 912 A.D.)

Hubaish ibn al-Hasan (nicknamed al-Asam, because of a lame hand) was the son of the sister of Hunain ibn Ishaq. Like his uncle in Bagdad, he flourished most probably in the second half of the ninth century. He was also a pupil and co-worker of Hunain in the translation of Greek works into Syriac and Arabic. He seems to have devoted most of his energy to the translation of Galen. Hunain credits him with the translation of three Galenic works into Syriac and of 35 into Arabic. Hubaish assisted his master in the translation of Dioscorides.

Many translations were made by him directly from Greek into Arabic. He completed a medical treatise ("Quaestiones Medicae"). His fame was of course eclipsed by that of his uncle. As a matter of fact, many translations made by him were ascribed to Hunain.[17]

ISA IBN YAHYA (c. 987 A.D.)

Another close disciple of Hunain was Isa ibn Yahya ibn Ibrahim, who translated various Galenic works: one into Syriac and 25 into Arabic. His Arabic versions are based primarily upon Hunain's Syriac versions. He also did a part of the translation of Oribasius. Some original writings are ascribed to him. According to Firhist, Isa ibn Yahya assisted Hunain in translating Hippocrates in 987 A.D.

ABU YAKUB IBN ISHAQ (c. 910 A.D.)

Abu Yakub ibn Ishaq (c. 910), a son of Hunain, also rendered Greek works into Arabic. This father-son combination has led to considerable confusion concerning the authorship of several works.

KOSTA IBN LUKA (864-923 A.D.)

A younger contemporary of Hunain was Kosta ibn Luka, a Christian philosopher and physician at Baalbec. He traveled extensively through Greece and Asia Minor, returning to Syria with a number of valuable manuscripts. He was then called to Bagdad by the Abbasid Caliphs to translate Greek works.

Kosta ibn Luka distinguished himself by his clarity of expression and brevity of style. He left a number of works. Among them was an Arabic translation of Hippocrates' "Aphorisms" (which had been originally translated into Syriac by Hunain) and "An Introduction to the Study of Medicine." He also wrote independent works on fever, diet, materia medica and on many other subjects. His practice was largely confined to the care of royalty, but his fame as a physician spread all through the Near East.

CHAPTER VIII

FAMOUS MEDICAL AUTHORS OF THE ARABIC PAST

No sooner were the classical works of the Greeks translated into the Arabic tongue than Arabic students, mostly outside of Arabia proper, rushed to read these works. Their reverence for the scientific works of ancient Greece was only second to their respect for the Koran. The greatest ambition of a student was to be able to understand the ancient masters in the original or in translations. Few dared to question ancient Greek authority. The opinion of the Greek masters was considered law. The additions that the Islamic physicians attempted to make to Greek medicine refer almost entirely to therapeutics. The theory and thought of the Greeks were left untouched. In such an atmosphere experimental medicine was practically impossible. Then too, since the Moslems were prohibited from performing any dissection on human bodies or on living animals, Galen's anatomical and physiological errors could not be corrected.

With reference to therapeutics, surgery, pharmacology and mineralogy the Arabians received some impetus from the experience of the Persians, Indians and Near East Scholars. Their own share in medicine was entirely in the realm of practical experience. Moslem scholars, although acute observers, were only thinkers in a restricted sense. In short, the legacy of the Islamic world to medicine and natural sciences is the legacy of Greece, not of Arabia.

Up to the beginning of the ninth century and even to the days of Rhazes, medicine was purely dogmatic in its conception. The best talent of the medical profession was directed to the study of the writings of Galen, Paul of Aegina, Aetius and other ancient writers. As a matter of fact, these pillars of medical wisdom were considered uncontradictable, even if practical experience showed that they had erred in particular instances.

It is not within the scope of this work even to name all the Arabic physicians who carried the banner of the medical profession throughout the early Middle Ages. Their number runs into the hundreds. It is our purpose, however, to deal with a few of the most celebrated Arabic medical writers.

YAHYA IBN SERABI (Serapion Senior 870-930)

Yahya ibn Serabi, known in Latin as Serapion Senior, was one of the most distinguished medical writers of the ninth century. He was also known as Janus Damascenus. A Christian physician from Damascus, Syria, his name has been often confused with ibn Masawaih (Mesue Senior) because of an error made by Constantinus Africanus. Yahya ibn Serabi wrote two books in the Syrian language: "Aphorisms" in twelve books and "Pandectae" in seven books. These works are largely derived from Alexander of Tralles. Both of these were translated into Arabic by Musa ben Abraham al Hodaith; and a Syrian Jew, Ebn Bahbul. "Pandectae" was translated into Latin by Gerard of Cremona and this edition is to be found in the Escurial Library under the title "Aggregator." This work appeared in various editions under different names, e.g., "Pandectae," "Therapeutica Methodus," and "Practica Siue Breviarum." The arrangement of the pathology in this work is faulty. Serapion advises venesection in most inflammatory affections and he gives a detailed description as to the choice of veins and the methods of technique. Up to the Renaissance, Yahya ibn Serabi was frequently quoted by medical writers.

According to Friend,[1] Serapion took his material chiefly from Aetius and Paul of Aegina. Rhazes, in his "Continens Medicinae," often quotes Yahya ibn Serabi verbatim.[2] A Latin translation of Serapion was published in Venice in the year 1479.[3]

ALI AL TABARI (died c. 875)

Ali al Tabari—more fully Abu-l-Hasan Ali ibn Sahl (ibn) Rabban al-Tabari—a native of Tabearistan (a Persian province south of the Caspian Sea) was born and educated at Rai where he practiced and taught medicine for a time. He embraced Islam and moved to Bagdad where he soon acquired an extensive practice and secured a position at the court of Caliph al Mutawakil (reigned 847-869). He was the son of a Persian Jew, Sahl al Tabari, and one of the teachers of Rhazes. His main work, "The Paradise of Wisdom" ("Firdawsu al-hikmat"), was completed in 850 during a brief residence in Sara-man-ras. This work deals chiefly with medicine, but also with philosophy, meteorology, zoology, embryology, psychology, and astronomy. It is based on Greek and Hindu sources and ends with a summary of Hindu medicine. Ali al Tabari also wrote a defense of Islam entitled, "The Book of Religion and Empire."[4]

SINAN IBN THABIT (860-943)

Sinan ibn Thabit, whose full name was Abu Said Sinan ibn Thabit ibn Qurra, was the son of the famous Thabit ibn Qurra. He flourished at Bagdad and died there in 943. Born a Harranian Christian, he embraced the Islamic religion in middle life. He became famous as a Moslem physician, mathematician and astronomer. Various mathematical and astronomical writings are ascribed to him. He was physician to three successive Caliphs: al-Muktadir, al-Kahir, and al-Radi who ruled from 908 to 940. His primary bid for fame rests on his brilliant administration of the Bagdad hospitals and his efforts to raise the scientific standards of the medical profession. In the year 931-32, the Bagdad healers were forbidden to practice unless they had received a diploma and had been examined for licensure. Sinan, who was in charge of this licensure, examined more than 800 applicants.[5]

RHAZES (865-929)

The classical period of Arabic medicine begins with Abu Bekr Muhammed ibn Zakariya al Razi, known in the Latin West as Rhazes or Albubator—the greatest physician Islam has ever produced. He was first in the Arabic countries to treat medicine in a comprehensive and encyclopedic manner. Although he followed the doctrines of Galen, he adequately demonstrated that he had learned much from Hippocrates.

Like Ali al Tabari, Rhazes was born in Tabaristan. He was a pupil of Ali al Tabari with whom he studied philosophy, physics, mathematics and alchemy. He was also interested in music. Up to his thirties he exhibited no interest in the science of medicine until he had occasion to travel to Bagdad. One day, while visiting the sick house of Bagdad, Rhazes was touched by the misery of the numerous sick and maimed persons he saw there. So impressed was he with this morbid spectacle that, upon leaving the hospital, he determined to devote the rest of his life to the study of the art of medicine so that he might in some measure alleviate the pain and suffering of mankind.

Rhazes remained in Bagdad for five years (902-907). It is not definitely known where he acquired his medical training although it is probable that he went back to Persia and entered the University of Jondisabur which was still the greatest medical center of the East. His great medical prowess soon became known all over the Near East and Caliph al Muktadir of Bagdad sent for him and appointed him chief physician and teacher at the hospital of Bagdad (918).

It was customary in those days for physicians to exchange knowledge by visiting the various medical centers. So, after practicing a number of years in Bagdad, he visited Palestine, Egypt and Spain where he discussed medical subjects with the distinguished physicians of his age.

Rhazes is regarded as an outstanding clinician as well as a brilliant diagnostician and therapeutist. As has been intimated, although he was a great admirer of Galen and accepted many of his theories, in practice he inclined towards Hippocrates. He became known as "the Arabian Hippocrates."

Rhazes was a prolific writer. His numerous works were zealously copied by later writers. He wrote several textbooks for his students on simple remedies and on substitute remedies. His large encyclopedias, the famous "Kitab al Mansuri" (*"Liber Medicinalis ad Almansorem"*) and the 24 volume "Kitab al Hawi Fi'l-Tibb" (*"Continens Medicinae"*), contain numerous original statements pertaining to medical science.

The *"Continens Medicinae"* is an enormous compilation and it includes all medical knowledge of the Mohammedan World at the beginning of the tenth century.[6] Rhazes, beyond doubt, was the greatest Arabian medical authority and some regard him as only second to Hippocrates. As a writer, he excelled Galen both in quantity and quality. He is credited with about 237 works, the greatest number of which are lost. The "Fihrist" credits Rhazes with 113 major works, 28 minor works and 2 poems.

Rhazes, like Hippocrates, based his diagnosis on observation of the course of the disease and he paid serious attention to dietetics and hygienic measures in association with simple drugs. "At the commencement of an illness," he states, "choose measures whereby strength may not be lessened; where thou canst cure by diet, use no drugs and where simple means suffice use no complex ones." Rhazes elsewhere declares: "Truth in medicine is an unattainable goal, and the art as described in books is far beneath the knowledge of the experienced and thoughtful physician."

In practice Rhazes was guided by independent experience, not only in his clinical descriptions, but also in his therapeutics. He relied much upon diagnosis and prognosis in the treatment of disease. His clinical histories exhibit his admirable powers of observation. The following case is typical of his clinical histories:

"Abdu'llah ibn Sawada used to suffer from attacks of mixed fever, sometimes quotidian, sometimes tertian, sometimes quartan, and sometimes recurring once in six days. These attacks, which were preceded by a slight rigour and micturition, were very frequent. I gave as my opinion that either these excesses of fever would turn into quartan, or else there was ulceration of the kidneys. Only a short time elapsed when the patient passed pus in his urine. I thereupon informed him that these feverish attacks would not recur, and so it was."

Rhazes warned physicians not to rely too much on uroscopy in seeking a diagnosis. It may be observed here that attempted diagnosis by uroscopy alone was employed by many "quacks" in Rhazes' day. It is related that as early as 760, a century before Rhazes' birth, Abu Koreish Isa was appointed court physician to the Caliph al Madi because he had diagnosed the sex of an unborn child by means of uroscopy. He predicted the birth of a son to the Caliph's pregnant wife and claimed that he did so by means of uroscopy.

In his *"Continens Medicinae,"* Rhazes presents precise methods for the treatment of various diseases. In this work, he cites a great number of cases from Graeco-Arabic and Indian literature—from Hippocrates down to Hunain—as well as numerous records from his own practice. These cases cover the whole range of medical science. This work also contains a collection of the therapies listed in all the medical texts that he was able to gather. For instance, in the fourth volume of this work,[7] in the chapter on colic, beginning with Hippocrates and Galen, he cites the following authors: Rufus, Philagrius, Alexander of Tralles, Oribasius, Paul of Aegina, the Byzantine Theodoceus, Sergius of Ras al Ayn (d. 536), Aaron the Priest (7th century), Masarjawaihi, ibn Masawaih (Mesue Major), Hunain, Hubaish, Thabit ibn Qurra, Ali al Tabari, Abu Guraig (the Egyptian Copt), Susruta the Hindu, and Qulhuman and many unknown authors.

After giving the opinion of authorities he presents his own practical experience under the heading of "My Opinion."

Rhazes' descriptions of smallpox and measles have become classics. He states that smallpox was known to Galen although the first mention of the disease by name was in the sixth century by Aaron the Priest.[8] Aaron, however, does not clearly differentiate between measles and smallpox. Rhazes ascribes smallpox to "a universal pestilence" arising from miasmatic influence, attacking especially those who have neglected venesection. Rhazes' description of the symptoms of smallpox is one of the best accounts in medical literature. It compares well with the account of the Plague of Athens described by Thucydides after the Peloponnesian War (404 b.c.) and the description of the Plague of Rome as described by the poet, Ovid (43 b.c.-17 a.d.).[9] Rhazes considers measles more dangerous than smallpox with the exception that blindness results more often from smallpox.

His treatise on smallpox and measles is headed as follows: "A specification of those habits of body which are most disposed to the smallpox: and of the seasons in which these habits of body mostly abound." Rhazes thereupon gives the following description which is here reproduced in full:[10]

(1) The bodies most disposed to the smallpox are in general such as are moist, pale, and fleshy; the well-coloured also, and ruddy, as likewise the swarthy when they are loaded with flesh; those who are frequently attacked by acute and continued fevers, bleeding of the nose, inflammation of the eyes, and white and red pustules, and vesicles; those that are very fond of sweet things, especially dates, honey, figs, and grapes, and of all those kinds of sweets in which there is a thick and dense substance, as thick gruel, and honey-cakes, or a great quantity of wine and milk.

(2) Bodies that are lean, bilious, hot, and dry, are more disposed to the measles than to the smallpox; and if they are seized with the smallpox, the pustules are necessarily either few in number, distinct, and favorable, or, on the contrary, very bad, numerous, sterile, and dry with putrefaction and no maturation.

(3) Lastly, those bodies that are lean and dry, and of a cold temperament, are neither disposed to the smallpox, nor to the measles; and if they are seized with the smallpox, the pustules are few, favorable, moderate, mild, without danger, and with a moderate light fever from first to last, because such constitutions extinguish the disease.

(4) I am now to mention the seasons of the year in which the

smallpox is most prevalent; which are, the latter end of the autumn, and the beginning of the spring; and when in the summer there are great and frequent rains with continued south winds, and when the winter is warm, and the winds southerly.

(5) When the summer is excessively hot and dry, and the autumn is also hot and dry, and the rains come on very late, then the measles quickly seize those who are disposed to them; that is, those who are of a hot, lean, and bilious habit of body.

(6) But all these things admit of great differences by reason of the diversity of countries and dwellings, and occult dispositions in the air, which necessarily cause these diseases, and predispose bodies to them; so that they happen in other seasons besides these. And therefore it is necessary to use great diligence in the preservation from them, as soon as you see them begin to prevail among the people; as I shall mention in the sequel.[11]

SYMPTOMS OF THE APPROACHING ERUPTION OF SMALLPOX AND MEASLES

(1) The eruption of the smallpox is preceded by a continued fever, pain in the back, itching in the nose, and terrors in sleep. These are the more peculiar symptoms of its approach, especially a pain in the back, with fever; then also a pricking which the patient feels all over his body; a fullness of the face, which at times goes and comes; an inflamed colour, and vehement redness in both the cheeks; a redness of both the eyes; a heaviness of the whole body; great uneasiness, the symptoms of which are stretching and yawning; a pain in the throat and chest, with a slight difficulty in breathing, and cough; a dryness of the mouth, thick spittle, and hoarseness of the voice; pain and heaviness of the head; inquietude, distress of mind, nausea, and anxiety; (with this difference, that the inquietude, nausea and anxiety are more frequent in the measles than in the smallpox; while, on the other hand, the pain in the back is more peculiar to the smallpox than to the measles) heat of the whole body, an inflamed colour, and shining redness, and especially an intense redness of the gums.

(2) When, therefore, you see these symptoms, or some of the worst of them, (such as the pain of the back, and the terrors in sleep, with the continued fever,) then you may be assured that the eruption of one of these diseases in the patient is nigh at hand; except that there is not in the measles so much pain of the back as in the smallpox, nor in the smallpox so much anxiety and nausea as in the measles, unless the smallpox be of a bad sort; and this shows that the measles come from a very bilious blood.

(3) With respect to the safer kind of the smallpox, in this, it is the quantity of the blood that is hurtful rather than its bad quality; and hence arises the pain of the back, from the distention of the large vein and artery which are situated by the vertebrae of the spine.[12]

Owing to Rhazes' theory that the cause of disease is fermentation of the blood, the remedy for smallpox, measles and for that matter, other diseases, is purification of the blood.

THERAPEUTICS

Rhazes' therapeutic measures are undoubtedly based on clinical experience. He maps out two different basic courses of treatment: One is to counteract the disease by antidotes and refrigerant measures (such as cold water, camphor mixtures, cold sponges, effusions, baths, venesection and purgatives) and the other is to effect a cure by remedies such as external heat and particularly steam, which stimulate the outbreak of the exanthemata. The treatment depends upon the degree of fever, the nature of the exanthemata and the conditions of the pulse, respirations and evacuations. Rhazes gives detailed instructions as to how to avoid complications and sequelae affecting the eyes, ears, nose and throat and he discusses the prevention of suppuration and cicatrization.

ANATOMY AND PHYSIOLOGY

There is little anatomy in Rhazes' "Continens Medicinae" beyond that taught by Galen. This is probably due to the fact that the Koran strictly prohibits dissection. Whatever knowledge Arabian physicians had on the subject of anatomy was learned from earlier writers. Notwithstanding the fact that Rhazes frequently took the liberty to modify or to add to the teaching of his masters, his knowledge of physiology is also very vague. After all, Galen on whom he depended so heavily, had few clear ideas on human physiology.[13]

ETIOLOGY, PATHOLOGY AND SYMPTOMATOLOGY

While Rhazes adhered to the humoral pathology of Hippocrates, he named sub-causes in discussing the etiology of disease. For example, jaundice is caused by obstruction of the bile and irregular fever can be caused by suppuration of the kidneys. The cause of most disease is fermentation of the blood.

He divides fever into symptomatic, essential, and inflammatory types. He disagrees with Hippocrates and Galen with respect to crisis. He believes that sweating per se does not indicate crisis but is merely a sign that nature has brought about a vicarious secretion.

TREATMENT

As stated, Rhazes was particularly learned in pharmacology and therapeutics. The treatment of fever depends upon the etiology of the disease. In inflammatory fever, he recommends the use of cold water applications. In putrid inflammation of the chest he advises the use of wine as a strengthening measure, and in phthisis, he suggests milk and sugar as a remedy. In indigestion, Rhazes recommends buttermilk and cold water. Rhazes prefers oil to mercury in cases of obstruction of the bowels. In melancholia he advises the playing of chess and music as diversionary measures. He lays great stress upon diet and bathing.

His pharmacopoeia is quite extensive. His prescription against colic, for example, is composed of quince seed, fenugreek (faenum graecum), fennel and camomile boiled together with bdellium resin. He states that if this remedy fails, resort should be had to an anodyne such as falunija.

According to Meyerhof, this remedy for colic is still being prepared according to the ancient Greek prescription in the drug bazaars of Cairo.

Rhazes represents in the Eastern part of the Islamic world the culminating point with regard to pharmacology. His successors added very little to his knowledge of drugs.[14]

He was acquainted with many drugs including nux vomica, senna, camphor, cardamum, musk, manna, amber, nutmeg, caryophyllus, sal-ammoniac, arock and various other alcoholic drinks. He used animal and mineral substances as well as vegetable products. He was familiar with decoctions, infusions, oils, powders, pills, syrups, liniments, plasters, suppositories, compresses, fumigations, clysters and collyria. He warns against the extensive use of purgation and he was not partial to emesis.

Venesection is recommended in a number of affections, but the time, the circumstances, the climate, the age, and the constitution of the patient must all be considered when using this therapeutic procedure. In geriatrics and pediatrics, blood letting is only to be performed in the most extenuating circumstances.

SURGERY

In surgery, Rhazes frequently follows Antyllus. In the twenty-third book, of his "Continens Medicinae," he gives a detailed description of the causes, symptoms and treatment of vesical calculi. In the seventh book he describes Antyllus' method of tracheotomy. In cases of intestinal obstruction he advises the application of fomentations over the distended intestines. If a portion of omentum becomes gangrenous, he recommends removal of the gangrenous portion after ligating the blood vessels with a fine thread.

He gives descriptions of spina ventosa, spina bifida, and various forms of hernia, and in treating these conditions, he borrows largely from Hippocrates, Galen, Aetius, and Paul of Aegina. He is against any excision of cancer unless the growth is limited, in which case the entire mass must be removed. He ordered cautery in case of rabid animal bites.

OBSTETRICS

Rhazes states that cephalic presentation is the only normal position for delivery and he recommends podalic version in all other positions regardless of whether the feet are presented or not. If extraction by head or feet is impossible embryotomy is indicated. In the event that a child is excessively large, he recommends exerting traction on it with a fillet (a loop for making traction).

RHAZES' ADVICE TO PHYSICIANS

In his treatise, "Upon the Circumstances which Turn the Head of Most Men from the Reputable Physician," Rhazes throws a stream of light upon the status of the physician as well as the character of the patients of his day. His keen sense of medical ethics as is evidenced by the sound, practical advice which he passes on to his fellow physicians shows how a doctor may retain the respect and confidence of his patients. Rhazes' words on this subject are no less applicable today.

Rhazes lists the factors which influence people to turn away from intelligent and learned physicians and place their trust in imposters. One is that the layman expects the physician to know everything: "If he inspects the urine or feels the pulse he is supposed to know what the patient has eaten and what he has been doing. This is lying and deception and is only brought about by trickery, by artful questions of speech through which the senses of the public are deceived. Many hire men or women to find out all the circumstances of the patient, and to report what is told by neighbors and by servants."

Another circumstance that leads to the contempt of legitimate physicians is that many diseases are but slightly removed from the border-line of health and are thus difficult to recognize and cure, whereas highly serious ones may externally appear trivial. When a layman with a border-line sickness sees that a physician is in doubt concerning his diagnosis or cure, he interprets such doubt as positive evidence that the physician is ignorant of even simple things and therefore will understand still less of more severe illnesses. This is a false analogy for the symptoms of such diseases are actually less obvious because there are only slight deviations from the normal and the cure is more difficult because no drastic remedies are indicated.[15]

Rhazes' advice to the medical profession is so sound that the writer feels it worthy of extensive reproduction. The following is taken from Max Neuburger's admirable "History of Medicine":

"Matters must be entrusted to him who is furthest from error, who errs most seldom . . . he who otherwise refuses to employ a physician would resemble him who would not ride a horse nor sleep in a canopied bed because horses stumble and the canopy might fall down—which are rare events. . . . A physician is sometimes undervalued who takes trouble over an incurable complaint; but the imperfection of the art should be considered, in this respect unlike other arts, of which men know more than is necessary, whilst in medicine men have not yet attained to the indispensable and do not possess a remedy for every ill. The fault is therefore with the art, not with the physician. The public demands that the physician should cure in a moment, like a magician, or that he should at least employ pleasant methods, which is not at all times and in all cases possible; to blame the physician on nature's account is a great injustice. Thus it is that sorcerers make their fortune, even though they behave iniquitously, and their incompetent works bring them a good livelihood, whilst the physician with utmost endeavor can hardly obtain the bare necessities."

Here Rhazes further explains the reasons why patients turn from capable physicians to ignorant healers: "The heart of man is further turned from the capable physician and toward fools because the ignorant and women sometimes succeed in curing complaints where this has not been done by the most famous physicians. The causes are manifold: luck, opportunity, etc. Sometimes the qualified physician effects an improvement which is not, however, yet visible; the patient is then placed under another doctor who rapidly brings about a cure and obtains the entire credit. If drastic measures are employed without knowledge and they are successful, their effects are plainly visible and are considered to be the result of great dexterity. If, however, they are unsuitable, they kill suddenly or lead the patient into danger. The public nevertheless applauds the sudden and visible effects and neglects those who do not adopt such measures; it talks much of the wonderful cures and forgets or conceals the failures."

In the following lines Rhazes writes of quacks who are often successful in treating diseases: "Many a quack is experienced in the treatment of a single complaint, or two or three, according to his practice, or because he has seen the treatment of an intelligent physician. Ignorant people, therefore, think that he has equal dexterity in everything and entrust themselves to him. It is a great mistake to think that, because he has a genuine remedy for one complaint, he has one for all. I have myself learnt remedies from women and herbalists who had no knowledge of medicine."

Rhazes makes note that fear often prevents physicians from employing drastic measures when attending a prominent personality: "The benefits of medicine may also be lessened through the fear that even experienced physicians have for drastic measures, whence they forsake the usual remedies and, if the patient be a king or an eminent, well-known man, suffering from a serious, hidden or doubtful complaint upon which physicians' opinions are divided, then the practitioner abandons strong remedies or even all medicine and employs foods of various kinds in order to avoid the wrath of princes or the hate of mankind."

Rhazes warns patients not to upset the doctor's equanimity when he examines them or administers remedies: "I would therefore remark that it is advisable for an intelligent ruler that he should not make his physician anxious, but should cheer him, be much in his society, and should make it known that he will not be held responsible for the cure of incurable complaints nor held to account for error or misunderstanding."[16]

Rhazes, in the following paragraph, urges the physician to read medical literature: "A thousand physicians, for probably a thousand years, have labored on the improvement of medicine; he who reads their writings with assiduity and reflection discovers in a short life more than if he should actually run after the sick a thousand years." Yet, on the other hand (like Paracelsus), he makes it clear that "reading does not make the physician, but a critical judgment, and the application of known truths to special cases."[17]

Rhazes was the first physician to apply the science of chemistry to the treatment of disease and he thus may be considered the founder of iatrochemistry.

He made investigations on specific gravity by means of the "al-mizan al tabii"—the hydrostatic balance. Various chemical treatises are ascribed to him, and one of these contains a list of 25 pieces of chemical apparatus. He also made an attempt to classify chemical substances.

It is said that Rhazes presented a book on chemistry to Prince Al-Mansur and that the prince was so pleased with this gift that he awarded Rhazes a purse of 1000 *dinars* and asked him to demonstrate one of the chemical experiments. The experiment, however, proved a failure, and this so enraged the Prince that he lashed the unfortunate author on the head with a whip and injured his eyes so that blindness ensued (traumatic cataract?). A surgeon offered to operate upon Rhazes, but when the latter asked him how many tunics the eye possessed, the surgeon admitted that he did not know. Thereupon it is said that Rhazes declared: "Whoever does not know that shall lay no instruments upon my eyes." Later Rhazes again declined operation, remarking that he had seen too much of the world already.

Rhazes died in 932 A.D., in abject poverty, having given away all his wealth to his poor patients.[18]

A complete list of Rhazes' works that is still extant was compiled by his students after he died.[19]

Rhazes was one of the six great physicians of the Islamic

world; the others were Hunain ben Ishak, Alhazan, Ali ibn al Abbas, Avenzoar and Avicenna.

ALI IBN AL ABBAS (died A.D. 994)

Of the greatest importance to the healing art of the Arabian countries was the comprehensive work of Ali ibn al Abbas, who was known in the West as Haly Abbas. Ali ibn al Abbas was a native of Ahwaz, Southwestern Persia, near Jondisabur. He flourished fifty years after Rhazes, who was also a native of Persia. It is not stated where he received his medical education, but it is assumed that he attended the University of Jondisabur which was in close proximity to Ahwaz. He was court physician to the Buwide Aahad ad-Danla.

His opus magnum was his *"Kitab al Maliki"* or "Royal Book," which became known in the Latin West as *"Liber Regius."* This work is a medical encyclopedia dealing with theoretical and practical medicine, the source of which may be traced in large measure to the "Continens Medicinae" of Rhazes. In the literature of the Arabian renaissance he is known as Ali ibn al Abbas Magusi, which signifies that he originated from a Persian family belonging to the faith of Zoroaster. The *"Kitab al Maliki"* was aimed by the author to be midway between the voluminous *"Continens Medicinae"* and the abridged *"Liber Medicinalis Almansorem"* of Rhazes.

"The Royal Book" consists of twenty volumes. The material is well organized and distinguished by a lucid and systematic description of the contemporary knowledge of medicine.

The first ten books cover the theory and the second ten the practice of medicine. The second and third books deal with anatomy and these have been translated into French by P. de Koning.[20] In the first three chapters of the first book, the works of Hippocrates, Galen, Oribasius, Paul of Aegina, Aaron the Priest, Serpion and Rhazes are discussed. The nineteenth book is the largest. It contains 110 chapters and is devoted to surgery. It was translated by Constantine Africanus into Latin and this gentleman neglects mentioning the true author's name.

"The Royal Book" was the standard textbook of Arabian medicine until it was displaced by the "Canon" of Avicenna a century later and it was the first book to be printed in Arabic at Cairo. The Latin editions which are still extant are the Venetian of 1492 and the Lyons of 1523. The former translation is that of Bishop Stephen of Antioch which was completed in 1127 and the latter was annotated by Michael de Capella.

Another work of Ali ibn al Abbas is "*Tractatus de Medicina*" which consists of three books: *Liber Sanitatis* (Sanitation), *Liber Morbi* (Diseases) and *Liber Signarum* (Symptoms). This work may be found in the library of the University of Gottingen.

Ali ibn Abbas advised young physicians to devote more time to practical instruction in hospitals. He emphasized the importance of studying the theory of medicine before engaging in medical practice and he avidly proclaimed that there is no substitute for clinical experience. He frequently formulated advanced opinions, particularly with regard to dietetics and materia medica.[21]

P. Brown states that he was the first to suggest the existence of the blood capillary system, when he stated that there are pores between the pulsating and the non-pulsating vessels (i.e., between the arteries and veins).

ALI BEN ISA (first half of the eleventh century)

Ali ben Isa, known in Latin as Jesu Haly, was the foremost Arabic ophthalmologist. He was the author of the "Tadhkirt" which is called in the Latin translation, "Liber Memorialis Ophthalmocorum." This "Book of Memoranda for Eye Doctors" was used for centuries as an ophthalmological textbook in Islam and in Christian countries. It is used among the Arabs even at the present time. In 1936, an English translation was issued by Casey Wood in Chicago. It is divided into three parts. Book I deals with the anatomy and physiology of the eye and this follows Galen. Book II deals with ocular diseases which can be diagnosed by ordinary examination (such as diseases of the aqueous and vitreous humors, nyctalopia, diseases of the lens, retina and nerves). Book III treats of internal diseases of the eye with descriptions of the remedies.

ISAAC ISRAELI (Isaac Judeus 832?-932)

Abu Ya'Kub Ishak ibn Sulaiman al-Isra'ili, popularly referred to as Isaac Israeli, physician and philosopher, was born in Egypt in the year 832 or shortly before this, and died at Kairawan (Tunisia) in 932.[22] According to Said ben Ahmad ben Said, "He lived over 100 years, never married and never sought wealth. He composed valuable works which cannot be weighed with gold and silver." Israeli studied natural history, medicine, mathematics and astronomy, and as a matter of fact he is reputed to have been a scholar of all the "seven sciences."[23] When he was already a centenarian, Israeli lost favor with his prince. He left about a dozen books. Most of these are on simple drugs and they are repeatedly quoted by al Ghafiki.[24]

Israeli first gained his reputation in Egypt as a skillful oculist. According to Hirsch, he was one of the most renowned ophthalmologists of his time and his observations on ophthalmology and particularly on trachoma are particularly valuable.[25]

After Israeli went to Kairawan, he became interested in general medicine and he studied under Ishaq ibn Amran al Baghdadi, with whom he is sometimes confused. At Kairawan his fame became widely disseminated and the works which he wrote in Arabic were considered by the Mohammedan physicians as "more valuable than gems." His lectures attracted a large number of pupils, of whom the two most prominent were Abu Yafar ibn al Yazzar, a Mohammedan, and Dunash ibn Tumin.[26]

Roger Bacon in 1268 listed Israeli with Hippocrates, Galen, Rhazes and Ali ibn al Abbas, as one of the best medical authorities of all times.[27] Campbell states that he enjoyed great fame in North Africa and exercised no little influence upon the medicine of the Middle Ages.[28]

In the year 904, or thereabouts, Israeli was nominated court physician to the last Aghlabite Prince, Ziyadet Allah. Five years later, when the Fatimid Caliph Ubaid Allah al Mahdi became master of North Africa with Kairawan as his capital, Israeli entered his service. The Caliph particularly enjoyed the company of his Jewish physician because of the latter's wit and because of the many times he outfoxed the clever Greek, al Hubaish, when they matched wits.

Israeli was a raconteur of note and he tells of his first meeting with the Caliph and his encounter with al Hubaish.

"I met the Caliph and his hosts at Arish (Larasa). I greeted him humbly in a manner befitting royalty and he invited me to see him. In the meantime he sent me 500 *dinars*.

"I found in his palace little of a serious atmosphere; he appears to have been in a jocular and laughing mood. I found him conversing with a Greek named al Hubaish, who drew me into conversation the moment he saw me. He asked me, 'Is there in salty sweet?' I assented. 'If so,' he continued, 'Sweet things are salty and salty things are sweet?' I replied, 'The sweet is sweet with pleasantness, but the salty is astringent.' I soon noticed that he tried to continue the conversation in order to embarrass me. Then I spoke to him and said, 'You certainly believe that you are a living being?' He answered, 'yes,' and I continued, 'Is a dog a living being?' He answered, 'yes,' and I concluded, 'If so, you are a dog and the dog is you.' The Prince, Ziyadat Allah, broke out with a hearty and loud laugh. I noticed that he was more pleased with the joke than with the substance of the conversation."

Israeli never married, and when one told him that it might have been wiser for him to have had children, he replied, "If I only leave my book on fever it is not necessary that I shall be remembered through descendants." He also is reported to have remarked, "I have four books through which I will be better and longer remembered than through descendants."[29]

At the request of the Fatimid Caliph Ubaid Allah al Mahdi (reigned 909-930), Israeli composed several medical works in Arabic which were translated into Latin by Gerard of Cremona (1114-1167) and later by the monk, Constantine Africanus (1087), who claimed their authorship for himself. It was only after more than four centuries (Leyden, 1515) that an editor of these works discovered the plagiarism and reissued them under the title *"Opera Omnia Isaci Judaei."* Israeli's works were also translated into Hebrew and Spanish by Jewish scribes.

Israeli was a contemporary of Rhazes and he has been classed by many historians as only second to him in medical knowledge. He wrote eight medical works, the best of which is said to be the book on fever. The Hebrew editions of his medical works were zealously studied by Jewish physicians. He wrote a collection of medical principles, proverbs and aphorisms, which is worthy of special mention. In this treatise entitled, "Guide to Physicians," he illuminates contemporary medical conditions and many of his views even now must command respect: "The chief task of the physician is to prevent disease. The majority of diseases are cured by nature. If thou hast the choice to effect cure by nourishment or by drugs, choose the former. Never employ more than one drug at a time.

"He whose business it is to bore pearls, must do this work carefully in order not to mar their beauty by haste. Even so, he who undertakes the cure of human bodies—the noblest creations on earth—should thoroughly consider the diseases with which he comes in contact and give his directions after careful reflection, so that he fall into no irremediable error.

"Comfort and soothe the patient, even if thou art in doubt, for by that means doest thou support nature.—If the patient does not follow thy directions, or if his servants and household do not carry out thy orders with dispatch or treat thee with disrespect, give up the case.

"Let not thy mouth condemn if an accusation is made against a physician, for to every man comes his hour.[30]

"Visit not the patient too often, nor remain too long with him, unless the treatment demand it, for it is only the fresh encounter which giveth pleasure.

"It is in keeping with the character of the physician that he should, in his mode of life, be content with well-prepared food in moderation and be no rioter or glutton. Also it is a shame that he (i.e. the physician) should suffer from a long drawn out disease, else the vulgar will say: 'If he cannot cure himself, how can he cure others?'

"Let thy deeds be thy praise, rather than find honour in another's shame.

"Demand thy fee of the patient when his illness is increasing or at its height; when he is healed he forgets what thou hast done for him. The more thou demandest for thy treatment, the more highly thou esteemest thy cure, the higher wilt thou stand in the eyes of the people. Thy art will be held of no account only by those whom thou treatest gratuitously."

Israeli's important work on fever is entitled, *"Kitab al-Hummayet"* (in Hebrew, *"Sefer ha-Kadahat"*), and this is a complete treatise, in five books, on the various kinds of fever.

"Kitab al-Adwiyah al-Mufradah wa'l-Aghdhiyah," is a work, in four sections, on ailments and their remedies. The first section, consisting of twenty chapters, was translated into Latin by Constantine Africanus under the title *"Diaetae Universales,"* and into Hebrew by an anonymous translator under the title *"Tib's ha-Mezonot."* The other three parts of the work are entitled in the Latin translation *"Diaetarae Particulares."* It appears that a Hebrew translation, entitled *"Sefer ha-Mis'adim"* or *"Sefer ha-Maakalim,"* was made from the Latin version.

"Kitab al-Baul" (in Hebrew, *"Sefer ha-Shetan"*) is a treatise on urine, of which the author himself later made an abridgment. Israeli also wrote the aforementioned "Guide to Physicians" of which the Arabic version is lost, but the Hebrew version is extant under the title of *"Manhag* (or *Musar) haRofeim."*

Israeli was the earliest Jewish philosopher (or one of the earliest) to publish a classification of the sciences. This classification was essentially the Aristotelian one as transmitted and modified by the Moslems.[31] He also wrote a monograph on medical and philosophical definitions.

"Kitab al Istiqsat" (in Hebrew, *"Sefer ha-Yesodot"*) is a medical and philosophical treatise on the elements, which the author

treats according to the ideas of Aristotle, Hippocrates and Galen. The Hebrew translation was made by Abraham ben Hasdai at the request of the grammarian, David Kimhi.

ABU SAHAL DUNASH BEN TAMIM (900-960)

Israeli's pupil, Abu Sahal Dunash ben Tamim, was born in Fez. He was physician to the third Fatimid Caliph, Ishmael Almansur ibn al Kaim, to whom he dedicated his work on astronomy. Ben Tamim, when a youth, studied medicine, languages and metaphysics under Isaac Israeli in Kairawan. He became accomplished in the whole range of sciences. He wrote books on medicine, astronomy and mathematics. In his opinion, mathematics, astronomy and music rank lowest among the sciences, physics and medicine came next, and metaphysics—the knowledge of God and the soul—ranks highest. In order that they might include Ben Tamim among their number, various Arab historians have claimed that he became a convert to Islam. The evidence indicates, however, that he remained faithful to Judaism to the end of his life. Ben Tamim kept up a correspondence with Chasdai ben Isaac ibn Shaprut, the Jewish statesman of Cordova, for whom he composed an astronomical work on the nature of spheres and various astronomical calculations on the courses of the stars.

AVICENNA (981-1037)

The most famous of Arabic physicians and philosophers, whose influence extended throughout the Islamic world and Europe and whose writings formed the principal reading of Christian scholastics, was Abu Ali Husain ibn Abdullah ibn Sina, commonly known as Avicenna ("Prince of Physicians"). He was born at Afsena in the district of Bokhara, then one of the chief cities of the Moslem world, and famous for culture. His father was a Persian tax collector in the neighboring town of Harmaitin. The family moved to Bokhara where Avicenna was placed under the charge of a tutor. As a boy of ten, it is said that he knew the Koran and much of the Arabic poetry by heart. Avicenna learned his arithmetic from a grocer and the higher branches of learning he derived from one of those wandering scholars who gained a livelihood by doctoring the sick and by giving lessons to the young.

According to his own account, Avicenna, by the time he was sixteen, not merely knew medical theory, but by gratuitous attendance of the sick, had discovered new methods of treatment. By the end of his seventeenth year, his period of medical apprenticeship had been concluded. He constantly studied higher philosophical problems. It is said that he read through the "Metaphysics" of Aristotle forty times, until the words were imprinted for all time in his memory.

Avicenna's first major medical appointment was as physician to the Emir, whom he cured of a dangerous illness in 997. His chief reward for this was that he was granted access to the Royal Library of the Samanids. When this library was destroyed by fire, Avicenna's enemies accused him of burning it in order to conceal the sources of his knowledge.

At the age of 22, Avicenna lost his father, and he wandered from place to place through the districts of Nishapur looking for a suitable place to practice his profession. He finally came to Jorjan, near the Caspian, where he met an old friend, through whose influence Avicenna got a position as lecturer on logic and astronomy. Several of his treatises were written in Jorjan and there he commenced writing his "Canon of Medicine."

He subsequently settled at Rai, in the vicinity of modern Teheran, where about thirty of his shorter works are said to have been composed. For some reason, the constant feuds which raged between the regent and her second son, Shams Addulah, compelled him to quit the place. He then went to Hamadan, where he established himself in the practice of medicine. There, the Emir, hearing of his arrival, called him in as medical attendant, and conferred upon him the rank of vizier.

During his sojourn in Hamadan, Avicenna pursued his studies

and his teaching. Every evening extracts from his great works, the "Canon" and the "Sanatio," were dictated and explained to his pupils. When the portions for the evening were completed, he spent much of the night with his pupils in festive enjoyment, with a band of singers and players, supplying the entertainment. However, with the death of the Emir, his influence faded and he was dismissed from his position. He left Hamadan very much disappointed that he could not carry on his work. Later he defied the new Emir and returned to this city and secretly pursued his literary labors. The fact of his return, however, soon became known and, to escape his apprehension by the authorities, his brother and a favorite pupil dressed him as a Sifi ascetic slave and took him out of town.

After a perilous journey, this group reached Isfahan, where he received an honorable welcome from the Prince of Isfahan. Soon the war that had raged continually between this country and Hamadan turned in favor of Isfahan. Hamadan was captured and Avicenna returned to Hamadan.

The remaining ten or twelve years of Avicenna's life were spent in the service of Abu Yafar ali Abdaulah, whom he accompanied as physician and general literary and scientific advisor. During these last years he began to study contemporaries and those closer to his period.

The chief quality of Avicenna was his ability to bring together the doctrines and theories of those who had preceded him and integrate and present them in a new form of his own. He may have lacked originality, but he had the faculty of impressing his opinions firmly on his listeners and readers.

Avicenna was a great pleasure lover and throughout his restless career, he never forgot his love of enjoyment. Unusual mental and physical vigor enabled him to combine devotion to work with indulgence in sensual pleasures. His passions for wine and women were almost as well known as his learning. Versatile, lighthearted, boastful and pleasure-loving, his personality contrasts with the nobler and more intellectual characters of Rhazes and Averroes.

Avicenna worked and played day and night, and he left his

own prescription for mental confusion and fatigue. In his autobiography, he says: "When I found a difficulty, I referred to my notes and prayed to the Creator. At night, when weak or sleepy, I strengthened myself with a glass of wine."[32]

His bouts of pleasure gradually weakened his constitution and an attack of "colic" seized him while he was in Hamadan which necessitated such drastic remedies that he could scarcely endure them. On another occasion the same condition recurred while he was on a pleasure trip and he reached Hamadan only with great difficulty. At home the condition continued to become worse and he refused to keep up the regimen imposed. Rather than stop his pleasure parties, he resigned himself to his fate. On his deathbed it is said that he was gripped by remorse. He bestowed his personal belongings on the poor, restored unjust gains, freed his slaves, and every third day until his death he listened to the reading of the Koran. He died in June, 1037, in his fifty-seventh year, and was buried in Hamadan.

Up to the Renaissance, the materia medica of Avicenna was considered classic. From the twelfth to the seventeenth centuries, his "Canon" was accepted in European universities as the most authoritative medical work, superseding the treatises of Rhazes, Ali Abbas and Avenzoar, although all of these authors used the same sources. Garrison asserts that the reason for this lies in the method and the train of reasoning of Avicenna, which appealed more to the physician of the Middle Ages than did the systems of his predecessors.[33] Campbell explains Avicenna's popularity as follows: "Those who could see the most small subtlety in a passage from the ancient writers were often more esteemed than the most learned so that passages that were obscure or unintelligible were considered sublime."[34] Some of Avicenna's contemporaries and those closer to his period as is so often the case, were disdainful of him. Avenzoar, for example, stated in no uncertain terms that the "Canon" was "useful only as waste paper." Arnold of Villanova (A.D. 1225-1312) stigmatizes Avicenna as "a professional scribbler" and declares his "Canon" is so full of misinterpretations of Galen as to nullify its value. Others, however, regard the "Canon" as a treasure of wisdom.

Avicenna was prompted to write the "Canon" because of the prevalent medieval idea that all medical knowledge reached its final culmination with the last Greek authority on the subject and that nothing could be added to what was already written down by the masters except perhaps some minor comment on indistinct ancient phraseology. According to this concept, knowledge of medicine, like knowledge of the Bible and the Koran, was fixed for all times. Avicenna therefore set out to codify all ancient authorities in one huge work, to save the physician the trouble of seeking out numerous different volumes, many of which were unavailable.

THE MEDICINE OF THE CANON

The "Canon" consists of five books: The first and second cover physiology and hygiene; the third and fourth deal with the methods of treating disease; and the fifth concerns itself with materia medica and the preparation of remedies. The last section also contains some personal observations.

Each book is again subdivided into tractates, chapters, and paragraphs. The first tractate (or fen) of the first book gives a definition of medicine, tells how it developed, and discusses the methods it employs as well as other fundamental doctrines. The material is mainly borrowed from the Hippocratic writings. The second tractate deals with pathology and the symptoms of disease and concerns itself particularly with the significance of the pulse and urine in the diagnosis of disease. The first chapter of the third tractate describes hygiene and prophylactic regulations. The last tractate deals mostly with drugs and non-medicinal therapeutics such as the use of the enema, venesection and cautery, and also covers various surgical diseases including fractures and dislocations.

ANATOMY AND PHYSIOLOGY

On the subject of anatomy and physiology, Avicenna was entirely influenced by Galen. He had no opportunity to dissect human bodies for this practice, as has been stated, was strictly prohibited by the Koran. His knowledge of physiology was based on the incorrect premises and faulty theories of Galen and others.

ETIOLOGY OF DISEASE

Avicenna follows ancient writers in discussing the causation of disease. The humoral theory is of first importance. He then mentions a number of secondary causes including climatic conditions, over-indulgence, surgical causes and contagion by drinking water. He views phthisis, smallpox, measles, and other epidemic diseases as contagious diseases.

DIAGNOSIS OF DISEASE

Avicenna decribes nineteen varieties of pain upon which he bases his diagnosis. He enlarges upon the value of the pulse and urine as diagnostic measures.

The symptoms of mania are delirium, violence, insomnia and unrest. "In some cases mania is aggressive, but in others it is cringing and submissive." Unconsumed bile and black bile will cause melancholia, the symptoms of which are fancies of sickness, fear, dread, inclination towards solitude, palpitation of the heart, despair, oppression and hypochondriasis. Psychic alterations depend upon qualitative and quantitative pathological changes in the humoral mixtures in the brain. In this concept, Avicenna has reference to the humoral theory of Hippocrates and Galen. Intellectual disturbances are caused by an abundance of black bile and result in anxiety and sadness. Abundance of yellow bile leads to irritability, confusion and violence. An increase of putrified phlegm causes a morose and serious mood.

Disturbances of perceptive power follow disease in the front of the brain. Abnormalities of the middle ventricles are responsible for weak-mindedness and imbecility. Failure of memory results when the posterior ventricle of the brain is affected.

Phrenitis is a mental derangement arising from acute febrile diseases and is characterized by forgetfulness of the immediate past, confusion and restlessness. It is caused by an accumulation of yellow bile in the meninges or brain.

Coma vigil, a stupor with delirium, wakefulness and semiconsciousness, is caused by an accumulation of phlegm and bile, with bile predominating. Lethargy is occasioned by intracranial phlegm and is manifested by a loss of memory with great exhaustion and profuse perspiration.

PATHOLOGY

In the section on pathology, Avicenna describes empyema, pleurisy, intestinal pathologies, venereal disease, diseases of the male genital organs, skin infections and diseases due to intestinal parasites. He describes the guinea worm (Dracunculus medinensis). In simple pleurisy, he states, the fever is continuous and there is a sharp pain beneath the ribs which is most marked upon deep inspiration; the breathing is difficult and the pulse is rapid; the patient is troubled by a painful cough which is first dry and then followed by sputum.

He gives an especially detailed description of nervous and mental diseases. He divides mental affections into elementary disturbances (of imagination and memory) and real psychoses which include melancholia, mania, and feeble-mindedness. Nightmare is a prodrome of apoplexy and mania.

In addition to discussing the symptoms and etiology of melancholia, the treatment of this condition is covered and this includes cheering the patient up by reading to him and entertaining him with music.

OBSTETRICS

To assist deliveries in cases of difficult labor, Avicenna mentions the administration of various drugs, vapors and baths, the use of pressure on the abdomen, and the employing of a knee-elbow position. The treatment varies with the nature of the case and its purpose is to bring the fetal head over the mouth of the womb. Avicenna states that the only normal presentation is cephalic and that pedal presentation is next common. He employs nooses to assist delivery when the child is very large. Before embryotomy is attempted, he recommends that a type of forceps be employed, but this method unfortunately is not described and it is not stated whether he recommends it to deliver living or dead children.

SURGERY

Avicenna describes the operation of intubation of the larynx, the technique of tracheotomy and the operation for empyema (with a knife or cautery). The operation for ascites is to be undertaken only in severe cases. He outlines a treatment for hernia which employs astringents and cautery and he covers an operation for lithotomy. He includes methods for arresting hemorrhage by ligature, tampon and caustics.

In the fifth tractate, Avicenna deals with fractures and dislocations. He describes a method for reducing the head of the femur when there is a dislocated thigh. He is said to have known and practiced the method of treating spinal deformities by forcible reduction which was reintroduced by Calot in 1896.[35]

Venesection has two purposes: the removal of superfluous matter and the elimination of morbid substances from the blood. He gives directions as to the choice of veins suitable for the practice of venesection: The cephalic veins are to be employed in affections of the upper half of the body and the saphenous veins in those of the lower half of the body.

Avicenna describes the manner of opening the vein, the amount of blood to be withdrawn, the position of the patient while the operation is being performed, and the indications and contraindications. He recommends venesection on the sound side of the body if the result is desired only after a lapse of time and its effect is to endure for a protracted period.

Avicenna lays down a seven point rule with reference to the administration of medicine:

(1) The remedy should be used in its natural state.
(2) The disease for which it is employed should be an uncomplicated one.
(3) The proof of the remedy's effectiveness should be made in two cases.
(4) The strength of the remedy should be inversely proportional to the severity of the complaint.
(5) The time of the commencement of the drug's action should be noted.
(6) Careful examination should be made to ascertain whether the remedy always or generally has the same effect.
(7) When drugs are employed on the human body, the patient's color and senses including taste and smell afford clues as to the therapeutic effects of the drugs.

Avicenna is said to have been the first to describe the preparation and properties of sulphuric acid and alcohol.

Avicenna wrote on all the sciences then known. In spite of those who belittle him, his "Canon" represents one of the highest achievements of Arabic culture. It became the medical textbook of choice in the European Universities and, until the year 1650, it was used in the schools of Louvain and Montpellier. Until very recent years, it was employed as the medical authority par excellence in Mohammedan countries.

About 100 treatises are credited to Avicenna. These range from tracts of a few pages to works taking up several volumes. Of course his great European reputation rests on the "Canon." A Latin edition of this work appeared in Rome in 1593, and a Hebrew version by Nathan Amathi (a scholar of Greek and Arabic) was published in Naples in 1491. There have been about thirty Latin editions based on the original translation by Gerard of Cremona. Other important medical works by Avicenna which have been translated into Latin are *"Medicamenta Cordialia"* and *"Canticum de Medicina."*[36]

The chief quality of Avicenna was his ability to bring together and synthesize the doctrines and theories of those who had preceded him and expound them in a new form as his own.

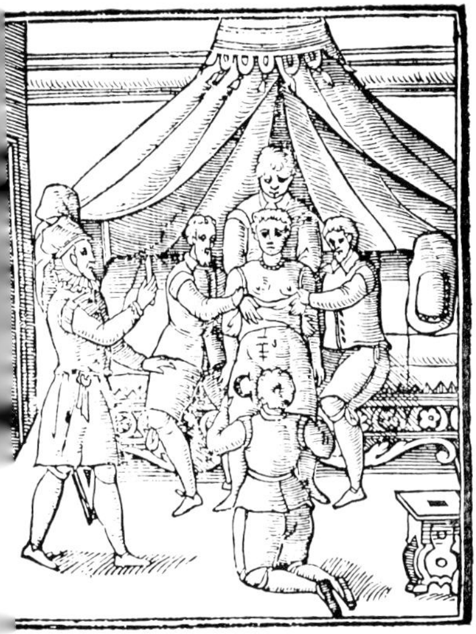

PLATE 45. Illustration of Caesarean section from Murcurio.

(Miller Library, Richmond Ac. Med.)

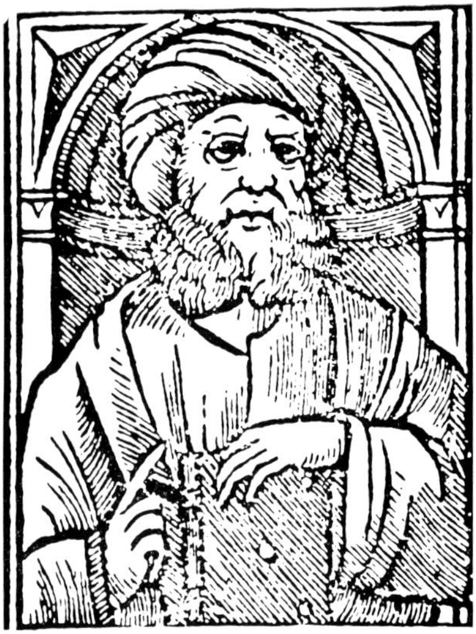

PLATE 46. Rhazes (c. 860-932)

(Courtesy New York Academy of Medicine)

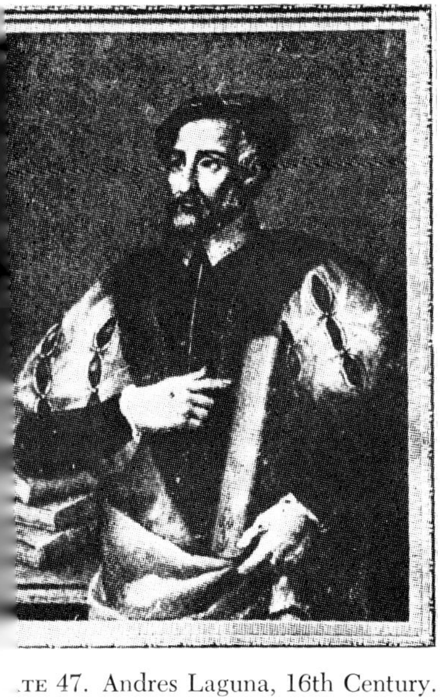

PLATE 47. Andres Laguna, 16th Century.

(Armed Forces Medical Library, Washington, D.C.)

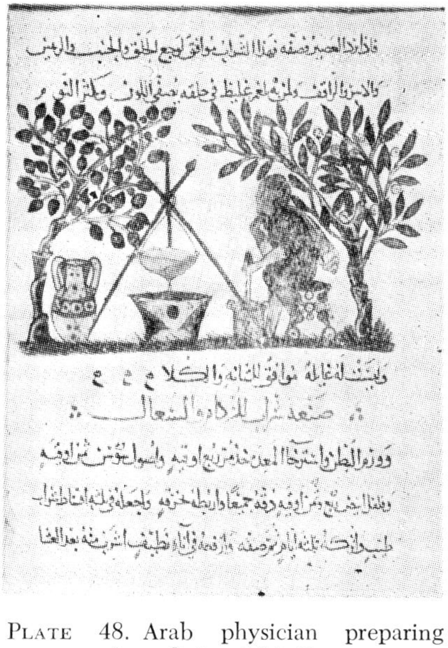

PLATE 48. Arab physician preparing cough medicine, 13th Century.

(Courtesy Metropolitan Museum of Art)

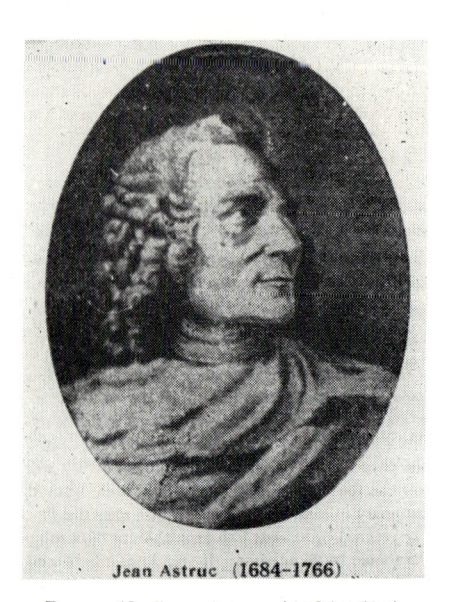

PLATE 49. Jean Astruc (1684-1766)
(Armed Forces Medical Library, Washington, D.C.)

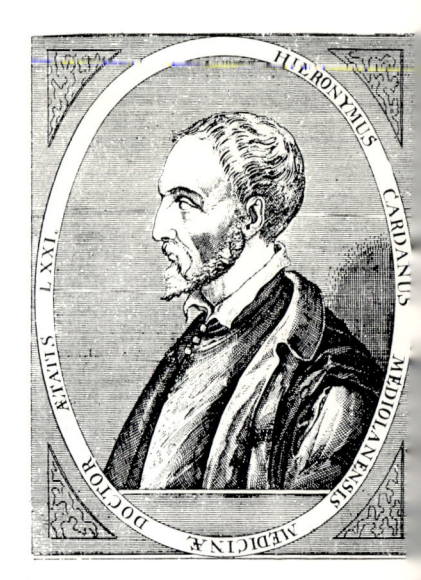

PLATE 50. Jerome Cardan (1501-1576) The great astrologer, physician a[nd] mathematician.

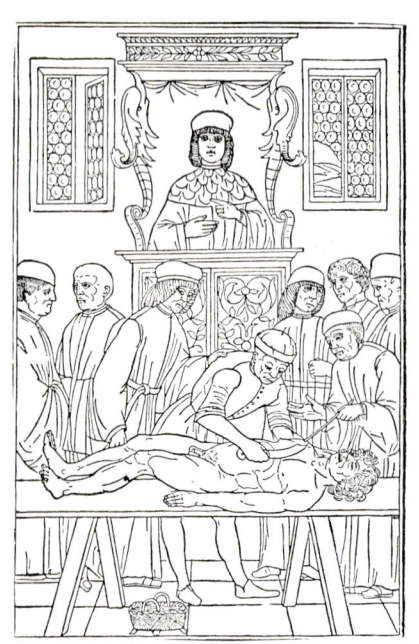

PLATE 51. From Ketcham's Edition of *Mundinus* published in 1494.
(Collection New York Academy of Medicine)

PLATE 52. Silhouette of Jesse Ben[nett] who performed the first Caesarean sect[ion] in the United States.
(Courtesy Richmond Academy of Medic[ine])

Although lacking in originality, he had the happy faculty of getting his material across effectively.

IBN AL HAITAM (Alhazen, 965-1039)

Perhaps the greatest scholar in Islam and one of the greatest students of optics of all times was Ibn al Haitam, known in the Latin West as Alhazen. He was a physicist, mathematician, physician and commentator on Aristotle and Galen. Alhazen was born in Basra in 965 and he flourished in Egypt until his death in 1039. The details of his life are obscure. He appears to have been one of those savants who was all but entirely absorbed in his scientific work. His work represents a great advance in the use of experimental methods. He vastly improved upon the current knowledge of the eye and the process of vision and he solved problems in optics mathematically. In Europe he is best known for his optical studies which have been translated into Latin.

He was the first to correct the Greek misconception of the nature of vision, by showing that the rays of light come from external objects to the eye, and do not issue forth from the eye and impinge on external things, as, up to his time, had been supposed. He determined that the retina is the seat of vision, and that impressions made by light upon it are conveyed along the optic nerve to the brain. He explains that we see single when we use both eyes, because of the formation of the visual images on symmetrical portions of the two retinas. It is impossible to conceive that Alhazen could have come to these conclusions unless he had engaged in the forbidden practice of dissection.

Alhazen shows that our sense of sight is by no means a trustworthy guide, and that there are illusions arising from the course which the rays of light may take when they suffer refraction or reflection. It is in the discussion of these physical problems that his scientific greatness becomes truly manifest. He is perfectly aware that the atmosphere decreases in density with increase of height. From this consideration he shows that a ray of light, entering the atmosphere obliquely, follows a curvilinear path which is concave toward the earth. Therefore, since the mind refers the position of an object to the direction in which the ray of light from it enters the eye, the result must be an illusion. Thus the stars and other heavenly bodies appear to us, to use the Arabic term, nearer to the *Zenith* than they actually are, and not in their true place. We see them in the direction of the tangent to the curve of refraction as it reaches the eye. Hence also, Alhazen shows that we actually see the stars, the sun, and the moon before they have risen and after they have set—truly a wonderful illusion. Alhazen demonstrates that in its passage through the air the curvature of a ray increases with the increasing density, and that its path does not depend on vapors that chance to be present, but on the variation of density in the medium. Alhazen used spherical mirrors and studied spherical aberration and the magnifying power of lenses.

Alhazen conceived the idea of applying mathematical and optical principles to explain animal function more than seven hundred years before Borelli (1608-1709) rediscovered this concept to explain the mechanism of the eye.

In his "Kitab al Manazar," Alhazen upheld those who said that man, in his progress through the ages, passed through a definite succession of states—a premonition of evolution. The Latin translation of his works on optics by Vitelo (1270) exerted a great influence on the development of modern science by Roger Bacon and Kepler.[37]

MASAWAIH AL-MARINDI (Mesue Junior, b. 1015)

Mesue Junior is in no way related to the distinguished physician bearing the name Mesue Senior who was previously discussed. It is highly probable that a Latin-writing author masqueraded under the name of Mesue with the idea of capitalizing on Mesue Senior's reputation, thus obtaining more readers for his works. The little that we do know of Mesue Junior comes from the unreliable pen of Leo Africanus who states that he was born in 1015 in the little town of Marindi on the Euphrates, that he was a Jacobite Christian and that he was educated in philosophy and medicine in Bagdad. His works are extant only in Latin and they are said to have been translated into that language from the Arabic by a Sicilian Jew. According to Steinschneider,[38] Mesue Junior's chief work is *"Canones Generales Simplicia Antidotarium Grabadin Medicinarum Particularium."* There are two Hebrew manuscripts of this work. Mesue's works were printed almost as frequently as Avicenna's. They were the subject of commentaries as late as the sixteenth century. Neuberger believes that his works were definitely originally written in Arabic.[39]

The aforementioned work on materia medica bearing the name of Mesue Junior was most popular in the Middle Ages, and was among the first medical works to be printed (Venice, 1471). The popularity of this work, says Campbell, and the idea that it was of Arabian origin, would indicate the position that Arabian medicine held in the minds of the Christians of Europe in the Middle Ages. It indicated the influence and position of Arabic teaching in Europe at this time, and suggests that in order to attract attention it was necessary to make believe that the work was of Arab origin, and that works of Latin origin were not considered worthy of the close attention of the scholastics of Europe.

ABDUL LATIF (1162-1231)

Among the most distinguished of the later Arabian physicians of the East was Abu Muhammad Abdul Latif ibn Jusuf, physician and historian. He was born in Bagdad, about the year 1162. In his youth he studied grammar, rhetoric, history, philosophy and philology and later alchemy, medicine, poetry and Mohammedan law. About the year 1189, when he was twenty-eight years of age, he commenced his travels. He visited Damascus where he taught medicine and philosophy and came out victorious in a debate with philosophers of high reputation. He then proceeded to Jerusalem, and afterwards to Egypt, where he formed a friendship with Maimonides (whose great scholarship obtained for him the title of "Eagle of Doctors"). While there, he delivered public lectures in the sciences and philosophy. Returning to Damascus, he gave lectures on a wide range of subjects, which were well attended. He then spent several years traveling in various countries, practicing medicine at a number of courts. In the year 1231, he died at Bagdad, the place of his nativity, which he had revisited for the purpose of presenting his works to the Caliph.

Withington relates an interesting anecdote: "When the physician Abdul Latif was in Egypt, the conversation turned one day upon the superiority of observation to mere reading; and someone remarked that there was a great heap of skeletons and dead bodies at Maks. So Abdul Latif went there, and found a hill consisting rather of corpses than of earth, and with more than 20,000 skeletons exposed on the surface. The delighted physician proceeded to examine these, and at once noticed that the lower jaw consists of one bone, and not of two as described by Galen. He tells us that he examined 200 lower jaws in every possible way and got others to examine them also, both in his presence and absence, and they all came to the same conclusion. Similarly he observes that the sacrum is composed of a single bone, and he expresses his intention, if Providence permits, of writing a book of revised anatomy comparing Galen with nature."[40]

Of the 150 works which he is said to have written on medicine and other subjects, his "Compendium Memorabilium Aegypt" is the only one extant which has survived the destructive hand of time. One Dr. Pococki brought the manuscript of this work to England and it was edited and published in Arabic along with a Latin translation by Joseph White in the year 1800 by the Clarendon Press. In 1810, a French translation was published in Paris.[41]

CHAPTER IX

ARABIAN CONTRIBUTIONS TO CHEMISTRY AND PHARMACOLOGY

"Islam has led the vanguard of progress and the Moslem has taught the world," said Emir Ali. This was not a vain boast on the part of an Arabian ruler. In large measure it is a fact.

The evolutionary process of the Arabian intellectual development did not stop with philosophy and medicine; its progress extended also into other fields. Thanks to the works of Yahya al Nahwe (John the grammarian, 7th century) and other linguistic writers[1] the Arabic language became a literary language. Arabia was the bridge by which universal knowledge passed from Persia and India to Europe and back from Alexandria to Persia and India. What Greece was to antiquity, Arabia was to the Middle Ages.

Syria, under the liberal rule of the Seleucides, became intensely Hellenized, and even during Roman days, it was considered a highly civilized province. In the larger towns, such as Antioch, Berytos and Palmyro[2] great institutions of learning existed. Students came from great distances—even outside the boundaries of Syria—to attend these schools and this had a great influence on the medical and educational centers of Haurran, Nesibit, and Edessa in the East. Nesibit[3] was for many centuries a great educational center. There was a talmudic academy in this city under the direction of Rabbi Judah ben Bathrai. Edessa received a strong impulse as a center of learning when the Nestorians were driven out from the Byzantine cities and sought refuge there. The refugees established schools in Edessa where grammar, rhetoric, arithmetic, geometry, music, astronomy and medicine were taught. The Nestorians, as has been previously shown, from the very beginning devoted themselves to the study of science.

Arabian progress, then, far from being limited to the sciences and philosophy, acquired a wider range as the Arabians came into contact with the system of knowledge of other peoples who were intellectually superior to them.

ALCHEMY

The chief claims of the Saracens to an important place in medical history is based on their progress in chemistry which they developed from the pseudo-science of Alchemy.

About 100 A.D. alchemy was practiced in Alexandria. It then spread to the Greek speaking world. The Nestorians and the Monophysites exiled from Byzantium were acquainted with the alchemical doctrine and carried this to Edessa in the North of Syria and through Syria to Persia (450-700 A.D.), whence, after the rise of Islam it was taken over by the Arabic speaking people.

Zosimos of Constantinople writing about 300 A.D., when Egyptian science and mythology were no longer a living tradition, tells us "that I have examined in detail furnaces in the ancient temple of Memphis . . ." and the context implies that these were the equal of those employed by the alchemists. Zosimos mentions the temple of Serapis of Alexandria which was destroyed in 390 A.D. Zosimos regards Democritus and Mary the Jewess as ancient authors. Democritus is often given credit for many alchemical writings around 250 B.C.

Papyri discovered about a century ago referred to as the papyri of Leyden and Stockholm indicate that they were written toward the end of the third century A.D., and contained about a hundred recipes for the preparation of gold, silver, asemos (a silver-like metal), precious stones and dyestuffs. The author of these papyri tried to make gold as follows: asemos, stater 1; copper of Cyprus, stater 3; gold, stater 4; melt them together.

The author of this papyrus gives the recipe to increase the weight of gold by mixing it with a fourth of cadmia (an impure mixture of oxide of base metals, copper, zinc, arsenic, etc.). The papyrus contains a great number of recipes for gold making.

It seems likely that the larger body of this writing was assembled by natural philosophers who went under the name of Ikwan al-safa, "Brethren of Purity" or "Faithful Friends" a sect that strongly believed in the power of science to purify the soul and they ascribed their works to this legendary Jabir. This society, while its theories and practices departed from the truth, for it included in science much that we would call magic, performed its tasks with sincerity and discovered some useful things without realizing their value.

The Arabian alchemists obtained their initial knowledge from two sources: the works of the Persian School and the writings of the Greeks of Alexandria. Syriac intermediaries and direct translations were employed to effect this. The Arabic-speaking peoples studied alchemy for 700 years; the chief centers of their labors appear to have been first in Iraq and later on in Spain. In the hands of these men, whose native tongue was Arabic, alchemy developed into chemistry, and from them, chiefly through the Spanish Moors, the European chemistry of the later Middle Ages was derived. While some Arabic writers and their European followers thus passed from alchemy to chemistry, others, not understanding the technical knowledge and the scientific view of the Alexandrian alchemists, degraded their work into a sordid search for gold, or a background for deceitful magic based on self-delusion or on outright chicanery.

The most famous Arabian alchemist was Abu-Musa-Jabir-ibn-Haiyan (Jabir or Geber) who flourished about 776 A.D. and is thought to have been the author of many writings which later appeared in Latin. This alchemist, who is said to have been one of the alumni of Harran, may be considered the father of modern chemistry.[4]

Jabir or Geber was undoubtedly acquainted with the Greek alchemy, perhaps in the Syrian translation. He divided alchemy into (1) spirits, volatile bodies, such as camphor, salammoniacs, mercury, arsenic and sulphur; (2) metallic bodies, the metals; (3) bodies non-volatile or pulverized solids, substances other than spirits or metallic bodies.

Jabir's theory of classification of metal is derived from Aristotle's views. The Greek alchemists spoke of several varieties of sulphur. It was a wide term for a fusible volatile combustible substance. However, sulphur in the modern sense was well known. The notion that metals are composed of mercury and sulphur was a part of alchemy and chemistry far into the eighteenth century.

Although Jabir held that metals were to be made from mercury and sulphur, he also supposed them to be composed of the four elements, earth, water, fire and air and to possess the qualities of these elements, dryness and cold, moisture and heat in varying degrees.

Galen attributed many diseases to excess of these qualities. If a patient suffered from heat, he prescribed a cold medicine. Jabir developed the idea of supreme elixir, the medicine of the metal.

According to "Kitab al Fihirst," the first Arabian writer on alchemy was Khalid ibn Yazid (c. 708) who was a pupil of the Syrian monk, Merianus. According to Paul of Aegina, the first ancient writer to treat the subject of alchemy was Fermicus III.[5]

Alchemy was originally developed in China. The devotees of the Taoist religion developed the so-called "science" of alchemy in their efforts to compound "the pill of immortality" and to concoct the "elixir vitae."

Wei Powei-Yang (c. 100-150 A.D.), known as "the Father of Alchemy," stated, "There are over 10,000 formulas employed in compounding the medicine of immortality. A profound subject like this is fit to be treated only by the wise. It is presumptuous for me to write about it, but I cannot hold my peace, for it would be a great sin on my part not to transmit 'the Tao way' which would otherwise be lost to the world forever." Wei Powei-Yang claimed to have a formula for prolonging life which he was disinclined to prescribe before first experimenting on a dog.[6]

In 133 B.C., alchemy, which was then an ancient art in China, received imperial sanction. The Chinese dynastic annals show that herbs and metals compounded in the crucibles of the Chinese alchemists very often led to disastrous results on those who bought the death-defying potions. How the Arabians came to borrow many of their ideas on alchemy from the Chinese still awaits investigation.

At the beginning of the Arabic period, many of the alchemists directed all their attention to the vain attempt to manufacture gold from base metals.[7] It is easy to see how frustration of work of this type could easily lead to self-delusion and even outright dishonesty.

How the Arabs were first lured into the pseudo-science of alchemy is not difficult to understand. To those who are not specifically instructed in chemistry, the very word is fascinating and calls to mind confused memories of colored liquids, rare odors—some exotic and some intolerable, glistening crystals, dazzling flames, suffocating fumes, startling explosions and a chaos of mystifying experiments. The polysyllabic jargon of the professional also served to arouse the interest of the early medieval Arabian. Anything so close to the border of the supernatural was bound to inspire feelings of awe and mystery.

The prefix "al" which starts the word "alchemy" is the Arabian article, and this shows that even the name of this pseudo-science is derived from the Arabic countries. "Alchemy" is believed by many to be derived from the Arabic "al-Kimija," which means, "an agent effecting transmutation." The Saracen name for alchemy was first "alembic" and this covered the process of distillation and analysis of substances of the three kingdoms of nature.[8] The Arabians zealously studied the properties, distinctions and affinities of various alkalies and acids. They converted various of the poisonous minerals into salutary remedies. However, their most eager search was for the transmutation of base metals into gold and silver.

This desire to transmute the base metals into gold and silver was the chief object of the early alchemists and their second most profound hope was to discover an "elixir vitae" (elixir of life), which could cure all diseases and bring eternal youth.

These two main avenues of investigation were connected for the specific was supposed to be in the nature of potable gold ("aurum potable").

We do not know how much chemistry the Arabs learned from the Greeks. We do not know how much they discovered themselves. Many of their works are still unstudied and we do not know how much of their work was handed down to Europe, but we do know that the Arabic works attributed to Jabir are a compilation made many years after the time when he is supposed to have lived and that this work is not identical with the earlier works which bear his name. Of this the most important text is the "Somma Perfecinis" which is the most important source for medical alchemy and chemistry. This book is certainly derived from Arabic sources, but it does not appear to be older than the thirteenth century. The most important feature of most of these texts is their advocacy of the sulphur-mercury theory of metals. Their description of alchemical methods and the beginnings of analysis consists of itemizing the methods for testing a metal to discover whether it is genuine gold. This discovery is of prime importance to the alchemists and chemists of the Middle Ages but the description of the furnace which is given by Jabir in a book of the seventeenth century is even of greater value.

The works of Jabir are very clear and free from mystery, but they did not enable the reader to make gold.

Alchemy was early combined with astrology. It was believed that there was an occult connection between the planets and the metals, as well as between the heavenly bodies and the various parts of the human body. In Latin Europe, the influence of this belief in medicine is seen in the terms "Lunar Caustic" and "Martian Preparations."

It was thought that the seven metals: gold, silver, iron, quicksilver (mercury), tin, lead, and copper, correspond in various ways with the seven planets and the seven days of the week. These metals were supposed to be generated in the bowels of the earth. Alchemy attempted to find the basic "fecundating" or "germinal" substances by which the baser of these metals could be transmuted into gold and by which the lives of men could be prolonged.

A number of basic chemical processes including distillation, sublimation, calcination, and filtration were known to the Arabs. To Geber falls the credit of having discovered nitric acid and aqua regia. Both of these were used some eight centuries ago. As a matter of fact, the greatest contribution of the Saracens to medicine was in the introduction of chemical compounds.

The Arabians invented the apothecary shop and introduced such valuable pharmaceutical preparations as syrups, juleps, alcohol, and tragacanth.[9] They also introduced scented waters such as those derived from the rose and orange. With the exception of Dioscorides and Pliny, the Saracens have contributed most of the early European pharmacopoeia. They collected and translated the materia medica of Dioscorides and other ancient writers. The Arabian pharmacologist, al Ghafiki made a list of a large number of medical and non-medical substances with terms coined by Arabs.[10]

Rhazes discusses in his writings the influence of the stars on the formation of metallic substances beneath the earth. He gives some theories concerning the formation of borax, orpiment (arsenic trisulphide), realgar[11] and certain combinations of sulphur, iron, and copper as well as some salts of mercury and compounds of arsenic. Rhazes believed in the transformation of metals and undertook to perform a transmutation before Emir al Mansur, Prince of Khorassan. After the latter had, at great expense, provided the necessary apparatus and materials for the accomplishment of the "magnum opus," the experiment failed miserably and al Mansur was furious. Rhazes subsequently died in poverty. Vincent (c. 1840) attributed to Rhazes the statement that copper is potentially silver and anyone who can successfully regulate the red color can bring it to a state of silver.

Avicenna was also a great believer in alchemy. Some of his countrymen believe that he found the "elixir vitae" and is enjoying the nectar of perpetual life and untold wealth to this very day as a result of the surcharged power of the philosopher's stone. Six or seven treatises on alchemy are ascribed to him. One of these, "Tractalibus Alchemiae," treats of the nature of mercury which Avicenna regarded as the universal vivifying spirit capable of penetrating, developing and fermenting. According to Waite, Avicenna describes several varieties of saltpeter and treats of the properties of common salt, sulphur, orpiment, vitriol and salammoniac. Sulphuric acid, silver nitrate, and bichloride of mercury were known previous to the Arabic Period.

Among other disciples of Geber may be mentioned Avenzoar, Averroes, and Abulkasim. Avenzoar is said to have made additions to the knowledge of medical preparations.

Abu Mansur, a north Persian physician, wrote a work on the principles of pharmacology from which may be inferred the chemical knowledge of the time. However, it appears that most of the Arabian alchemists of the eleventh, twelfth and thirteenth centuries devoted themselves primarily to attempts at transmuting the base metals into gold.

The returning Crusaders aided the spread of Eastern learning throughout Europe. The European nobles, who were impoverished and desired to replenish their treasuries, evinced particular interest in the transmuting of base metals into gold.

During the thirteenth century, learned men gave their attention to the study of alchemy and consequently the art reached a high degree of development. These scholars considered that the transmutation of the metals was a settled fact and avidly maintained the existence of the philosophers' stone. Some of their number—including Albertus Magnus, Thomas Aquinas, Arnold of Villanova and Raymondus Lullius—greatly influenced the development of chemistry by their pursuit of alchemy with a scientific spirit.

Albertus Magnus mentions alum caustic, alkali, red lead, arsenic, green vitriol (iron sulphate), iron pyrites, and various compounds of sulphur. He knew that arsenic renders copper white and he was familiar with the method of purifying the precious metals with lead. He found that sulphur attacks all the metals except gold and designated the cause of this combination by the term "affinities."

Roger Bacon was among the few scholastics who denied the possibility of transmutation of metals by existing means and who denied the very existence of the "philosophers' stone" (in his "Speculum Secretorum"). He states that to claim to make silver out of lead or gold or copper is as absurd as to pretend to create anything out of nothing. "The truth never held such a pretense . . . as this means which the alchemists call indifferently the 'elixir vitae,' the 'philosophers' stone' . . . (by which the fake claim is made that) with the help of Aristotle's 'secret of secrets,' experimental science has manufactured not only gold of twenty-four degrees, but of thirty, forty, and onward, according to pleasure."

The theory of transmutation of metals is founded upon the ancient Greek alchemists' concept that all substances are composed of one primitive matter ("prima materia") and that their differences are due to the presence of different qualities imposed on it. The alchemists hoped that by taking away the divergent qualities, they would obtain the basic "prima materia" itself. The "prima materia" was early identified with mercury. "The mercury of the philosopher" was not ordinary mercury, but the essence or the soul of mercury which was freed from the Aristotelian elements: wind, fire, water and earth. Thus the alchemists attempted to remove the four elements from ordinary mercury. It was thought that once "prima materia" had been attained, it would have to be treated with sulphur to confer upon it the desired qualities. The underlying idea, then, was that all metals are composed of mercury and sulphur. This concept persisted in one form or another up to the seventeenth century.

The Saracens were great travelers and conducted investigations in many strange lands. They penetrated as far east as Borneo and China and introduced a large number of new, non-chemical medicaments into their materia medica. These medicinal agents included alum, ambergris, borax, camphor, cassia, cloves, myrrh, nutmeg, senna, sandalwood, musk, clover, aconite, tamarind, syrup of julep, nitre and soda. The words alchemy, alcohol, algebra, chemise, cotton, admiral, alfalfa, arsenal, azure, cipher, zero, zenith and hundreds of other modern English words are vestiges from the Saracens.

The Arabs established hospitals and lecture-rooms at Damascus, Cairo, and Cordova,[12] and they commenced the application of chemistry to the practice of medicine offering explanations of the actions of the various drugs on the human body in health and in disease.

The Arabians exhibited great energy and skill not only in conquest, but also in many other fields of human endeavor. They are credited with the introduction of many discoveries. First and foremost is the system of Arabic numerals which we still employ and which was orginally derived from India by the Arabians. With this came Indian geometry and various basic astronomical tables. The Arabic word for "naught" or "zero" is "Sifir" from which our word "cipher" is derived. The Arabic numerals, operating on a decimal system, revolutionized arithmetic. It had previously been necessary to keep separate columns for units, tens, hundreds, etc. The abacus system employing beads strung on wires or rods set in a frame for keeping accounts is still met with in China. With the introduction of Arabic naughts, figures could be kept in a row in the series of units, tens, hundreds, etc. and the need for separate columns for each was obviated. The Arabic system found its way into Europe during the twelfth century after having been employed among the Arabs for a period of 250 years. Numerous terms as "cipher" and "algebra" witness the part played by the Arabs in developing our system of calculation.

A certain number of Greek tales derived from India can be traced directly through Arabia. The game of chess, although Indian by origin and Persian by name, came to Europe via the Moors.

It introduced a great number of new and active remedies from the vegetable kingdom into medical practice. It may fairly be stated that it created the modern science of chemistry and revived the pharmacies to an extent that the practice of medicine was definitely advanced. It contributed directly to the reform of practical medicine by the scientific preparation of various chemical remedies and indirectly by the union of the natural sciences with medicine. "Here and there," says Ward, "a flicker of inventive genius flashed up, as when the Saracen, ibn Junis, at the end of the tenth century, invented the pendulum; as when the compass, perhaps invented by the Chinese—and certainly used by them in traveling overland—found its way to Europe and was applied to water navigation."

The Arabians were extremely well versed in chemistry and technology. They were acquainted with the use of gunpowder and of artillery before the West. Even as early as the eleventh century, "The ship of the king of Tunis carried with it a number of iron tubes, from which were thrown much thundering fire." The Arabians derived from China a knowledge of paper, and, as early as 650, made silk paper for themselves in Samarcand, and by 706, cotton paper in Mecca. The latter was introduced into Spain in the twelfth century. At the same period, and about 500 years before the West, the Arabians made woodcuts for the ornamentation of paper manuscripts. Even the great art of printing, which had been independently invented in China, was actually brought to Europe by Arabian navigators.

Almost all the luxury of Europe came in by way of the East. Fine materials, including silk, cotton, velvet, satin (from the Arabic "zayton"), damask, cashmere, muslin (from "Masul"), chintz, moire, taffeta, gingham, chiffon, serge, cramoisy (Arabic "girmazi") and mohair came from the East as did such articles of dress as the sash, shawl, chemise, tiara, mask and turban.

In house decoration, such items as carpets, tapestries, mattresses, sofas, alcoves, and baldaquins (from Bagdad where cloth for canopies was made) are Arabic in origin. The names of utensils such as "carafe" (Arabic "qharafa") and jar (Arabic "jarrah") are Arabic in origin. Among table fruits we owe to the Arabs mulberries, pistachios, figs, citrons, watermelons, apricots, damsons (plums of Damascus), oranges, peaches, lemons and limes; among vegetables, artichokes, asparagus, spinach, and eschalot (introduced from Ascalon, Syria); among flowers, tulips, lilacs, roses, and jasmine.

All-spice, pomade, cosmetics, and many dyes including indigo (from India), are Eastern in origin.[13] Some of the more domestic musical instruments such as the lute, the tambourine, and the rebec (Arabic "rabab"; an early medieval stringed instrument), come from the same source as do various precious stones including the ruby, turquoise, amber, jasper, jade and lapislazuli.

Joseph Jacobs has compiled a list of a large number of objects whose names, in the various European languages, are derived from Oriental tongues.[14] Many of these objects were undoubtedly introduced into Europe after the Crusades, but some of them can be shown to have been used in Europe before the twelfth century, in which case their introduction was probably via the Radanites who conveyed them from Arabia.

Arabian medicine, with Arabian culture, reached its zenith at the period of the greatest power and greatest wealth of the Caliphates in the ninth and tenth centuries. At that time intellectual life was deeply rooted in the Arabian universities, which the great caliphs were zealous in founding. Such Arabian universities arose at Bagdad, Bassora, Cufa, Samarcand, Ispahan, Damascus, Bokhara, Firuzabad, Khurdistan, and, under the scholastic Fatimids (909-1171), in Alexandria. Some persisted even as late as the fourteenth century. After the settlement of the Arabians in Spain, under the Omayyad Caliphs (755-1031), famous universities sprung up at Cordova (possessing in the tenth century a library of 250,000 volumes), Seville, Toledo, Almeria and Murcia. The Caliphs, Abderrahman and al Hakem were particularly responsible for these institutions. Less important universities also developed in Granada and Valencia.

In spite of all these institutions the Arabian civilization always bore the stamp of its foreign origin. Even the basic Arabian religion was a mixture of Jewish, Christian and even pagan ideas. The chief claim of the Saracens to an important place in medical history is the warm reception they gave to Greek medicine at a time when it was banished from its original soil and forgotten by the Western World. During the long centuries that the West was veiled in a mist of ignorance and superstition the priceless tenets of Greek medicine were guarded and preserved by the Arabians.

The academies of the Arabians were imitations of the schools of Alexandria, and indirect successors of the old Egyptian sacerdotal schools as well as forerunners of our modern universities. They often included large blocks of buildings—indeed miniature cities—as must have been the case at Bagdad. Here were collected at one time, and from all portions of the world, 6000 teachers and students. The Arabian academies were associated with hospitals and pharmacies, and included residences for teachers and dormitories for students. Many of them had excellent library facilities. Some of these institutions, especially the later Spanish universities, enjoyed so great a reputation for erudition that many students attended them even from Christian countries, in order to acquire a higher education. Jewish students particularly, came from the scattered corners of Europe to attend these schools.

The medical departments in these schools, however, were only secondary affairs. Theology, philosophy, mathematics, physics, astronomy and astrology were the chief subjects in the Arabian curriculum; and medicine was nowhere taught independently of these branches.

When a student passed his final examinations, he was granted the "venia legendi igaze"—the right to teach.

As already pointed out, practical anatomy was utterly excluded by religious belief, and midwifery and gynecology were forbidden fields for men. The practice of operative surgery, too, was considered unworthy of a man of honor. It was permitted only to lithotomists, cataract gougers, and similar persons of the lower class. The fatalism of the Arabians also discouraged recourse to the knife. Even venesection and cauterization were not considered becoming practices for a physician of respectability. Such procedures were performed by his assistants only. These servants of the physicians performed various operative techniques including incision of the eyelids, removing the veins from the whites of the eye and extracting cataracts. An honorable physician actually did nothing more than to impart to the patient his professional advice with reference to food and medicine. Even the extraction of teeth was avoided, and, although dentistry was cultivated, as among the ancients, it was practiced only by the lower class of medical men. There are a few exceptional cases where the better physicians engaged in surgery. It is recorded that Thabit ibn Senan cured the stump of an arm that had been cut off.

There must have been a number of female practitioners, since certain operations on women, such as lithotomy, and replacing a prolapsed uterus, could only be performed by women. All the covered portions of the female body were prohibited from being stripped by strange men, and, of course, least of all could the sexual organs be touched or examined by them. Possibly, however, these female physicians were merely midwives.

Midwives were the only obstetricians and they did not shrink from performing the bloodiest operations, such as embryotomy and even lithotomy, on female patients.

There were apothecaries in the hospitals, as well as others who practiced independently and had no connection with these institutions. Male and female nurses were also employed. The better physicians existed for the rulers and the wealthy classes only. The common people, in the great majority of cases, employed ignorant popular physicians ("tubib"), conjurors, jugglers, and the like, for, according to the Koran, actual medical treatment, as well as the study of medicine, was simply tolerated, and to the most devout believers, the practice of medicine was regarded as an outright infringement upon the sphere of Allah. Even from the better physicians of the rulers, miraculous and immediate cures were expected rather than regular medical treatment.[15]

Cordova had 40 hospitals, but the greatest was one at Cairo. It was founded in 1283 by El Milik al Mansur Gilavun. It was directed by a physician-in-chief and had male and female nurses. Special wards were reserved for wound cases, those afflicted with diseases of the eye, dysentery cases and patients with fevers. There was a gynecological ward and another for convalescents.

The hospital admitted all diseased persons regardless of race, creed, color or social status.

These hospitals stimulated the spread of medical knowledge —nurtured by the indefatigable efforts of Arabic and Jewish scholars who translated the Hellenic works from the original sources in the true spirit of learned antiquity—throughout the Arab countries and later throughout Europe. The Arabian schools kept alive the memory of Greek learning and made various original contributions to our knowledge of nature.

Arabian medicine, entirely independent of its introduction into nosology of a few and important diseases, rendered essential services to the advance of general medicine in the following directions:

It cultivated the works of the Greeks and made them accessible to the West (though in a more or less corrupted form), until, after the revival of learning, when the Greek writers could once more be studied in their original language. This transfer of Greek science, including medicine, to the West was accomplished via Italy and Spain, and even as early as the age of Charlemagne, although it became more marked in the following centuries. By performing this function, the Arabians acquired a very high importance in the intellectual development of the West, particularly with regard to its medical culture. Hence the popular scorn of the Arabians, manifested by those who proclaim that only new facts are important in medicine, seems entirely out of place.[16]

Indirectly the Arabian civilization and culture was of further advantage in that it awakened, by its own too servile imitation, an opposition against its teachers, and even against itself.

CHAPTER X

THE ARABO-SPANISH PERIOD

The spread of Islam westward resulted in the capture of Egypt, North Africa, Sicily, and a portion of Italy and Spain. When the victorious armies of Islam reached Alexandria in 640, they found the ancient city no longer the great intellectual center it had been for one thousand years. The Academy which had housed the famous school of great medical teachers including Herophilus and Erasistratus was no longer in existence. The medical school had but few students and was eclipsed by the academies of Jondisabur of Persia and those of Bagdad. The once great library contained little more than sixteen books of Galen which had been translated by Hunain and his gifted nephew Hubaish (whom Wittington describes as the Erasmus of the Arabic Renaissance). The famous Alexandrian library had been destroyed before the Arabs took possession of Alexandria by zealous Christian fanatics at the order of Bishop Theophilus of Alexandria, but a few Greek classics were left which had been turned over by the Byzantines to the Alexandrian library when Egypt was dominated by the Eastern Roman Empire.

All available records show that the story that the invading Arabs destroyed the great Alexandrian library is not based on facts. The Arabian general who captured Alexandria is supposed to have been told by Caliph Omar: "If the books confirm the Koran they are superfluous; if contradictory they are pernicious; let them be burned." The general then is supposed to have ordered the books used as fuel for the four hundred public bath houses that existed in Alexandria. Like most good stories, this one has little if any foundation.

The caliphs were all disposed towards learning, and none of the valuable books were destroyed by them. To the contrary, the caliphs cultivated the arts and sciences at a time when the rest of the world was sunk in ignorance and superstition.

The fact is that the aforementioned Theophilus who was archbishop of Alexandria, and to whom Gibbon refers as "the perpetual enemy of peace and virtue, a bald bad man whose hands were alternately polluted with gold and blood," after demolishing the temple of Serapis, betook himself to destroy the library in the year 389. "The valuable library of Alexandria was pillaged or destroyed and nearly twenty years afterwards the appearance of the empty shelves existed to the regret and indignation of every spectator whose mind was not totally darkened by religious prejudice." [1]

Scarcely had the Ommayyad dynasty of Damascus, Syria, firmly settled in Spain when it embarked on a cultural program.

The commanders of the faithful, the Emirs of Cordova, distinguished themselves as patrons of learning. They set an example of culture and refinement that was indeed in strong contrast to the policies of the native European princes. Granada, which site the Saracen armies first occupied, developed into a wealthy and most beautiful city. No nation has ever excelled the Spanish Arabs in the beauty and costliness of their pleasure gardens and to these we owe the introduction of many of our most valuable cultivated fruits.

From the ninth to the twelfth centuries the Arabic West raised the dignity of learning in Europe. Many scientific works were written by Christians, Jews and Moslems at the express wish of the Ommayyad Caliphs of Cordova.

The greatest and most liberal Caliph was Abd al Rahman the Third (912-961). It is related that when Prince Abd al Rahman reached Spain after escaping from Bagdad because of a plot to assassinate him by the Abbassides, he proclaimed himself Caliph in Cordova on January 9, 929. Abd al Rahman adorned his capital with magnificent buildings and schools in his ambition to outdo the Abbassides in spreading the arts and sciences to Spain. He established a university which for centuries was the center of learning in the West.² He was followed by Caliph al Hakham II, another liberal ruler (961-976).

The period covering the reigns of the Ommayyad Caliphs was the Golden Age of Moslem Spain. Cordova, Toledo, Granada and Seville became the principal cities of European learning. Caliph al Hakham II was noted for his aversion to war and political intrigues and for his love of literature and culture. He established a library of 400,000 superbly bound and illuminated volumes. He personally supervised the copyists and binderies in his palace. It is reported that he made personal annotations on many of the volumes. During his reign, learned men of every faith were welcome at Cordova and he succeeded in making the town of Cordova "the Bagdad of the West."

His successor, Caliph al Hakham III, built the famous Mazquito on the site of the Christian Visigothic Church. This monument of Arabic civilization was only second to the Caaba of Mecca. The reigns of the al Hakhams were marked by the encouragement of scientific and philosophical studies. The science of medicine was particularly encouraged and became widely disseminated throughout the Moslem West. The literary competition brought forth a number of great philosophers and distinguished physicians.

It was in Spain—the most distant province of the Mohammedan Conquest—that the best of the Arabian, Jewish and Christian civilizations merged, and that the foundation for the revival of learning was laid. The Spanish Jews, originally fugitives from Palestine after this land was captured by Titus, had brought Alexandrian culture along with them. Many of them were learned in the arts and sciences of the ancient Greeks. They were among the first to appreciate the cultural disposition of the liberal caliphs. They kept up communications with the Arabic East and embarked upon the task of translating Greek classics into the Arabic vernacular.

Orthodox Moslem scholasticism with its rational philosophic theology, which was founded by the Persian philosopher, al Ghazzali, was transported to Spain and found there a fertile field for development.

Among the literary savants of Arabic Spain, may be mentioned the poet and philosopher, Solomon ibn Gabirol (Avicebrone). This great scholar was among the early representatives of speculative thought in Spain. He was followed by Averroes, who avidly opposed the combination of religion and science.

Medicine was preserved and raised in Arabic Spain to a position of dignity largely by the efforts of four distinguished physicians: Abulkasim, Avenzoar, Averroes and Maimonides. The literary and medical fame of each of these demands individual description.

ABULKASIM (c. 936-1110)

The most distinguished Arabo-Spanish physician was Abu 'L-Qasim uz-Zahrawi better known as Abulkasim (Abul Casim). He was born of Spanish parentage at El-Zahra, near Cordova, where he probably received his education. His medical reputation was brought to the attention of Caliph Abd al Rahman III (912-961) who named him as his court physician.

His *opus magnum* was his "al-Tasrif," a comprehensive work upon medicine and surgery in 30 parts. This encyclopedic medico-chirurgical work is subdivided into two main parts, each containing fifteen sections. His surgical tract,[3] which was translated into Latin by Gerard of Cremona, was the leading textbook on surgery for about 500 years, up to the time of Saliceto. The material of his "al-Tasrif" was largely borrowed from the "Epitome" of Paul of Aegina as well as from Oribasius and Aetius. This work has the merit of including personal observations and good practical judgment in selecting the best of the texts which he consulted.

Abulkasim's surgical treatise is divided into three books.[4] The first book deals with the indications for and contraindications against surgical operations and with surgical technique. Descriptions and illustrations of proper surgical instruments are included—a rather rare phenomenon in the textbooks of those days. There is a description of cautery and its use in surgery. Cautery was extensively employed by Mohammedan surgeons instead of the knife, the use of which was forbidden in the Koran. The second book deals with general, ophthalmic and dental surgery and the third book is devoted to fractures, dislocations and the management of paralysis following fractures of the spine. The third book contains methods of treating wounds and ends with remarks on suppuration. The third book is largely a translation of Paul of Aegina. The parts of "al-Tasrif" dealing with pathology and diagnosis have not survived in the Arabic text.

In the twenty-seventh, twenty-eighth and twenty-ninth sections of "al-Tasrif," Abulkasim deals with materia medica and gives an alphabetical list of simple drugs. This part is frequently quoted by writers of the East and West, most notably by the Arabian pharmacologist, al-Ghafiki. The eighteenth section deals with preparations and remedies derived from the mineral, vegetable and animal kingdoms. The nineteenth section, which deals with synonyms and substitutes, is known in Latin as "Liber Seroitoris." Abulkasim represents an early author employing chemistry in the practice of medicine.

The anatomy, physiology and dietetics of Abulkasim are borrowed from Galen and Rhazes. With reference to anatomy, he admits that his knowledge on this subject was derived from books and not from practical dissection. "He that would devote himself to surgery," he states, "must be versed in the science of anatomy which Galen has transmitted." In the introduction of his "al-Tasrif," Abulkasim complains of the insufficient anatomical knowledge of his contemporaries. He points out a number of errors made by ignorant surgeons. He criticizes the barber-surgeons and the traveling mountebanks who retarded the science of surgery in Western Europe. It seems that he did not realize that his own inexperience with dissection might also have a similar effect on surgery in the Latin West where his book was very popular with medical students.

SURGERY

The surgical writings of Abulkasim, however, definitely eclipsed the "Epitome" of Paul of Aegina and the "Liber Almansorem" of Rhazes as a surgical text because of its lucid descriptions and its illustrations of text and instruments. It was adopted in almost all European schools.

In the aforementioned second book, he gives a detailed description of lithotomy, lithotrity (the crushing of a vesical calculus within the bladder by means of an instrument) and circumcision.

Amputation, he states, should not be performed above the elbow or above the knee joints, for if mortification extends from these points, death is inevitable. The indication for amputation is gangrene, which can arise from external and internal causes.

Abulkasim performed an operation on the thyroid. He describes a "tripod" trephining instrument which was provided with a thread and a sharp point. He also devised a deep rectal syringe. He states that he knows no one who has performed the tracheotomy operation.

In the third book, Abulkasim condemns badly set fractures. In case of fracture of the spine, he points out that the resulting paralysis depends upon the seat of the lesion. For fractures of the pelvis in women, he recommends the passing of a sheep bladder into the vagina and distending the bladder by blowing air through the tube in order to assist reposition. He was first to write of the treatment of deformities of the mouth and dental arches (second book).

The last chapter of the first book is devoted to the stoppage of hemorrhage and cauterization plays an important part in doing this. Other methods of stopping hemorrhage include styptics, digital pressure and complete severance of the injured artery.

OBSTETRICS

With regard to obstetrics, Abulkasim suggests methods of treatment in prolapse of the hand or foot, presentation of the knees, and transverse positions. He also mentions face presentation. In presentation of both feet the delivery should be effected by the breech, after the reposition of the feet. His description of the position of the parturient woman during delivery is similar to what is presently known as "Walcher's position." He also mentions instrumental deliveries. The works of Abulkasim in manuscript form contain accurate, although inartistic, sketches of a variety of surgical instruments employed in obstetrics.

Martin Spink reproduced sketches of some twenty-five instruments from two manuscripts in the British Museum.[5] He expressed the opinion that the text in question was "the most fully illustrated early surgical treatise in any language." He believes that the sketches were made from actual instruments, and that these were similar to those used by the ancient Greeks and Romans. He also is of the opinion that the sketches were copied into the Western manuscripts of the Latinized Abulkasim.

Abulkasim writes much, and ably, on the delivery of women, and he gives the details of an unusual case which came under his personal observation, in which the fetus died without delivery and the mother became pregnant a second time. The second fetus also died and remained unexpressed. Soon after, an abscess formed at the navel, ripened and discharged. To his great surprise, not only pus, but bones poured out through the abscess. He felt that these were unquestionably from the dead fetuses (tubal pregnancies?). The mother lived many years after this event, but continued for the rest of her days to have an open ulcer at the site of the abscess from which there was a continual discharge.

Abulkasim gives a detailed description of the removal of foreign bodies from the ear. The first requisite is a bright light. The removal of foreign bodies which have penetrated into the external auditory meatus depends upon the nature of the substance of which the foreign body is composed. For hard substances such as iron or glass, oily instillations and sternutators (substances which cause sneezing) should be used. For beans, suction, extraction by forceps, or a probe covered with adhesive material, should be used. A swollen foreign body should be reduced in size with a knife. Insects in the ear should be removed by suction or oily injections.

In his book on fractures and dislocations, he states, "This part of surgery has passed into the hands of vulgar and uncultured minds for which reason it has fallen into contempt."

Although Abulkasim is no great advocate of employing incision in case of hydrocephalus, he does recommend this procedure in other tumors of the head which are cutaneous and circumscribed, and especially when they are encysted. He strongly advocates this procedure as being unattended with danger provided nerves and arteries are preserved from injury. He adds that the danger is even further lessened when the substance of the tumor is compact and solid, since in such cases, the chance of hemorrhage is greatly lessened.

Abulkasim follows Paul of Aegina in his method of treating swellings of the tonsils which undergo suppuration. He explains how the tonsils themselves, when so enlarged as to impede respiration, should be extirpated. He declares that this operation is difficult to perform but is not attended with any danger. Abulkasim is nevertheless of the opinion that this operation should only be performed when the base of the swollen tonsil is small, and the enlargement itself has a round form and is white in color. When the base is large, he declares that the ensuing hemorrhage may be excessive and productive of danger and inconvenience.

In the same chapter he treats of other tumors in the cavity of the fauces, which occasionally arise and demand extirpation in the same manner as enlarged tonsils. He presents the history of a woman who had such a growth which was of a livid color, but unattended by pain. Since it impeded both deglutition and respiration to a marked degree, he declares that it would prove speedily fatal without surgical intervention. This growth sent two branches into the cavities of the nose. He describes the operation of excision with the greatest minuteness. However, when he noted that when one tumor was removed by means of the knife, a fresh one grew in its place, he had recourse to the use of cautery. He felt that cautery would effectually check the tumor's further growth, but, at the same time, he candidly admits that he did not follow up this case.

Abulkasim describes an unusual case which came under his observation, in his ninety-third chapter. This patient was a woman of spare habit, with very prominent veins. On examining her hand, he found a tumor in one of the veins, accompanied by inflammation. After the lapse of an hour, this tumor started to climb up the arm with a kind of vermicular motion, the pain shifting its seat along with the movement of the tumor. In the space of another hour, it traversed the body, and reached the other hand, where it exhibited the same appearance as it did at first. What surprised Abulkasim most was the rapidity of its passage from one limb to the other.

Abulkasim gives, from his own practice, many accurate descriptions of wounds from arrows, together with his plan of cure, and an account of his surprising success in several cases. Among other cases, he mentions having extracted the head of an arrow from the nose, in which it had been lodged for a considerable time, with the recovery of the patient by the end of the fourth week. From his experience in this case, he contends that it is an error to suppose that the cartilage of the nose cannot be made to reunite after it has been divided.

In his account of the operation for extracting stone from the bladder, he is much more accurate and copious than either Celsus or Paul of Aegina. He particularly describes the mode of extraction by incision in female patients. It would appear, however, that where such complaints occurred in female subjects, surgeons had few opportunities of operating, for they were prevented from interfering when the patients were either unmarried girls, or married women with any pretensions of modesty. In such cases, female operators were employed to act under the direction of the surgeon, who was not himself permitted to be present. The surgeon could be solely guided in his judgment by the reports of these female operators and he had no opportunity of examining the patient first hand. Hence, we can be at no loss to account for the usual silence of the early surgeons on such matters, and we may easily conclude, that what Abulkasim gives us on the subject, is the result of secondary description, rather than primary observation.[6]

"I have detailed briefly the methods of operations," says Abulkasim. "I have described the necessary instruments and I have presented their forms by means of drawings. In short, I have omitted nothing which can shed light for the profession. The apprenticeship of this branch of knowledge is very long, and he who devotes himself (to surgery) must be versed in the science of anatomy of which Galen has transmitted us the knowledge."

As intimated previously, Abulkasim complains in the introduction of his book of the insufficient anatomical knowledge of his contemporaries and points out a number of errors made by ignorant surgeons. "Operative skill has vanished without leaving a trace behind it. One can find only in the ancient writers a few references to it but even they are incomplete and useless through bad translations and mistakes. The bulk that is contained in literature is borrowed from the Greeks, especially that of Paul of Aegina."[7]

Abulkasim was not followed, however, to any great extent, by the Arabian physicians. They preferred Rhazes and Avicenna as medical teachers. The chief influence of Abulkasim was in Latin Europe. The Europeans liked his lucidity and his method of presentation. There can be little question that his method of presentation surpassed that of Galen. He maintained a dominant position in Europe for five hundred years.

The Latin translation of "al-Tasrif" by Abulkasim was first printed in Venice in 1497. "Al-Tasrif" contains an almost verbatim account of Rhazes on smallpox.[8] Another medical work of Abulkasim is entitled in Latin, "Libre Servitoris." This book contains twenty-eight of his treatises and was published in Venice in 1479 by Nicholas Jenson. This last mentioned compilation describes medical preparations obtained from mineral, vegetable and animal materials. It represents an early example of the science of chemistry employed in medicine. He also wrote a work on gynecology called "Collectio Gynaecorium."

AVENZOAR (c. 1113-1162 or 1199)

One of the most distinguished physicians of Arabic Spain was Abū Mervān Abd ul-Malik ibn Zuhr (Avenzoar)—who flourished at the beginning of the twelfth century. He was born in Seville, the capital of Andalusia, where he exercised his profession and built up his great reputation. His ancestors had been celebrated as physicians for several generations, and his son, Abu Bekr Muhammed ben Abd al-Malik ibn Zuhr, was held by the Arabians to be an even more eminent physician than himself.

Imbued through ancient family tradition with the spirit of medicine, he determined to be a physician from his early childhood, and, after many years of studies, he dedicated all his abilities to the practice of medicine, in which endeavor he was inspired by the highest ideals.

Avenzoar was not dependent upon his profession for a living. He inherited a large fortune from his ancestors. He gratuitously attended the poor and people of small income, but accepted fees from the rich. "He was charitable as he was skilled, and liberal as he was enlightened." He was a foe to every kind of quackery be it medical or religious, and he ridiculed the faith placed in old wives' prescriptions. He loathed the superstition of astrology. He may have lived to an old age, and some historians believe that he lived to the advanced age of 135 years.[9] His favorite maxim is to the effect that experience is the best guide and test of practice and that every physician conforming to this test will be acquitted both here and in the hereafter. "It is not by logical distinctions and sophistical refinements that the art of healing is to be acquired, but by the union of daily experience with requisite powers of discrimination."

He was thus like Rhazes, who also believed that the advance of medicine does not lie in theory but in practice, and in bedside observation. While he revered his predecessors, he freed himself from all medical sophistry and blind adherence to authority and tradition. He was considered the most celebrated physician of his time and was employed at the court where rich gifts were showered upon him.

Avenzoar belonged to the *Dogmatists* or *Rational School*, rather than to the *Empirics*. He was a great admirer of Galen but reserved his independence. On one occasion he appears to have been persecuted for his independence and free thought. He states himself that he was once unjustly fined and thrown into prison by a certain Count Haly of the Royal Stables, notwithstanding the fact that he cured Haly's son of jaundice.

Avenzoar was a contemporary or tutor of Averroes, who, according to Leo Africanus, heard his lectures, and learned medicine from him. From his writings it would appear that the offices of physician, surgeon and apothecary were already considered distinct professions.

Avenzoar's "Theisir" ("The Alleviation of Disease") abounds with interesting clinical reports and rational practices. This work makes every effort to exclude preconceived ideas and to capitalize on his own independent observation and judgments based on clinical experience.

He evinces a considerable knowledge of anatomy in his remarkable description of his own personal case of inflammation and abscess of the mediastinum and in his differential diagnosis of common pleurisy from abscess or dropsy of the pericardium. His mode of self treatment in the aforementioned case is interesting. While he was on a journey he was seized with a severe inflammation terminating in abscess of the mediastinum which was marked by agonizing pains which increased upon coughing, a strong, rapid pulse and a high temperature. He bled himself on the fourth evening, and removed a pound of blood, after which he assiduously bandaged the part of the body where he had performed the phlebotomy and fell asleep. While asleep, the bandage worked loose and further hemorrhage ensued. Awakening, he found his bed soaked through with blood and his strength much reduced. He placed a tight bandage over the blood vessel and the bleeding stopped. He ascribed his recovery to his great loss of blood. Avenzoar also was afflicted at various times with sciatica and dysentery.

Avenzoar studied cases of thickening of the pericardium, and dropsy in the pericardial chamber. In patients who died of this ailment, he noted that the pericardium frequently was found distended and containing from half a pound to a pound of water (postmortem examination?). In cases of tuberculosis, Avenzoar substituted goat's milk for ass's milk which had been recommended by Galen. (The Arabs were forbidden to drink ass's milk.)

Avenzoar believed in the noxious influence of miasmata upon health. He distinguishes between primary and secondary diseases of the heart. He describes serious pericarditis, paralysis of the pharynx and inflammation of the middle ear. He expresses himself strongly upon the indications for certain surgical operations with a thoroughness which could only have been acquired through practical experience. His therapeutics betray an extensive knowledge of pharmacy.

Avenzoar is the only Arabic writer who speaks of bronchotomy in dangerous cases of inflammation of the tonsils where breathing is interfered with. He readily admits that this is a hazardous operation which he never personally performed or even witnessed.

In obstruction of the esophagus he suggests three modes of treatment: (1) the introduction of food into the stomach by means of a silver tube; (2) immersing the patient in a bath containing a nutrient fluid which thus can enter the body through the skin; and (3) employing nutrient enemas (proctoclysis).

Avenzoar excelled all of his contemporaries in his pharmaceutical skill. His book on pharmaceutical preparations abounds both in simple and compound medicines. He is particularly explicit on the subject of poisonous plants and antidotes. He discusses solvents of stones favoring "oil of Alquiscemus" which his father had brought from the East. He employs drying evacuant remedies including black hellebore in treating a bony excrescence from the spine which resembled a horn in its form and texture. He personally suffered from such an excrescence himself which gave him severe pain. He succeeded in removing it in its entirety by the use of such remedies. He recommends

PLATE 53. Facsimile of title page.

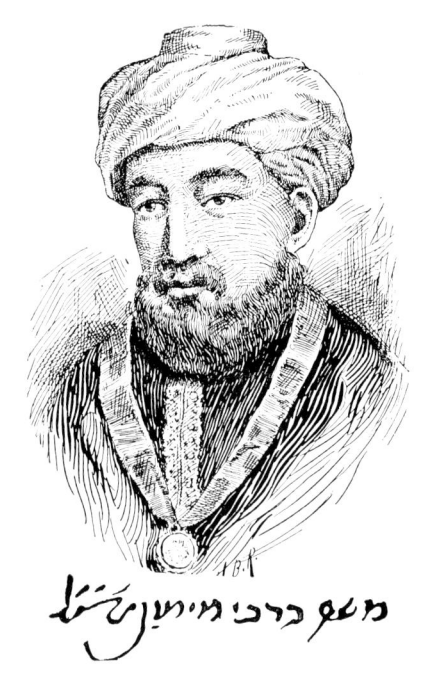

PLATE 54. Traditional Portrait of Moses Ben Maimon, with autograph. Born Cardova 1135, died Cairo 1204.

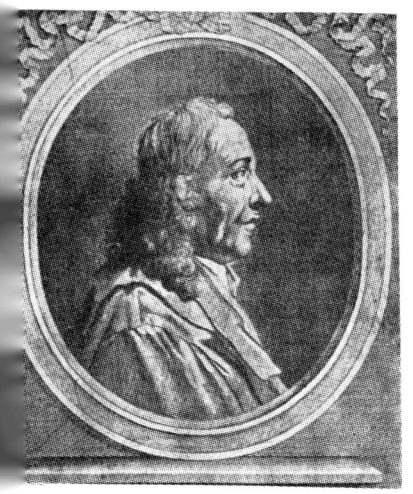

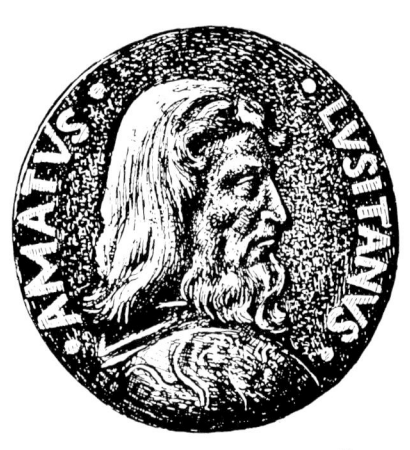

PLATE 55. Marcellus Malpighi (1628-1694)

PLATE 56. João Rodrigues de Castelo Branco (1511-1568)
(Courtesy Armed Forces Medical Library, Washington, D.C.)

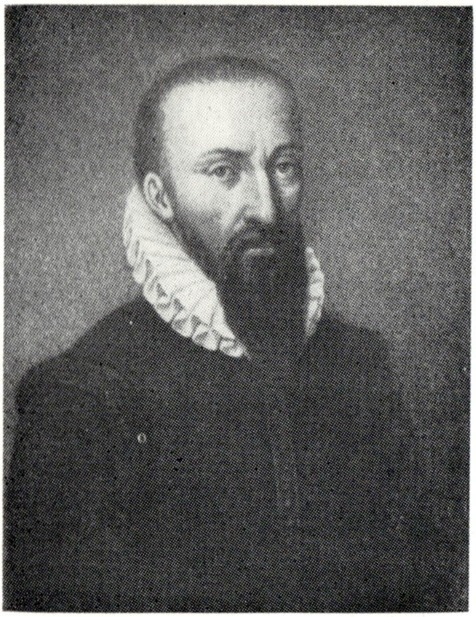

PLATE 57. Ambroise Paré

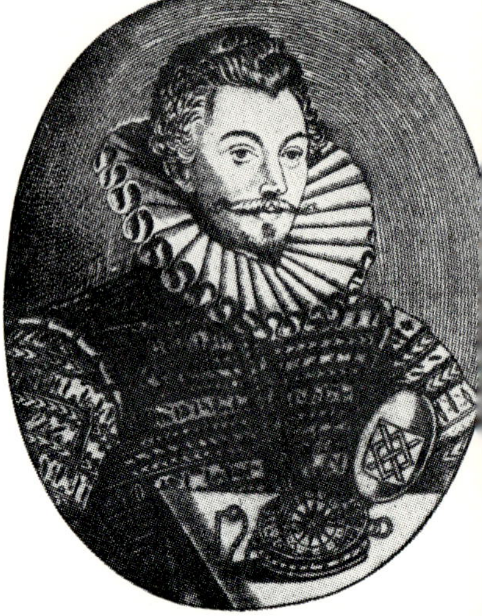

PLATE 58. John Haryngton (1561-1612)

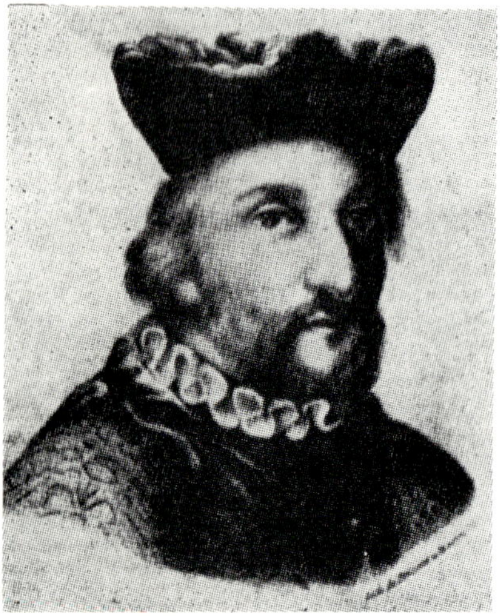

PLATE 59. Arnold of Villa Nova

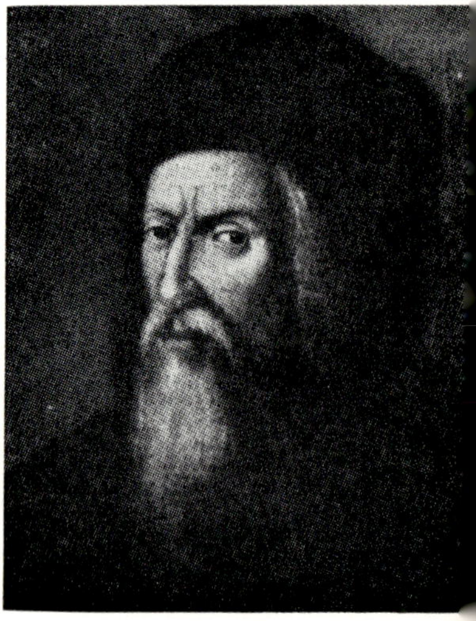

PLATE 60. Berengario de Carpi (1470-1530)

hellebore as being the most active (although not safest) purgative.

Hellebore was employed by ancients in large doses. Aretaeus prescribed it in 2 drachm doses. This drug was thought effective in carrying off the black bile. Avenzoar's father observed the diuretic properties of black hellebore.

Avenzoar recommends the Bezoar stone in various diseases. "The best Bezoar is found in the East where it is produced from the eyes of a deer. In these countries, the deers eat serpents for the purpose of improving their strength, and before they have sustained any injury from them, they run down the rivers and plunge themselves in water up to the head: a practice taught them by instinct. Here they remain immersed without drinking (which would be instantly fatal) until their eyes begin to water: this humour continues to exude under their eyelids, and coagulate there until it acquires the size of a chestnut."

In Avenzoar's time, it was considered beneath a physician's dignity to practice operative surgery. Nevertheless he, like Abulkasim, practiced surgery with marked distinction. He drew the line, however, at lithotomy for even the Greeks had disdained to perform this operation. He advocated removing stones from the bladder by the internal use of the oil of dates. He is credited with the first total extirpation of the uterus, although this operation developed because he accidentally confused the uterus with an internal abscess. Avenzoar also engaged in experimental operations on the lower animals. He performed a tracheotomy on a goat.[10] Avenzoar theoretically proposed the removal of exostosis by the magnet.

In physiology, on the subject of the relative importance of the organs, Avenzoar calls attention to the fact that no organ can perform its functions properly without the aid of another (e.g., the brain or lungs are helpless without the liver), and that one cannot, therefore, distinguish any one organ as the most important. Furthermore, in opposition to Galen, he assigns sensibility to the teeth and the bones, and holds that the continuance of life depends upon a correct balance of the humors.

As far as the etiology of disease is concerned, he lays stress upon the deleterious qualities of the air around swamps. His special pathology mentions pericarditis and pericardial exudation, consumption, abscess and growths of the stomach, mediastinitis, salivary concretions under the tongue, quinsy, and paralysis of the pharyngeal muscles.

Avenzoar's therapeutics recommends that in inflammatory cases venesection be performed on the sound side only. In opposition to Galen he considers amaurosis to be curable.

It should be stressed that Avenzoar's book "Theisir," in which he records the foregoing results of his experience, avoids all subtleties, and emphasizes experience as being the best guide of the physicians.[11]

Avenzoar is averse to the use of purgatives but is strongly in favor of venesection, using it even upon his own three year old son. In consumption he advocates the use of goat's milk. He mentions the itch mite (sarcoptes scabiei).[12]

His book, "Fi' Ladwiyat Wa'laugh Dyat" ("The Methods of Preparing Medicine and Diet"), was translated into Hebrew in the year 1280 by a Jewish physician named Jacob and thence into Latin by Paravicius, whose version, first printed at Venice in 1490, passed through several editions. The Latin version is entitled, "Adjumentum de Medale et Regimine" ("The Methods of Preparing Medicine and Diet").[13]

This book indicates that Avenzoar was in charge of a hospital and was frequently consulted for advice by the state. Throughout this work he exposes the doctrines of the *Empirics*. He generally follows Galen although this work has considerable material not found in Galen.

Avenzoar speaks of several eminent schools of medicine which existed contemporary with him in Spain. The medical school at Toledo enjoyed the highest reputation. Avenzoar praises the several professors who taught at these schools, and, upon all occasions, gives the greatest deference to their opinions. Avenzoar appears to have had little or no acquaintance with those Arabian authors who wrote in Asia, since he neither speaks of them in his works, nor avails himself of their labors.

Avenzoar's son, Abu Bekr Muhammed ben Abd al-Malik ibn Zuhr, was distinguished not only as a physician but also as a grammarian and poet. In one of his verses, he expresses his thoughts concerning Galen's work, "The Medical Art."

"The Medical Art encourages the sick with life and hope,
When death is near the Medical Art says, 'I give up.'"

The Mauritanian King, el-Malik el-Mansur Jacub ben Jusuf, summoned the young Avenzoar from Seville to the capital of Morocco to serve as his body physician. On one occasion the King perchance picked up a few of his poems in which young Avenzoar expresses concern for his family. The King immediately ordered the doctor to bring his entire family from Seville to Morocco. His main medical contribution was "De Cura Ocularum," a book of therapeutics of the eye. The younger Avenzoar died in October 1199, and his son was the last of the Avenzoars.

The Avenzoar family was renowned for many generations for its learning in politics, science, law and medicine. The first ibn Zuhr (Muhammad ibn Zuhr al Ijadi) emigrated to Spain in the year 912, following which the descendants adopted the old family designation "ibn Zuhr al Ijadi" in addition to their own names.

The great grandfather of the famous physician was a prominent lawyer who was greatly respected by the Spanish community for his piety, charity and scholarship. He died in Talahira in the year 1031 at the age of 86. There are six generations of famous descendants of this ibn Zuhr.

His son, Abu Mervan Abd ul-Malik ben Mervan ibn Zuhr, set out on a long journey to the Orient where he spent a lengthy period studying medicine. He practiced first in Bagdad and then in Cairo. After practicing for sometime in Kairowan, he went to Dania, whence his fame reached Spain and Mauritania. He was consulted on medical problems by the royalty and people of both countries.

His son, Abul Allah Zuhr ben abu Mervan abd ul-Malik, the second medical generation of the Avenzoar family, was a famous physician. He received his first medical instructions from his father and from Abul Aina el-Misri under whom he also studied philosophy and the other sciences. He studied medicine and philosophy at the University of Seville.

When quite young, he had already attained a fine reputation in medicine and the other sciences. This brought him to the attention of the Caliph who appointed him vizier of Islamic Spain.

It is related that the famous Avenzoar, when he was presented by a merchant from Iraq with a copy of Avicenna's "Canon," remarked: "It does not deserve to be placed in my library." He thought so little of the "Canon" that he cut off the margins of the manuscript to write prescriptions for his office patients.[14]

Baas, Garrison[15] and other historians state that the Avenzoars were racially Jews. This is questioned by Steinschneider[16] and Wustenfeld.[17] The last bases his argument that Avenzoar was not a Jew, on the fact that the name of the first ibn Zuhr was Muhammad, a name which Jews and Christians would hesitate to adopt. This argument is not convincing. The fact that the family adopted that name from the chain of names as soon as they reached Spain more likely is an indication that the name Muhammad was used in North Africa to hide their racial identity because of persecution. Such a change of names was common in Spain among the Moranos.

AVERROES (1126-1198)

One of the greatest of all personalities that Arabic Spain has produced was Abul Walid Muhammad ibn-Ahmed ibn-Muhammad ibn Ruschd, who became known in Latin Europe as Averroes. This man exercised a very great influence upon his own times and succeeding generations. Averroes was born at Cordova where his father and grandfather were judges. Following the tradition of his family his early education was in jurisprudence.

Having completed his studies, Averroes succeeded, on the death of his father, to the posts he had held. Notwithstanding the handsome income which he derived from these sources plus the receipts of his private professional practice, his generous and liberal disposition kept him perpetually poor. He was a man of sound judgment and great talent, and he excelled particularly in the acuteness of his powers of reasoning.

He realized that his interest was more inclined to the sciences, philosophy and mathematics and he set out to pursue these studies, under well known instructors. He soon acquired a wide reputation as scholar and philosopher. His great learning reached the ears of the philosophical vizier, ibn Tufail (Abubacer), and the latter introduced him to Prince Jusuf. The latter, having discovered that Averroes also possessed a full knowledge of the Melakite system of laws (from his early training), appointed him to the office of *Cadi* in the city of Seville (1169). He was later appointed governor of Andalusia, a position which he did not hold for long because his outspoken adherence to Aristotelian philosophy and his expressions of free thought aroused doubts as to his adherence to Islam, and gave his enemies the chance to accuse him of heresy. He was expelled from the community and banished to an-Nisaba, a Jewish settlement near Cordova. Through the intervention of friends, the successor of al-Mansur sent him to Morocco where he served in various capacities for the government.

Averroes informs us in his works that he was acquainted with the sons of Avenzoar, but he says nothing concerning any acquaintance with their father. From this we may fairly presume that, since he lived in the same town as Avenzoar, and was too distinguished to be passed without notice, that the elder Avenzoar must have been dead by that time. It is related that while in Cordova he met the physician and philosopher, Avenzoar (ibn Zuhr)—probably referring to the son. These two philosophers became fast friends and it appears that Averroes was influenced by the younger Avenzoar to study medicine.

Averroes' medical work is embodied in seven books entitled "Kitab-al Kullyyat," known in the Latin West as "Colliget." This "Compendium of the Science of Medicine" was translated into Latin in the year 1255 by a Jewish physician, Banacasa of

Padua. Although this opus reveals a great knowledge of the subject, it is not, in the ordinary sense, a medical textbook. It rather represents the efforts of a philosopher who mastered a subject not of his own choice, to bring back philosophy to the medical art—after Hippocrates had succeeded in separating them.

The "Colliget" offers little that was new in medicine and still less of medical experience. It impresses the reader that the author had read much about medicine but had little practical experience. The "Colliget" is, in reality, a commentary on the "Canon" of Avicenna. In the opening paragraph of his "Colliget," Averroes appeals to only those readers who are learned in natural philosophy and dialectics.

It was at the personal request of the Emperor of Morocco that Averroes wrote this work on medicine, and he admits that it is only a compilation of the observations of others, with some additions of his own. In this work he arranges the whole science of medicine under seven general divisions. Commencing with the general precepts of the art, he gradually develops the subject and a thorough acquaintance with logic and natural philosophy are necessary to enable the reader to comprehend him. He furnishes nothing new on the subject of anatomy, contenting himself with simple transcribing.

With Aristotle, he claimed sensibility for the heart; in other respects he held that the heart was merely the place of origin of the arteries. He considered the ethereal principle inherent in the semen to be the only essential agent in propagation. He stated that a woman might become impregnated merely by bathing in water in which a man had just had a seminal emission. He was prompted to adopt this opinion by his gullible acceptance of the oath of a cunning wife, who swore that she had in this manner become impregnated without the aid of her husband.[18]

Averroes was of the opinion that the sense of sight originates in the lens of the eye. Smallpox, according to his teaching, never befalls the same individual more than once. In therapeutics he rejects the employment of mathematical formulas in the compounding of remedies, and holds that the duty of the physician consists chiefly in the application of general principles to special cases.

Averroes appears to have been particularly anxious, in the compilation of his great work on medicine, to rectify the conflicting theories of former writers, and, particularly, to reconcile the conflicting opinions of Aristotle and of Galen. To Averroes, Aristotle was supreme and Galen was secondary. One may observe his partiality to Aristotle as against Galen for, whenever there is a difference of opinion between these two savants, he sides with Aristotle. He mentions Alkindus in his writings whose work on the proportions and doses of medicines, is yet extant. Alkindus makes an absurd attempt to explain the powers of medicines by the laws of arithmetic and music. This is justly ridiculed by Averroes. Alkindus' notion, that "the activity of a medicine always increases in a double ratio when compounded with others," is visionary and unfounded.

Averroes surpasses Avicenna in applying Aristotelian principles of philosophy to the art of medicine. He often appears guilty of misjudging facts and he certainly did not personally advance the science of medicine. He taught that the physical causes of disease and epidemics must be sought, as those of other natural phenomena, beyond the patient himself.

What Averroes lacked in medical acumen he made up in full measure in philosophy. A disciple of Aristotle, his philosophical system was adopted in the Arabic language by Spanish Jewish thinkers and through them was carried over to the Christian countries.

His greatest ambition was to obtain the reputation of being *the* commentator of Aristotle. However, his combination of religious beliefs, Aristotelian doctrine and neo-Platonism prevented him from fulfilling this ambition. The result was that he created a new system of philosophy which became known as *Averroism*. His doctrine exercised an important influence upon the learning of Latin Europe up to the seventeenth century.

His doctrine that the individual soul, at death, retreats again to the Universal Soul whence it came, caused him to be charged with denying personal immortality of the soul of man.

In his commentary on the works of Aristotle he combines the theosophy of India, with the dogmas of Erigena and others and he presents the doctrine of *emanation* and the return of the soul to the Universal Soul. His conception of God and nature shook the foundations of Islam and Christianity, so his doctrines were vigorously opposed by both religions. His pantheistic doctrine that the soul or the nature of man is absorbed into the universal nature at death, thus denying personal immortality, led to his persecution by both the Moslem and the Christian Churches.

He became a sceptic in the faith in which he had been brought up and in which he had held so sacred an office as that of High Priest. His honesty and sincerity greatly outweighed his prudence and he would not suppress his opinions. Because of this he was deprived of all of his offices, charged with heresy and imprisoned. However, he was soon released and restored to his offices in consequence of the misconduct and extortion of the person who had been appointed to succeed him.

Two of the principal charges leveled against Averroes were that he taught there is no creation *ex nihilo* (no making of anything out of nothing) and that there is a creation, from moment to moment, whereby the world is maintained and changed. According to Averroes, the creative power is always at work maintaining, moving and directing the world. This premonition of the doctrine of evolution appears sound to our modern ears, but in his time the theologians cried out, "Sacrilege! The author has no soul!"

It is related that when the Christians and Moslems relegated his book to the index expurgatorius and his soul to spiritual flames, Averroes uttered the Arabic equivalent of: "Sit anima mea cum philosophis!" ("Let my soul be with the philosophers!")[19]

The learned Jews of Spain took up the philosophy of Averroes with great enthusiasm and, when they were expelled from Spain, they spread his doctrine in the south of France and Italy. In the fourteenth century many commentaries on Averroes appeared. In the fifteenth century Averroism among Jews began to decline and in the next century Spinoza practically ignored the writings of Averroes. He was a religious free-thinker, who, hiding himself behind the precepts of philosophy, awakened doubts as to the creed of the Church, and the Church accordingly hated him bitterly. He died in Morocco in the year 1198 at an advanced age. To recapitulate, he passed away after having suffered bitter persecution at the hands of his fellow-believers in consequence of the pantheistic views awakened in him by the study of Aristotle, whose most worthy follower he was among all the Arabians. His loss marked the end of the cultural and scientific era of the Arabs in Spain and with it a decline of Arabian medicine and learning ensued. Averroes' fame among the Moslems vanished with his death by the end of the twelfth century. However, his renown in Latin Europe continued.

MAIMONIDES (1135-1204)[20]

One of the most learned physicians of the Arabo-Spanish Period was Abu Imran Musa ben Maimum ibn Abd Allah, known in Europe as Maimonides, and among Jews as "Rambam" (a contraction of Rabbi Moses ben Maimuni). He came from a family noted for their prominent men for seven generations. His father was a judge (*dayan*) in Cordova, well learned in the Jewish lore, from whom Moses got his early Hebrew education. For his early secular education, his father employed distinguished Arabic teachers. Thus, when Moses was thirteen years of age, he was initiated in all the fundamental branches of learning of that time.

In 1148, his native town of Cordova fell into the hands of the fanatical Almohades and the Maimuni family as all their co-religionists were compelled to choose between the acceptance of the Islamic religion and exile. The Maimuni family chose the latter and harder course. For a period of twelve years they were obliged to live an errant life in southern Spain and North Africa, traveling from place to place and leading the life of Moslems in the open and Jews at home. During these years, however, Moses was able to compose a number of his philosophic and rabbinic works.

In the year 1158, Maimonides settled with his family in Fez, Morocco, where being unknown, he hoped to pass as a Moslem. In his writings, he relates that while in Fez he discussed with medical men of Maghrib various medical subjects. He seldom refers to Andalusian physicians.[21]

Leo Africanus states that while Maimonides lived in Spain, he became a disciple of Avenzoar in medicine and of Averroes in philosophy. Of course these represent two of the greatest medical and philosophical authorities of the thirteenth century, but this statement appears improbable for Maimonides was only ten years old when he left Spain. It seems more likely that he studied medicine during his seven year stay with his family in Fez (c. 1158-65).

As the reputation of young Moses was steadily growing in the city of Fez, authorities began to inquire into the religious disposition of this highly gifted young man, and his dual life became increasingly dangerous. He was forced to leave Fez and wander from city to city to escape the informers who openly charged him of having relapsed from Islam into Judaism. The crime of relapsing from Islam into Judaism after conversion was punishable by death. Under the law of *force majeure*, no plea was admissible. The famous scholar Judah ibn Shoshan was seized and executed on charges of returning to Judaism. Indeed Maimonides had one time saved himself from a similar fate by the intercession of his friend, the Moslem poet and theologian, 'Abdu'l-Arab ibn-Muisha. Maimonides and his family later migrated to Maghrib, the extreme west of the Mohammedan world, but even there he found no peace. In fact, his position there became so hazardous that the Maimuni family resolved to leave Maghrib.

In the darkness of the night on the 18th of April, 1165, the family boarded a vessel bound for Palestine. For six days their voyage was calm, but on Saturday, the 24th of April, a terrific storm assailed the vessel, and shipwreck seemed imminent. When the danger passed, Maimonides, after the manner of the time, solemnly vowed that he would annually observe the 10th day of Iyar (i.e. April 24) as a fast day: "As on this occasion we were desolate and destitute of all succor but God's, so year by year on this day will I sit solitary, apart from all my fellow-men, to pour out my innermost soul before the Lord alone."

The boat finally landed at the port of Acre whence the family departed for Jerusalem. They stopped in the Holy City but a short time, and at the end of the same year (1165), they went to Cairo.

Soon after his arrival in Egypt, Maimonides' father died. "Following this physical sufferings threw young Maimonides in a bed of sickness; heavy losses diminished his fortune; informers appeared against him, and brought him to the brink of death." The final blow fell when his brother David perished in the Indian Ocean, and with him was lost not only their own capital, but also the money placed with the brothers by other traders. The loss of his brother affected him so much that he did not recover from this loss for many years. His letter to his friend, Rabbi Japhet of Acco (Acre), written long after the catastrophe, bears touching tribute to the close feeling that had united the brothers.[22] The letter reads:

"It is the heaviest evil that has befallen me. His little daughter and his widow were left with me. For a full year I lay on my couch, stricken with fever and despair. Many years have now gone over me; yet still I mourn, for there is no consolation possible. He grew up on my knees; he was my brother, my pupil; he went abroad to trade that I might remain at home and continue my studies; he was well versed in Talmud and Bible, and an accomplished grammarian. My one joy was to see him. He has gone to his eternal home, and has left me confounded in a strange land. Whenever I come across his handwriting or one of his books, my heart turns within me, and my grief reawakens. I should have died in my affliction but for the law which is my delight, and but for philosophy which makes me forget to moan."

After the death of his brother, Maimonides decided in favor of medicine as a means of earning a livelihood. At first he was unknown and his practice was not extensive. Alkifti informs us that he gave public lectures on philosophical subjects, but neither his medical nor his tutorial pursuits kept him from occupying his mind with the literary work which he had begun in his tender years in Spain and which had been continued off and on by land and sea during the vicissitudes of his troubled life.

After several years of practice, Maimonides' authority in medical matters became firmly established, and he was appointed private physician to Saladin's vizier. He was recommended to this high position by al-Kadi al Fadil al Baisami, a high officer of the state. Saladin, recognizing Maimonides' skill, bestowed upon him many distinctions. According to the Arabic historian al-Kifti, Maimonides declined a similar position offered to him by "the King of the Franks in Ascalon."[23]

In Egypt, Maimonides acquired exceptional renown on account of his profound erudition, and his great medical knowledge. Not only was he highly gifted, but he was a tireless worker with an inexhaustible zeal. He amassed an exceptional amount of knowledge in all branches of science. He particularly mastered Greek medicine and Aristotelian philosophy as is attested by his many-sided literary activities. As a religious teacher he endeavored to reconcile the fundamentals of religious belief with the dictates of reason and thought as is so amply demonstrated in his celebrated "The Guide for the Perplexed."

As a physician, Maimonides was both independent and practical, a soberly observing clinician, free from misconception and mysticism. He displayed in his diagnosis and therapeutics the Hippocratic spirit of "vis medicatrix naturae." He had a decided preference for dietetics as a form of treatment. Theoretically he was inclined to Galen, but he often manifested independence of the "Pergamen." He did not hesitate to criticize Galen when he disagreed with him.

In his "Treatise on Asthma," he refers to a discussion on the death of a royal patient, the Almoiavide Prince Ali ibn Yusuf ibn Tashfin, who died in the year 1142 after having been inadequately treated for an attack of asthma. Maimonides states that Abu Bekr Muhammad ibn Zuhr, son of the famous Avenzoar, and Abu Yusuf, son of the famous physician and poet, ibn al Maulim, conveyed to him the opinions of their fathers who had taken part in the consultation on the case of the Prince in the town of Marakesh.

It is certain that, in addition to his great theoretical knowledge obtained from the writings of Hippocrates and Galen, he also obtained in Morocco a large practical experience in medicine. It is doubtful whether Maimonides had access to the original Greek sources, and Galen was made available to him in the Arabic translations prepared in the ninth century by Hunain ibn Ishaq.

Perhaps Maimonides gained some of his clinical experience by accompanying his medical masters in Morocco, when they visited their patients. Maimonides was well acquainted with the writings of Rhazes whom he often quotes in his book, on "Ailments and Protection against their Dangers." The numerous Greek names of drugs and plants in his works are probably copied from Hunain's translation of the materia medica of Dioscorides, as revised in the tenth century by Hasdai ibn Shaprut. Maimonides refers to ibn Sina whose encyclopedic work, "Canon Medicinae," had been brought from the East. Other authorities often cited in Maimonides' works are Avenzoar, ibn Wafid, ibn Julful al Tamimi, al Ghafiki and ibn Janah.

Maimonides had no hospital at his disposal and presumably he did not have the facilities to give clinical instructions to his students. Evidently his lectures were largely of a theoretical nature but they unquestionably included his personal observations and experience.

In his day, the poor of the Egyptian capital were attended in the cellars of mosques and synagogues, reminiscent of the practice in the old temples of Aesculapius. The patients were brought in and left in the cellar under the main part of the house of prayer to sleep. This practice is a relic of ancient "temple sleep," known as "incubation."

When the present writer visited the synagogue of Rabbi Moshe of Fustat (named after Maimonides) in the year 1909, the sexton called his attention to an anteroom of the synagogue where patients were still brought to be cured.[24]

Among Maimonides' most devoted pupils was young Joseph Aknin of Aleppo, who, like many other of his kinsmen, had remained true to Judaism despite his superficial conformity to the dominant religion. Joseph was about thirty years old when the fame of Maimonides reached him. He hastened to leave his home to present himself before the master. On reaching Alexandria, he wrote to Maimonides, explaining his ardent ambition to learn from the lips of the teacher whose books had already gained such a wide reputation. Maimonides recognized in his correspondent a kindred mind, and welcomed Aknin with a cordiality that soon ripened into genuine affection. "If I had none but thee in the world, my world would be full," said Maimonides. Master poured out his heart to pupil, and when Aknin was forced to leave Cairo for Aleppo, the bond of affection between "father" and "son" was so firmly tied that their intellectual kinship endured unto death. It was for Aknin that Maimonides wrote his third great work, "The Guide to the Perplexed."

Arabic authors of unquestioned veracity have left records of Maimonides' medical activities in Cairo. The testimony of ibn al Qifti is particularly interesting.

"He settled in Fustat amongst the Jews, manifested his faith and inhabited a place called al-Masisa." Ibn al Qifti is evidently mistaken when he states that Maimonides earned his livelihood by commerce in precious stones. It was his brother, David, who had engaged in the jewelry business.

Maimonides and his students were in the habit of gathering together and reading the science and philosophy of the ancients. Offers came in seeking his medical services at the courts of kings. It is even believed that the Frankish King at Ascalon—probably Richard Coeur de Lion—sought out the good doctor, but Maimonides refused to accept this offer and persisted in his refusal. When al Muizz (i.e., Sultan Nur ad-Din) became the master of Egypt and the Alide (Fatimid) rule was overthrown, Qadi al-Fadil 'Abd ar-Rahim ibn 'Ail al-Baisani employed him as his personal physician and set a generous fee for his services.[25]

The famous medical practitioner, Abd al-Latif of Bagdad, to

whom reference has previously been made, undertook the journey to Cairo specially to make the acquaintance of three prominent men: One of these was Maimonides and the others were ibn al-Qifti (c. 1248), who was a personal friend of Maimonides' favorite pupil, Joseph ben Yehuda, and the famous medical historian, ibn Abi Usaybi's (c. 1270), who was a colleague of Maimonides' son, Abraham, at the Nasiri Hospital in Cairo.

Writing of his medical career in a letter addressed to his pupil Joseph ibn Aknin, Maimonides states: "You know how difficult this profession is for one who is conscientious and exact and who states only that which he can support by argument and authority."[26]

Maimonides derides medical superstition in the following words: "Fools have composed thousands of books vain and vacuous. . . . It is a fatal mischief that whatever is found in books is instantly accepted as truth, especially if the books are ancient." He further states: "Regard not all that you see in books as convincing proof. The liar lies with his pen as readily as with his tongue."[27] Elsewhere he remarks: "Astrology is a disease, not a science; a tree under the shadow of which all sorts of superstitions thrive, and which must be uprooted in order to give way to the tree of knowledge and the tree of life."[28]

Maimonides also declares: "Many pious Jews believe in the reality of witches and demons, but fail to realize that the Law commands all such things to be banished from sight because they are all falsehood and deceit as is the idolatry with which they are connected."[29]

Maimonides' deep sense of responsibility and devotion to his profession may be derived from the Prayer and Oath of the "Sage of Fustat," which reads:

"The Eternal Providence has appointed me to watch over the life and health of thy creatures. May the love for my art actuate me at all times: May neither avarice, nor miserliness, nor the thirst for glory, nor for a great reputation engage my mind; for the enemies of truth and philanthropy could easily deceive me and make me forgetful of my lofty aim of doing good to thy children. May I never see in the patient anything but a fellow creature in pain. Grant me strength, time, and opportunity always to correct what I have acquired, always to extend its domain: For knowledge is immense and the spirit of man can extend infinitely to enrich itself daily with new requirements. Today he can discover his errors of yesterday and tomorrow he may obtain a new light on what he thinks himself sure of today. O God, thou hast appointed me to watch over the life and death of thy creatures; Here I am ready for my vocation.

And now I turn unto my calling:

"O stand by me, my God, in this truly important task: Grant me success: For without thy loving counsel and support, man can avail but naught. Inspire me with true love for this my art and for thy creatures. O, grant that neither greed for gain, nor thirst for fame, nor vain ambition, may interfere with my activity. For these I know are enemies of truth and love of men, and might beguile one in the profession from furthering the welfare of thy creatures. O strengthen me. Grant energy unto both body and soul that I might ever unhindered ready be to mitigate their woes. Sustain and help the rich and poor, the good and bad, enemy and friend. O let me ever behold in the afflicted and suffering, only the human being."

With regard to his medical writings, with which we are presently concerned, it should be stated that he studied medicine from the same textbooks as did al Rhazes, ibn Sina, Avenzoar and Abulkasim. None of this famous group had access to original Greek sources and all of them followed the translations of Hunain Ibn Ishag and his school of translators.

Maimonides, like Rhazes, tempered ancient teaching with rational criticism based on direct observation. His methods of observation influenced later Christian physicians such as, for example, Henri de Mondeville and Guy de Chauliac. What Rhazes was in the East, Maimonides was in the West and what Abulkasim was to Arabic surgery, Maimonides was to Arabic medicine. He was the most distinguished physician of the Western Caliphate.

He carefully selected his material and his subject matter is systematically arranged. He showed great independence and originality in his practice. His medical works are written in the general style of Avicenna and Averroes.

He composed all of his medical works in the Arabic language and these were introduced to the Latin world largely via Hebrew translations. The most popular of his medical writings is the "Kitab al-Fusul fi-l-tibb" ("Medical Principles"), more often called "Fusul Musa" ("Moses' Aphorisms"; Hebrew: "Pirke Mosha"). This work is a collection of 1500 aphorisms extracted from Galen's writings, together with 42 critical remarks. Galen's thoughts are classified in 24 out of the 25 chapters devoted respectively: (1-3) to anatomy, physiology and general pathology; (4-6) to symptomatology and diagnosis, with special reference to pulse and urine; (7) to etiology; (8-9) to general and special therapeutics; (10-11) to fevers and crises; (12-14) to bloodletting, cathartics and emetics; (15) to surgery; (16) to gynecology; (17) to further etiology; (18) to gymnastics, massage, etc.; (19) to bathing; (20) to dietetics; (21-22) to drugs; (23) to Galenic ideas which are often misunderstood; and (24) to rare cases. In a final chapter (25), the author shows his independence. He does not hesitate to outline a general criticism of Galenic medicine and philosophy. In this work Maimonides shows his great ability as a systematizer of knowledge as is exemplified in the "Mishna Torah" ("Code of Jewish Law"). Thus while his medical writings are mostly summaries of other writers, he has selected his material according to his own liking and he has added his own experiences.

In the last chapter, he indicates some forty topics about which Galen contradicted himself and he ends this chapter with a discussion of Galen's teleological ideas from the biblical standpoint. This last chapter, the most important of the work, was apparently unfinished at the time of Maimonides' death. It was edited by his nephew, Yusuf ibn 'Abdallah Abu-l-Maali, in 1204-1205. The "Fusul" was translated into Hebrew under the title, "Pirke Mosha," by Zerahiah ben Isaac ben Shealtiel in Rome in 1277, and again by Nathan ha-Meati in Rome in 1279-1283.[30] It was reprinted in Vilna in 1885. The Latin translation which contains 260 pages is marked by the brevity that characterizes all his works.

Another work, "The Extracts" ("al-Mukhtasardt"), is a series of selections from the "Sixteen Books of Galen" and from five other books. Maimonides adopted the rule of not changing anything more than a conjunction or a participle in the wording of the books from which he made extracts. He contents himself with the mere selection of texts which he wished to insert in his "Extracts." He expressly states in the introduction to his "Aphorisms" that in "The Extracts," he had intended to prepare a selection from Galen's works for students, without any change in the text. There is no complete Arabic manuscript of these "Extracts" in existence, but several unpublished Hebrew translations are available.[31]

Hippocrates' "Aphorisms" had been translated into Arabic by Hunain ibn Ishaq (d. 873). Maimonides wrote a commentary to this translation, "Sharh Fusul Abu-Qrat," as many other Arab medical writers had done before him. Maimonides' professed intention was to follow generally the commentaries of Galen on this work, but from time to time he voices his own opinions. He reveals himself in this work as a severe critic. He does not accept all the sayings of the "divine" Hippocrates as sacred, but distinguished between the useful and the useless, the clear and the obscure, the true and the false aphorisms. This work was written in Arabic between 1182 and 1190 and was translated into Hebrew by Nathan ha-Mathi. A Latin translation was published in Bologna in 1489 under the title "Brevarium."

Maimonides' work on hemorrhoids ("Fi 'il Bawdsir") is a short treatise and was composed by Maimonides for the use of a young man of a noble family in Cairo. Maimonides divides his abstract into seven chapters, which deal with normal digestion, foods harmful to sufferers from hemorrhoids, foods beneficial to sufferers from hemorrhoids, and general and local (e.g. baths, oils, and fumigations) treatment. He disapproves of bleeding or operation except in cases of great severity. Maimonides emphasizes the causative effect of poor digestion and particularly constipation on hemorrhoids and he prescribes an efficacious diet, mostly of a vegetable nature. Tamarinds, myrobalans, spinach, and marshmallow are among the therapeutic agents recommended. In this work Maimonides cites Rhazes, Avicenna and ibn Wafid.[32]

The treatise on sexual intercourse ("Fi'l-Jima") written by Maimonides at the request of a nephew of Saladin, the Sultan al-Muzaffar 'Umar ibn Nur ad-Din, comprises nineteen chapters on the nature of man, on the utility and harmfulness of sexual intercourse, on the remedies to create and inhibit the desire for sexual intercourse and on all kinds of cosmetics. The text includes numerous prescriptions, mainly aphrodisiac and narcotic, and the number and variety of these are surprisingly great. The Hebrew translation of this treatise was made by Zerahiah ben Isaac ben Shealtiel. It was also translated, during the Middle Ages, into Latin.

The treatise, "Discourse on Asthma" ("Maqala fi'r-Rabw;" Latin: "Tractatus Contra Passionen Asthmatis"), was composed by Maimonides in about 1190 for a patient of high rank. In the introduction, Maimonides gives the complaints of the patient, which include angina and such violent headache that he was prevented from wearing a turban. The patient asked whether or not "a change of air" from Alexandria to Cairo would benefit him. Maimonides explains, in thirteen chapters, first, the general rules regarding diet and climatic conditions, and then the special diet suitable for sufferers from asthma. This is followed by prescriptions and a review of the effects on asthma of the climates of different countries of the Near East. He insists on the danger of the use of strong remedies for asthma, referring to the previously mentioned case of Emir 'Ali ibn Yusuf ibn Tashfin of Morocco, who died in 1142 because he took too strong a dose of theriac administered by his doctors.

The book on poisons and antidotes ("Kitab as-Sumum wa'l-Mutaharriz min al-Adwiya al-Quttala") is a treatise composed by Maimonides in 1199 at the request of his noble protector, the Vizier Al-Qadi al-Fadhil and Supreme Judge 'Abd ar-Rahim 'Ali al-Baysani. It was translated into Hebrew by Moses ben Samuel ibn Tibbon and (probably) by Zerahiah ben Isaac. From

Hebrew, it was translated into Latin, under the title, "Tractatus de Venenis," by Armengaud de Blaise, who also translated the treatise on asthma. A French translation was made by J. M. Robmonatz (Paris, 1865).

"In the month of Ramadan, 595 A. H. (corresponding to July, 1199 A.D.), al-Fadhil asked Maimonides to compose a short treatise on the treatment of cases of poisoning by venomous animals before the arrival of the physician or until the patient might reach the dispensary where the theriacs were kept. Maimonides reminds his patron of the great number of treatises on poisons, written by Arab authors, and proposes to give extracts from them, while mentioning a limited number of remedies only in order to make possible quick help in urgent cases."[33]

The first section containing six chapters, deals with the bites of snakes, the stings of scorpions, bees, wasps, spiders, tarantulas, and the bites of mad dogs. Maimonides warns against dressing the wounds immediately and advises letting the blood flow from them in order to carry away as much of the poison as possible. He also recommends a vegetable diet and the drinking of strong wine—treatment which is not at great variance with our present-day conceptions. He emphasizes that the length of the period of incubation of canine hydrophobia may deceive the doctor and patient, and he lays stress on the danger of the bite of man. The second section, in four chapters, treats of poisons and poisonous remedies, referring particularly to copper acetate, arsenic, yellow oxide of lead, hyoscyamus, the Solanaceae, poisonous narcotics, mushrooms and cantharides.

He gives very good descriptions of the symptoms of poisoning. For example, overdosage of Spanish fly produces hematuria and belladonna poisoning produces redness of the face. He states that the very complicated theriacs are not now esteemed as efficacious remedies.

Maimonides wrote his treatise "On the Regulation of Health" ("Fi Tadbir as-Sihba") a few months before his treatise "On Poisons," in the first year of the reign of Sultan Al-Afdal, at the request of the ruler himself. The Sultan was a frivolous and pleasure-seeking man of thirty, subject to fits of melancholia, due to his life of inordinate luxury, his intrigues, and his warlike adventures with his own relatives and the Crusaders. He complained to his physician, Maimonides, of constipation, dejection, evil thoughts, premonition of death, and bad digestion. Maimonides then produced the treatise in question, which very soon acquired a great reputation. Moses ben Samuel ibn Tibbon made a Hebrew translation from the Arabic in 1244. Two Latin versions were also made, one of them by the famous translator, John of Capua, a converted Jew (thirteenth century).

Maimonides composed this treatise in four chapters. The first is a short abstract of dietetics, mostly derived from Hippocrates and Galen. He discusses the qualities of various foods, especially different kinds of meats. He does not agree with Galen who advised against the use of fruits because they had apparently produced fever on himself. "What is good for one individual may be bad for another," says Maimonides. In Chapter II, he gives advice concerning hygiene, diet, and remedies for patients in the absence of the physician. Chapter III is the most interesting, as it shows Maimonides, as doctor, in the new capacity of "hygienist of the soul." After having dealt with laxative remedies and diet, according to Galen and Avenzoar, Maimonides describes in vivid language the erratic behavior pattern of individuals of an unsteady mind.[34]

Maimonides plaintively explains: "How often does there fall to someone's share a great fortune or a powerful position, and it is this that causes the decay of his body and the deterioration of his soul and character, shortens his life, and alienates him from his Creator, the Most High! What an eternal misfortune is this for him! On the other hand, how often does someone lose his fortune or his power, and it is this that strengthens his body, perfects his soul with moral qualities, prolongs his life, brings him nearer to the Lord, and incites him to devotion to His service. What an eternal happiness is this for him! (Your Majesty's) humble servant utters this according to the opinion of some ancient physicians, philosophers, and propounders of divine laws before the rise of Islam. Generally speaking, most of what the common people think to be happiness is in reality misfortune, and what is thought to be misfortune is happiness."[35]

In the fourth chapter, Maimonides devotes seventeen paragraphs to the hygiene of climate, dwelling-place, occupation, baths, sexual intercourse, wine-drinking, susceptibility to colds, and spoiled meat. The whole treatise is a short, but complete abstract of hygiene in an easily understandable form. It is no wonder, therefore, that this medical book of Maimonides met with such great success.

Probably the last of Maimonides' medical writings was his "Discourse on the Explanation of Fits" ("Magala fi Bayan al-A'rad"). It was composed in the year 1200, shortly before the Sultan Al-Afdal was deposed and four years before Maimonides' death. Evidently the ruler had not changed his vicarious mode of life and continued to suffer from fits of melancholia and dejection. He sent to Maimonides, who was ill in Cairo, a detailed report of the results of the consultations of his other physicians and he asked for his opinion and advice. Maimonides' answer is contained in a short abstract, which he addressed to "The King of Riqqa." It may be concluded from this title that the sultan had taken up his residence in a palace at or near the village of Riqqa in Upper Egypt, not far from the oasis of Al-Fayyum. Dr. Kroner has edited the Arabic text of this little treatise and a fragmentary Hebrew translation, with a German version and commentary.

Maimonides has written on a large variety of subjects in various books and letters addressed to his medical colleagues, royalty or lay friends. Many of his letters have been collected and published in Hebrew by Samuel ibn Tibbon (Vienna, 1874) under the title, "Iggereth Teman." Maimonides prided himself that he never failed to reply to any letter, except when he was too ill to write. He moreover tells us that he always answered with his own hand, and declined the use of a secretary, lest he be suspected of arrogance. This statement coincides with the discoveries in the Cairo *Geniza* where many questions addressed to him have been found with his autographed answer attached. His replies are as clear as they are terse. One cannot help but perceive in them the author's great qualities.[36]

It is due to his many letters that all the details of his active life are known. He was not a translator, but from the letter he had written to his friend Samuel ibn Tibbon (1198), he shows that he was familiar with the proper rules of translation:

"Let me premise one canon. Whoever wishes to translate, and purposes to render each word literally, and at the same time to adhere slavishly to the order of the words and sentences in the original, will meet with much difficulty. This is not the right method. The translator should first try to grasp the sense of the subject thoroughly, and then state the theme with perfect clearness in the other language. This, however, cannot be done without changing the order of words, putting many words for one word, or vice versa, so that the subject be perfectly intelligible in the language into which he translates." Maimonides then advises ibn Tibbon as to his course of philosophical reading. But the most fascinating passage is the one in which Maimonides describes his own manner of life:

"Now God knows that in order to write this to you I have escaped to a secluded spot, where people would not think to find me, sometimes leaning for support against the wall, sometimes lying down on account of my excessive weakness, for I have grown old and feeble.

"But with respect to your wish to come here to me, I cannot but say how greatly your visit would delight me, for I truly long to commune with you, and would anticipate our meeting with even greater joy than you. Yet, I must advise you not to expose yourself to the perils of the voyage, for beyond seeing me, and my doing all I could to honor you, you would not derive any advantage from your visit. Do not expect to be able to confer with me on any scientific subject for even one hour either by day or by night, for the following is my daily occupation: I dwell at Misr (Fustat) and the Sultan resides at Kahira (Cairo); these two places are two Sabbath days' journey (about one mile and a half) distant from each other. My duties to the Sultan are very heavy. I am obliged to visit him every day, early in the morning; and when he or any of his children, or any of the inmates of his harem, are indisposed, I dare not quit Kahira, but must stay during the greater part of the day in the palace. It also frequently happens that one or two of the royal officers fall sick, and I must attend to their healing. Hence, as a rule, I repair to Kahira very early in the day, and even if nothing unusual happens, I do not return to Misr until the afternoon. Then I am almost dying with hunger. I find the antechambers filled with people, both Jews and Gentiles, nobles and common people, judges and bailiffs, friends and foes—a mixed multitude, who await the time of my return.

"I dismount from my animal, wash my hands, go forth to my patients, and entreat them to bear with me while I partake of some slight refreshment, the only meal I take in the twenty-four hours. Then I attend to my patients, write prescriptions and directions for their various ailments. Patients go in and out until nightfall, and sometimes even, I solemnly assure you, until two hours and more in the night. I converse with and prescribe for them while lying down from sheer fatigue, and when night falls I am so exhausted that I can scarcely speak.

"In consequence of this, no Israelite can have any private interview with me except on the Sabbath. On that day the whole congregation, or at least the majority of the members, come to me after the morning service, when I instruct them as to their proceedings during the whole week; we study together a little until noon, when they depart. Some of them return, and read with me after the afternoon service until evening prayers. In this manner I spend that day. I have here related to you only a part of what you would see if you were to visit me.

"Now, when you have completed for our brethren the translation you have commenced, I beg that you will come to me, but not with the hope of deriving any advantage from your visit as regards your studies; for my time is, as I have shown you, excessively occupied."[37]

According to the Arabic medical historian, ibn Abi Usaibia (who served as physician at the hospital of Cairo where Abraham Maimonides was his colleague), the poet Alsaid ibn Sina wrote of Maimonides' greatness as a doctor in the following ecstatic verse:

"Galen's art heals only the body,
But Abu-Amran's the body and the soul
His knowledge made him the physician of the century.
He could heal with his wisdom the sickness of ignorance.
If the moon would submit to his art,
He would free her of her spots at the time of full moon,
Would deliver her of her periodic defects,
And at the time of her conjunction save her from her waning."[38]

The following of Maimonides' descendants were physicians: his son Abraham (1185-1254), his grandsons, David (1212-1300), and Obadiah, and the two sons of David, Abraham (Maimonides II) and Solomon Maimonides; also Obadiah's two sons, Isaac and Jacob and Abraham's son Moses; also Isaac's son Obadiah and Jacob's son Joshua. All of these physicians held the office of *Nagid*.

Maimonides' most famous pupil was Yusuf al-Saliti (c. 1226) of Aleppo. The contemporaries of Maimonides in Cairo were Imram al Isra Ali (1165-1239), Samuel abu al Nasr ibn Abbas (c. 1165), abu al Hasan (c. 1251), Jacob ben Ishaq (1250) and the pharmacologist, Abu al Muna al Kuhim (c. 1325).[39]

Although there was little unfavorable criticism of his medical works from his medical colleagues, his philosophical work, "The Guide for the Perplexed," created a severe tempest among theologians—particularly those of his own faith. This book brought Maimonides into conflict with religious leaders at home and abroad although the perplexities which Maimonides had derived are definitely not those of a sceptic. Maimonides remained firm in his religious thought although he was bewildered "on account of the ambiguous and figurative expressions employed in the Scripture." In a sense the problem before Maimonides was the same that faces all those who cannot serve two masters: reason and faith. Wherever possible, he tries to explain difficult passages in a rational sense. "Employ your reason," he says, "and you will be able to discern what is said figuratively, hyperbolically and what is meant in a literary sense."[40] He also affirms: "Those passages in Scripture which in their literal sense contain statements that cannot be proven must and can be interpreted otherwise."[41]

"The Guide for the Perplexed" (in Arabic: "Dalatat al-Ha-irin") was written for his beloved friend, Joseph ben Indah ibn Aknin, when Maimonides was 55 years old or 14 years before he died. It was translated into Hebrew by Samuel ibn Tibbon (c. 1204) under the title, "Moreh Nebuchim." The Arabic text of the "Guide" was edited by S. Munk and published in Paris (1856) from which the English translation was made by M. Friedlander, London, 1851, and reprinted in 1904.

The Latin translation of "The Guide for the Perplexed" was eagerly read in the universities during the Middle Ages. It had a great effect on the development of scholasticism.

The esteem in which Maimonides was and is held by his people may be inferred from the maxim: "From Moses (of the Scripture) to Moses (Maimonides) there arose no one like Moses."

CHAPTER XI

JEWISH CONTRIBUTIONS TO MEDICINE
IN THE MIDDLE AGES

It is difficult to differentiate between Jewish and Saracenic contributions to medieval medicine.[1] Both groups of contributors bore the same names, both wrote in the Arabic language and both used the same sources of information in their writings and in their practices. It is a fact that Jews have always taken a great interest in the arts and sciences and particularly in the science of medicine. Their contributions were not confined to one period, one country, or even one language. In every land where they have been scattered they have evinced a deep interest in medicine, but their activities were never more pronounced in proportion to the rest of the population than in the Middle Ages.

The tendency of the medieval Jews to enter the medical profession was unquestionably enhanced by the fact that they were excluded from most other occupations and from public office. Medicine was the only dignified calling that could be pursued by them independent of the state—even though, of course, even this occupation was not free of handicaps. Prejudice against Jewish physicians and bans against those using them often resulted in cruel persecution. There were numerous decrees forbidding Jews from practicing medicine and many ordinances prohibiting Christians from patronizing Jewish physicians. The maxim, "It is better to die than to owe one's life to a Jew" was widely quoted. Yet it is apparent that even in high places these restrictions were more often violated than observed.

Mohammedan and Christian rulers, when in need, frequently sought the advice of Jewish physicians. Caliphs usually maintained Jewish physicians at their courts and often preferred them to Islamic doctors who depended more largely on spiritual healing, astrology, and magic, in the treatment of disease.

In attempting to appraise the Jewish share in the catalysis of medieval European thought, it is important to distinguish between the activities of the Jews as translators or intermediaries and their direct and original contributions to learning and medical progress. In the latter category, the Jewish physicians were on no higher level than their non-Jewish confreres. It is largely as intermediaries or translators between Islam and Christiandom that the Jews effected their greatest service to civilization during the Middle Ages. Their knowledge of languages enabled them to translate from Arabic into Hebrew and from Arabic and Hebrew into Latin.

Even the Rabbis of the East employed Arabic when dealing with secular subjects. Rabbi Saadyah ben Yusuf (882-942), the dean of the Academy of Sura, wrote his philosophical work in Arabic, as did his younger contemporary, the physician, Isaac ben Solomon Israeli. Later, during the Spanish-Arabic period, the Jews of Spain spoke Arabic as their dominant language and cultivated Latin, the cultured language of the nearby European countries. They frequently translated the Arabic and Hebrew medical classics into Latin.

The Jews formed the intermediaries between the East and the West—between the Moslems and the Christians who were generally very antagonistic to each other. In their antagonism, both religious groups frequently let up from time to time in their persecution of the politically feeble Jews and permitted them to travel from one country to another. When the Jews were persecuted, this further stimulated them to travel. In consequence of these factors, the Jews carried not only merchandise from East to West and vice versa but also ideas.

In 847, Ibn Khordadhbeh, the Postmaster-General of the Caliphate of Bagdad, wrote his "Book of Ways," in which he gives a description of the routes taken by such Jewish intermediaries.

His account conveys a glimpse of the history of the Jews in the Middle Ages:

Routes of the Jewish Merchants Called Radanites

"These merchants speak Arabic, Persian, Roman, Greek, the languages of the Franks, Andalusians, and Slavs. They journey from West to East, from East to West partly on land, partly on sea. They transport from the West eunuchs, female and male slaves, silk, castor, marten and other furs and swords. They take ship in the land of the Franks, on the Western Sea, and steer for Farama (Pelusium). There they load their goods on the backs of camels and go by land to Kolzum (Suez) in five days' journey over a distance of twenty-five parasangs. They embark in the East Sea (Red Sea), and sail from Kolzum to El-Jar (Port of Medina) and Jeddah (Port of Mecca); then they go to Sind, India, and China. On their return they carry back musk, aloes, camphor, cinnamon, and other products of the Eastern countries to Kolzum and bring them to Farama, where they again embark on the Western Sea. Some make sail for Constantinople to sell their goods to the Romans; others go to the palace of the King of the Franks to place their goods." [2]

That these Radanites (Jews) acted as intermediaries in ideas as well as in commerce may be derived from a passage in the work of Abraham ibn Ezra (1092-1167)[3] which reads as follows:

"In olden times there was neither science nor religion among the sons of Ishmael . . . until the great King by the name Es-Saffiah (c. 70) arose who heard that there were many sciences to be found in India . . . and there came men saying that there was in India a very mighty book on the secrets of governments in the form of a fable . . . and the name of the book was 'Kalilah and Dimnah' . . . He sent for a Jew who knew both languages and ordered him to translate the book . . . and when he saw that the contents of the book was extraordinary—he desired to know the science of the Indians and accordingly sent the Jew to Arin, whence he brought back one who knew the Indian numerals and besides many astronomic writings."

Thus, according to ibn Ezra, a Jew was instrumental in bringing the so-called "Arabic numerals" from India to Arabia. Another Jew named John of Seville (c.1110-1180; known as Aven Deuth or Abraham ibn Daud) rendered the works of Mohammed al Khwarzimi on practical Indian arithmetic into Latin thus bringing this branch of mathematics within the grasp of Christian Europe.[4] Another Jew, Plato of Tripoli, who was Aven Deuth's friend, translated Abraham bar Hiyya's (1065-1136) geometrical work "Liber Embadorum," from Hebrew into Latin.

The "Toledo Astronomical Tables" (the so-called "Alfonsine tables"), edited by Abraham al Zarkali were worked out by Isaac ibn Sid (Don Zag) and other Jewish astronomers who translated them into Spanish for Alfonso of Castile. These tables were again adopted for use by the famous Jewish physician and astronomer, Isaac Israeli.[5]

During the fifth and sixth centuries A.D., under Byzantine domination, owing in part to disturbed political conditions and in part to superstition and the attention given to pseudo-sciences, medicine sank to a very low state. The persecution of the Jews under Honorius in 404-419, under Theodosius the Great (493) and under Kobad of Persia (520) culminated in the promulgation of widespread laws forbidding Jews to hold any public office or follow any handicraft. This influenced many young Jews to pursue a medical training.

With the spread of Mohammedanism, a great revival of the sciences took place in Western Asia. The Caliphs established colleges which included medical schools in Bagdad, Kufah and Basra and these were open to students and teachers of all races. Among the teachers and students of these schools, many bore Jewish names. At least one of the teachers at Bagdad was definitely a Jew (Joshua ben Nun). Even after a law was promulgated in Bagdad which prohibited Jews from teaching or studying medicine in any language except Hebrew or Syriac, the schools still continued to be attended by Jewish students.

The earliest known Jewish physicians during the Arabic Golden Age were Abu Hafsah Yazid (c. 643), physician to Caliph

Omar; Ishaq ibn Amram (c. 799), who wrote a treatise on poison; Masarjawaih of Basra (c. 883), physician to Caliph Muawiyyah I, who was induced by the Caliph to procure translations of works written in foreign languages. Masarjawaih personally translated from Syriac into Arabic, "The Pandects of Aaron," dealing with medicinal plants and foods. According to Sarton, Aaron Harun himself was a Jew.

The works of Masarjawaih, which are now lost, are frequently quoted by later Arabic writers. Masarjawaih wrote an original work "Ailments and Simple Drugs" which is quoted by the Arabian pharmacologist al Ghafik and other writers. Rhazes Aaron Harun himself was a Jew.[6]

Long before the decline of Alexandria, Cairo and Kairawan became the seats of colleges and medical schools where Jewish physicians flourished. At Kairawan (c. 793) lived the Jewish physician Shammakh. To his eternal professional discredit, it was he who poisoned Imam Idris by order of Harun al-Rashid.

At Algiers (ninth century), Ishaq ibn Imran was court physician to the Emir Ziyadat Allah II, and Ishaq ibn Imran the Younger, was court physician to the last Aghlabite Emir, Ziyadat III. Ishaq ibn Imran was born at Kairawan, the chief city of the Arabs in Barbary. He was a student at Bagdad and he translated the works of Aristotle, Galen and Ptolemy. It is related that one time he declined to treat the Emir when the latter was dissatisfied with his Christian physician. When the Emir indignantly demanded to know the reason of this refusal, the doctor replied: "The disagreement of two physicians is more deadly to the patient than tertian fever." Apparently this was the disease from which Emir Ziyadat Allah III was suffering. Imran the Younger's successor was the distinguished physician Issac ben Solomon Israeli (c. 832-932), who later became oculist and physician to the Fatimid Caliph Ubaid Allah al Mahdi al Kairawani.[8]

Sahl, or Rabban al Tabari (c. 800), who lived at Tabaristan on the Caspian Sea, was an eminent physician and mathematician. It was he who translated into Arabic the "Almagest" of the Greek astronomer Ptolemy. In about 850, his son, Ali ibn

Sahl ibn Rabban al Tabari (Abu al Hasan), lived in Iraq, where he became a convert to Mohammedanism. He was court physician to the Caliphs, al Mutasim and al Mutawakkil.

Ibn Abi Usaibia of Damascus (1203-70) enumerates fifty Jewish medical authors of Arabic countries. Chief among these were Isaac Israeli and Moses Maimonides. The former's contribution on fever and the latter's treatise on diet are particularly noteworthy. Both of these works were early translated into Latin and had a great influence on European medicine. They were used as textbooks in schools and were quoted by later writers as authoritative.

Jews played a particularly prominent part as translators, first from Syriac into Arabic, then from Arabic into Hebrew and finally from Arabic and Hebrew into Latin. The Jews were exceptionally active in adapting the Arabic medical works into Latin. The great medical work by Rhazes, "The Continens," was translated at Naples in 1280 by Moses ben Salomo Faraj (Farragut) at the request of Charles Anjou, King of Italy; and the "Colliget" of Averroes was translated by another Jew of Padua (1255) named Jacob Bonacosa. Jews also aided in the translation of Abulkasim's "al-Tasrif" and Avenzoar's "The Book of Simples and the Rules of Health" (1281).

The work of Maimonides on diet, "Regimen Sanitatis", written for the son of Saladin, may have no treatment value in the light of modern scientific therapeutics, but is of great value from the points of view of hygiene and preventive medicine. His doctrine of preservation of the soul is rational and forms an historical link with modern psychology.

The so-called psychosomatic approach of the modern physician is in reality only a rediscovery of what has been known to all great teachers from Hippocrates down to Charcot.

Maimonides recognized the relationship that exists between the psyche and the soma and the true interdependence of mind and body. He noted that a healthy person is cheerful and contented and that a sick person is depressed and displeased.

His book, "Regimen Sanitatis", served for many years as a textbook in the Academies and Universities and received the

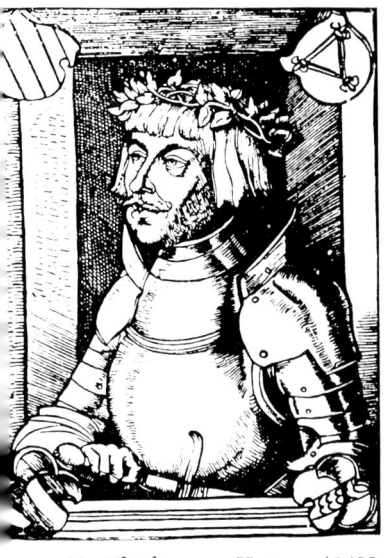

PLATE 61. Ulrich von Hutten (1488-1523). From a woodcut in Von Hutten's *Gesprachbuchlein*, 1519.
(Courtesy Armed Forces Medical Library, Washington, D.C.)

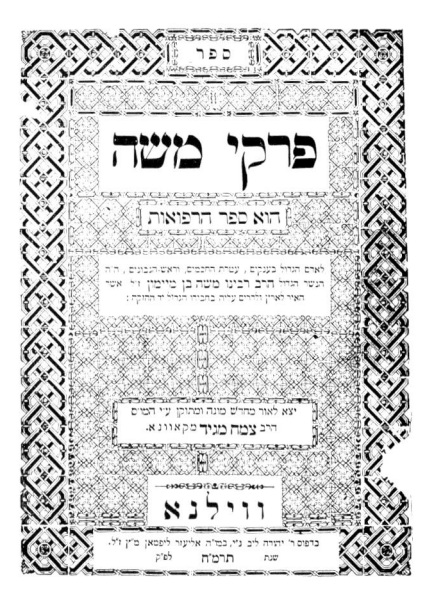

PLATE 62. Frontispiece of the Hebrew text of Kitab-al Fusul fi-l-Tibb under the title of Pirke Moshe Wilno in 1888.

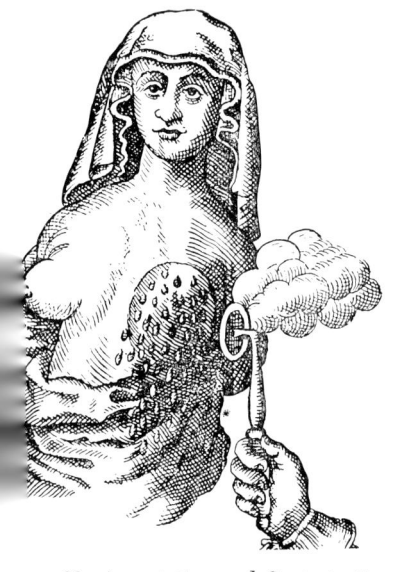

PLATE 63. Amputation and Cauterization of Breast, after Johann Schultes, 17th Century.

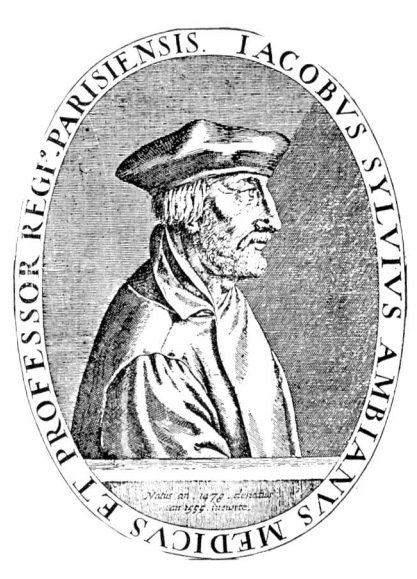

PLATE 64. Jacobus Sylvius, Teacher of Vesalius (1478-1555).

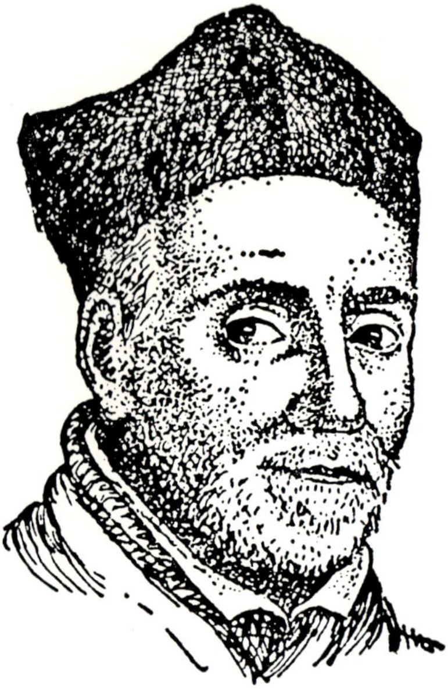

PLATE 65. Athanasius Kircher
(1602-1680)

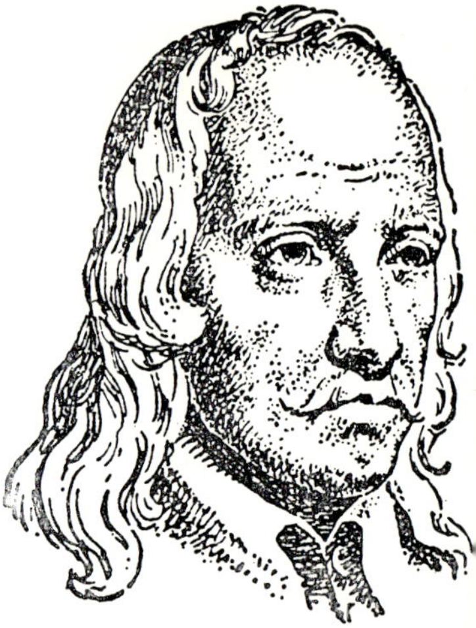

PLATE 66. Giovanni Alfonso Bore
(1608-1679). He evaluated the force
the heart beat at 180,000 pounds.

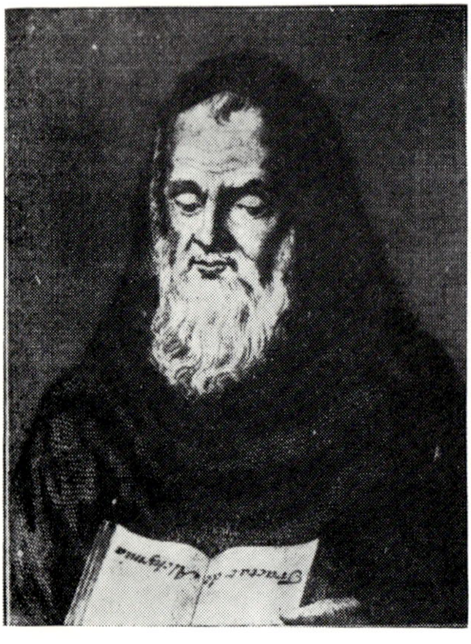

PLATE 67. Roger Bacon
(Courtesy Armed Forces Medical Library,
Washington, D.C.)

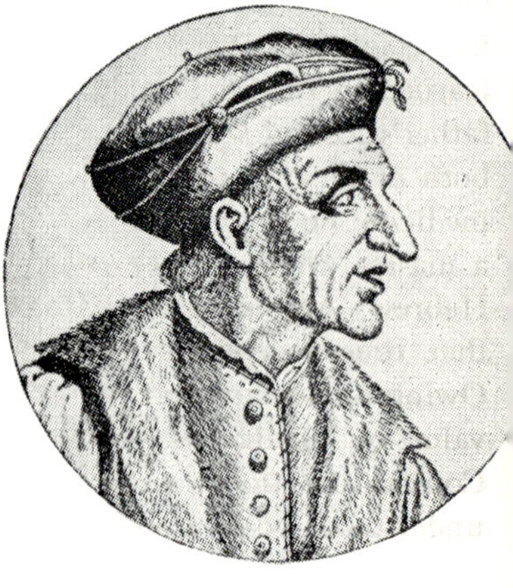

PLATE 68. Thomas Linacre (1460-15

recommendations of such men as Jehuda ben Samuel ben Abbas. In the fifteenth chapter of Jehuda's book, "Yair Nativ", he speaks of the "Regimen Sanitatis" as a most suitable book for the student. He considers Maimonides to be of the caliber of Avicenna, Galen, Rhazes, Averroes and Isaac Israeli. Sam Tob Falaquere (1260) in his "Ha-Mebakesh," mentions among many noted books the "Regimen Sanitatis" as a most valued book for students.

Among Saladin's physicians may be mentioned Nathaniel Israeli (c. 1150) known as "the Egyptian." He was also court physician to the last Fatimid Caliph of Egypt, Abu al Bayzan al Undawwar (c. 1184), as was Abu al Maali, brother-in-law of Maimonides. David ben Solomon (1161-1241) was connected with the hospital of Nasari in Cairo. Abu Mansur (c. 1125) was one of the physicians of Caliph al-Hafiz. Solomon ben Joseph (c. 1481), *Nagid* of Egypt (c. 1481), was physician to Sultan al-Milik al Ashraf.

When the Arabs crossed the Straits of Gibraltar and conquered Spain, Jewish physicians were found in the principal cities of Cordova, Seville and Toledo. One of the most noted of the Jewish doctors was Abu Yussuf Chasdai ben Isaac ibn Shaprut (915-970), a member of the learned family of ibn-Ezra. Chasdai was definitely a modern in his attitude. His easy-going and genial nature was free both from the heaviness of the Orientals and the gloomy earnestness of the Jews. His ancestors had come from Jaen. His father, Isaac, was wealthy, liberal and learned in the sciences. The son was constantly exposed to the father's love of science and his worthy application of riches and both of these attributes became part and parcel of Chasdai. In medicine he attained only a theoretical knowledge, but he was a master when it came to literature and diplomacy. He knew Hebrew, Arabic and Latin excellently. The last language at that time was understood primarily by the Christian clergy. Owing to the fact that the Arabic physicians placed such a high value on medical textbooks, Caliph Abdul-Rahman III asked Constantine, the Byzantine Emperor, to send him a scholar who understood both Greek and Latin to translate Dioscorides' materia medica. Constantine, who wished to show his good will to the Mohammedan court, sent a monk named Nicholas as translator. Of all the physicians of Cordova, Chasdai was the only one who understood Latin, and he was, therefore, requested by the Caliph to take part in the translation. Nicholas translated the original Greek version into Latin, and Chasdai retranslated Nicholas' version into Arabic. Abdul-Rahman was pleased with the completion of a work, which according to his own idea, added great splendor to his reign.

Caliph Abdul-Rahman III, appreciating Chasdai's value and usefulness, appointed him interpreter and diplomat. At first Chasdai accompanied the principal ambassadors to the Spanish Christian courts. Soon the Caliph rewarded him by appointing him to various high offices. Chasdai became minister of foreign affairs and at the same time held the posts of minister of trade and minister of finance—yet he had no official title. He was neither *nagid* (vizier) nor *katib* (secretary of state).

Chasdai, through his diplomatic facilities, was able to verify the persistent rumor of the existence of a Jewish state in the land of the Chazars. His letter to King Joseph is very interesting from an historical point of view.

Other distinguished physicians were Abu al Walid Merwan ibn Gasmah of Cordova (995-1045), and his grandson, Abu Merwan ibn Zuhr, who lived in Bagdad, Cairo and Spain. Abu al Walid Merwan ibn Gasmah, born in Cordova, was a famous physician of Saragossa, who was also known as a Hebrew grammarian. He had an excellent knowledge of the Hebrew and Arabic languages and spoke both fluently. He is the author of "Expositia Succinta" which treats of common remedies and of weights and measures used in medicine.[9] He died in 1121.

There were a number of physicians among the descendants of Maimonides including his son Abraham (1155-1254) and his grandson David (1212-1300). All of these occupied the exalted position of *nagid* (vizier).

The importance of the Jews in relation to Western scholasticism may be said to date from Caliph Abdul-Rahman, during whose reign Jewish scholarship was transferred from the East to Cordova. One of the most eminent of the Spanish Jews was the poet and philosopher Avencebrol (1022), otherwise known as ibn Gabrirol, or Jabirul. He is the author of "Fons Vitae" (Hebrew: "Mekor Hayyim") and is said to have introduced Neo-Platonism in the West. Avenpace (c. 1138), also known as ibn Bayya, author of "The Hermit's Guide," developed the Neo-Platonic interpretation of Aristotle which was used by Averroes. The Neo-Platonic philosophy that was developed in the Latin West was an adaptation of the teachings of Averroes. Averroes had no influence on the Arabians of the East.

Other Jewish physicians of note in Spain were the lyric poet, Judah ha-Levi (b. 1085); Sulaiman ibn al Musallim, court physician to Caliph Ali of Seville (1106-45); Abraham ibn Ezra (1092-1167) of Toledo who translated some works on astronomy; Judah ben Joseph ibn al-Fakhkhar of Saragossa, court physician to Ferdinand III; and Samuel ibn Wakar (died c. 1333), physician to King Alfonso XI.[10]

After the Arabs lost Spain, the intolerance of the Christian rulers forced many Jewish physicians to leave that country. Among the celebrated physicians that left Spain to escape persecution were the translator and physician, Moses ibn Tibbon (c. 1240-1283); and the philosopher and medical authority, Moses ibn al-Jazzar, author of "Zedat ha-Derakim" and translator of Hunain's "Introduction to Medical Science," and Rhazes' works on the classification of maladies and on antidotes.

Nathan ha-Meati of Cento, "the Italian Tibbonide," who lived in Rome (1279-1283), translated the following medical works: Ammar ben Ali al Mausuli's "Al-Muntahib fi'Ilaj al-Ain" on the treatment of diseases of the eye; the "Canon" of Avicenna and the "Aphorisms" of Maimonides. Many anonymous translations are attributed to Nathan ha-Meati including those of ibn al-Jazzar's "Memory and Amnesia," Abul Qasim's al-Zahrawi's "Tsarif," Galen's "On Ailments," Hippocrates' "On Airs, Waters and Places," and "Regimen in Acute Diseases" and Avenzoar's "Lamp of Health." All of these are reported to have been translated into Hebrew by Nathan ha-Meati or his son Solomon. The works of Avenzoar were translated into Latin by John of Capua, a Jewish convert to Islam.

Zerahiah ben Isaac ben Shealtiel who was born in Spain but lived in Rome (1277-1288), translated the first two books of Avicenna's "Canon," a medical work of Galen from the Arabic of Hunain ibn Ishaq, three chapters of Galen's "Katagne" and the "Aphorisms" of Maimonides.

Other important translations were those of Isaac ben Shem-Tob, who translated Rhazes' "Al-Mansure" and Zahrawi's "Al-Tasrif." Solomon ben Joseph ben Ayyub, who was born in Granada and flourished in Beziers, translated Avicenna's "Ardjuza." [11]

In 1412, when John II prohibited Jews from practicing medicine in Spain, some famous Jewish physicians migrated to France. This group included Judah ibn Tibbon, Joseph ben Isaac ben Kimhi, Isaac ben Shem-Tob and Solomon ben Joseph ben Ayyub. Others went to Algiers including Simon bar Zemah Duran. Still others sought refuge in Italy, including Joshua ben Joseph ibn Vives Al-Lorqui, who became physician to Pope Benedict XIII after he was converted to Christianity and assumed the name, Hieronymus de Santa Fe. It was this physician who arranged for the famous disputation at Tortosa between Christian and Jewish scholars in 1414.

In Portugal the following Jewish doctors flourished: Moses Solomon, physician to Ferdinand I and John I; Gedaliah ibn Yahya the Elder (c. 1300), physician to King Diniz; Gedaliah ibn Yahya the Younger (c. 1476), physician to Alfonso V, who later emigrated to Turkey because of religious persecution; and Drs. Joseph Vizisch and Rodriquez, physicians to John II of Portugal (1481-90), who were members of the commission appointed by the King to examine and to pass upon the request of Columbus for ships. Amatus Lusitanus, a prominent Portugese Jewish physician towards the end of the fourteenth century who was driven out of Portugal by the inquisition, became famous in Antwerp. As the inventor of an obturator for cleft palate and a bougie, he enjoyed a great reputation as a surgeon in Lisbon. He performed a successful operation for emphysema.[12]

In his "Memoirs," Jean Astruc (1684-1766), who had studied medicine in Montpellier, where he had taken his medical degree in 1703, and where he had become professor in 1715, lauded the Jewish participation in the early years of that University. He states: "Numerous Arabs and Jews mingled with the native population and joined with them in contributing physicians, for they were then the two nations most learned especially in medicine and in natural sciences."[13] He cites early references to Jewish physicians[14] and says: "We must also acknowledge that it is to them (i.e., the Jews) that the Faculty of Montpellier owes much of its reputation which it had in its beginning, because they were, during the tenth, eleventh and twelfth centuries, almost the sole depositories of this science in Europe and it is through them that it was communicated from the Arabs to the Christian World."[15]

At the beginning of the fourteenth century, the center of Mohammedan learning moved westward and no more Jewish physicians are met with in Iraq after that date. The sciences followed the conquering armies of the Arabs from Asia Minor through Egypt, and the Mediterranean countries to Spain, southern France, Sicily, and to Italy, where they became crystallized in the School of Salerno.

From this School proceeded Hananeel of Amalfi, Abu al-Hakim of Turin, and Faraj ben Salim (Faragut). The last lived in Salerno about 1250, and was physician to Charles of Anjou, King of Sicily. He was one of the first physicians to translate medical works into Latin. Capho, another Jewish doctor of Salerno, in the twelfth century wrote a primer on the dissection of the pig ("Anatomia Porci") which was reprinted in the little anatomic manual of Dryander in 1537.[16]

While the University of Salerno was flourishing, Jewish schools, where medicine was taught, existed in the south of France. About the year 1000 Rabbi Abon was principal of the Jewish school at Narbonne and one of his pupils founded the Jewish medical school at Montpellier (c. 1025). Such unimportant schools as these developed into the great universities of France —Paris, Narbonne, and Montpellier—which soon were to eclipse Salerno. Paris University was always a seat of orthodox Christian theology and only a few Jewish physicians are met with there at the end of the thirteenth century. These include the physicians Copin and Moses, Rabbi Isaac and his son Vital. The University of Paris was closed to Jews in 1301.

In 1350, Jews were permitted to return to France and we soon meet with names of Jewish doctors and especially court physicians (e.g., Samuel and Meshullam ben Avigdor at Montpellier; Elias of Arles (c. 1407) at Valence; Jacob Lunel, the Surgeon Dolan and the physician Bellan at Carcassonne).

The Jewish physicians were among the first to profit by the decrees of William VII, Lord of Montpellier (1181), which led to the opening of a school for teaching medicine in Montpellier. There is nothing in the statutes of the University to indicate that it refused to accept Jews as students or to grant them diplomas, but laws were, from time to time, promulgated against Jews as teachers and practitioners of medicine (e.g., the edicts of Count William in 1180, of the Council of Beziers in 1246 and of Alby in 1254). In 1293 a law was enacted punishing with three months' imprisonment Christian patients who accepted treatment from Jewish physicians. In 1306, Philip of Arlois expelled all Jewish physicians from the city of Montpellier.

Notwithstanding this repressive legislation, the University of Montpellier was celebrated for its great liberality, and Christians, Jews and Moslems taught and studied in this institution together. In marked contrast to the scholasticism of the University of Paris, Montpellier from its very inception had on its teaching staff instructors from Spain who were imbued with the philosophy of Averroes.

The Universities of Italy appear frequently to have been especially liberal towards Jewish professors and students and Jews were frequently called upon to lecture on medicine and philosophy. Despite the Constitution of the University of Padua, which contained the "irrevocable and unchangeable" clause to the effect that no Jew may be admitted to any examinations for the doctorate or any other honorable degree,[17] Jewish students were admitted to the University of Padua.

In the latter half of the fifteenth century the great Jewish philosopher and physician, Elijah Delmedigo (1460-1497), by reason of his high reputation, "was chosen by the University of Padua, with the approval of the Venetian Senate, as umpire in a dispute on some philosophic subject between the professors and students of the university."

It is recorded that Rabbi Abraham de Balmes (?-1523), physician to Cardinal Grimani in Padua and noted author and translator (both into Hebrew and Latin), held lectures on philosophy before Christian audiences at Padua. He had taken his degree of Doctor of Philosophy and Medicine in Naples in 1492.

Parenthetically, it may be stated here that the students of Padua customarily stole Jewish corpses for anatomical purposes from the burial places. The Jews paid large sums of graft to prevent the bodies of their revered dead from being snatched from the cemeteries. Later grave snatchers were severely punished and students were obliged to submit to the will of the authorities.

(Jacob Mantino (b. 1490), a distinguished papal physician, lectured on medicine in Bologna in 1529 and at the Sapienza in Rome in 1539, during the pontificate of Paul III).

Before the graduation at various Italian universities, Jewish students were required to deliver 170 pounds of confetti to the Christian students. It is interesting to note, however, that students were compelled to invite the whole student body to dinner. Their graduation fees were larger than those of the Christian students. It is interesting to note, however, that Jewish students were exempted from wearing the Jewish hat, but were forbidden to practice medicine among either Jews or Christians.

Following an old custom, when the first snow of winter had fallen, all citizens were required to pay a certain tax to the students (six ducats). Even when this "celebration of the first snow" was abolished in 1633, Jews were still compelled to continue payment of the tax.

The reader may have observed that the Hebrew physicians who participated in the various translations, first from Syriac into Arabic, then from Arabic into Hebrew, and finally from Arabic and Hebrew into Latin, employed Hebrew as a medium of translation but not as a vehicle for original work. There are two Hebrew authors who are exceptions to this rule and who used Hebrew in original works: Asaf Judaeus and Sabbatho ben Abraham ben Joel (Donnolo). Because of the great historical value of their works these physicians will be discussed herein in some detail.

ASAF JUDAEUS

One of the most distinguished medical authors during the early Arabic Period is Asaf Judaeus. Very little is known of his life. Sarton dates his birth to the ninth and tenth century.[18] Venetianer maintains that Asaf flourished in the seventh century.[19] Recent studies by Muntner show that his birth took place a century earlier (sixth century), soon after the closure of the Jerusalem Talmud. Muntner also states that Asaf lived in Israel (Palestine) in the neighborhood of Tiberias (a great literary center at that time) and that he studied in Alexandria.[20]

His work "Sefer Asaf" is probably the earliest medical work written in Hebrew (Mishnaic). It is variously known as "Sefer Asaf," "Midrash Asaf" or "Midrash Rephuah."

Four different copies of this manuscript are extant. The contents of these manuscripts vary in minor detail, but in main, they all contain treatises on anatomy, physiology, embryology, diseases of various organs, hygiene, medicinal plants, antidotes for various poisons and urinoscopy. This work also contains aphorisms and names of medical plants. According to Steinschneider, the aphorisms are those of Hippocrates and the medicinal plants bear a resemblance to those described by Dioscorides.

The Munich manuscript is the most complete, containing 396 pages. This manuscript deals with the blood, bones, brain, bile, heart, kidneys, liver and spleen, and with diseases of these organs. Embryology occupies an important place. The etiology of disease is ascribed to an imbalance of the four humors. The body is described as being composed of four elements.

The significance of the pulse, urine and fever in various diseases is discussed and prognosis finds a prominent place in this book. Antidotes to various poisons are listed. One hundred and twenty-three different herbs are mentioned, and their therapeutic uses are noted.

The Munich manuscript cites two authorities: "The Book of Wisdom of India" and "A Book of the Ancients." The latter work may be the "Corpus Hippocraticum." The Oxford manuscript names such authorities as Mar Mor, a Christian of Salerno; Mar Joseph, a physician; Rudolph, a physician of Worms, and Samuel the physician. According to the names cited, the authorship of the book was as late as the thirteenth century, but some authorities are certain that these names were added many centuries after the book was composed.

The author's name varies in the various manuscripts: He is known as "Asaf he-Hakam" (Asaf the Wise). In the Bodleian manuscript, the author is called Johanan ha-Jericho. In another place, in the same manuscript, he is referred to as Judah ha-Jerichoni and in a still later section he is called Samuel Yarhinai. The last name evidently refers to the famous physician and astronomer, Mar Samuel (second century, A.D.). The author is elsewhere referred to as Asaf ben Berechiah ha-Yarhoni (Asaf, the Astronomer).

All through the work it becomes evident that Asaf was acquainted with the medical works of the Greek masters as well as the medical dicta of the Talmud.

In anatomy he did not always follow the Greek masters. He differed from Hippocrates and Galen as to the number of bones in the human skeleton. According to Asaf there are 248 bones as are enumerated in the Mishna;[21] Hippocrates finds 92 bones while Galen counts about 200. Asaf follows the Talmud with reference to the blood vessels. He knows the difference between the veins and the arteries, and he counts both as 360.[22]

Asaf knew the position of the internal organs and their relationship to each other. He gives a description of the blood vessels, and how they ramify to the internal organs and all over the body. Of course, he has erroneous ideas about the circulation of the blood. He understands the phenomena of the respiratory and digestive systems and he gives a good description of the latter (Galenic).

PHYSIOLOGY

He premised the entire function of the human body upon the four elements (fire, earth, air and water), the four humors (blood, yellow bile, black bile and phlegm) and the four properties (warmth, moisture, coldness and dryness). As to the four elements, Asaf states: "Fire could not burn without air and has no basis without earth. The earth could not exist with too much water without having the fire to dry it out. . . . Through the air the fire burns into flames. . . . Water extinguishes the fire: They cannot tolerate each other but water agrees with earth. The earth subdues fire and is effected by air." Thus, if the four elements in the human body have counterbalance of opposing elements, a person is well. A disturbance of the elements is the cause of disease.

The brain is located in the head and is compared to a king in his palace who rules over his state.[23] The phlegm rules the person, from the brain, whence it extends through the spinal canal to the sacrum and to the ribs where it is localized in the chest cavity. Because phlegm originates from the brain it is more powerful than the three other humors. The intellect is in the brain and is supported by the living soul. It is conveyed via the blood vessels over the entire body.

The primary life-giving element of the body is the blood which originates in the liver where the red gall bladder is situated. The gall bladder has two openings; through one the red gall goes up to the brain and through the other to the lower parts of the body. Close to the kidneys, the black gall is mixed with the red gall and predominates.

Asaf appears to have been a follower of the *Pneumatics*. He believes with Mar Samuel that disease originates from the *"pneuma"* (air). His concept of embryology is largely Talmudic (some of which may also be traced to the Greeks): A union of the male sperm with that of the female egg takes place in the uterus. In 40 days the embryo may be detected.[24] The embryo is matured in 9 lunar months of 28 days each.[25] There are three partners in the child: The nerves, blood vessels, bones, membranes and brain, are derived from the father. The flesh, skin and blood from the mother. The spirit, soul and wisdom from God.[26] The identity of the fetus' sex may be recognized in 90 days.[27]

To the modern physician, Asaf's physiology and pathology appear to be jumbled. However, if one considers the author's time and locale, he will find that his descriptions of diseases and their remedies are far superior not only to those of his contemporaries but also to his successors for many centuries after him.

Asaf gives us vital information on the physician's art and ethics. His ethical concepts on every page of his work challenge our thinking. He admonishes his pupils to attend to the poor and disabled without fee. He believes that before a physician enters his profession he should carefully study the causes of disease. He warns physicians that, in treating a case, a careful examination should be made of local climatic and health conditions. Asaf states: "It befits the sage when he sees the man, to know and discern the signs of the diseases and the pains according to the deviation of the four elements and to arrange the therapy so that he may be strengthened. And it is befitting to the sage to be careful and to know the signs of the diseases according to their periods, to heal their infections according to their periods and also to cure with a selection of medicines which are suitable for healing."[28]

The Oath of Asaf the Physician

And this is the covenant which Asaf the son of Berekyahu and Johanan the son of Zavda made with their disciples and caused them to swear in the words of the vow:

Do not be a party to killing a soul by an abortifacient, nor give a woman who has conceived illicitly to drink (thereof) so that she may abort. Do not covet beauty among women to commit adultery with them. Do not reveal the secret of a man who has confided in you. Do not take any bribe to ruin or destroy. Do not harden your heart to the point of refusing to heal the poor and needy. Do not say "bad" of the good, nor "good" of the bad. Do not walk in the rules of sorcerers to bewitch, enchant and cast spells so as to separate a man from the woman of his bosom or a woman from the husband of her youth; nor so as to covet any wealth or bribe to promote lewdness; nor so as to participate in any worship of idols to cure thereby, nor to inspire confidence in the healing power of any part of their worship; but instead to detest, abominate, and to loathe all of their devotees and those who trust in them and those who inspire confidence in them. For all of them are vanity and cannot help. For they do not exist. Satyrs, dead spirits are they. They will not save their corpses, so how can they save the living? So now believe in the Lord your God, the God of truth, the living God, for he kills and quickens, smites and heals, teaches man to know and also to be of avail, smites in righteousness and judgment, heals in kindness and mercy. Crafty schemes cannot be hidden from him, nor is anything concealed from his eyes. He grows curative plants, and puts in the heart of the wise, ability to heal, in the multitude of his kindnesses, and to relate wonders in the assemblage of many. So that all living may know that he is his maker, nor is there a savior beside him. The nations trust in their images who cannot save them from their difficulties nor rescue them from their troubles. For their hope and prospect are for the dead. Therefore it behooves you to separate from them and to turn aside and be distant from all the abominations of their idols and to cling to the name of the Lord, God of the spirits of all flesh, in whose hand is the soul of all living to kill and to quicken, nor can any rescue from his hand. Remember him at all times and seek him in truth, uprightness and perfection of way, so that you may prosper in all your deeds and he will grant to you help to prosper by your hand and be congratulated in the mouth of all flesh, and so that all the nations may abandon their idols and desire to worship the Lord like you. For they will recognize that their confidence is vanity, and in vain is their toil for they cry to a god that can do no good or save. But you, be strong and do not let drop your hands for there is a reward for your work and the Lord is with you as long as you are with Him. If you keep his covenant and walk in his statutes to cling to them, you will be reckoned as his holy ones in the eyes of all flesh, and they will say: "Happy is the people for whom it is thus; happy the people whose God is the Lord."

And their disciples answered and said:

All you have admonished us and commanded us, we will do. For it is a commandment of the law, and we must perform it with all our heart, and all our soul and all our might; to do, to hearken, and not to swerve aside nor turn right or left.

And they blessed them in the name of God the Most High, Creator of Heaven and Earth. And they further adjured them and said to them: "Behold the Lord God and his Holy Ones and his Law are witnesses against you that you shall fear Him and not deviate from His commandments, but walk in His statutes and rightness of heart; not to incline after gain to aid the godless against innocent blood, nor to mix deadly poison for any man or woman to kill his neighbor; nor to tell their ingredients nor to transmit them to anybody, nor relate any of their words, nor to put bloodshed in any work of healing, nor to be a party of stirring up illness against anyone, nor to inflict a blemish on a person by hastily cutting human flesh with an iron instrument or cauterizing with fire until it has been tested two or three times— (only) then shall you give your counsel. A haughty spirit shall not dominate you for the uplifting of your eyes and heart. You shall not bear the grudge of any enmity against a sick person, nor change your word by anything the Lord our God hates to do, but keep His orders and commandments to go in all His ways, to find grace in His eyes, to be innocent, faithful and right.

Thus did Asaf and Johanan make their disciples swear.

DONNOLO (c. 913-982)

One of the famous physicians of the Middle Ages was Sabbatho ben Abraham ben Joel, commonly known as Donnolo. He was born in Uria, near Otranto, Italy.[29] At the age of twelve he was captured by a band of Saracens and taken off to Palermo. He was redeemed by his father who had been banished with his family to the same city. According to Sarton he was a keen student of the Arabic language.[30]

Donnolo was the first Jewish medical author in the West to write in Hebrew (Asaf Judaeus wrote in Hebrew also but he was probably from the East). According to his own statement, he studied medicine for forty years before he considered himself qualified to teach Jewish physicians the art and practice of medicine.[31]

It is not known where he received his medical education. There were few lay physicians at that period in Italy and medicine was largely in the hands of clerics and administered from the monasteries. He probably obtained his first knowledge of medicine from the books that had been translated from the Greek into Arabic by Hunain ibn Ishaq. In accordance with the custom for physicians in those days, he traveled first to medical centers of his own country (Italy) in search of medical knowledge. It is known that he lived for a time in Salerno which was then a young institution but it is not known whether he was a student or a teacher there. Aside from Uria (near Otranto) he practiced in Martis near Russano, and in the province of Calabria.[32]

Contemporary writers refer to Donnolo as "learned and exceptionally wise in medicine." In the biography of St. Nilus, reference is made to Donnolo in the following paragraph:

"On the next day the Saint came down from that place, and when he had entered into the city, there came to him a certain Jew, Donnulus (Donnolo) by name, who had been known to him from his boyhood, because he was studious to a very high degree, and was learned in the medical art in no common way. He therefore began to speak to the Father thus: 'I have heard of your severe mode of life in which you train yourself, and of your great abstinence, and I was surprised, knowing the habit of your body, that you have not fallen into a decline. Therefore if you are willing, I will give you a drug befitting your temperament, so that after that in your whole life you may fear no sickness.' And the great Father said: 'One of you Hebrews said to us: "It is better to trust in God than to trust in man." We, therefore, do not need drugs made by you. You indeed would not otherwise have been better able to make sport of more simple Christians than if you had boasted that you had given Nilus of your drugs.' The physician, hearing this, answered nothing." [33]

Donnolo's work, which was written in 946, enumerates 120 remedies which, according to Steinschneider,[34] are based upon Greek sources—mainly Dioscorides—and are fairly free from Arabic influence which in his day dominated over medical science. It is possible, however, that he consulted the Arabic translations of Hasdai ibn Shaprut and it is certain that he saw the book of Asaf. Donnolo often uses Asaf's Hebrew terminology in both of his works, notwithstanding the fact that he does not mention Asaf by name.[35] The writing contains a description of the medicinal plants and their preparation made up "according to the wisdom of Isias and the Greeks" and "according to his own (i.e. Donnolo's) experiments in the practice of medicine during forty years."

The other medical book by Donnolo is the "Antidotarium" which is extant in manuscript, but apparently has never been published.

In his commentary on the "Book of Creation," Donnolo refers to anatomy and physiology. His works as have been stated, represent the very first medical treatises in the West written in Hebrew and are distinguished for their originality and independence.

The next Jewish medical author of note to write in Latin was Alcandurs (Alexander) who flourished in the middle of the tenth century. His occasional use of Hebrew script and repeated use of Hebrew equivalents of the names of constellations and planets indicates that he was definitely a Jew.[36]

There were also Jewish women physicians in the late Middle Ages. Prominent among this group was Sarah la Mirgesse, a Jewess living in Paris in 1292, who practiced medicine. One of the most interesting notes on medieval Jewish women physicians is found in the early records of Marseille which testify to an agreement in the year 1326 between one Sarah de Saint Gilles, widow of Abraham, and Salvet de Bourgneuf, the son of David. Sarah agreed to teach Salvet the "artem medicine et phisice" for the period of seven months; and she further agreed to board, lodge and clothe Salvet. In return the pupil guaranteed to relinquish all fees, which he might receive during his apprenticeship, and turn them over to his instructress.[37]

Another record testifies to the fact that the wife of Pasquale, a physician of Catania, in Sicily, was examined in 1376 by the physicians of the Royal Court and obtained permission to practice medicine throughout the kingdom and to devote herself to the treatment of the poor who were unable to pay the large fees of other physicians.

In the German states, Jewesses were often found engaged in the practice of medicine—especially as oculists. Kunrat von Ammenhausen, a Swiss poet of the fourteenth century, complained that Christians are so foolish that they call in a Jew or Jewess in case of illness.[38]

The Jewish women physicians were no less the object of opposition than their brothers; as an instance may be mentioned the complaints of a Doctor Roslin, who protested, in 1511, against granting licenses to "disgraceful Jews and Jewesses."

Archbishop John II, of Wurzburg, in 1419, granted a license to one Jewess, Sarah of Wurzburg, to practice medicine throughout the bishopric. The terms of this document are interesting: "Concerning the Jewess, the doctoress, franchised for (the past) three years; 1419. We, John, etc., make known, etc., as heretofore agreed upon, that Sarah the Jewess, the doctoress, is to pay annually four golden pence, two florins, and in addition also ten florins for taxes and as a voluntary contribution (*"lipniss"*). Thus we shall let it stand for the time as thus agreed upon for the next three full years so that she may practice her profession without interference on our part or of those belonging to us, unconditionally, and should anyone intend to prosecute her or actually do so, against such one we shall take action to the best of our ability so that he be stopped, unconditionally. Dated the spring of 1419." [39]

Another case is narrated by Rabbi Judah ben Asher (1270-1349), who was born in Germany: "When I was three months old I suffered with my eyes and did not get better.... When I was three years old I was confined to the house for one year because I could not see my way, until a Jewess came, skilled in the healing of the eyes and she treated me for two months. But for the two months she treated me I might never have seen any more." [40]

In the Archives of Frankfort-on-the-Main there is recorded the payment of one florin to Barbara, the daughter of a deceased physician, for the medical attention she administered to the soldiers who had fallen at Wissenkirchen in 1394.[41]

In 1439, in this same city, we learn that "Judenartzin" were ordered to leave the city or "pay the taxes like other Jews." A Jewish doctress, in 1457, was forbidden to remain in Frankfort unless she paid the "Nachtgeld." [42]

In closing our discussion of medieval Jewish contributions to medicine, and science, the present author is tempted to cite the view of an eminent modern historian on the subject. Matthias Jacob Schleiden (1804-1881), the famous German philosopher, scientist and originator of the cellular theory, writes: "All Europe had its Middle Ages, a period of barbarism, of intellectual and moral decay as deplorable as any that can be conceived. Only the Jews formed an exception, despite depression and oppression which often robbed them of fortunes. Every affliction, however bitter and severe, only served to enable them to quicken their higher mental and moral efforts. . . . They continued to develop their intellectual life without interruption to the end of the Middle Ages, preserving and translating for other nations the bases of morality and of mental life. Like all nobly endowed nations, they were stimulated now and then during happy moments when the burden of existence was lightened, but every reverse of fortune, every affliction, however bitter and severe, only served to stimulate them to higher moral and mental levels." [43]

Rudolf Virchow, the founder of cellular pathology, said:

"In early medieval times it was the Jews and the Arabs who made a definite impression upon the progress of medical science. In our times Hebrew manuscripts have been brought to light which show with what zeal and learning Jewish physicians of early medieval times were active in the preservation and advancement of medicine. We may in truth say that down to these times the hereditary talent of Jews, which has contributed so much that is great to science, can often be discerned." [44]

Colonel F. H. Garrison remarked:

"The Hebrew and Mohammedan physicians, with their peculiar analytic cast of mind, their intensive modes of thought and their appreciation of 'values', soon acquired a right materialistic way of looking at concrete things. Thus while medical men under Christianity were still trifling with charms, amulets, saintly relics, the Cabala, and other superstitions, many of the Jewish and Mohammedan physicians were beginning to look upon these things with a certain secret contempt." [45]

CHAPTER XII

SCHOLASTICISM AND MEDICINE

Scholasticism is a term usually employed to denote the system of philosophy and theology of the schoolmen in the Middle Ages, whose knowledge was based on the authority of books and on abstract theory rather than on life. This method of thought, after centuries of intellectual darkness, appears to have dawned in Western Europe contemporaneously with the consolidation of the Empire of Charlemagne. This liberal monarch attracted to his court the most learned men of Western Europe for the purpose of enhancing the spread of education among the peoples of his Empire. In 787, he ordered the establishment of schools in every abbey of his realm. Among his most prominent advisers were the two scholars, Peter of Pisa and Alcuin of York (735-804), who endeavored to obliterate the wide gap existing between religious and secular learning.

Charlemagne's schools eventually developed into centers of medieval learning and speculation. The pupils were instructed in the seven liberal arts: the trivium—grammar, rhetoric and logic; and the quadrivium—arithmetic, geometry, astronomy and music. The title "doctoris scholasticus" was applied originally to any teacher of such a school. Gradually dialectics and logic eclipsed the elementary discipline and the designation "doctor" was bestowed on anyone who occupied himself with logic, theology and philosophy by the dialectics method of reasoning.

The founders of scholasticism were Johannes Scotus Erigena (known as John the Scot, 800-879) and Gerbert (died 1003), who affirmed that all authority came from reason, but reason never from authority. After an acquaintance had been formed with the writings of Aristotle and his Arabian interpreters, Bishops Lanfranc (1005-1089) and Anselm of Canterbury (1035-1109) became promoters of the scholastic philosophy. Alexander of Hales (died 1245) was the first to make philosophy subservient to theology, a thing which had not been done by the earlier scholastics.

Scholasticism reached its highest development during the twelfth, thirteenth and fourteenth centuries. It began to decline with the rise of the universities, even though the universities themselves had generally been a product of scholasticism and many eminent scholastics were among their first teachers.

The aim of scholasticism was to harmonize theologic doctrines with secular learning and particularly with the philosophy of the ancient Greeks. This really was not a new project for it had been begun centuries earlier in Greece and continued later in Alexandria. In the last named place Philo Judeus had endeavored to harmonize the Mosaic teachings with the philosophies of Aristotle and Plato. Mohammedan and Jewish scholars tried to instill Hellenistic ideas into their religious doctrines in the later Middle Ages.

Moslem scholasticism had a rational philosophical background. It was founded by the Persian, al Ghazzali of Bagdad (451-505), in the fifth century. The tolerance of thought accorded by some Caliphs as soon as their supremacy remained unquestioned, permitted the teaching of such doctrines in schools and colleges.

The Arabo-Spanish schools developed scholasticism on the same lines as did the Christian schools a century later. There was the same attempt to harmonize the sacred literature of the Koran with the teachings of Greek philosophy and the same contest existed between those who relied on reason and rational authority and those who put their trust either in pure revelation or in mystic religious experiences and denied the basic validity of reason in matters of faith.

It should be emphasized that both Jewish and Arabian philosophies were advocated not by priests, but by laymen who were interested in rationalizing their religious teachings. Among the Arabo-Jewish scholastics of outstanding importance were Avicenna (980-1037), Averroes (1126-1198) and Maimonides (1135-1204). These three savants constructed systems of religious philosophy which had been begun by the Moslem scholastic, al Ghazzali, and which were later modified by the Christian scholastic, Thomas Aquinas (c. 1227-1274). "The Guide for the Perplexed," of Maimonides, had influence in the later Middle Ages on Judaism, Christianity and Mohammedanism.

Christian scholastic philosophers at the outset subordinated reason to faith in their attempt to incorporate their philosophic arguments into the doctrine of the Church. In their discussion, they frequently included material from the sciences of medicine and law, for they concerned themselves more with the so-called "logical" formulation of problems than with their solution or even true understanding. Of course to attain a knowledge of natural phenomena it was necessary to study the processes of nature. Yet the scholastics refused to do this and instead resorted to wild mental gymnastics and speculation.

The teachings of Averroes and other thinkers came into severe conflict with Christian theologians and were met with strong opposition, especially from the Dominican school. None-the-less, by the thirteenth century, Averroes was recognized as an authority in the universities of South Italy, Paris and Oxford. Roger Bacon and Duns Scotus (1265 or 1275-1308) thought his teachings worthy "to be placed with Aristotle as a master of science and proof."

The schoolmen discussed a large variety of subjects outside the realm of religion and even in their theological discussions they exhibited freedom of thought within certain well-defined limits. They were guided not only by the concepts of Aristotle but also by the doctrines of the Neo-Platonists and St. Augustine as interpreted by Johannes Scotus Erigena. St. Augustine, a man of real learning in his generation, was one of the greatest of all Christian philosophers. Some of his followers expressed their views to the extent as to regard the whole biblical history as symbolic. This naturally aroused a storm of controversy which is far from dead even at this date.[1] Yet the very idea that the universe is understandable to the human mind prompted students to observe facts and analyze them rather than accept ancient tradition uncritically. Consequently, in time, inductive logic from observation of nature replaced pure deduction from ancient or more recent authority.

The solutions offered by the schoolmen for the many absorbing natural problems, however, were inadequate, for scholasticism was based upon these four general assumptions: (1) The universe is homocentric and the whole of nature is made for man. The world is only to be thought of in terms of human sensation and human psychology. (2) Absolute objective truth can only be attained by the human mind. (3) The basic principle of truth was first revealed in Scripture and has been developed by the Fathers of the Church. When philosophy extends beyond theology, truth may be ascertained by reflection on the teachings of Aristotle. (4) Every principle must be worked out to its full logical issue.

The central theme of the scholastic debates was the doctrine of "universals" or "intelligible forms." This concept represents one of the two main tendencies of medieval philosophy. The controversy between Plato and Aristotle on the nature of "universals" or "intelligible forms" found its way into the writings of Porphyry and into the commentaries of Boethius, and so reached the medieval mind.

With the name of Anselm (c. 1033-1109) is associated the founding of the philosophical sect of *realists* which taught that an object and its conception are one and the same thing. The opponents of the realists were the *nominalists,* whose leader was the monk Roscellinus (end of the eleventh century). This latter group affirmed that conceptions are obtained solely from perception of existing objects and that perception must precede conception. Realists and nominalists fought it out tooth and nail until the latter group succumbed. The most famous champion of realism was Pierre Abelard of Palet, near Nantes (1079-1142).[2] Abelard considered doubt profitable, since it often leads to the proving of truth.

Anselm found in the universals the only means by which he could rationalize religious dogma. To him universals were real and active principles.

Questions such as this were discussed: Are individuals the only realities, classes or universals existing merely as mental concepts or names as Aristotle taught? Or do the universals possess quite separate an existence and a reality apart from the phenomena of the isolated beings, as Plato held in his idealistic philosophy, which had come to be called realism? For instance, are Democritus and Socrates realities, and humanity only a name? Or is man a species with a reality of its own, receiving here and there certain forms which make it Democritus or Socrates who are thus merely accidents of the real substance, humanity?

The controversy between the nominalists and realists arose over the problem of genera and species: (1) Do such really subsist in themselves or are they only products of the mind? (2) If they truly are subsistent, are they corporeal or incorporeal? and (3) Are they separated from sensible things or placed in them?

The realists held that universals alone have substantial reality, existing *ante res*. The nominalists held that universals are mere names invented to express the qualities of particular things, existing *post res*. The *conceptualists*, mediating between the two extremes, held that universals are concepts which exist in our minds and express real similarities in things themselves.

With much vain subtlety the controversy about universals involved issues of the greatest speculative and practical importance. Realism represented a spiritual, and nominalism an antispiritual view of the world. Realism was favorable to and nominalism unfavorable to the teachings of the Church. Nominalism became a doctrine of sceptics and suspected heretics, such as Berengar of Tours (d. 1088) and Roscellinus (c. 1050-1122). Even Abelard's mediating doctrine of conceptualism was sufficiently heretical to involve him in lifelong persecution. This controversy, started in the eleventh century, lasted until the middle of the twelfth century when the first period of scholastic philosophy ended.

The main orthodox philosophers of the later scholastic period (in the thirteenth century) who supported moderate realism were Albertus Magnus and Thomas Aquinas (1227-1274), and the chief supporter of later nominalism was the fourteenth century English Franciscan, William of Occam (d. 1340). Nominalism stimulated a new tendency in thought—a distrust of abstractions and an impulse towards direct observation and inductive research—a tendency which had its fulfillment in the scientific movement of the Renaissance.[3]

To the realists, any irregularly formed syllogism carried conviction with it, regardless of the premises on which it rested. Many premises were assumed without any attempt to verify their truth. Their methods of argumentation consisted of three propositions: the first one was called the major premise; the second, the minor premise; and the third, the conclusion. For example, taking as the first proposition, "No finite being is exempt from error"; as the second, "All men are finite beings"; the conclusion is, "Therefore no man is exempt from error." Such intellectual gymnastics resulted not in the discovery of any truth but in a victory gained in a combat of words aided by subtle and hair-splitting discussions in a language comprehensible only to the initiated.

The subjects which the scholastic philosophers selected to express their mental acuity ranged from the sublime to the amusing and even to the ridiculous. Petrus Lombardus, Bishop of Paris, devoted much serious discussion to the problem of whether the bowels move or not in Paradise. He was also interested in deciding how many angels can comfortably dance upon the point of a needle.

Other schoolmen wasted their time and energies in futile arguments as to whether a spirit can live in a vacuum or whether Adam and Eve, not being born in the natural manner, possessed umbilical marks. The schoolmen, more often than not, were reluctant to investigate earthly subjects.[4]

It would be unjust, however, to look upon scholasticism in general as philosophically barren and entirely devoid of reality. Even though the schoolmen were dominated by a religious spirit, they did not completely exclude rational thought. Indeed, many of them actually searched for truth with a scientific eagerness. As a rule, the scholastics were not antagonistic to reason *per se*; on the contrary, they often fought battles in the name of reason. It should be vehemently and emphatically emphasized that reason, if admitted at all, has a way of ultimately claiming the whole of man.

The form of scholasticism that has outlived its day may be justly identified with *obscurantism*, but not so the systems of those who, by their intellectual force alone, held all the minds of Europe in subjection. The medieval schoolmen, although exhibiting some original speculations, in the main blindly followed Aristotle and other ancient authorities.

The scholastics as a class were intellectually highly cultured men who would reflect credit on any historic age. Their finespun dialectical discussions sharpened their wits and prepared them for the dawning period of the Renaissance and Reformation.

While scholasticism as a whole may be regarded as a precursor of the emancipation of reason, its effect on medicine was definitely destructive. The Hippocratic method of bedside study was replaced by the words which ancient authors had written about disease and disease itself ceased to be studied. The best doctor was the one who could quote the greatest number of authorities, especially in the classic languages. Since the qualification of a medical man hinged chiefly upon a knowledge of the Greek and Arabic texts and commentaries thereon, anyone who could read Greek or Arabic texts was considered a doctor of medicine and ecclesiastics who had never attended a patient became writers of medical texts.

Instead of reading medical texts as they were written and as the author wanted them to be understood, the scholastics tried to find hidden ideas between the lines and profuse and pointless discussions and interpretations ensued. The scholastics felt certain that they were reducing the science of medicine to the art of reasoning, but they obviously would have done better to study the patients at the bedside and observe the signs and symptoms first hand.

The therapy of the scholastic doctors was essentially monastic in character, but perhaps the vegetable, animal and mineral substances employed outweighed the prayers, incantations, charms and relics of saints which had been so commonly used in the monasteries. Synthetic drugs, of course, were not known and the therapeutic use of metallic drugs such as those made from gold, silver, copper and mercury was poorly understood.

According to the scholastics, technical dexterity was attained from argumentation, disputation, and the use of commentaries rather than from straightforward clinical investigations. For every newly-risen problem arguments were cunningly drawn from the book-wisdom of Aristotle, Galen and Avicenna. "The dialectic method, which was fundamentally confined within a vicious circle of preconceived opinions based only upon authority, could be of little service to a science where much if not everything, should be dependent upon experience. Medicine was bound from its very nature to suffer more than other technical subjects under the oppression of scholasticism." [5]

The activity of scholasticism is mainly confined within the limits of the eleventh and the fourteenth centuries. It may be divided into two well demarcated periods: the first extending to the end of the twelfth century and embracing as its chief exponents Roscellinus (c. 1050-1122), Anselm, William of Champeaux, Thomas Aquinas (c. 1225-1274) and Duns Scotus; and the second period extending to the fourteenth century and including such stalwarts as Roger Bacon, Albertus Magnus, Peter de Abbano, Petrus Hispanus, Arnold of Villanova, Bernard de Gordon and Robert de Grosseteste. It is with the latter group of scholastics with which we are presently most concerned because of their deep interest in medicine.

ROGER BACON (c. 1214-1292)

One of the most eminent scholastics was the English Franciscan, philosopher and scientist, Roger Bacon, often referred to as "Doctor Mirabilis." Born at Ilchester, Somerset, he studied in Oxford under Grosseteste and possibly also under Adam Marsh. In the year 1236 he went to Paris; then he traveled to Italy where he dedicated a book to Pope Innocent IV (1243-1254). Following this he returned to Paris where he lectured as a regent master at the University. He returned to Oxford in about 1251 and here he assumed the Franciscan habit from this year until 1257.

Apparently he got into difficulties with his superiors, soon after his first publication in 1254. The growing suspicion of his doctrines, however, soon caused him to be sent back to Paris, apparently for more strict supervision by his Order, and he was forbidden to write or to teach his doctrines. An actual censorship of all his writings was established by the Franciscan Order. In 1266, he was ordered by Pope Clement IV, who had heard of him in France and England, to secretly send him copies of his writings. This papal request, which was made over the head of Bacon's superiors, made him doubly obnoxious to them. Bacon sent three of his books to the Pope, but unfortunately the latter died before he could intercede on his behalf.

The Franciscan censorship became more severe after the condemnation of Averroism in 1277 and in the following year Bacon was condemned for teaching "suspected novelties." According to a Franciscan chronicle ("Chronica Viginti Quattuor Generalium"), he was imprisoned from 1278 to 1292 and he died soon afterwards.

Bacon blamed the prevailing unhealthy conditions existing with regard to theology, medicine and philosophy on the ignorance that existed of the original tongues of the great classics. He pointed out how corruptions crept into the original texts through carelessness and ignorance, or by outright tampering—especially by the Dominicans.

Bacon insisted that experimental methods alone give a certainty in science and this represented a revolutionary change in the mental attitude of his day. Bacon read all the books he could obtain, Arabic (probably in Latin translations) as well as Greek, but instead of accepting their authors' views as facts, Bacon insisted upon verifying their statements by personal observation and experimentation.

Roger Bacon and Cardinal Nicholas of Cusa are perhaps the only two who can be specified, within a whole thousand years in Western Europe, who combined both the essentials of original observation and bold synthesis.

Bacon testified concerning one Peter (Peter de Abano?) who was a researcher in magnetism: "I know of only one person who deserves praise for his work in experimental philosophy, for he does not care for the discourses of men and their wordy warfare, but quietly and diligently pursues the works of wisdom. Therefore what others grope after blindly, as bats in the evening twilight, this man contemplates in their brilliancy, because he is a master of experiment."

Most of the experments which Bacon conducted were in optics, on which he spent time and considerable money. As a friar, Bacon was pledged to poverty, but, by borrowing from friends, he got together enough funds to conduct his experiments and publish his books. He is renowned for his "Opus Majus," containing his views at length; his "Opus Minor," an epitome of his works; and his "Opus Tertium." His scientific work is chiefly known from these books although various of his works still remain in manuscript form.

A part of the "Opus Majus" is devoted to experimental science. He distinguishes between external and internal experience ("scientia experimentalis, per sensus exteriores; scientia interior, intuitiva")—a distinction which was unfortunately lost by many of the later philosophers. Bacon was primarily interested in external or objective experiences.

It should be mentioned that some of his experiments were fantastic, and in spite of his efforts to separate experimentation from magic, he did not always succeed. However, he was always ready to sacrifice theories for facts and to confess his own ignorance.[6]

His interest in light was probably aroused by his study of the Latin version of the works of the Arabian physicist Ibn al Haitham. Bacon describes the laws of reflection and the general phenomena of refraction. He understands the properties of mirrors and lenses and describes a telescope, although he does not claim to have made one. He gives a theory as to the causation of rainbows as an example of inductive reasoning.

Roger Bacon describes many mechanical inventions, some actually known to him, and some as possibilities for the future. Among the latter group is included mechanically driven ships, carriages and flying machines. He discusses magic mirrors, burning glasses, gunpowder, the magnet, artificial gold and the Philosopher's stone, in a hodge-podge of confused fact, prediction and credulity. In the "Mirror of Alchemy," he adheres to the Alexandrian theory that all things strive toward improvement. "Nature," he writes, "tries ceaselessly to reach perfection—that is, gold."

"There is one science," he says, "more perfect than others, which is needed to verify the others, the science of experiment, surpassing the sciences dependent on argument, since these sciences do not bring certainty, however strong the reasoning, unless experiment be added to test their conclusions. Experimental science alone is able to ascertain what can be effected by nature, what by art, what by fraud. It alone teaches how to judge all the follies of the magicians, just as logic can be used to test argument."

Bacon, with the courage of his convictions, proclaimed that mathematics and optics must underlie all other scientific studies. Both these sciences, he says, are understood by Robert of Lincoln. Mathematical tables and instruments are necessary, although they are costly and easily destroyed. He pointed out the errors of the current calendar method and calculated that one extra day was gained each 130 years. He also gave a lengthy description of the countries of the known world, and estimated its size. He supported the theory of its sphericity, long before Columbus came to that conclusion.

However, his agreement with the scholastic view that the end of all science and philosophy is to elucidate and adorn their queen, theology, hampered his work as did his admonition to physicians that they do not study the heavenly bodies upon which all changes in the bodies of man depend.

There is much that we can learn from his work, "De Erroribus Medicorum Secundum Fratrem Rogerum Bacon de Ordine Minorum," translated by Withington.[7] A few of his characteristic statements follow in a condensed form:

"Physicians foolishly trust to ignorant apothecaries who overcharge, substitute and dispense stale drugs . . . Physicians are further in error with regard to compound medicines. There are 36 great and radical defects, some of which have as much to do with simple as with compound medicines . . . Haly says there are nine kinds of black bile, and he says that from each of these humors when they become maladjusted arise many diseases, such as anthrax, fistula, cancer, lupus, St. Anthony's fire and the like, for which physicians have no sufficient remedy . . . Another defect is a great one, that although simple laxatives containing harmful ingredients ought to be prepared by separating the harmful from the helpful—as in the viper the poisonous activity is separated from the flesh which is an antidote to all poisons—no method for this is given in the books of the Latins, except in a very few, and so many dangers arise."

According to Professor Newbold, Bacon is the true discoverer of the microscope, the animal cell and many other things ascribed to a far later time.[8] Bacon has been credited with the invention of spectacles.[9]

ALBERTUS MAGNUS (1193-1280)

The most eminent naturalist of the thirteenth century was the Dominican priest, Albert von Bollstadt, commonly referred to as Albertus Magnus or Albert of Cologne. He was born at Lauingen in Suabia, and was educated principally at Padua, where he received instruction in Aristotle's writings. In 1221 or 1223, he became a member of the Dominican order and studied theology under its rules at Bologna and elsewhere. He taught for several years at Bologna, Regensburg, Freiburg, Strassburg and Hildesheim. In 1245, he went to Paris where he received his doctorate, and taught there for some time.

He wrote on botany which in those days included materia medica. During the period that he lectured in Paris he had among his students Roger Bacon, Petrus Hispanus and Thomas Aquinas.

In 1254, he was made a provincial of his order and he answered the errors of the Arabian philosopher, Averroes. In 1260, the pope made him Bishop of Regensburg, which office he resigned three years later. The remainder of his life was spent partly in preaching throughout Bavaria and the adjoining districts and partly in retirement in the various houses of his order. Almost the last of his labors was his defense of the orthodoxy of his former pupil, Thomas Aquinas. He died in 1280 at the age of eighty-seven.

In a theological treatise he commits himself to the remarkable statement that while in doctrine of fact and morals, Augustine is to be considered a higher authority than the philosophers, in questions of medicine, Galen and Hippocrates are more reliable and in questions of natural philosophy, Aristotle is a better authority.

Albertus Magnus was the most widely read and most learned man of his time. The whole of Aristotle's works, presented in the Latin translations, the works of Maimonides and notes of the Arabian commentators, were digested, interpreted and systematized by him in accordance with Church doctrine. His activity, however, was more philosophical than theological. The philosophical works, occupying the first six and the last of his twenty-one volumes, are divided according to the Stagyrites scheme of the sciences, and actually consist of interpretations and condensations of Aristotle's works, with supplementary discussions and occasional divergences from the opinions of the master.

His large encyclopedia "Vincentius Bellovacensis" earned him the title of "Doctor Universalis." "My purpose in regard to natural science," says Albertus Magnus in the introduction to his physics, "is, to the best of my ability, to comply with the request of the members of my order to write them a book upon nature, wherein they may at the same time correctly understand the writings of Aristotle."

His knowledge of medicine and of physical science, considering the age, is quite accurate, although we find in his system many of those gaps and futile discussions which are characteristic of scholastic philosophy. For example, in his commentary on the "Textus Sententiarum" of Petrus Lombardus, he discusses the question as to whether Adam, in the removal of the rib out of which Eve was formed, really experienced pain and whether at the day of judgment that loss of a rib would be compensated by the gift of another.

Magnus' long study of Aristotle endowed him with great power of systematic thought and exposition. The results of that study, as left to us, by no means warrant the contemptuous title sometimes given him—"the ape of Aristotle." They rather lead us to appreciate the motives which caused his contemporaries to bestow upon him the honorable surname—"The Great" and "Doctor Universalis."

His works, "De Vegetabilibus" and "De Virtutibus Herbarum," were based upon original observations. He does not write on medical practice, a subject forbidden by the Dominican Order. His work on cosmetics, "De Secretis Muliorum," was in reality written by his pupil, Henry of Saxony. He also wrote a commentary on Isaac Judeus' book, "On Special Diets."

Albertus Magnus, in the tenth book of his "Summa," in which he catalogues and describes all the trees, plants, and herbs known in his time, declares: "All that is here set down is the result of our own experience, or has been borrowed from authors whom we know to have written what their personal experience has confirmed; for in these matters experience alone can be of certainty."

In another place, he even casts doubt upon the general value of authority in the profane sciences and he rejects it in favor of experience as the only reliable criterion. In relation to medical subjects the extracts scattered throughout many of his works dealing with anatomy, physiology and psychology are of interest. Albertus Magnus also wrote upon the healing virtues of plants and stones but he dealt little with practical medicine. Nevertheless his influence as the reintroducer of Aristotle as the cornerstone of science and medical education was a great one.[10]

He frankly confesses that he takes much of this "experience" from books and some of these books are now known to be most inaccurate. Even the greatest medieval schoolmen constantly based their works on the respectable "hearsay of classical writers and the popular traditions of hoary antiquity." Dr. Singer states that Albertus Magnus is "among the few medieval writers who were real observers of nature."

In spite of his confessed adherence to the main views of Aristotle "the master," Albertus Magnus succeeds in a surprising manner in manifesting a certain independence such as is seen (in his "Digressiones") from his criticisms upon abstract elucidations and his original experiences and observations gained during his wanderings throughout Germany as a provincial of his order. This independence in observation—an uncommon phenomenon in an age of purely book-learning—was especially beneficial to zoology and botany and to a lesser degree also to climatology, mineralogy, chemistry and physics.

ROBERT GROSSETESTE (c. 1175-1253)

Robert Grosseteste or Greathead (Robert, Bishop of Lincoln) was born of humble parentage at Stradbrook, Suffolk and was educated in Oxford where he became the first chancellor. He was the first lecturer to the Oxford Franciscans (1224) and bishop of Lincoln from 1235 to his death in 1253.

He was the main organizer of philosophical studies at Oxford and he was famous as a mathematician, astronomer, physicist, philosopher and translator from the Greek into Latin. His influence was strongly felt in England for several centuries. He was clearly the forerunner of his most famous pupil, Roger Bacon. Grosseteste invited Greek scholars to England and imported Greek books while his pupil, Roger Bacon, wrote a grammar of the Greek language. The aim of both was to find the key to the enigma of Aristotle and other Greek classical authors and the septuagint[11] in their original tongue.

Robert Grosseteste's literary activity must have been tremendous. He wrote various commentaries on the analytics and on the physics of Aristotle.[12] His astronomical ideas were partly Ptolemaic. He wrote various astronomical and astrological treatises including "De Generatione Stellarum" and "De Cometis." The majority of his scientific treatises deal with physical and meteorological questions. He was much concerned with that complex subject called "perspective" and with optical questions in general. He was well aware of the magnifying properties of lenses, a knowledge which he probably transmitted to Bacon. Grosseteste was one of the earliest English authors to be acquainted with the writings of the Salerno School. Notwithstanding his interest in astrology and alchemy he was remarkably free from magical fancies. His relation to medicine is based on his studies of light and refraction which were probably derived from his studies of the works of al Haitam in the Latin translation.[13]

PETRUS HISPANUS (b. 1213)

The first and only physician to become Pope was Petrus Hispanus of Lisbon, Portugal. He was born in the year 1213 (before Portugal was separated from Spain). His medical education was received in Paris where he studied under the supervision of Albertus Magnus. He also was a student for a short time at the University of Montpellier.

He received his ecclesiastical training after he was appointed body physician to Pope Gregory X. His advancement was phenomenally rapid and when Pope Adrian V died, Petrus Hispanus succeeded him taking the name of John XXI.[14] It is not clear where he practiced medicine after he received his degree. He appears to have practiced for a short time in Siena.

Petrus Hispanus is the author of several works. His "Thesaurus Pauperum" (Treasury of the Poor) deals with dietetics and therapy and contains comments on Hippocrates, Galen and other ancient physicians. According to Thorndike,[15] this book was highly popular in the late Middle Ages.

His "Liber de Oculo" ("Book of the Eye") is said to have served as an ophthalmological textbook for two centuries. He is quoted by many famous medical writers including Guy de Chauliac. Michelangelo copied one of his prescriptions for his own use.

His "Aquae Merabilis" ("The Wonder Water"), which he claimed "elevates the physician who can prepare it to the rank of prophet," contains filings of silver, copper, gold, etc., suspended in the urine of a boy. This prescription was very famous and Arnold of Villanova mentions it in his "Brevarium." Despite the fact that Petrus Hispanus strove to exclude superstition from his work, it is full of nostrums. In his "Salernitan Medicae," he mentions a valuable ointment for hemorrhoids which is prepared by boiling "a little worm found under a rough stone" in linseed oil. One has to be careful in preparing this salve that the worm rolls up like a ball when it is removed from under the stone.[16] In his superstitious practices and sympathetic remedies Petrus Hispanus was a true son of his period.

His work on logic, "Sumulae Logicales," has appeared in forty-eight different editions since the invention of the printing press. Petrus Hispanus' occupancy of the Vatican was short. He died a tragic death after the ceiling of his palace fell in on him. He was not popular in Rome and the people did not approve of his scholastic inclinations. In fact, they vilified his name by declaring that he had sold himself to the devil for which his violent death was retribution.

ARNOLD OF VILLANOVA (the Catalonian, c. 1225-1311)

One of the most extraordinary personalities among the scholastics of the Middle Ages was Arnoldus de Villa Nova (near Valencia in Spain). He received his medical education at Naples and traveled extensively. He practiced medicine in Paris, Montpellier, Barcelona and Rome and died at sea on the way from Naples to Genoa, where he was buried.

His knowledge was of an encyclopedic nature. He was physician, alchemist, astrologer, diplomat, social reformer and translator of medical works from Arabic into Latin. He had some knowledge of Greek and Hebrew. He emphasized the importance of the natural sciences and their great value to education. He often professed opposition to magic and sorcery and he wrote "Let us return to nature;" yet his works are full of superstitious ideas. His medical knowledge was sought by kings and by popes.

He was a favorite of Pope Boniface VIII, whom he is said to have successfully treated for stone in the kidney. On several occasions, he was accused of heresy but was always acquitted through the intervention of Pope Boniface. Because of Pope Boniface's friendship with Arnold, he himself was accused of heresy after his death.

Arnold practiced as a physician in various towns of Italy, France and Spain. He appears to have aroused the admiration of his contemporaries as a medical author and alchemist; yet his main sphere of action was as a diplomat in the interest of the state of Aragon. He strenuously endeavored to effect social reform. In the year 1299, while serving as ambassador from Aragon to the court of Phillippe le Bel, he came into conflict with the clerics of Paris because of his free expression of religious views. He was summoned before the inquisition which compelled him, after brief imprisonment, to recant his unorthodox views.

Arnold of Villanova played an influential part in the history of ecclesiastical policies in the late thirteenth and early fourteenth centuries. The threatened Knights Templars and the distressed Monks of Mount Athens sought his influence.

Arnold of Villanova was a prolific writer. His best known treatise was the "Breviarium" which deals with diseases "from head to foot" ("a capita ad dulcem"). His books deal especially with surgery, gynecology and poisons.

The best insight into the capacity of the great Catalonian is afforded by his work "Parabola Medicationes." This work deals to some extent with internal medicine, but largely with surgical diseases.

His commentary on "Regimen Salernitanum" is considered the best on that poem. He also wrote a good monograph that offers sound advice on diet in old age and also various rejuvenatory remedies.

In addition to his rational basis in the art of healing, Arnold presents a high moral conception of the medical profession. There is scattered throughout his writings humane ideals inspired by true piety and a deep sense of responsibility.

Although he was a product of the age of scholasticism, he opposed scholastic method and engaged in chemical experiments with the alchemists. He evinces in his writings the conviction that dialectics, despite their deceptive glamor, are barren and empty and can in no way satisfy either the spiritual need or the real demand of science.

In anatomy, physiology and pathology, he has very little to offer that can be considered any advance over Galen and the Arabs, but he excels in his method of handling various medical subjects. He starts out with a definition of the disease. He then discusses minutely the predisposing and exciting causes as well as the physiology and pathology. This is followed by a careful and detailed description of the symptoms. Next comes the diagnosis and prognosis and, finally, he deals at length with the methods of treatment.

Arnold stresses diet and hygiene as prophylactic measures against disease. He frequently prescribes wine with the diet for its therapeutic virtues. In prescribing medicaments, he pays careful attention to the patient's age, temperament and habits of life. He favors the use of mild medical preparations as long as the diagnosis is in doubt. He is opposed to the use of drugs which have not been sufficiently tested. He favors bloodletting in the form of leeching, cupping and venesection. His materia medica consists largely of vegetables, but he also uses some animal and mineral substances.

Arnold is considered one of the orginators of medical chemistry. He distilled alcohol from red wine, volatile oils and aromatic waters. He prepared volatile and aromatic water and various metallic preparations.

Von Storchs quotes Arnold as saying: "I hold that epilepsy is an occlusion of the chief ventricles of the brain, with loss of sensation and motion; epilepsy is a noncontinuous spasm of the whole body. This disease takes rise from different causes, such as superfluous foods, drinks or poisons, the bites of mad dogs or reptiles, and poisoned, corrupt, and pestiferous air. When the pores are constricted, and superfluities are retained, the natural heat is lessened and there follows a filling up of the chief ventricles of the brain. And these are the three causes which principally induce epilepsy."

For epilepsy, Arnold recommends the flesh of birds (except those living in the marshes), and the flesh of yearling lambs, swine, and goats, flavored with strong-smelling wine. Fish which live in rivers can only be eaten if cooked dry on hot coals. The epileptic is permitted to eat spinach, parsley, fennel, asparagus, and wheat bread—all well-cooked. He may drink yellow wine and white wine of good odor. The therapeutic measures prescribed by Arnold consist of mineral baths at midnight, purges, and cauterizations—a course of treatment almost as distressing to the epileptic as the seizures themselves. Foods to be avoided by the epileptic are cabbage, lentils, beans, brains of animals and celery. Celery should be avoided because of its tendency to induce epilepsy.[17]

Some of Arnold's aphorisms sound very modern:[18] "He who in his chosen branch educates himself not for science but for gain, becomes an abortionist . . . A knowledge of names is essential to science, but no cure is ever achieved by a mere formula . . . That mode of treatment is best which achieves the desired end with the fewest means. . . . An intelligent and pious physician makes every effort to cure disease with proper foods rather than with drugs."[19] Arnold also recommends various amulets and a liberal quantity of yellow or white wine of good odor.

Arnold warns the physician: "Always do something when you come into a patient's presence lest they say you can do nothing without your books."

Arnold's therapeutics seem modern in an age when it was the practice of the (medieval) physician to mix a large number of herbs and drugs in one prescription. Polypharmacy added to the difficulty of preparing remedies. To the mind of the layman, the more complex the mixtures, the better the doctor and the more erudite the pharmacist.

HILDEGARD OF BINGEN (1098-1179)

The most celebrated medieval monastic physician was the Benedictine Abbess, Hildegard von Bingen. She was born in the year 1098 at Böckelheim, a village in the county of Sponheim, a district between the rivers Moselle and Nahe. The daughter of a soldier named Hildebert of the petty nobility, she was but eight years old when placed in the Benedictine convent of Disibodenberg on the Nahe River. She became a nun when she was of the canonical age. She learned some Latin, but was never proficient in that language. She admitted that she knew how to write only "rude Latin."

She founded and was Abbess of the convent of Rupertsberg, near Bingen, for 35 years. She died at this institution at the age of 81. She was in ill health all of her life and perhaps this is what led her to observe and study various diseases and remedies.

Hildegard's medical writings consist primarily of two works; "Liber Simplicis Medicinae" and "Liber Compositae Medicinae" which were written between the years 1151-1159. The first book deals with the simple, natural sources of medical treatment: chiefly various foods and common herbs. This book covers the effects of various diets on health and disease and discusses the value of wheat, barley, beans, ginger, pepper, mint, aloes, mushrooms, radishes and many kinds of *myntza*. It lists the merits of milk, honey, salt and myrrh and 213 varieties of plants that may be used in disease.

Hildegard of Bingen discusses the medicinal values of air, water and earth. With reference to the medicinal value of air, she says: "Sometimes disturbances of the air and other elements mount to the brain and cause an interchange of its humors, creating a milky frothing through the nose and throat so that an inflammation is set up like the froth of milky water."

She enumerates 55 kinds of trees and 26 precious stones (including beryl, sapphire, topaz, chrysolite and pearl) which can be employed in making various marvelous medicines. She enumerates 37 varieties of fish (beginning with the whale which she recognizes as a mammal), 68 kinds of birds, 43 kinds of animals (beginning with the elephant), 18 types of reptiles and eight metals (gold, silver, tin, copper, lead, brass, iron and mercury). She recognizes lead and brass as poisons and emphasizes the tonic values of copper and iron.

In the second book she deals with all sorts of diseases from insanity to halitosis and the common cold. She offers her own theories as to etiology and therapy. She gives considerable space to procreation and birth and discusses venesection, fever, asthma, painful urination, toothache and problems of menstruation.

In one of her smaller works, the subjects of melancholic headache, migraine and amentia are discussed. Then she takes up the eye, ear, nose and throat followed by the heart, liver and kidneys. She follows these with surveys of nerve pain, bone tumors, sterility in men and women, fistulas, ulcers and gout. Next she presents a topical plan of diseases proceeding from the head to the foot.

Hildegard devotes a smaller work to colds, difficult birth, amenorrhea, menorrhagia, epilepsy, leprosy, fever (acute, quotidian, tertian and quartan) and, for good measure, she describes diseases of sheep, horses, asses, pigs and goats.

In a pamphlet entitled, "De Coriza," Hildegard makes the following statement:

"If the distress of a great discharge from the nose becomes too annoying to a man, let him take four parts of anise to one part of fennel and put them on a heated tile or thin brick and stir them together whilst they vaporize and inhale the vapor, and eat some fennel and anise with bread. Do this for three or four or five days until the discharge from the head and nose be eased. For the heat and moisture of fennel gathers the ill-adjusted humors and the dry coldness of the anise dries them up, when these two are tempered together on a heated brick, as has been said."

There is no evidence that Hildegard ever attended a medical school because there were ecclesiastical restrictions against priests and monks attending lectures on either law or medicine because these subjects tended to withdraw them from their spiritual duties. As a matter of fact, the fourth Lateran Council, in 1215, restricted clerics from the practice of medicine when such involved "cutting or burning" for these procedures were inconsistent with the gentleness of their calling. Surgery was not practiced in the monastic infirmaries. For this reason, Hildegard's medical writings ignore surgery completely, and she seems to be vague in her handling of anatomy.

Although there is nothing new in her books and she was obviously a product of her age in many ways, Singer points out that she was acquainted with the Hippocratic doctrines of miasma and the humors, and most likely with other ancient works that were preserved in the Benedictine convents.[20]

BERNARD GORDON (13th century)

One of the most prominent teachers of the University of Montpellier was Bernardus Gordonus (Bernard de Gordon), who flourished during the closing years of the thirteenth and the beginning of the fourteenth centuries. He appears to have been a Frenchman, although he claims to have had Scottish ancestry.

His "Lilium Medicinae," which still exists in several rare

manuscripts, was first published in Venice in the year 1496. It is a typical Arabist textbook of medical practice characteristic of the Middle Ages, marked by scholastic subtlety and rigid adherence to dogma. The subject matter, however, is well arranged and reads well.

Bernard Gordon believes in the contagious nature of acute fevers, consumption, anthrax, St. Anthony's fire, scabies and leprosy. He tells of a countess afflicted with leprosy who came to Montpellier to be treated. There she met a bachelor of medicine who fell in love with her and was promptly attacked with the disease.

He gives a graphic description of the Plague as described by the English physician Mirfield. He published his studies on diet, fevers, prognostics, general therapy and blood.

Bernard Gordon gives the first description of the two most momentous medical inventions of the Middle Ages: the modern form of truss which seems to have been invented by Salvino Armati about 20 years earlier, and most important, the invention of spectacles. The history of spectacles will be given in the next chapter.

Gordon made a great impression upon the students of Montpellier and his "Lilium Medicinae" became very popular. Eight editions appeared before the year 1500. He was well thought of among his contemporaries. According to Dupony[21] Gordon identified syphilitic chancre and his findings were corroborated by the famous French surgeons, Lanfranc and Saliceto.

Baas does not throw bouquets at the author of the "Lilium." He evaluates him as a sensible Englishman who regulated his fees according to the wealth of his patient. But it is only fair to add that there were physicians in Gordon's day in Montpellier who made no discrimination between rich and poor and between laymen and ecclesiastics. All were charged to the limit.

Gordon himself relates[22] that in 1153 the Bishop of Lyons, having fallen seriously ill on a trip to Rome, was brought to Montpellier where he spent all he possessed, and even that which he did not possess, on physicians there.

GILBERTUS ANGLICUS (1180-1250)

Gilbert the Englishman, also known as "Doctor Desideralissimus," was the leading exponent of Anglo-Norman medicine. His work resembles Gordon's in style, content, and arrangement of material. Gilbert's principal work is usually referred to as "Laurea Angelica" (also termed "Compendium Medicinae"). Even this reference to a flower in the title is analogous to "Lilium Medicinae."

It might be mentioned here that medieval authors were in the habit of naming their works after attractive flowers and luscious fruits. Gilbert, however, admits that his "rose" was plucked from other gardens, including those of Pythagoras, Hippocrates, Plato, Aristotle, Galen, Rufus, Boethius, Alexander of Tralles, Theophilus, Haly Abbas, Rhazes, Isaac Judeus, Averroes, Constantine Africanus and Avicenna.[23]

Gilbert's medical compendium is a mixture of Salernitan and Arabic medicine. It contains some interesting descriptions of various diseases including leprosy, measles and smallpox. He is said to have recognized smallpox as being contagious. During the year 1250, Gilbert was chancellor of Montpellier University.

Gilbert's medical compendium covers a wide range of subjects including general diseases, physiology, neurology, ophthalmology, gynecology, obstetrics, embryology, dietetics, urinary and venereal disease, therapeutics, toxicology and operative surgery. His discussions are of the scholastic-dialectic type, based on humoral pathology. The best chapter (and the first by an Englishman on this subject) is the one on gout, "De Arthritica Passione" with which Gilbert was evidently very familiar.

Gilbert's therapies are characterized by the crude polypharmacy and superstition of his age. For example, his remedies for apoplexy include the flesh of a lion, the gall of a scorpion and the eggs of ants. His ointment for gout must have been well known for it is noted by Petrus Hispanus. Gilbert lists an "infallible" remedy for sterility applicable to either sex. His chief remedy for epilepsy is a potion containing the liver and blood of a vulture. In treating epilepsy, he also recommends the recitation of a gibberish of meaningless words, or the writing of an incantation and the tying of it on the patient. He recommends the gall of a vulture as the basis of an ointment for an inflamed eye.

In his work the author attempts to establish on a broad basis a synthesis between Salernitan and Arabic medicine, but unfortunately he is too ready to make concessions to the latter regardless of his own convictions.

Gilbert gives much space to two hundred complicated antidotes. He covers dietetics and he apologizes for his surgical speculations, saying that he mentions them only for the sake of completeness. He diagnoses leprosy in an early stage. He differentiates smallpox from measles by the elevation of the lesion above the level of the skin in the former condition. His therapy for measles and smallpox includes wrapping the patient in a red cloth. For sea sickness, he recommends the purification of drinking water by distillation. For scrofula which was known as "king's evil" ("morbus regnis"), he recommends "king's touch." He refers to spectacles under the term "oculo sorenilius."

It is evident from certain passages that Gilbert was constrained by the spirit of the time to yield to various methods which he did not whole-heartedly support. In some passages the author tends to follow Hippocrates in his simple method of treatment, but at the same time, he warns his readers that such treatments may appear highly peculiar to his contemporaries. His own observations are literally lost in a mass of hair-splitting theoretical discussions.[24]

Some of Gilbert's aphorisms are as follows:

He who laughs frequently is kind and genial in all things and is not worried over trifles.
He who laughs rarely is contrary and critical.
He who has large ears is stolid and long-lived. He who has a large mouth is gluttonous and daring.
He whose teeth are defective and small is weak in his whole body. He whose canine teeth are long and straight is a glutton and a rascal.

Gilbert was undoubtedly recognized as a famous physician in his time. His name is included in the well-known list of Chaucer which gives the "authorities" of his "Doctor of Phisik."[25]

Gilbert received his early education in England; then he visited a number of foreign countries in search of higher learning. He practiced in France for a time. After he returned to his native England, he composed the aforementioned "Laurea Anglica" (published in Lyons in 1500). His work created quite a stir in medical circles, but not because of its originality. With all its faults, the "Laurea Anglica" was accepted in England with great enthusiasm because it was the first medical work produced in England for several centuries, because it was written in a lucid style, and arranged in a systematic form and because its contents were much improved over the hitherto popular leechdom of Bald.

George Stubbs (1724-1806), one of the most noted English historians, summarized the scholastics in the following words: "They benefited mankind by exercising and training subtle wits, and they reduced dialectics, almost, we might say, logic itself, to absurdity. I do not undervalue them, because the great men among them were so great that even a method did not destroy them: in reading St. Thomas Aquinas, for instance, one is constantly provoked to say, what could not such a mind have done if it had not been fettered by such a method?"[26]

CHAPTER XIII

THE INVENTION OF SPECTACLES

At least one great contribution to medical science has been credited to the scholastics by many historians and this is the invention of spectacles. The present writer is inclined to the opinion that if Roger Bacon was not the first to utilize this great discovery that has so aided the student, the artist and the craftsman, he was certainly the first European to describe it.

The science of optics is older than the Middle Ages. The fact that for a knowledge of external things man is more indebted to the sense of vision than to any other sense caused the ancients to be more familiar with optics than with any other branch of physics. None-the-less one searches in vain to find a practical device so simple as spectacles to come down to us from antiquity. One is amazed that the enlightened ancients—brilliant as they were—did not go one step further and make use of the convex glass to aid vision, at least for the aged. It is difficult to understand why the burning-glass was not applied to the eye, either by accident or curiosity, and found to improve sight.

The lens, as an instrument for magnifying objects or for concentrating rays to effect combustion, was known at an early period of history. Aristophanes, in his "Clouds" (c. 424 B.C.), mentions the use of the burning-glass to destroy the writing on a waxed tablet. Much later, Pliny describes such glasses as "solid balls of rock-crystal" or "hollow glasses."

The ancient Greeks were acquainted with the fundamental law that light travels in straight lines and that an object is seen in the direction in which it really lies. The antiquity of mirrors points to an acquaintance with the phenomena of reflection.

A treatise on optics, assigned to Euclid by Proclus, (411-485) and Marinus, (c. 100) shows that the Greeks were acquainted with the production of images by plane, cylindrical, concave and convex spherical mirrors.

The English archeologist, Sir John Layard, while excavating in Nineveh about a century ago, discovered a plano-convex lens of rock crystal among the ruins of the palace of Nimrud. This, of course, implies a knowledge of the burning and/or magnifying power of the crystal.

Certain elementary phenomena of refraction were also noted in deep antiquity. These include the apparent bending of an oar at the point where it meets the water, and the apparent elevation of a coin or other object in a basin when more water is added.

Books on the subject of refraction date back to the beginning of the Christian Era. Early in the second century A.D., the great astronomer and physicist, Claudius Ptolemy, wrote a work on "optics" which has come down to us via imperfect manuscripts in Paris and Oxford. Ptolemy's opus on optics consists of five books, and for our present purpose, the fifth book is most interesting.[1] It deals with the refraction of luminous rays in their passage through media of different densities, and also with astronomical refractions.

The subjects discussed in Ptolemy's work include the nature of light and color, the formation of images by various types of mirrors and refractions at the surface of glass and of water. Tables of the angles of refraction corresponding to given angles of incidence, with rays passing from air to glass and from air to water, are included as are also astronomical refractions such as the apparent displacement of a heavenly body due to the refraction of light in its passage through the atmosphere.[2] Yet, with all this theoretical knowledge, the ancient Greeks apparently never employed spectacles.

There is no reasonable evidence that either the ancient Egyptians or the Hebrews had any knowledge of spectacles. Some biblical scholars point to the following verse in the book of Psalms: "Mine eye is consumed because of grief."[3] The commentator Rashi (contraction of "Rabbi Solomon Yizhaki") interprets the Hebrew word "*Oshesho*" in the sentence as meaning "looking through a glass before the eyes," thus inferring that at least in the time of Rashi in the year 1175 spectacles were in use.

The Talmud refers to a magnifying glass as "*ispeclaria hameira*" ("lucid specularum"). "All prophets looked through an *ispeclaria* that did not increase the light, but Moses looked through an *ispeclaria* that increased the light."[4] It is doubtful whether these references could have applied to spectacles or whether they were uttered in a metaphorical sense.

Doubt may also be cast on the statement of Plinius Secundus to the effect that Nero watched the combat of the gladiators through a convex lens. He used the word "*smaragadus*" which also applies to certain precious stones.[5] It is thus far from certain whether Pliny referred to spectacles, to a magnifying glass or something else entirely. Furthermore, according to Pliny himself, Nero was near-sighted and consequently a magnifying glass would have been of no use in aiding him to see from a distance.

The Chinese appear to have been first to have definitely employed spectacles. Marco Polo recorded that when he visited China in 1270 he found the people using lenses to aid their sight. The Chinese, according to many historians, were the only people of antiquity who developed a knowledge of scientific appliances,[6] but spectacles, unlike other Chinese discoveries, never reached Europe.

The experimental study of refraction, which had been almost entirely neglected by the early Greeks, received more attention during the opening centuries of the Christian era. Cleomedes, in his "Cyclical Theory of Meteors" (c. A.D. 50), alludes to the apparent bending of a stick partially immersed in water, and to the rendering visible of coins in basins by filling the basins with water. He also remarks that the air may refract the sun's rays so as to render the sun visible even though it actually has sunken beneath the horizon.

The analysis of white light into the continuous spectrum of rainbow colors by transmission through a prism was observed by Lucius Aennaeus Seneca (c. 4 B.C.-65 A.D.), who regarded the colors as fictitious, placing them in the same category as the iridescent appearance of the feathers on a pigeon's neck.

The Arabs, as the tenth century was approaching, were on the verge of discovering the use of spectacle lenses to aid vision, but somehow they missed it. Abu al Haitam (966-1020), known in the West as Alhazen, perhaps the greatest original scholar in Islam and one of the greatest students of optics of all times, showed great advance in his experimental methods relating to sight. His optical studies[7] have been translated into Latin.

He was the first to correct the Greek misconception as to the nature of vision, by proving conclusively that the rays of light come from external objects to the eye, and do not issue forth from the eye and impinge on external things—a concept widely held up to his time. He determined that the retina is the seat of vision, and that impressions made by light upon it are conveyed along the optic nerve to the brain.

No one could come to these conclusions, nor, indeed, know anything about these facts, unless he had engaged in the forbidden practice of dissection. He explained the phenomenon as to how we see one picture while using both eyes, on the basis of the formation of the visual images on corresponding portions of the two retinas.

Alhazen demonstrated that our sense of sight is by no means a completely trustworthy guide, and that optical illusions arise from the course which rays of light may take when they undergo refraction or reflection. He was aware that the atmosphere decreases in density with an increase in height; and from this consideration he reasoned that a ray of light descending upon the earth enters it obliquely and follows a curvilinear path which is concave toward the earth. He noted that since the mind refers the position of an object to the direction in which the ray of light from it enters the eye, the result must be an illusion. He demonstrated that in its passage through the air the curvature of a ray increases with the increasing density, and that its path does not depend on vapors that chance to be present, but on the variation of density in the medium. Alhazen used spherical mirrors and studied optical aberration and the magnifying power of lenses. Yet he did not hit upon the idea of spectacles.

Roger Bacon, known as "Doctor Mirabilis" (1214-1292), one of the greatest men that England has produced, is frequently credited with the invention of spectacles. Bacon, despite the ecclesiastical discipline to which he had to submit, was fearless and outspoken in his principles. Although he was incarcerated for 14 years in prison and his books were banned by the Church, he did not divert one iota from his convictions. He stands out as the first great experimental philosopher, not only of his own time, but for many centuries to follow as well.

In his "Optical Science" which was written shortly before he was imprisoned, he states: "If a man looks at letters or other small objects through the medium of a crystal of glass or of some other transparent body placed above the letters, and it is the smaller part of the sphere whose convexity is toward the eye, and the eye is in the air, he will see the letters much better and they will appear larger to him. . . . Therefore this instrument is useful to the aged and to those with weak eyes. . . . The wonders of refracted vision are still greater; for it is easily shown by the rules stated above that very large objects can be made to appear very small, and the reverse, and very distant objects will seem very close at hand, and conversely." [8]

With all his great theoretical and experimental knowledge, Bacon's alleged discovery of convex lenses to assist vision has not been positively substantiated.

The history of science, and more particularly the history of inventions, constantly confronts us with problems such as are presented by such writings as Friar Bacon's. Rarely has it been given to one man to promote an entirely new theory or to devise an entirely original instrument; it is more generally the case that, in the evolution of a single idea, there comes some stage which arrests our attention, and to which we assign the dignity of the term "invention."

The obscurity that surrounds the history of spectacles, the magic lantern, the telescope and the microscope, may find a partial solution in the spirit of the Middle Ages. The natural philosopher who was bold enough to present to a prince a pair of spectacles or a telescope would be in imminent danger of being regarded by the Church as a powerful and dangerous magician of satanic origin. It is also conceivable that the maker of such an instrument would jealously guard the secret of its actual construction, however much he might advertise its potentialities. Particularly the former factor might have applied to Roger Bacon. While others claimed the credit of inventing spectacles he, for reasons noted, might have been afraid to renounce their claims.

Spectacles were first used by the public at the end of the thirteenth century. The Italian dictionary of the "Accademici della Crusca" (1612) mentions a sermon delivered by Jardeno di Rivalto in 1285 (published in 1305) which refers to the invention of spectacles. Part of the sermon reads: "It is hardly twenty years since the art of making spectacles which enables us to see better was invented: One of the most useful in the world, I have myself seen and spoken to the man who first made them." There is little doubt that Jardeno di Rivalto refers to the Friar Alessandro della Spina who was at the Monastery of Florence with him in the year 1285.[9] In the archives of the monastery of Florence where Spina died in the year 1313 the following words are recorded: "He (Spina) was a good man of retiring disposition who reproduced anything he saw and which he had heard about. He made spectacles himself which were first made by someone who would not divulge the secret of their manufacture. With kind heart and willing hands he imparted what knowledge he had to his followers." The archives seem to indicate that the date of the invention was the year 1305 and that the person who would not divulge the secret was none other than Salvinus de Armatus of Florence who, as we will see, came into possession of this secret device through the worthy Spina via an indiscreet friend of Roger Bacon from whom he learned the technique of making spectacles.

William Molyneux, in his "Dioptic Nova," declared that Bacon understood all kinds of optical glasses and knew likewise the methods of constructing them. He quoted Bacon as saying: "Glasses may be formed that the most remote object may appear just at hand, and the contrary so that we may read the remotest letters at an incredible distance and may number things though ever so small." [10] This passage certainly shows that Bacon had very nearly, if not completely arrived at a theoretical proof of the invention of spectacles, even though his writings give no account of their actual construction.

In 1276 or thirty-one years before spectacles were accepted by the people at large as an aid to vision, the English Friar, Roger Bacon, was probably ready with his invention when he writes, "How useful this glass must be for those who are old and have weak eyes."

The story of how Salvinus de Armatus came into possession of Bacon's invention is recorded as follows: While in the monastery of Monte Cassino where he spent a period of 15 years, Bacon confided his device for making glass lenses for magnifying purposes to his friend Heinrich Goethals. The latter was commissioned to go to Rome to interview Pope Martin IV. When Goethals landed in Florence he heard that the Pope had died and during his sojourn in this city he met Alessandro della Spina, a friar to whom he confided Bacon's device for persons with impaired vision. The worthy Spina, to whom we have previously referred, repeated the secret of the invention to his friend, Salvinus de Armatus. The latter did not lose much time in introducing convex spectacles to the public. (Concave spectacles were introduced two centuries later.)

Peter Von Muschenbroek (1692-1761) states that on the tombstone of Salvinus de Armatus, who died in the year 1317, there is an inscription assigning the invention of spectacles to him:

"Here lies Salvinus de Armatus of the Armati of Florence, inventor of spectacles. God pardon him his sins."[11] The last phrase shows how the Church viewed with suspicion inventions designed to aid weakened organs of the body. The clerical attitude was: "God's work is perfect and cannot be aided by the hands of man." Isaac D' Israeli relates that because teleologically speaking fingers were designed for manipulating objects, the use of forks was denounced by the clergy as an insult to the Creator:

"When God in his wisdom has provided man with natural forks (fingers) it is impious to substitute metallic artificial forks for them when eating."

In Germany and Flanders glasses were apparently in use towards the close of the fifteenth century.

Francesco Redi of Arezzo (1627-1797) writes to Falconieri at Rome in 1676 stating that he had seen an old manuscript dated 1285 in which the writer had stated: "I find myself so oppressed with years that without the glasses known as spectacles I have strength neither to read nor write. These have been lately invented for the convenience of poor old people who are weak sighted." He did not name the inventor, but the famous Italian surgeon, Albertotti who flourished at the time of Salvinus de Armatus, stated that the latter's claim to the discovery had not been proven.

Bernardus Gordonus (Bernard de Gordon), professor at the University of Montpellier, who flourished during the closing years of the thirteenth and early years of the fourteenth century, in his book "Lilium Medicinae" (1305) was the first physician to mention spectacles as "Oculus Berellinus." He credited this invention as well as the invention of the modern form of truss to Salvinus de Armatus.

Another celebrated surgeon, Guy de Chauliac (1298-1368), professor at the University of Paris, while praising his own eye lotion, also alluded to spectacles. "If this (his lotion) does not relieve you then try eye-glasses." This would imply that the medical profession was not in a hurry to heed the public clamor for spectacles and perhaps entertained grave doubts as to their real value.

Both the makers and wearers of spectacles were often men of profound learning. Among them were theologians, philosophers, mathematicians, and astronomers. Some of the spectacle makers have already been mentioned. The great mathematician, astronomer and physicist, Isaac Newton (1642-1727), who was also interested in optics, wrote about the subject and constructed spectacles. The astronomer Galileo Galilei (1564-1642), the inventor of the microscope Anton van Leeuwenhoek (1632-1723), and the philosopher, Baruch Spinoza (1632-1677), all supported themselves by grinding lenses.

The users of glasses included elderly scholars, theologians and monks, who occupied themselves with copying manuscripts. The wearers of glasses were greatly respected and spectacles came to be the symbol of scholarship and educational superiority.

In St. Mark's Convent in Florence, there is a miniature of St. Matthew sitting in front of a table with spectacles on the tip of his nose. A similar picture is seen in a fourteenth century manuscript at the Bibliotheque Nationale of Paris. There St. Paul is depicted as wearing spectacles. These illustrations show the respect bestowed upon the wearer of spectacles.

Lydgate, in his "Life of our Ladye" (written about 1430), tells of a festival in connection with the marriage of the daughter of Juta of Austria. One Pietro Bonapart, who was ambassador to the Austrian court, caused a great sensation by appearing with glasses across his nose which were said to have been made by the Florentine Salvinus de Armatus.

In Spain, in 1659, spectacles were already very popular. The wearers were supposed to be important and dignified personages who belonged to high society. The spectacles were an emblem of elegance, distinction and superiority.[12]

A single eye glass (monocle) was worn in England and Germany by the aristocracy, more for show than for utility. Up to the nineteenth century, German aristocrats, evidently eager to assume a regal and scholarly aspect, wore frames without glasses. An inferior frame was worn in the presence of a superior. Persons of lesser rank did not possess the temerity to be seen in glasses. The present writer recalls the day when abroad, and to some extent here in the United States in the rural districts, the so-called common man seldom wore glasses in public lest he become a laughing stock. He recalls one case in which the nickname "professor" stuck to a bricklayer who was guilty of an infraction of this rule throughout his life.

Until Donder's time,[13] even in the case of eye sickness, glasses were not fitted by specialists. There were no scientific means of estimating the degree of refractive error or for that matter, of determining whether the patient was far-sighted (hyperopic), near-sighted (myopic) or old sighted (presbyopic). Only trial and error methods by the patient himself were employed.

In the early part of the nineteenth century refraction was still not an essential part of the oculist's speciality. Dr. Littell[14] states: "Oculists are often consulted about the selection of glasses (i.e., the quality of glasses) . . . properly selected glasses afford greatest aid and comfort . . . without diminishing the sight, although the contrary is vulgarly imagined."

The actual sale of glasses was in the hands of peddlers, who walked from house to house exhibiting their wares on trays—a sight which older physicians still may recall. Even after the spectacle hucksters were outlawed, spectacles have been and still are sold on the counters of five and ten cent stores.

Before the middle of the last century there were no trial lenses with which to estimate refraction errors. The first box of trial lenses was made by Mr. A. Nacht, and the first physician to construct such an outfit for his own use was C. F. Arlt in the year 1843.[15] The early trial cases had no cylindrical lenses to correct astigmatic errors notwithstanding the fact that cylindrical lenses had been used by Thomas Young as far back as in 1793. This gentleman corrected his own astigmatism by grinding himself such lenses. In 1827 the English mathematician and astronomer, Sir J. B. Airy (1801-1892), repeated the same feat for his own personal use.[16]

In 1803 Dr. William H. Wallastan introduced the periscopic lens, and finally in 1847 Donders conceived the idea of prismatic lenses. Their usefulness was tested out later by Von Graefe.

Küchler in 1843 and Arlt in 1844 were the first to introduce letters of different size as standards for determining visual acuity. Ten years later Jaeger published his scale of types which received general acceptance. Finally Snellen emerged with his test cards.

The first American contribution to the perfection of spectacles was by Benjamin Franklin, who, in 1794, conceived the idea of splitting two lenses, and fixing them in a frame—the upper section to be used for distant sight and the lower section for near sight. This invention has finally resulted in the manufacture of invisible bifocal lenses.

W. C. Posey[17] is authority for the statement that Dr. Isaac Hays of Philadelphia was the first ophthalmologist in America (1854) to prescribe cylindrical lenses to correct astigmatism.

CHAPTER XIV

THE RISE OF THE UNIVERSITIES

Scholasticism helped develop the greatest contribution of the Middle Ages to civilization—the founding of the universities.[1] Of course higher schools of learning were not a medieval creation for great schools of learning had thrived previously: There was the Lyceum in Athens, the Museum in Alexandria, the Bayt al Hakimah in Bagdad, the Dar al Kakimah in Cairo, the highly rated school of learning in Jondisabur, the many academies in Mesopotamia which had been established by the Jews and Arabs, and the great schools that had existed for ages in India. Nevertheless, the establishing of the medieval universities deserves our undying praise because these institutions formed a bridge by which the basic tenets of civilization were transferred from antiquity to the age of enlightenment.

The medieval Latin term *universitas* was originally employed to denote a community, guild or corporation of students and teachers organized for mutual protection without any prearranged curriculum. Experts on any given subject taught novices who were anxious to learn. In the course of the thirteenth and fourteenth centuries, such guilds sprang up in most of the great European centers where monastic schools were not sufficient to satisfy the growing needs of the population.

What we now call a "university" was originally known as a "studium generale"—a term which was applied to higher institutions of learning. The latter were authorized by a papal document issued in 1244-45 by Innocent IV. In the course of time, the term "university" began to be applied to a community of teachers and scholars of higher education whose corporate existence had been recognized and sanctioned by civil or ecclesiastical authorities, or both.

These higher schools of education became extraordinarily popular and the highways became more and more frequented by poor boys who, coming from near and far sought to reach the universities so that they could secure a higher education.

In the dormitories students, in the name of knowledge, slept on straw piled on the floor. The average student who was very poor often had to earn his precarious livelihood by begging—a profession which in those days was respectable. The schools of the monasteries were maintained in a similar way. Monks went around from door to door collecting bread and other articles of food and clothing for their students. Frequently the student found his way to the university by stealing on the wayside anything that was not locked or nailed down.

Private instruction on a fee basis was also frequently given in the houses of the masters. Naturally enough, such students were of the wealthier class and these often lived with their masters.

Oxford and Cambridge Universities were among the first (fourteenth century) to arrange for special quarters (hostel) for students. Such facilities were supervised by a member of the faculty or a prominent citizen and students were furnished with food, lodging and books.

In 1271, the six regents and the dean, comprising the faculty of Paris University, promulgated a rule to the effect that students were required to wear a square cap and a silver medallion.

Students were identified by the country and nation from which they came. In the "studium generale" or "university," all students were compelled to speak Latin which was considered the literary language. Students who absentmindedly spoke in their native tongue in public were punished. Some universities actually employed spies (*"lupi"*) to detect those foreigners who by design or mistake tried to use their own language.

At times innocent games in which the students were accustomed to indulge, were considered sacrilegious—even chess. Students were permitted only "manly" exercises such as practice with the sword, bow and arrow and lance. A common illicit sport of students was to heckle the hangman while he was performing his duties.

The school buildings were somber one or two story stone structures, unheated, and lighted with torches, with no window at all or only one.

The entrance examination to the university often consisted in answering some questions proffered by the rector in acceptable Latin. Since few men in Western Europe had mastered even the rudiments of an education, the entrance examination was most likely a test of the applicant's ability to read and write in the Latin language. Many of the applicants probably first attended monastic "preparatory" schools where Latin exclusively was spoken.

In the classrooms at first it was customary for students to sit on sacks of straw on the floor, and for the master to sit in the center on a higher sack of straw in order to dominate his listeners. This custom was changed in the year 1366 when students were ordered to sit on the ground "so that they might have no reason to be proud." [2]

The curriculum of the university comprised, besides the seven liberal arts and sciences (i.e. grammar, dialectics, geometry, arithmetic, astronomy, rhetoric and music), various other subjects. During the reigns of Charlemagne, Theodoric and Alfred, men were encouraged to devote their time to studies, but there were no first rate schools or academies with curriculums that embraced all sciences, nor were outstanding scholars especially encouraged to disseminate their learning.

In the earlier Middle Ages a university could not exist in Western Europe because there was not enough learning to justify its existence. As a matter of fact, up to the eleventh century, learning was almost entirely confined to the seven liberal arts of the traditional curriculum. It might be fairly stated that in 1000 A.D., scholastically speaking, Latin Europe possessed scarcely more than a fraction of what had been known in Alexandria in the year 200 A.D.

The wide acceptance of the Christian doctrine that the body

was of little importance in comparison with the soul was especially lethal to the study of medicine.[3] At first, "all the universities stood under the jurisdiction of the Church; the teaching was performed under Church regulations, and the books read were chosen by the Church; therefore education, especially in medicine, was purely theoretical and dogmatic and quite impractical, consisting merely in the recitation of a Greek or Arabian writer in Latin translation, with the professor's interpretation."[4]

Although medical books are often found in monastic libraries, the preponderance of evidence suggests that little was known or practiced in the monastic infirmary beyond the traditional leechdoms and old wives' remedies. As pointed out in a previous chapter, medical practice was expressly forbidden to monks as offering too great a temptation for private property and covetousness. Rashdall ventures the opinion that the development of the universities in Europe was not due to the initiative of any pope and that no university was a direct outgrowth of any cathedral school or was founded by monks.[5]

The university made a physical impression upon the student. The student could easily be distinguished from the artisan and peasant youth by the pallor of his face (due to undernourishment and poor living conditions), his manner of speech, and other traits which he acquired by virtue of his living in an educational atmosphere and his spending so much time indoors absorbed in study.

The earliest academic degree was "master." The privilege attached to this degree was authorization to teach. The teachers of Bologna later chose the title "doctor" for their guild. Some teachers preferred to be called "professor" or "domini." In the University of Paris the teachers of philosophy, medicine and art were known as "magister." Frequently they were addressed as professors and seldom as doctors.

In Oxford, the title "doctor" was adopted for all graduates of the superior faculty (i.e. philosophy, medicine and theology) and "magister" for all graduates of the inferior faculty (i.e. law and the arts). In Oxford as in most universities of Western

Europe, there were three degrees: "bachelor," "licentiate" and "doctor."

At Montpellier, the titles of "bachelor," "licentiate" and "master" were conferred upon students in the various grades of progress. Only the teachers at Montpellier were styled "doctors."

The word "doctor" is derived from the Latin "*docere*" meaning "to teach." This designation originally signified a teacher with the highest degree conferred by the universities. Its use by physicians arose from the fact that medical men were looked upon as learned men—perhaps the most learned men in the community. The title "doctor" was probably used for the first time in the twelfth century.

The most difficult task in the early days of the universities was to procure good manuscripts. The records of the faculty of the University of Paris of 1295 contain a list of 20 volumes of medical books possessed by the university, nearly all by Arabian writers. Louis XI, worrying about his health, was anxious to have the works of Rhazes in his personal library. The only copy of this work available in the medical school was thereupon lent to this monarch.

In the early days of the universities, little importance was given to the teaching of medicine and no definite program of medical education was offered. In Paris, the faculties of the learned professions of theology, medicine and law eventually elected a dean at their head. In Bologna, the medical students obtained the right to elect a rector of their own, the "collegium doctorum" who had the authority to confer the medical title and to grant the license to practice medicine. The parceling of medicine into a separate faculty came during the twelfth century.[6]

In medical schools the favorite textbooks included "Tegni" by Galen, the "Aphorisms" by Hippocrates, "Liber Febrium" by Isaac Judeus and "Antidotarium" by Nicholas of Salerno.

One of the special advantages of Montpellier University over Paris was the fact that it possessed many manuscripts of the Arabian writers.

In Bologna and Padua, the price of manuscripts was regulated and the universities controlled their literary productions. Any bookstore was liable to punishment for selling inaccurate copies. According to Rashdall,[7] there were in 1323 more than 28 booksellers in Paris besides the keepers of open air book stalls. Bologna had the distinction of being the first university where medicine was taught. Paris was the second. Both universities were founded in 1180.

Medicine become a popular profession largely because its practitioners could amass large fortunes. One who disliked the attention paid to the medical profession wrote: "With coppers and silvers they received for their poisons they (i.e. the doctors) built themselves fine houses in Paris." Nor was surgery spared from the wrath of the critics: "She (Chirurgery) has such a bold hand that she spares no one from whom she may be able to get money."

There are few changes in the modern universities from the original plans. The customs, ceremonies, titles, and degrees have been carried down to modern times. The differences are only in the increase of knowledge and in the methods with which it is imparted.

The medieval university regulations pertaining to graduate physicians were very strict and the final examinations lasted many hours. The fact that the candidate had to swear in the examination that in case of failure he would not take revenge on the faculty throws light upon the character of the student at that period.

The leading medieval universities to be covered in the present volume include Salerno, Naples, Pavia, Bologna and Padua (in Italy); Montpellier and Paris (in France); and Oxford and Cambridge (in England). Of course these institutions are investigated primarily for their medical curricula. Chapters are also presented which contain information concerning the status of medical education in medieval Germany and Russia.

It is of special interest to devote several pages to a consideration of the medieval medical curriculum.

The following course of study was required to practice medicine and receive a Bachelor of Medicine (M.B.) degree:[9]
Bachelor of Medicine:
For License and Inception:
  For M.A. candidate, six years' study (in all).
  To have lectured cursorily, for theory, on the "Liber Tegni" of Galen, or "Aphorismi" of Hippocrates, *pro majori parte*.
  To have lectured cursorily, for practice, on the "Regimenta Acutorum" of Hippocrates or the "Liber Febrium" of Isaac Judaeus, or the "Antidotarium" of Nicholas.
  To have responded in the schools of the regents for two years.
  For others, to have been admitted to practice, as above: eight years' study (in all): to have given the above lectures.
For admission *ad practicandum* in Oxford:
  For M.A. candidates, four years' study.
  To pass an examination conducted by the regent doctors.
  For others, eight years' study and examination.[10]

An eight year period of study was required to complete the medical course, most of which time was spent on the theory of medicine. The books usually employed as texts were the "Regimenta Acutorum" of Hippocrates, the "Isagogue" of Johannitus (809-873), "De Urinis" and "De Pulsibus" of Theophilus Protospatharius, the "Liber Febrium" of Isaac Judeus and the "Antidotarium" of Nicholas of Salerno (twelfth century). The last two years were spent in discussions, disputations and lectures.

No mention is made of clinical experience or dissection and nothing is said about surgery. It was possible for the fully qualified doctor to leave Oxford without ever having laid hand upon a patient. It seems that neither Oxford nor Cambridge were particularly interested in surgery, although there were some surgeons in thirteenth century England who had studied at Oxford. One was Magister Regerus Chirurgius who testified at a coroner's inquest for the University on a surgical subject.

Physicians skilled in medicine were considered the most learned and to their discretion was entrusted the cure of the sick. Great care was exercised to ascertain that only competent persons were allowed to practice or appointed to the medical faculty.

The teaching consisted of lectures, reading of books and disputations. To this day certain teachers of English universities are known as "readers."

While the common aim of all the universities of the Middle Ages was to spread knowledge, the different institutions differed from each other in accordance with the state of culture at the site of origin and various immediate needs. Some schools, as, for example, Salerno and Montpellier, were securely established and the professors and students remained there more or less permanently. At other universities such as Bologna and Padua, both teachers and students were constantly coming and going from and to other universities always seeking to improve their status. Most of the universities were more or less under the control of the clerics. The lectures, the textbooks and the discussions were at first in conformity with the methods of the Arabs and later with the procedures of the scholastics who aimed rather at dialectic versatility than at depth of knowledge. The educational methods employed adequately demonstrated whether the students had mastered the contents of the lecture and also served to test the students' general knowledge.

Unfortunately educational discussions frequently degenerated into an empty display of words which only satisfied the personal vanity of those so engaged. John of Salisbury (15th Century) wryly declared: "The young people pride themselves on their knowledge of Hippocrates and Galen, make use of unfamiliar expressions and introduce their aphorisms on every occasion."

In medicine, the Italian schools were more advanced than those of the other countries. Bologna was the first university to develop the study of anatomy. There the old religious prejudice against dissection gradually succumbed to the advance of the scientific spirit. Dissection was practised in Bologna at least since the time of Thaddeus of Florence (1223-1302), who was responsible for the securing of more "anatomia" than at other universities. Mondino da Luzzi (1276-1325), sometimes called "the father of modern surgery," was one of the earliest teachers of surgery in Bologna. His "Anatomia" remained the standard textbook for two centuries.

It was customary, in the Italian universities, for a medical doctor to read the proper sections of the anatomical treatises while the professor of surgery performed the dissection. Yet another doctor pointed out the bones, muscles, etc., as they were named by the reader.

Bologna endeavored to have the best medical teaching staff. Hugh of Lucca was induced to come to Bologna as a military and public surgeon by an offer of 600 libra.

A statute of Florence provided that food, wine and spices were to be provided to keep up the spirit of the professor and students during the anatomical ordeal.

It was arranged at Bologna that every medical student of two years' standing could attend an anatomical dissection at least once a year. Twenty students were admitted at a time to see the dissection of a man and thirty to see that of a woman.[11]

The plan of instruction and organization at the universities tended more and more to the freeing of scientific investigation and to the acquisition of scientific knowledge.

The University of Montpellier was practically independent of retrogressive control. The favorite medical textbooks at this institution were the "Canon" of Avicenna, the "Isagogue" of Johannitus, the "Aphorisms," "Regimen" and "Prognostics" of Hippocrates, the "Ars Parva" of Galen and the "Liber Medicinalis" of Rhazes. No work in the original Greek was available. Later the works of Soranus, Paul of Aegina, Aetius, Alexander of Tralles and Dioscorides became available.

Medical teaching at the medieval universities consisted chiefly of theoretical discussions. The medical writings of the ancients and their Arabian and Italian commentators formed the foundation of the discussions. The teacher added his explanations to the available texts and gave his students the benefit of his practical experience. There were different teachers who taught various medical subjects and the curriculum included anatomy, pathology (humoral), materia medica, fevers, surgery, and phlebotomy. The lecture rooms, as they appear in contemporary pictorial representation, show the teacher on a raised platform reading out of a bulky volume to his pupils who are seated below him and are engaged in taking notes.

Concerning the daily schedule of study, Haeser (1871-1884) has prepared a list of the studies of the medical student at the University of Leipzig (founded in 1409) at the end of the fifteenth century:

Hour	First Year	Second Year	Third Year
6-7 A.M.	First book of "Canon" of Avicenna with the explanations of Jacob of Forli.	The "Ars Parva" of Galen, with exposition of Torrigiano.	The "Aphorisms" of Hippocrates with commentaries of Galen and Jacque.
1 P.M.	Book IX of Rhazes' "ad Almansorem" with the exposition of Arculanus.	Further books of the "Canon" of Avicenna.	Further books of the "Canon" of Avicenna with commentaries of Dinus de Garbo e Hugo.
3 P.M.	During this period the "doctors" read various works aloud—especially the "Prognostics" of Hippocrates.		

The curriculum also included *"anatomia seu corporis insectio singulis annis, corpore."* [12]

The first lecture began in winter at seven o'clock in the morning and in summer at six. It dealt with theoretical medicine. A total of three years were spent on these subjects. At one o'clock the lectures on practical medicine began. Three years were also consumed in completing this course of study. The *"Liber Medicinalis ad Almansorem"* by Rhazes with the commentaries of Johannes Arculanus (d. 1484) was covered during the first year. During this year some attention was also given to the book "On Fevers" written by Isaac Israeli. The various books of the "Canon" of Avicenna were covered in the second and third years.

Students were advised to study together in order that they might iron out difficulties of the members of their group. Before going to sleep every student must, "like an ox, chew the cud of what he has learned during the day." [13]

After obtaining the degree of bachelor, the student occupied himself with lectures on special subjects, taking part in the discussions which took place every week under the guidance of the professor. The students also assisted in anatomical dissections and visited hospitals.

To receive the degree of Doctor of Medicine the candidate was required to be twenty years of age and to have attended five years of school. If he had ever previously been licensed, four years of study was sufficient. The student also had to attend lectures on some medical tractate and to have responded in a dispute at least twice during the school term. In some schools it was required for the graduate to have practiced for a year under the supervision of some famous doctor.

In Paris it was established that at least fifty lectures be given on the "Aphorisms" of Hippocrates, thirty on the "Regimenta Acutorum," and thirty-six upon "Prognostics."

In Bologna, physicians were allowed to practice surgery which was looked down upon by the Paris doctors as degrading and entirely beneath the dignity of one learned in the wisdom of Hippocrates, Aristotle and Galen. To be respected even at Bologna, however, the surgeon had to be a physician. He who was not also a physician was in an inferior position.

Examination in surgery was given by the medical faculty and license to practice was granted to those who passed the examination. However, qualified surgeons did not rank as doctors of surgery.

At the University of Tubingen, the following curriculum was employed in 1481:

our	*First Year*	*Second Year*	*Third Year*
A.M.	Galen's "Ars Medica."	First book of Avicenna (anatomy and physiology).	"Aphorisms" of Hippocrates.
P.M.	First and second sections of Avicenna's "Treatise on Fevers."	Ninth book of Rhazes (local pathology).	Galen

In almost all medical curricula, Avicenna or some other Arabian physician's work was used as a textbook of surgery, although practical surgery had been almost entirely foreign to these authors. Besides the ordinary course of instruction, lectures were frequently give on Mesue, Aegidius Corboliensis (c. 1170) and Constantine Africanus (1011-1085).

Anyone who had studied in a University for three years and had attained the age of 21, might become a teacher. First, such a novitiate had to lecture upon the preparatory branches. After three years' further study, he became a "Magister in Physica." To be a "doctor," he had to complete a course of study of six years.

According to documents discovered some years ago, physicians at first were known under the title of "magister." At the beginning of the eleventh century a doctor was called a "medicus vulgerum," and during the second half of the thirteenth century, the title "doctor" is first met with.

In the northern universities, medicine ranked with theology and law and was included in the Superior Faculty. Bologna did not become important as a school of medicine until the School of Salerno declined in the thirteenth century. At that time, the popularity of the Arabic writers was at its height. Arabian teaching, however, contaminated the pure Greek teaching with a mass of astrologic superstition. The physician had to modify his treatment in accordance with the aspect of the heavenly bodies. Astrology was for a time included as one of the regular studies in Bologna.

The position of the astrologic professor was a delicate one for the Church looked upon astrology as a most perverse and satanic science. Cecco d'Ascali, a prominent astrologist, ended his days at the stake (1327).

Although astrology, from a medical point of view, was definitely retrogressive, it must not be entirely despised, for it was at Bologna that Copernicus developed his astrological calculations which resulted in modern astronomy.

Rashdall states: "The rapid multiplication of Universities during the fourteenth and fifteenth centuries was largely due to a direct demand for highly educated lawyers and administrators ... It (i.e. the university) trained pure intellect, encouraged habits of laborious subtlety, heroic industry, and intense application, while it left uncultured the imagination, the taste, the sense of beauty—in a word, all the amenities and refinements of the civilized intellect. It taught man to think and to work rather than to enjoy. Most of what we understand by 'culture,' much of what Aristotle understood by the 'noble use of leisure,' was unappreciated by the medieval intellect. On the speculative side of the Universities were ... 'the schools of the modern spirit.' They taught men to reason and to speculate, to doubt and to inquire, to find a pleasure in the things of the intellect both for their own sake and for the sake of their applications to life. They dispelled forever the obscurantism of the Dark Ages. From a practical point of view their greatest service to mankind was simply this, that they placed the administration of human affairs—in short, the government of the world—in the hands of educated men. The actual rulers—the kings or the aristocrats—might often be as uneducated or more uneducated than the leaders of modern democracies, but they had to rule through the instrumentality of a highly educated class."[14]

It is obviously impossible in the present work to discuss the merits of all the universities founded in the Middle Ages. Such a task would require a huge volume in itself. Many such works are available in the libraries[15] even though these special works do not cover all of the eighty universities that were founded during the Middle Ages.[16]

The present work will discuss those higher schools of learning that have contributed to our medical knowledge. The small universities founded in the Middle Ages will be mentioned only by name: Siena (1241), Salamanca (1243), Piacenza (1248), Palermo (1312), Florence (1320), Grenoble (1339), Pisa (1343), and Valladolid (1346). The fourteenth and fifteenth centuries witnessed the rise of the principal German and Slavic universities: Prague (1347), Cracow (1364), Erfurt (1379), Wurzburg (1402), Leipzig (1409), Rostock (1419), Greifswald (1448), Freiburg in Breisgau (1455), Basel (1460), Budapest (1465),

Ingolstadt (1472), and Tubingen (1477). Scandinavian universities originated in Copenhagen (1475), and Upsala (1477). In Scotland universities were founded in St. Andrew (1411), Glasgow (1453) and Aberdeen (1494).[17]

Medicine attained a scientific position and came under the domination of serious thinkers as soon as the universities succeeded in freeing themselves from the control of the clerics. Though not comparable to our modern medical luminaries, the university medical professors were nonetheless far in advance of medicine's previous guardians who were for the most part empirics and ignorant clergy.[18]

CHAPTER XV

MEDICINE IN MEDIEVAL ITALY

It is one of the whims of destiny that the revival of learning in the later Middle Ages began in Italy in the very country where, after the fall of the great Roman Empire, classical knowledge was first extinguished and ancient tradition forgotten.

Italian medicine up to the opening of the universities (about the tenth century) was purely of a religious nature.[1] It took refuge in the monasteries where it found safe asylum among the studious monks who studied the classical languages by glimmering candlelight. In the monastery founded by St. Benedict at Mount Cassino in 539, medicine occupied a prominent place—at least in its theoretical aspects. From Mount Cassino medical knowledge and practices extended to other Benedictine monasteries and convents.

It is related that King Theodoric through his minister of state, Cassiodorus, urged the monks to read the works of Dioscorides including his description of medicinal plants and herbs and the classical works of Hippocrates and Galen which were long preserved in the archives of the cloisters. Later the monks cultivated gardens around the monasteries where medicinal plants were cultivated.

Another contribution of the Church to medicine was the opening of hospices erected in the vicinity of the monasteries, where strangers, the sick and disabled, found peace and succor under the friendly care of the monks, in whom the human misery caused by wars and epidemic diseases, stimulated a feeling of compassion and self-sacrifice.

Italian medicine up to the ninth century was to all intents

and purposes Church medicine. A new era dawned with the establishment of the medical school at Salerno. There, medicine for the first time in the Middle Ages, assumed a lay trend. It is interesting to note that Salerno, the first university, was founded as a medical school. The second (Bologna) was established as a law school, and the third (Paris) was first opened as a school of theology and philosophy. This succession of events may be taken metaphorically to symbolize the relative importance of man's personal interests. His first interest is in his body, then his possessions and finally his religion. Salerno tried to free itelf from religious bonds and, in doing so, assumed a distinctly scientific character. One can well imagine the struggle that took place at this institution between the new scientific tendencies and the old hair-splitting scholastic theses.

SALERNO

To Salerno belongs the credit of having sheltered the first medieval medical school. For several centuries, this institution enjoyed a reputation second only to Alexandria. Salerno's historical reputation rests not so much on its advances in theoretical or practical medical knowledge but on the fact that it served as a connecting link between the medicine of antiquity and that of the Renaissance in the Christian West.

Salerno, where the university was located, is situated 35 miles southeast of Naples. It was a popular Roman health resort as early as 200 B.C. Its charming location, its mild and salubrious climate, its mountain air and, above all, its proximity to Naples, attracted people who needed medical care from all over Italy.

Salerno became a common meeting ground for Jews, Christians and Mohammedans. In this town, lay physicians as well as monastic healers, found an outlet for their professional skills. Three hundred years before the College of Salerno was founded, hospitals and nurseries with women attendants were thriving in Salerno. Among the more famous early sojourners to Salerno was the famous poet, Horace, who tarried there between 68 and

65 B.C. There is a tradition that the medical school at Salerno was founded by four different physicians; a Jew, a Greek, a Saracen, and a Roman.

The tradition of Greek medicine in Southern Italy was never really entirely interrupted. That the medical men of Salerno had some knowledge of Greek medicine in the seventh, eighth and ninth centuries is apparent. The presence of Donnolo[2] in Salerno during the second half of the ninth century suggests the probability that Salerno at that period was already an educational center.

The University of Salerno is said to have been founded by the Benedictine monks of Mount Cassino. The monks were priests and physicians as the rabbis of old were ecclesiastics and physicians.

So notable a medical historian as Haeser[3] maintains that it is beyond doubt that the schools of Salerno and Montpellier were founded with the help of the Jews. Jews were also among the teaching staffs of these institutions. Renzi (1800-1872) mentions Jewish physicians who taught at Salerno in the years 848-855. These include Joseph who taught in 848 and Joshua who taught in 855. Among the Jews who taught at Salerno, may be mentioned Donnolo. In the judgment of Sarton, "Donnolo's personality is of considerable interest because it enables us to realize how the so-called 'School of Salerno' gradually came into existence. It is just such men as Donnolo who, by their very presence, created that focus in southern Italy of medical syncretism and eventually of medical teaching."

Steinschneider, in his elaborate work on Donnolo (913-982?) whose medical tractate he had discovered, points out that while there is nothing known of Donnolo having lived in Salerno or having had any relation with the school there, it is natural to seek some connection; for Donnolo's work is the earliest in lower Italy after the fall of Rome and shows that Donnolo was under Greek medical influence, which the School of Salerno likewise represented.

In the ninth century, Salerno rose to prominence. It became for the Occident what Bagdad had been for the Orient—the leading medical school. In the eleventh century lectures were delivered in Greek, Arabic, Hebrew and Latin. The medical school of Salerno became celebrated under the name of "Civitas Hippocratica."

The first teachers of Salerno were probably local physicians (with a sprinkling of ecclesiastical healers) who customarily attended their patients at the local sanitaria and hospitals. The instructors include Copho (c. 1110), Garipontus (c. 1015), **Petrocellus or Petronius (1035), Constantine Africanus (1015-1085),** Nicholas of Salerno (c. 1140), Abbela (c. 11th century), and Aegidius Corboliensis (c. 11th century), from Corbeil near Paris. He wrote several books, (De Pulsibus) on the pulse and (De Urinus) on the urine, Elinus[4] and his assistant, Zarach, are said to have taught in Hebrew. Among the professors of Salerno was a physician named Grapheus or Grassus (11th or 12th century), a native Jew of Jerusalem, who was the author of one of the first books on ophthalmology, *Practica Oculorum* or *Ars Probatissima Ocularum II*, the most popular Latin textbook. There were also women physicians including Trotula, the wife of a famous physician of Salerno, Johannes Platearius (c. 1125), who was probably an obstetrician.

According to Steinschneider, Faraguth or Faragrius (c. 1300), was among the first authors of Salerno. He translated the works of Rhazes into Latin.

Gariopontus (died c. 1050) is the author of an encyclopedic work, *Passionarius*, the material of which is apparently taken from the Latin translations of Galen, Paul of Aegina, Alexander of Tralles and Theodorus Priscianus (c. 380) author of *Rerum Medicorum Libri IV*. (Published Basel, 1532). This book was popular among the physicians of the eleventh century.

"Passionarius" is particularly interesting from a linguistic point of view for Gariopontus' terminology is more or less modern. The therapy of this work is based upon practical experience. His rules about the choosing of a wet nurse are worthy of note: "She should not be too far from nor too near to her last childbirth; she must abstain from highly salted food or an excess of pepper." His special diet for the wet nurse prohibited the use of garlic and onions. His frequent quotations from Greek, Roman and Arabic medical authorities shows that he and the School of Salerno followed the teachings of Greek and Roman, as well as Arabian physicians.

The two chief works of the School of Salerno are the "Compendium Salernitanum" and the "Regimen Sanitatis Salernitanum." The former is the first example of a complete textbook of medicine and surgery in which many authors participate under a responsible editor. On this standard work seven writers cooperated: Afflaccius (president of the School of Salerno), Bartolomeus, Copho, Ferrarius, Petronius, Johannes Platearius and Trotula. Especially interesting are the sections relating to venesection, pulse, urine, and fever. All of these subjects are treated according to the principles of Hippocrates.

The structure of the second work consists of a group of Latin poems. One poem begins:[5]

> Thou to health and vigor wouldst attain
> Shun mighty cares, all anger deem profane;
> From heavy suppers and much wine abstain;
> Nor trivial count it after pompous fare
> To rise from table and take to the air.
> Spurn idle noonday slumbers, nor delay
> The urgent call of nature to obey.
> These rules if thou wilt follow to the end
> Thy life to greater length thou may extend.

The second important work, "Regimen Sanitatis Salernitanum," was the backbone of the practice of medicine for a long period. The best text was written by Arnold of Villanova; it passed through 240 separate editions and has been translated into almost every language.[6]

It was generally ascribed to John of Milan who was supposed to have been head of the faculty of the school at the time it was written. Indeed some manuscripts bear his name. Arnold of Villanova, who copied the text, appears to have been the most reliable physician in Salerno.

Sudhoff traces the origin of the *Regimen Sanitatis Salernitanum* to Aristotle's *Conservatione Corporis Humanis* which was translated by John of Toledo, a baptized Jew.

Another popular work was the *Antidotarium* of the famous Nicholas of Salerno (1140); this is the first formulary for compounding medicines on record and the first medical work to be printed (Venice, 1471). It contains many of the then newly introduced Eastern drugs and a table of apothecaries weights and measures.

$$20 \text{ grana} = 1 \text{ scrupulus}$$
$$3 \text{ scrupuli} = 1 \text{ drachma}$$
$$1\frac{1}{2} \text{ drachmae} = 1 \text{ hexagium}$$
$$6 \text{ hexagia} = 1 \text{ uncia}$$
$$12 \text{ uncia} = 1 \text{ libra}$$
$$2\frac{1}{2} \text{ librae} = 1 \text{ sextarius}$$

Nicholas was also the author of *Quid pro Quo*—an alphabetically arranged catalogue of equivalent drugs, capable of replacing each other, when, for any reason, any particular drug was not available.[6a]

An important production of the Salerno School is "Practica Chirurgerie" by Roger Frugardi of Palermo or Roger of Palermo (c. 1210) as taken down by his student Giudo Aretino, partly from lectures and partly from private conversations and written in the year 1180. Roger was a student and teacher at Salerno. In about 1230, a famous pupil of his, Roland of Parma (c. 1250), edited and added to the *Practica*, producing a book which soon became well known as the *Rogerina*. At Salerno, Bologna, and other medical centers, copies of the *Rogerina* were annotated by different surgeons. Finally, in about 1270, there was written at Salerno the *Glossulae Quatuor Magistrorum Super Chirurgium Rogerii et Rolandi*. This commentary by the "four masters," whose names are known as Archimattaeus, Petrocellus or Petroneus (1055), Platearius and Ferrarius, was for generations regarded as the most authoritative surgical work in existence. In about the year 1100, Archimattaeus wrote two works, one on

318

the practice of medicine and the other a guide to the physician on his relations with his patients.

As far as its surgical section was concerned, the *Practica* displaced the *Pantegni* of Haly ibn al Abbas, which Constantine Africanus had translated. The *Practica* is divided into four parts. Of these, the first is concerned with wounds of the head and fractures of the skull; the second deals with diseases of the neck; the third with conditions affecting the upper limbs, the chest, and the abdomen; and the last section covers diseases of the lower limbs, the use of the cautery, and the treatment of leprosy and convulsions. Roger of Palermo is the first to suggest that perforated intestines, which had hitherto presented insurmountable difficulties to surgeons, might be more readily sutured over a hollow of elderwood. Roger recommends ligation of ruptured blood vessels when cauterization and styptics fail to check the bleeding. Like Abulkasim, he favors the re-fracture and resetting of bones which have been broken and united in bad position. One of the most remarkable sections of Roger's "Practica" is the part which describes clearly and rationally the treatment of scalp wounds and fractures of the skull.

Roger describes cancer and syphilis. He presents a case of hernia of the lungs. He administers sponges and seaweed (containing iodides) in the treatment of goiter. He employs styptics, sutures and ligatures. He recommends the healing of wounds by second intention.

Roger does not believe that clean healing, by first intention, is even possible. He states that it is only natural for wounds to become infected and suppurate before finally healing. He insists that wet dressings and ointments should be applied to wounds in order to produce "laudable pus." His authority in later years restrained surgeons from permitting wounds to heal by themselves without any interference.

Roger knew the surgery of war well enough to realize the limitations of his art. "If a man is wounded in the heart, lung, liver, or diaphragm, we do not undertake his treatment." Also hopeless were spinal injuries which he believed were "scarcely or never cured by surgery." Worst of all were wounds of the kidneys, which were committed, without comment, "to the grace and goodness of God."[7]

Salerno made no major contribution to anatomy. The work on the subject of anatomy was taught by Copho the younger, author of *De Anatomia Porci*[8]—anatomy of the pig. Another book by Copho was *Artis Medendi*, a treatise on the practice of medicine.

A medical work entitled *"Tractatus Aegritudinum Curatione"* was very popular. It divides fevers into quotidian, ephemeral, intermediate, and continuous types. Psychosis is treated in this book with diet, purges, bleeding, some drugs, and with music. This book offers the following curious observation on the prognosis of phthisis: "When the hemorrhage occurs at the beginning of the disease, it is a good omen."[9]

It is quite certain that Salerno was never anything else but a medical school. Although, according to De Renzi, of the thirty doctors connected with the Salerno medical school, seven were ecclesiastics, there is not the slightest allusion in the text of "Passionarius" to mysticism or priestly therapeutics. The fact that the professors were allowed to marry shows that ecclesiasticism had little influence on the school. There can be no question, however, that the school was influenced by the Mohammedan physicians of Spain and the Islamic doctors of the East.

The curriculum was so complete and democratic that it attracted students from all over the world. No distinctions were made with regard to race, creed, sex or nationality. It was Salerno that initiated for the first time in centuries a truly scientific method of studying medical science.

The oldest document extant from Salerno is the charter granted by Emperor Frederick II in 1231. By this time, the glorious days of Salerno had already been eclipsed by the younger institutions.

Before the close of the twelfth century, the Salernitan school added to its many laurels entitling her to fame, the re-establishment at long last of the art of surgery, which, during early medieval times, had sunk to a very low level. Cleric-physicians had held themselves aloof from operative manipulations and this field had been left to the uneducated empirics and barbers.

Salerno never developed into a real university. It was a medical college in the modern sense. The Salernitans made concessions to the teachings of Rhazes, Haly Abbas and Avenzoar.

Salerno was a secular institution surrounded on all sides by monastic schools. The school of Salerno must be credited with having arrested the decline of science in the West.

The best known physicians connected with the revival of medicine are Arnold of Villanova and Constantine Africanus. The former is a compiler of the *Regimen Sanitatis Salernitanum* which was considered one of the best Salernitan books. The short verses of clinical instruction activated the study of therapeutics. Originally (1311) the medical poems of Arnold contained 362 pages, but later commentators kept adding to their number until this work eventually became over 3,000 pages in length. The story of Arnold of Villanova will be presented in connection with the University of Montpellier. At present a short description of the life and works of Constantine Africanus is in order.

CONSTANTINE AFRICANUS (A.D. 1010-1087)

Constantine Africanus or Constantine the Moor was born in Carthage. His extensive travels enabled him to learn many languages, among them Arabic and Latin. After many years of wandering throughout the East, he arrived at Mount Cassino Monastery in 1072, bringing with him the works of Rhazes and Avicenna. He spent the remaining 15 years of his life in translating as many as 40 Greek classics from Arabic into Latin.

Constantine's translations into Latin as medical texts, were to the Western World, superior to any it had yet known. Some go so far as to rate Constantine as the herald of the Revival of Learning.

It is not known for certain whether Constantine Africanus taught in Salerno Medical School, but it is quite likely that he mingled with the masters of that school and that he influenced its learning greatly. Shortly before his migration to Mount Cassino, he obtained employment as secretary to Robert Guiscard, the Norman ruler of the Sicilies, but he did not find the court life congenial so he resigned.

Through his translations he became one of the most important figures in the history of Mount Cassino and in the development of medicine in Europe.

Among his Latin translations are the "Pantegni," which was a portion of the "Royal Book" of Haly Abbas, the book "On Diet" of Isaac Judaeus, and various of the writings of Hippocrates and Galen. Constantine Africanus' works stimulated the studies of medicine, materia medica and pharmacy. Despite the fact that he never gave his sources, his works succeeded in reviving interest in the Greek medical classics, in Salerno.

Salerno differed from contemporary centers of learning in that it was not under monastic control; lay physicians flourished and they attempted—at first feebly to be sure—to return to originality in medicine. These lay physicians, untrammeled by religious duties and unhindered by monastic ordinances, extensively and laboriously transcribed the Greek masters into Latin, which action was the main contribution of the School of Salerno to the history of medicine.[10]

Salerno began to decline soon after Frederick II (1194-1250) founded the University of Naples (1225). His successor, Charles of Anjou (1226-1285), favored Naples and brought in to this institution famous teachers from the Universities of Paris and Orleans. After the founding of the Universities of Palermo and Montpellier, the prestige of Salerno rapidly declined, but it persisted until 1811 when Napoleon finally abolished it.[11] Derenberg visited Salerno in 1848. He found no trace of the Medical School which had once been its glory.

UNIVERSITY OF NAPLES

The University of Naples was founded by the Emperor Frederick II in the year 1225, as a school of theology, jurisprudence, the arts and medicine. Frederick's design was that his subjects in the Kingdom of Naples should find in the capital adequate facilities for instruction in every branch of learning, and that they "not be compelled in the pursuit of knowledge to have recourse to foreign nations or to beg in other lands." In the year 1231, however, he decreed that the faculty of medicine should cease to exist, and that medical studies should be pursued nowhere in the kingdom but at Salerno. The University of Naples never attained great eminence, and for a time was closed altogether, but it was reopened in 1258 by King Manfred. In 1266 its faculty of medicine was reconstituted, and from 1272-74, Thomas Aquinas was one of its teachers of theology.

UNIVERSITY OF PAVIA

Pavia had become widely known as a seat of legal studies even before Irnerius (12th century) taught at Bologna. There is no evidence, however, to establish a direct connection between this early school and the University which was founded there in 1261 by virtue of the charter granted by Emperor Charles IV.

The new *studium* included faculties of jurisprudence, philosophy, medicine, and the arts. Its students were formally under imperial protection and were endowed with privileges identical with those which had been granted to students of Paris, Bologna, Oxford, Orleans and Montpellier. The studium in Pavia was temporarily closed and the students transferred to Piacenza. With the decline of the University of Piacenza after the death of Giovanni Galeazzi, however, Pavia again prospered. Its professors throughout the fifteenth century were men of distinguished ability and received munificent salaries such as few of the other universities could offer. Pavia became especially famous for the study of the civil law. With the exception of Padua, Pavia, had no rival in Italy.

Like most of the universities of Italy, Pavia attracted many foreign students, who were arranged in the classes according to their nationalities. The student body does not seem to have controlled the university as occurred in Bologna.

Pavia presented quite a range of subjects in its curriculum. In 1433, it had 20 medical teachers. There were special morning, afternoon and evening lectures on medicine, practical medicine, surgery, physics, metaphysics, logic, astrology, and rhetoric. The most striking omission on the roster is anatomy which does not appear even as late as 1467.

The textbooks consisted largely of the works of Arabian authors. In 1447, lectures were given on the "Almansor" of Rhazes. In the catalogue of Ferrari's library more than half of the works are Arabian commentaries on Greek medicine. In Ferrari's textbooks printed in 1471, which were previously circulated as manuscripts, the great influence which the Arabic works had over the students of Pavia is evident.

The Pavian physicians practiced polypharmacy. Osler aptly states: "I have the records of an elaborate consultation written in his (Professor Ferrari's) own handwriting from which one may gather what a formidable thing it was to fall in the hands of a medieval physician." [12]

In one of his case histories, Dr. Ferrari discusses the case of Sir John de Calabria who had a digestive weakness in his stomach and rheumatic cerebral disease combined with superfluous heat and dryness of the liver. After diagnosing the case, Ferrari presents an elaborate discussion on the patient's diet and general mode of life. It must have taken a fully stocked apothecary's shop to compound the 22 prescriptions listed by Ferrari in treating this case and designed to meet every possible contingency.

Dr. Ferrari plays an important part in the history of Pavia between the years 1432 and 1472 as is evident from the documents relating to the Ferrari family.

UNIVERSITY OF BOLOGNA

The oldest complete university in Europe was Bologna (Salerno was only a medical school). If the archives of the town of Bologna can be relied upon, Bologna was founded in the year 1123. The people of Bologna in 1923 celebrated the eight hundredth anniversary of the University. The origin of the University, however, really goes back to the year 1088 when a guild of law students was formed for their mutual protection.

From the very beginning, the students, rather than the masters, were in administrative control of the university. They were a privileged class. Emperor Barbarosa (in 1158) accorded to them the privilege of freedom to travel and relieved them from all civil jurisdiction.

About the year 1200 the faculties of medicine and philosophy were established and the former slightly antedated the latter. The university developed slowly and there was a long succession of able teachers, among whom Thaddeus Alderotti and Mundinus were the most eminent. The Faculty of Arts, down to the fourteenth century, scarcely attained eminence. The teaching of theology remained for a long time exclusively in the hands of the Dominicans. It was not until the year 1360 that Innocent VI recognized Bologna as a *"studium generale"* or an institution of general education for all students with the power of conferring degrees of universal validity.

Only the professors who were in receipt of salaries from the municipality are mentioned in connection with the University. Of these, there were twelve teachers of civil law and six of canon law (evidently the law department was the largest), three of medicine, three of practical medicine, one of surgery, two of logic, and one each of astrology, rhetoric and notarial practice.

The University came to include the College of Doctors of Civil Law, the College of Doctors of Canon Law, the College of Doctors in Medicine and Arts and, from 1352 on, the College of Doctors in Theology. Though the professors were largely dependent upon the students, they had separate organizations of their own. The colleges alone—not the University itself—were concerned with the conferment of degrees. Each faculty in Bologna was entirely independent of every other (except for the union of Medicine and Arts). The only connecting link between the colleges was the necessity of having their degrees approved (after 1219) by the same chancellor who was the Archdeacon of Bologna.[13]

In 1219, Honorius III ordered that no promotion to the doctorate should take place without the consent of the Archdeacon of Bologna. Perhaps it was partially this particular restriction of their rights that influenced a large number of students to secede from Bologna and found the school in Padua. In 1295, the Medical College of Bologna was established under an independent rector who was recognized by the city. The College of Medicine obtained control over the liberal arts.

Since the professors were selected by the students at Bologna, they were held strictly accountable to the students for the proper performance of their duties. A teacher who refused to vow obedience to the representative of the students had no means of collecting his lecture fees and was liable to further punishment at the will of the rector. The usual penalty for displeasing the students was dismissal. Even the ordinary social amenities were denied to such a discharged professor.

The masters for a time gave lectures in their own houses and helped support themselves by renting out rooms to their students. In 1405, the College of Medicine and Arts issued an order prohibiting lecturing in noisy business districts.[14]

After five years of study for a civilian and four years for a canonist, the rector raised the student to the dignity of a bachelor by permitting him to give extraordinary lectures. After two years in this capacity, he was ready to proceed to the doctorate —an elaborate and expensive ceremony during which the degree was granted.[15]

The doctoral candidate's thesis was examined by two professors who questioned him on its contents. If he passed the examination, he was finally presented by the promoters to the chancellor, who conferred upon him the right to teach everywhere. This ceremony ended with a banquet which the candidate gave to friends after he was conducted through the town in triumphal procession. The banquet was so elaborate and costly that the students requested that it be dropped. They also requested that the graduate be not required to wear any other costume except an ordinary black gown.

The University of Bologna gained much prestige when Thaddeus Alderotti joined the staff of teachers in 1260. He was regarded by his contemporaries as the most famous physician in Italy. He was immortalized in verse by Dante, who called him, "the Hippocratist." Alderotti is considered the founder of dialectic medicine.

The University of Bologna occupies a most important position in the history of scholastic medicine. Bologna was already a seat of scholastics and dialecticians when the University opened its doors.

The University of Bologna's real bid for fame rests on the part it played in the revival of modern surgery and anatomy.

THADDEUS ALDEROTTI (c. 1223-1303)

Among the famous physicians of Italy was Thaddeus Alderotti of Florence. Owing to the impoverished condition of his home, his education began when he was twenty-two years of age. He quickly learned the elementary subjects. In the year 1260, when he reached the age of 37, he was well learned in medicine and philosophy and occupied a prominent position at the University of Bologna. Nine years later he began to write.

Thaddeus Alderotti taught medicine after the manner of the scholastics. He paid much attention to the logical elaboration of the subject, but in spite of his adherence to the hair-splitting method of the scholastics, he may be considered a scientific physician.

His anatomical knowledge was primarily derived from the Greek and Arabic physicians although it is probable that he on occasion engaged in dissection upon cadavers. His statement to the effect that he could not, with certainty, answer a question relating to pregnancy because he had not the means of making dissections on pregnant women, leads to the inference that he had dissected other cadavers. It appears that under the influence of Thaddeus occasional dissections were performed in Bologna. There are also hints in his works that postmortem examinations were occasionally conducted.

In his "Consili Medicinalia," he incorporates many interesting clinical observations from his own practice. He wrote commentaries on Hippocrates, Galen and on the "Isagogue" of Hunain ibn Ishak. He also authored a short treatise on hygiene, "De Conservanta Sanitate." His library contained, among other books, the "Canon" of Avicenna and the "Liber Almansor" of Rhazes. He translated the ethics of Aristotle into Latin. He was very famous among physicians and medical authors and his students included Bartolomeus da Variganana (13th century), Henry Mondeville and Mondino de Luzzi.

He acquired great wealth from his medical practice. It is said that he exacted enormous fees from certain patients. Pope Honorius XII (1285-1287) paid him 200 florins a day besides a stipend of 6,000 florins.[16] Various physicians of the Middle Ages had little difficulty in collecting higher fees than modern physicians can command. Gabriel Bactishua (referred to earlier in this work), a favorite of Harun al Rashid, received $1500 for bleeding and purging the commander of the faithful, besides his regular monthly salary of $6,200. It is estimated that during his professional life his total fees amounted to about $10,000,000. When he was called to treat Caliph al-Mamun, he received $125,000 for this consultation.[17] Abu Nasr, an Arabic physician, received more than $60,000 for curing a certain Caliph.

Thaddeus' treatise on fever was translated into Hebrew under the title, "Klal Kizur al Minhag Hakadahat."

WILLIAM OF SALICETO (c. 1210-1275)

Another famous teacher of Bologna University was Guglielmo de Saliceto, better known as William of Saliceto. He was born in the town of Saliceto, near Piacenza, Italy. He studied medicine and surgery at the University of Bologna, where he subsequently lectured on surgery. Saliceto was considered the greatest surgeon of the thirteenth century.

In 1275, he moved to Verona where he was appointed chief of the local hospital. His opus magnum, "Chyrurgia," served as a textbook on surgery. He began writing this book in the year 1271 and completed it in the year 1275. Saliceto dedicated this work to his master, Bruno del Carbo, father of Dino del Carbo (d. 1327), a famous physician of Florence. The senior Carbo was a prominent surgeon and professor at Bologna.

Saliceto divided his "Chyrurgia" into five parts. Part one deals with miscellaneous surgical subjects. Part two concerns itself with injuries and contusions of the various parts of the body. Part three covers fractures and dislocations. Part four includes a survey of surgical anatomy—the first attempted by any surgeon. Topographical anatomy was a new science in those days. Part five surveys various operations and the instruments employed in performing them.

The anatomy of Saliceto was not based on personal dissection, but on the anatomical descriptions of Galen and the Latin translations of the Arabs. He, however, manifested independence in subscribing to or rejecting the teachings of the ancient anatomists.

Saliceto treats injuries of the skull by applying a heavy dressing to prevent a harmful excess of air from entering the wound and he lays stress upon the gravity of paralysis on the opposite side. He prescribes treatment for arrow wounds and other penetrating wounds of the chest and abdomen. He diagnoses fractures of bones by crepitus. He treats insect wounds with applications of oil. He arrests hemorrhage with sutures, pressure on the bleeding part, rest and suitable diet. The instruments used for cauterization were made of gold, silver, brass or iron. At times he advises the local application of caustic drugs.

He describes a typical case of a syndrome which he believes to be the first indication of a group of symptoms presently associated with nephritis.

His work, "Summa Conservationis et Curationis," contains good advice with regard to bedside manners, diagnostic enquiries, obstetrical judgment and hygiene for every age.

Some of his wise sayings are as follows:

"The physician should be reflective with downcast countenance, giving the impression that all his wisdom is contained in the mind." . . . "Very little conversation should be indulged in with friends and relatives of the patient for the chain of foolish speech is not attributed to silence." ... "The physician should hold himself aloof from all that might damage his reputation with the public." ... "Visits to patients should not be over frequent, but only upon the desire of the patient." ... "Great care should be taken in supplying narcotics, ordering abortifacients or employing measures to prevent conception if this last is contrary to religion."

His teachings on diet and hygiene are wise and thorough. He recommends especially careful hygienic regulations during pregnancy and for the newly born child, during the first year of life. To facilitate a constipated child's defecation he recommends lubricating the anus with oil. Crying of a baby should not arouse anxiety as this expands its lungs and assists its metabolism. The child should be bathed daily. Wine is forbidden to all children. At the end of the sixth year, consideration should be given to the child's training. After fourteen years of age, more freedom may be given as to choice and quality of food. All children require good and proper exercise, a healthy dwelling-place and a suitable sleeping apartment.

Saliceto was aware of the contagious character of certain diseases and indicated proper prophylaxis. His "Chyrurgia" was translated into Italian, French, English, Hebrew and other languages. The author most often quotes Hippocrates, Galen, Rhazes, and Avicenna.

Among the famous surgeons who studied or taught at Bologna were Hugh of Lucca (d. 1252-1268), Hugh Borgognoni (c. 1180) and his son Theodoric (1205-1296). Hugh of Lucca emphasized simple devices for healing lesions of the extremities and fractures. Although he has left no written manuscripts, his ideas are known, through his son Friar Theodoric Borgognoni.

THEODORIC BORGOGNONI (1205-1296)

Theodoric of Cervia (Theodoric Borgognoni) was the most original surgeon of his time. He was the son of Hugh of Lucca who was also famous for his surgical skill and sound judgment.

He received the appellation, Theodoric of Cervia, because of the bishopric he occupied in that diocese under the Dominican Order. He became especially noted for his innovations in the treatment of wounds. If he is not the discoverer of aseptic surgery, he at least anticipated Lister's treatment with the extreme cleanliness he insisted upon and the avoidance of salves and plasters. He washed the wound with wine before approximating the edges and employed lint soaked in wine to facilitate union. He was strongly of the opinion that the formation of pus ("laudable pus") interferes with natural union and is harmful.

In his surgical anthology, "Chirurgia" (1498-1499), he states: "It is not necessary, as Roger and Roland have written, as many other of their disciples declare and as all modern surgeons teach, that pus should be generated in a wound; no error can be greater than this. Such a practice hinders nature, provokes the disease and prevents the coagulation and consolidation of the wound."[18]

Hugh and Theodoric, father and son, are also remembered for their use of soporific sponges which were steeped in a mixture of opium, hyoscyamus, hemlock, lettuce and mulberry juice. These sponges were applied to the nose and to the site of operation and were similar to those mentioned in the "Antidotorium" of Nicholas of Salerno. Theodoric suggested the use of mercury until salivation ensued in treating various skin diseases. Theodoric was bitterly attacked by Guy de Chauliac as a plagiarist. The antagonism existing between these two authorities was undoubtedly fanned by the fact that Theodoric violently contradicted the pseudo-Galenic doctrine of "coction."[19]

Another distinguished physician of Bologna was Lombardo Bertuccio (d. 1347), who, if for no other reason, is entitled to fame for numbering among his pupils the great surgeon Guy de Chauliac and Pietro di Azzolino of Argelata.

MUNDINUS DE LUZZI (1270-1326)

The most famous teacher during the first quarter of the fourteenth century at the University of Bologna was Mundinus de

Luzzi, son of the apothecary, Merino. He was the first to revive the study of practical anatomy. Before him, dissection was largely practiced on animals. He was the first to introduce human dissection at Bologna. He was associated with Bologna from 1306-1326.

Mundinus was born at Bologna in the year 1270 and it was at Bologna that he received his first instruction and where he gave the first public lectures on anatomy. He performed the first autopsy in his early days at Bologna on a male cadaver. According to Singer, this may have been done to discover the cause of death. An autopsy on a female body, according to Ciasca, was performed by Mundinus in January, 1315.

His work, "Anathomia," although full of Galenic errors, was the first real anatomical textbook written and it shows that he conducted regular dissections. He is said to have been the first physician to descend from his rostrum to watch the students dissect from close range in order to verify the statements made by Galen with reference to anatomy. His "Anathomia," first written in 1316 passed through twenty-five editions and it remained standard in the Italian schools until the time of Vesalius. The first printed edition was published in Padua in the year 1478.

Despite the fact that through the influence of Mundinus it became quite common to practice dissection in every medical school using the "Anathomia" as a guide, the science of medicine did not advance much in the fourteenth century.

Public dissections were decreed at the universities of Montpellier in 1366, at Venice in 1368, at Florence in 1388, at Lerida in 1391, at Vienna in 1414, at Bologna in 1405, at Padua in 1478 and at Tubingen in 1485.[20]

In the "Anathomia," Mundinus quotes Galen's reasons why a man should write books:

(1) To satisfy his own friends.
(2) To exercise his own mental powers.
(3) To be saved from obliviation, incident to old age.

It is reported that in the year 1319, Mundinus assisted a young girl student named Alesandra Galioni. She became an enthusiastic dissector and is reported to have been the first to practice the injection of colored fluid into the blood vessels of the dissected body so as to trace their distribution.

UNIVERSITY OF PADUA

The University of Padua was unquestionably the direct result of the migration of a considerable number of students from Bologna (in 1222). In the year 1228, the students of Padua were compelled by circumstances to transfer their residence to Vercelli, and in the latter part of the thirteenth century grammar, rhetoric and medicine were incorporated into the curriculum. During the oppressive tyranny of Ezzelin (1237-1260), the university maintained its existence with some difficulty. Later it became one of the most flourishing schools of Italy—a great center of Dominical and other learning.

The fame of the University of Padua received a great impetus when Pietro d'Abano was appointed a teacher there in 1306. His eminence as a physician and philosopher was so great that students from far and wide came to listen to his discourses.

PIETRO D'ABANO (1250-1316)

Pietro D'Abano, known also as Petrus De Apono or Aponensis, Italian physician and philosopher, was born at the Italian town from which he takes his name in 1250. After studying medicine and philosophy at Paris, where he also taught medicine for some time, he settled at Padua, where he attained the reputation as the most celebrated teacher and the most skillful physician of his time.

Pietro's *opus magnum* covered the entire field of current knowledge including theoretical and practical medicine. In this work, he strived to reconcile divergent views so that all schools could derive a knowledge of natural philosophy which he believed to be the cornerstone of all sciences, including medicine.

He was an Averroist in his philosophy and a dialectician in his ideas. This book, "Conciliator Controversiarum quae inter Philosophos et Medicos Versantur," published in Mantua in 1472 and Venice in 1476, made his name famous and led to his being known as "the conciliator." In this work, he presented all problems as dialectical queries and solved them so that in almost every case the empirical proof was overcome by syllogism. His true master in medicine was Avicenna although in his studies on the soul, Pietro was generally faithful to the ideas of Averroes. He was not, however, slavishly bound to his masters and often manifested his independence. Because of his adherence to the philosophy of Averroes, Padua acquired the reputation of being a heretical university.

He was called by the city of Padua in 1306 and he became professor of medicine at the University in that year, although his name was already well known to scholars. He very soon became a celebrated practitioner and was often consulted by Pope Honorius IV and Marquis Azzo d'Este. Students came from far and wide to attend his lectures. It is said that when Gentile da Foligno (d. 1348), one of the greatest surgeons of this time, came before the hall where the master was teaching, he fell on his knees and cried out: "Hail, O holy temple!" Among his pupils were Gentile da Foligno and Dino Del Carlo.

"The influence," states Castiglioni, "exercised by Pietro through his teaching and his books, some of which were considered authoritative till the end of the fifteenth century, was certainly deep and vast, and even Dante, who lived at Padua at this time and probably was one of his pupils, felt his influence."[21]

Pietro also wrote "De Venenis Corumque Remediis" (1472), of which a French translation was published at Lyons in 1593.[22]

Pietro's simple and natural therapeutics shows that he was against all complicated measures of treatment. He prescribed cold water in many cases as the best remedy.

As intimated, with reference to the existence and function of the soul, he followed Averroes,[23] but his general philosophy was not bound to either Averroes or Aristotle.

Pietro d'Abano translated some of Aristotle's and Galen's writings from Greek into Latin. He was a firm believer in astrology as applied to medicine, but he was by no means an exception in this belief. Many physicians of his time had faith in astrology. He translated the astrologic works of Abraham ibn Ezra into Latin.

These are some of the questions brought up in his famous work, "Conciliator," which remained unanswered:

"Is the number of elements four or otherwise? . . . Has air weight in its own sphere? . . . Does blood alone nourish? . . . Does the marrow nourish the bones? . . . Is there a mean between health and sickness? . . . Is a smaller head a better sign than a larger one? . . . Are the arteries dilated when the heart is, and contracted also when it is? . . . Can a worm be generated in the stomach? . . . Should one take exercise before or after meals? . . . Should heavy food be taken before light food? . . . Should one eat twice or several times a day? . . . Should the main meal be at noon or at night? . . . Should one drink after eating fruit? . . . Should one sleep on the right or on the left side? . . . Does confidence of the patient in the doctor assist the cure? . . . Should treatment begin with strong or weak medicine? . . . Is cold water good in fevers? . . . Can fever coincide with apoplexy? . . . Is paralysis of the right side harder to cure than that of the left? . . . Can consumption be cured? . . . Does milk agree with consumptives? . . . Is a narcotic good for colic? . . . Is bloodletting from the left a proper treatment for gout in the right foot?"

Pietro lists the following fundamental qualities necessary for a good physician: "He must be logical, intelligent, of good memory, an attentive reader, diligent, expert, truthful, faithful, strong, modest, courteous and sympathetic."

Legend has it that before he died, Pietro told his students who had gathered around him that he had devoted his life especially to three noble sciences: The science of philosophy made him subtle; the science of medicine made him rich; and the science of astrology made him a liar.

Pietro was considered the most scientific and literary man of his age. As intimated previously, with regard to medicine, Pietro's master was Avicenna. He accepted the latter's four phases of disease; onset, increase, fastigium, and decline. According to Pietro, natural philosophy is the basis of all science including medicine and materia medica. He tried particularly to reconcile Arabian medicine with the speculative philosophy of the West as taught by Averroes. Puccineoti's (1784-1822) reference to "the pestiferous Arabic seeds" scattered in the University of Padua and Venice by Pietro d'Abano is unjust, for it is precisely because of Pietro that Padua had a more liberal trend than other schools of learning in Italy.

One of the accusations brought against Pietro was that he refused to visit patients except for exorbitant fees. Perhaps it was his mercenary tendencies coupled with his meddling into astrology, that caused him to be charged with practicing magic. He was openly accused of possessing the "philosopher's stone" and of bringing back into his purse, with the aid of the devil, all the money he had ever spent.

In 1315, the Dominicans accused him of being a heretic because of his adherence to Averroism. He was twice brought to trial by the Inquisition. On the first occasion he was acquitted. He died in 1316 before the second trial was completed, but nonetheless, was found guilty. His body was ordered to be exhumed and burned. However, a friend secretly removed the body and the Inquisition had to content itself with the public proclamation of its sentence and the burning of Pietro d'Abano in effigy. His fame as a scholar and his zeal as a teacher could not leave indifferent those who saw in him a destroyer of medieval scholasticism.

Castiglioni, referring to Pietro d'Abano, says: "He was one of the most eminent scholars of his time who, with his vast literary and scientific lore dominated the whole learning of his epoch. He attempted to solve with philosophic arguments the contradiction which arose between medicine of the Arabic authors and speculative philosophy. He endeavored to prepare nine treatises covering completely theoretical and practical medicine in which all tendencies would be reconciled and through which scholars could be informed about natural philosophy, which in his opinion, was the pivot of science as well as diseases and their remedies."[24]

Among the prominent physicians of later generations who studied at Padua were Vesalius, the great anatomist; William Harvey, the discoverer of the circulation of the blood; Richard Mead (1673-1754); and the two Jewish physicians, Capilius Pector and L'Ebreo Solomon Lazzi. Thanks to the academic freedom enjoyed in this university, Protestants and Jews were able to obtain their degrees there despite the injunctions of the popes prohibiting instruction and certification to non-Catholics.

The liberality of the people of Venice which was in the Suzerain of Padua, combined with the extensive commerce carried on with many countries, made the Paduans more tolerant than the citizenry of other Italian cities. Their motto was: "We are Venetians first and Christians after."[25]

CHAPTER XVI

MEDIEVAL FRENCH MEDICINE

Medicine in France during the early Middle Ages was under priestly domination. The idea that diseases are demonic in origin and that natural means are most ineffectual in combating them, was most popular. Only religious measures could combat the occult forces successfully. Prayer, making the sign of the cross over the affected area, sprinkling the diseased parts with holy water and other such spiritual remedies, afforded the only efficient means of curing the sick.

Remedies such as the blood of animals, the juices of plants and herbs and the excreta of animals and humans were often added to the religious ritual to bring about a cure. Astrological concepts which were scientific in name, but purely magical in fact, were also used in combating disease both prophylactically and therapeutically.

There were no great medical personalities in France in the early Middle Ages—certainly no one to even compare with Galen, Aetius, Paul of Aegina and Rhazes. Marcellus, the Empiric of Bordeaux (fifth century), court physician of Emperor Theodosius and author of "de Medicamento" was the most celebrated physician of the early French medieval period. His work (first printed in 1536), however, does not display any originality. It contains the names of some diseases, a few prescriptions and a large amount of superstition.

Marcellus Empiricus lived during or shortly before the reign of King Clovis (466-511 A.D.), the monarch who at his coronation (A.D. 498) inaugurated the practice of "royal touch" as a cure for those afflicted with scrofula.

338

Gregory of Tours (538-595 A.D.) in his writings has preserved the names of some Gallic physicians of his day: Reoval, physician of Badegona; Maribif, physician of Chilperic; Apollonair, his own physician, and Sedicus, the court physician of Charles the Bald,[1] but these are merely names and nothing is known of their accomplishments.

From the eighth to the thirteenth century, French medical instruction was dominated by oriental influences. Jewish physicians were in great demand. Charlemagne maintained two of them at his court: Farragus and Bubalya Pengestus (L'Meunier) who composed the "Tacuin" or table of health. Charles the Bald also had a Jewish physician at his court. The Jewish doctors were in demand largely because they were believed to possess the secrets of the Arabs. They read Arabic and studied the Arabic versions of the commentaries of Hippocrates and Galen.

When the Jews were banished from France, the monks were permitted to practice the medical art. To the monks we are indebted for preserving some of the works of the Greek masters, thus supplying the potential fuel for future generations to emerge from the shadow of medievalism.

At the close of the ninth century an oculist by the name of Gerbert enjoyed a wide reputation. Other Gallic physicians named Baudouin and Grimbald were famous for they were called in consultation by the King of England during his illness. It is not known whether they were ecclesiastics who practiced medicine or lay physicians. Bishop Gilbert Maninot of Lisieux was the first physician of William the Conqueror. It is likely that his medicine was of a religious nature.

The monastery of St. Benignus imparted a considerable knowledge of medicine to the monks, and some of them enjoyed a wide medical reputation. However, monkish medicine was not always popular and as a matter of fact it was against the rules of their monastic order for monks to practice medicine outside of the monastery.

The practice of surgery up to the twelfth century was always in the hands of laymen. The Church was opposed to the shedding of blood in any manner or form. The type of lay physicians of those days may be inferred from the advice given by one of them to King Baldwin of Flanders in 1205. Abbot Guibert de Nogent tells us, in special admiration of King Baldwin's generous and humane character, that, when he was severely wounded, and dangerous internal suppuration supervened under a treacherous film of growing flesh, he refused to save himself at the expense of a fellow-creature's life. His physician had recommended that he command one of his Saracen prisoners (for it was criminal to ask it of any Christian) of his own stature to be wounded in the same place where he himself had been smitten, and, after the infliction of this wound, to be slain for postmortem study. Baldwin's "extreme piety" was shocked at this suggestion. He permitted the experiment to be made upon a bear, "a beast that is useless except as food or sport."[2]

Other great men were not so scrupulous. Frederick II, "the marvel of the world," had strong if ruthless scientific interests, with the power of gratifying every whim. On one occasion, the chronicler Salimbene tells us, he fed two men sumptuously at dinner, and then sent one to sleep and forced the other to take vigorous exercise. After a sufficient interval, he caused both to be opened, in order to judge which had digested best. On another occasion, he enclosed a living man in a sealed casket. Since, when the casket was opened no soul appeared, but only the corpse, this strengthened his disbelief in survival after death.

Under stringent legal restrictions in medieval times, the surgeon worked daily and hourly in jeopardy of life and limb. In the seventh century Guntram, King of Burgundy, had two physicians executed upon his wife's tomb because the queen died of plague in spite of their treatment. In 1337, a traveling eye surgeon was thrown into the Oder because he failed to cure John of Bohemia of his blindness. In 1464, Mathias, King of Hungary, issued a proclamation that whoever cured him of an arrow wound would be richly rewarded, but he who failed would be put to death. This barbarity is living evidence of the status of medicine in those days. Traveling quack surgeons, in couching a cataract, often put out an eye; in cutting for stone, often mangled the viscera; repairing a hernia, often nicked the gut—all with catastrophic results.

The traveling inguinal hernia surgeon usually believed that castration was a necessary part of his operation because he thought that the intestines and testicles are enclosed in the same sac which must be removed in its entirety to effect a cure and prevent relapse and faulty healing of the peritoneum.[3]

Albutt gives a striking example of a medieval "cutter" who in ligating an artery, paralyzed his patient's arm by severing a nerve. The doctor was ever afterwards chased and cursed by his miserable victim whenever the two chanced to meet.

The hospital was an early French institution. It was first built for isolating lepers, but afterwards its use was extended to offer hospitality to strangers, to the poor and to the sick. The Hotel Dieu of Paris was, for a time, the only place that would admit sick persons. It gradually grew into a large institution and, although its rooms were small and inadequate, it was kept clean. It is stated that 1300 brooms were used up annually in the cleaning of this institution.

The administration of hospitals in France was under the charge of the bishop of the diocese and various prominent citizens. The medical staffs were recruited from various religious Orders—especially the Augustine Order. The medical service of the Hotel Dieu at Paris was under the control of a senior physician ("*docteur regent*") of the medical faculty of Paris University. Surgeons were placed under the authority of physicians for the art of surgery had fallen into the hands of the unlettered. The inferiority of surgeons retarded the development of surgery to an immeasurable degree.

Prior to Jean Pitard (thirteenth century), surgeons in France were not subject to any restraints or regulations. Pitard established the rule that no one of the surgical corporation could practice surgery unless he had previously submitted to a rigorous examination. Prior to Pitard, the surgeons had the right to conduct examinations and to confer various lower degrees, but not that of "doctor." Jean Pitard, founder of the College Saint de Come, therefore, may be considered to be the Father of French surgery.[4]

The medieval surgeons' lot in France was not a happy one.

They were engaged in constant quarrels with the members of the next lower order—the barber surgeons. The medical faculty apparently favored the barbers whenever possible. The reason why the medical doctors favored the barbers over the surgeons was obviously because the barbers were much less their competitors. The doctors even gave the barbers courses in dissection, as well as lectures although most of this instruction was given in secret. The instruction to the barbers was given in French and the surgeons also used the French vernacular. However, the Faculty of Medicine officially spoke only Latin. It was compulsory for a medical student to speak Latin in all public places as well as in the class-room.

For a long time, the Faculty of Medicine refused to recognize the surgeon and vice versa. Eventually, however, the medical faculty was forced to acknowledge the authority of the surgeons.

Just as the medical faculty suffered, or thought they suffered, at the hands of the surgeons, so the latter had to constantly combat the machinations and demands of the barbers who tried their best to be incorporated into the surgeon guild and to conduct anatomical demonstrations. Finally, in 1423, the surgeons secured a decree from the provost of Paris prohibiting the barbers from exercising any of the functions of the surgeons.

UNIVERSITY OF MONTPELLIER

The University of Montpellier or Mons Pesulanus (named so for its commerce with spices) is perhaps the oldest school of general education in Western Europe. Salerno was older, but it devoted itself only to medicine. Montpellier had medical teachers ("magister physic") since the tenth century. The medical school is said to have been first frequented by Jewish students and physicians.

About the middle of the twelfth century, the Almabades of African origin forced the Jews of Spain to leave the country. Many settled in the commercial Mediterranean city of Montpellier, France, which is close to the Italian border. There they established a great center of learning.[5] In its early days there were heated controversies between the Jewish physicians of Spain who followed the Arabic medical teachers and the Christian physicians of Spain who had been educated in Salerno. William IV, Lord of Montpellier, in the year 1181, stopped the strife among the masters of the Jewish and Christian physicians, when he proclaimed Montpellier to be a school of free resort, where any teacher of medical science from any country, might give instruction. Montpellier was a recognized school of medical science within the boundaries of modern France as early as the twelfth century.

Before the end of this century, the University of Montpellier also possessed a faculty of jurisprudence—a branch of learning for which Montpellier afterwards became famous. The schools of medicine and of law continued, however, to be totally distinct bodies with different constitutions. Both schools were free of ecclesiastic and scholastic influence although the masters were enjoined to live in celibacy.

Among the students and teachers were the famous Jewish physicians Samuel ibn Tibbon (1160-1230) and Jacob ibn Machir (1236-1304). Barring the very infrequent temporary periods of intolerance, Jewish persons were allowed to study and teach in Montpellier.[6]

On the twenty-sixth of October, 1289, Montpellier was raised by Nicholas IV to the rank of a "studium generale," a mark of favor which, in a region where papal influence was so potent, resulted in considerable prosperity. The University by this time also included a faculty of arts. There is reliable evidence of the existence of a faculty of theology before the close of the fourteenth century, although this school was not formally recognized.

Like at Salerno, medicine remained the chief glory of Montpellier, and Montpellier cultivated the study of the classical medical writers especially Hippocrates.

In 1220, the conduct of the masters and teachers was regulated. One of the most important rules was to the effect that no one could teach in the school unless he had been examined and received a license from the Bishops of Maguelone and Avignon. The Bishops, with three senior masters, selected the chancellor, whose primary duty was to preserve discipline. Throughout the entire medieval period, the medical faculty of Montpellier enjoyed the benevolence and protection of both the ecclesiastical and lay powers.

It was required of the medical student to attend medical lectures for at least five years and to engage in medical practice in a hospital or as an apprentice to an older physician for seven months. After the first three years of study, an examination was conducted by the masters of the school. Each master proposed various questions. A judge was always chosen from among the teaching physicians to adjudicate disputes between teachers and students. Three kinds of diplomas were granted, the baccalaureate, the licentiate and the degree of "magister." If the student passed the examination satisfactorily, he received his baccalaureate degree. After two years of further study, he received the masters' degree. The doctorate followed after the candidate delivered a discussion on a medical topic for one hour on three succeeding days.[7]

Many students who desired to interrupt their studies at the University to start in practice later returned to school to continue their studies. The students paid their fees directly to their masters. The young doctor who became the recipient of a medical degree received the insignia of his rank, a cap of black cloth surmounted with crimson silk, a gold ring, a golden girdle and a book of Hippocrates. The chancellor then bade the new doctor sit near him and gave him the benediction following which the new physician pronounced his customary oath.

It is estimated that the cost of the five year course in medicine amounted to the equivalent of several thousand dollars.

The chancellor had a dean directly under him who was, as a rule, a senior master and two procurates or preceptors chosen from among the faculty. A medical student who practiced medicine without first submitting to the final examination was promptly expelled, but surgical students were not forced to submit to an examination.

Montpellier, being situated not far from the Spanish border, had a large number of students under Judeo-Arabic influence.

Jean Astruc (1684-1766) gives the names of four consecutive generations of Jewish physicians with family name of Saporta, beginning with Louis and including his son of the same name, his grandson Antoine and his great-grandson, Jean. The first Louis Saporta had a position on the teaching staff of Montpellier. He gave up that position in the year 1490 to accept the position of municipal physician at Marseilles. He returned to Montpellier in 1506. Charles VIII, whose physician he was, presented him with a coral dish encrusted with the coat of arms of France. He lived to the ripe old age of 106.[8]

The second Louis Saporta and his son Antoine also studied in Montpellier. The latter took his medical degree from this university in 1531. He was appointed professor in 1540, dean in 1551 and chancellor in 1560. He wrote a work on tumors which was published in Lyons in 1624. He died at the age of 90.

Jean, the fourth generation of the Saporta family, graduated from Montpellier in 1572, became a professor in 1577 and vice-chancellor in 1603. He died in 1605 and left a work on venereal diseases.[9]

Barthelemy describes the Saporta family as a medical dynasty which included some of the most prominent members of the faculty of Montpellier.[10]

In 1340 dissection of at least one human body a year was permitted at Montpellier. The body was always that of an executed criminal obtained from the authorities. The dissection was done by a surgeon in the presence of a physican. Among the eminent students and masters of Montpellier were Petrus Hispanus, the Catalan, Arnold of Villanova, Henry de Mondeville, Guy de Chauliac, Gilbertus Anglicus, Bernard Gordon, John of Gaddesten, Balescan de Tarante and François Rabelais. Even in later years, Montpellier was attended by eminent physicians, including Sydenham (1624-1684), Barbeyrac, Sylvius, Bauhin (1560-1624), Barthez (1811-91), Grasset, Vieussens (1614-1716), and others.

Montpellier reached its zenith in the thirteenth and fourteenth centuries after which it became eclipsed by the University of Paris.

THE UNIVERSITY OF PARIS

The beginning of the history of the University of Paris is obscure. Some claim that it goes back to Alcuin, and that Charlemagne was its real founder. Be this as it may, there can be no question that the University of Paris developed in response to new French educational demands.

The study of logic in Paris started about the year 1100, engendered by the controversies between Lanfranc (d. 1350) and Berangar (c. 1470-1550) and between Anselm and Roscellinus. These quarrels convinced the intelligentsia that spiritual truths depend upon the correct use of prescribed methods of argumentation and dialectics came to be looked upon as "the science of sciences." As a result of this, William of Champeaux opened a Parisian school for the advanced study of dialectics as an art in the first decade of the twelfth century.

The University of Paris had no buildings of its own and all lectures were given in private homes. Unlike the University of Bologna, which was started and controlled by students, the University of Paris was developed entirely by teachers who taught by virtue of the license conferred on them by the chancellor of the cathedral.

Among the early pupils in the newly founded school was the Scotchman, Peter Abelard, (1079-1142), in whose hands the study of dialectics made notable advance. Abelard's popularity was extraordinary and he became surrounded by 3,000 students. He was also interested in medicine and told the nuns in the convent of Champaigne to devote themselves to surgical practices. By the middle of the century, John of Salisbury, on returning from the French capital to England, related with astonishment how all learned Paris had gone well-nigh mad in its pursuit and practice of dialectics.

Abelard's stormy life, his endless conflicts with the clergy and his tragic punishment perhaps contributed more than anything else to the founding of the University.

Paris was the first university with a complete cooperative constitution under ecclesiastical control. During the thirteenth century, it was the most famous school in Europe. Students from distant lands came here to be instructed by monkish teachers in the seven liberal arts.

The University was under scholastic control. On all formal occasions the pope was represented by the chancellor of Notre Dame in whose parish the University had its origin. Masters and scholars were treated alike, wore clerical garb, maintained priestly tonsure and enjoyed the privileges of clerics. Like the ecclesiastics, they also had to live a life of celibacy. This community of teachers of recognized fitness did not in itself suffice to constitute a university.

Sometime between the years 1150 and 1170, the period when the "sentences" of Peter Lombard were given to the world, the University of Paris came formally into being. Its first written statutes were not, however, compiled until about the year 1208, and it was not until long after that date that it was dignified with the presence of a rector. Its earliest recognition as a legal corporation came about the year 1211, when a brief of Innocent III empowered it to elect a proctor to be its representative at the papal court.

When the word "medicine" is used in connection with the University of Paris, it always refers strictly to medicine and never includes surgery. Since surgery was forbidden to clerics, and the students and masters were clerics, surgery was entirely excluded from the curriculum. This prohibition not only applies to the University of Paris, but also to the institutions at Oxford and Cambridge. Such was not the case in the Italian universities, and apparently not in Montpellier, where Guy de Chauliac, although a cleric, was a far-famed teacher of the surgical art.

Members of the Medical Faculty of Paris were privileged to wear the long robe. Surgeons, on state occasions, were permitted to wear only a short robe. The barbers, an auxiliary body, were not permitted to wear any robe at all.

The professor, when demonstrating anatomy at Paris, made use of the services of a barber-surgeon. Several lay nurses were attached to the medical staff, one of whom was a midwife. Patients in dying condition were placed in special beds and given the last sacrament. In the general hospitals of medieval France insane patients were admitted together with the physically sick. Presumably they were placed in special rooms.

No one could graduate from the University of Paris until the age of twenty-two. When one entered the study of medicine he had to relinquish all other scholastic pursuits. The dean was chosen by all the doctors of the Faculty, was elected for one year and was inducted into office with elaborate ceremonies.

The course of instruction was long and trying. In winter, the classes began at six A.M. and in the summer at five. Four degrees or grades were given: bachelor, licentiate, master and doctor. In the early years it was not necessary to have a Master of Arts degree to become a doctor. By an edict of Pope Martin V, in 1426, this, however, became a definite requirement and no one was allowed to matriculate for the medical course who had not studied at least two years with the Faculty. The total length of study was usually six years, but the exact time was controlled by a series of examinations. Before being admitted to the examinations, the candidate had to swear that in case of failure, he would not avenge himself on the Masters. This precautionary measure throws light on the turbulent character of the medieval medical student. The principal examinations led to the degrees of *baccalaureus* and *docteur*. A treatise was an essential requisite. Finally came the administration of the Hippocratic Oath.

The grade above bachelor was that of licentiate. In order to take this next step the student was required to take four special courses—each on a particular book. One non-medical book was permitted: Aristotle's work on animals and meteors might be substituted for a medical book. The bachelor was finally admitted to the examination for license after the presentation of testimony as to his fitness.

The examination consisted chiefly of questions on Hippocrates and Avicenna, and the presentation of various dialectical arguments. All the professors were permitted to ask questions of the candidates for doctor and master. Some of the questions asked were: Is the loud voice warm? Which is more important: air, food, or drink? Is the necessity of death innate? Does the fetus resemble the mother more than the father? Is water healthier than wine? Is living on bread and water healthy? Is it healthy to get drunk once a month? Is woman an imperfect work of nature? Does a libertine life lead to baldness? Which is the most healthy, wine mixed with water, pure water or pure wine? Should literary men marry?

The licentiate was not permitted to practice as soon as he received his certificate. A regulation of the Faculty demanded that for a period of two years he must accompany the doctors in their practice at the Hotel Dieu or elsewhere.

After passing the examination and performing the various ceremonies pertaining to his rank, the candidate had to take an oath to observe faithfully the secrets, practices, customs and duties of the profession and honor the Faculty at all times. The candidate also had to swear to honor and respect the dean and all the masters of the Faculty, to come to the aid of the Faculty against anyone who violated the statutes of the profession or the honor of the Faculty, to prosecute those who practice illegally and to submit to the punishments inflicted by the Faculty. The candidate had to promise to be present in academic costume at all masses ordered by the Faculty, at all exercises of the Faculty and at all debates for a period of two years. The candidate also had to maintain a thesis upon one question of medicine or hygiene and he had to guarantee that he would always conduct himself and his affairs in peaceful fashion. The oath was read in Latin by the dean and the candidates responded by "I swear" to the recitation of each article.[11]

The favorite medical textbooks used in the early days of the University were the "Canon" of Avicenna, the "Aphorisms," "Dietetics" and "Prognostics" of Hippocrates, the "Ars Parva" of Galen, the "Isagogue" of Johannitus and the works of Dioscorides and Rhazes. In the centuries that followed, further medical works were employed including those of Soranus, Paul of Aegina, and Alexander of Tralles. Among the distinguished students and professors of the University of Paris were the Franciscan Englishman Roger Bacon (Dr. Mirabilis), Gilbertus Anglicus, Thomas Aquinas and Albertus Magnus.

What France lacked in the early Middle Ages it made up in good measure in the later years. It produced an array of great physicians and surgeons including Lanfranc of Milan, Henry de Mondeville (c. 1354), Jean Yperman (1295-1351), and Guy de Chauliac (1300-1370). French medicine was greatly influenced by the medical school of Salerno which was instrumental in the introduction of the lay spirit in French medicine. The greatest boon to medical knowledge in France were the Universities of Montpellier and Paris.

LANFRANC (d. c. 1315)

Lanfranc (Lanfranchi or Lanfrancus Mediolanensis) of Milan was the most gifted student of Saliceto. He practiced in his native city until the year 1290 when he was banished as a result of political disturbance. He found asylum in Lyons, France, where he wrote his "Chirurgia Parva," for the use of his sons. In 1295, he reached Paris where he acquired considerable success as a medical practitioner and as a teacher of surgery in which field he achieved a great reputation that enabled him to be admitted to the "College de St. Come."

His method of teaching surgery consisted in holding public clinics. He elevated the status of French surgery by insisting that surgeons possess a good knowledge of medicine.

His great work "Chirurgia Magna" was dedicated to King Philippe le Bel (reigned 1285-1314). This treatise is divided into five parts. The first part is in the nature of an introduction, and gives a definition of surgery and a brief description of anatomy. Part two treats of the various parts of the body describing wounds and the anatomy of the parts. Part three discusses various treatments which are not necessarily surgical. This section includes a detailed description of hair and skin diseases, apostemata, eye, ear, nose and throat ailments, hernia, stones, lithotomy, sexual malformation, dropsy, hemorrhoids, and venesection. Part four covers fractures and dislocations, and part five is an antidotary.

His "Chirurgia Parva" is a surgical compendium dealing with wounds and ulcers divided into sixteen chapters. For wounds, he orders a dressing in which an application of "red powder" is directly applied to the wound. Large incised wounds must be closed by sutures. He controls bleeding by digital pressure and ligatures. He states that open wounds tend to produce pus. The success of healing an ulcer depends upon the seat of the lesion as well as the ailment that has produced it. Cancer is to be treated only with the knife or actual cautery when complete removal is possible.

Fracture of the skull may be diagnosed by the harsh rattling sound produced when percussing over the fractured area with a small stick. Another diagnostic method recommended is to pluck a thread held taut between the teeth with a finger nail. In case of fracture of the skull, this will cause pain to the patient at the site of the fracture. Lanfranc recommends trephining only in skull fractures with depression of the fragments and consequent cerebral pressure effects.

He warns to be extremely cautious in performing paracentesis of the abdomen for ascites. He says that performance of this procedure in a routine fashion regardless of the underlying disease and the individual condition is a menace to the patient. He rejects nephro-lithotomy, but advises cystotomy when external measures such as baths, etc., fail. In the rationale behind his treatment of abscesses, the humoral theory plays an important role.

He indicates thirty different veins useful for venesection in children, the aged, and pregnant women.

The "Chirurgia Magna" was translated twice into English before the middle of the fifteenth century. Both of his works were translated into Hebrew.[12]

HENRI DE MONDEVILLE (1260?-1320)

The most distinguished pupil of Lanfranchi was Henri de Mondeville, who became recognized as one of the greatest surgeons of the thirteenth century. He was born in the second half of the thirteenth century, most likely in Normandy. The exact date of his birth is not known. He received his medical training at the Universities of Paris, Bologna and Montpellier. He was one of the four body physicians of King Philippe le Bel, whom he accompanied on tours and military campaigns. He was a great teacher and attracted many students to his classes.

His "Chirurgia" which he began in 1306, remained unfinished because of his manifold public and private activities. The completed parts of this unfinished work show that the author was unbiased in his observations and that his conclusions are based on his own experience. He retired from public life in 1316, but he was not able to complete his work during the last four years of his life. He died of a lung infection.

De Mondeville's "Chirurgia" demonstrates that he possessed a great book knowledge and that he followed the best authorities in choosing his surgical technique, his instruments; his dietetics, and his therapeutics. In cranial injuries he recommended great conservatism, although he was not afraid of surgery of the head. He believed in non-suppurative methods of wound treatment. He was rational in his practice and free from superstition.

GUY DE CHAULIAC (1300-1370)

Another surgeon of note connected with the University of Paris was Guy de Chauliac. He was born in Anverne near Lyons, France, of a poor peasant family and received his education in Toulouse, Montpellier and Paris. After receiving his medical degree at the University of Paris, he went to the University of Bologna to study anatomy, this being the only place at that time where anatomy was studied directly from the human cadaver. His theological studies attracted the attention of the dignitaries of the Church and he became canon and prior of the Church of St. Justus.

His medical career began in 1345, when he settled at Avignon to practice the medical profession. During a deadly plague of black death, which broke out in this town, he remained on duty although many of his colleagues fled to escape this dread scourge. Guy de Chauliac, describing the contagious nature of this plague, states: "So great was the contagion that one caught it from the other not only by being with him, but by simply looking at him."

Guy de Chauliac became the greatest authority in Europe during his time. "He was a writer of rare learning, endowed with a fine critical and historic sense, and indeed, the only medical historian of consequence between Celsus and Haller (1708-1773)."

His famous work "Chirurgia Magna" which appeared soon after 1363, is an exhaustive and critically inspired collection of surgical knowledge. It was used as a textbook centuries after his death. To this day, this book makes good reading and reveals the author as an exceptionally careful student in both branches of medicine, but especially in surgery. He displays a wide knowledge of Greek and Arabic authors. He does not hesitate to criticize his authorities and to recommend recent medical advances as being more advantageous than various hallowed ancient practices.

Speaking of recent writers, he remarks: "We are like children sitting on the neck of a giant who see all that he (the giant) sees and something besides."[13]

Guy de Chauliac definitely surpassed his teachers Saliceto, Theodoric, Lanfranc and Henri de Mondeville, but he felt privileged to draw from their works. None of his predecessors exceeded him in surgical technique and theory. He is recognized as having laid the real foundation of modern French surgery and his influence upon the neighboring countries was marked.

Guy de Chauliac's technique in treating fractures and dislocations was far in advance of his time. He set fractures with a splint and bandage and employed weights and pulleys in overcoming the over-riding of the fragments in hip fractures. He advocated the use of narcotics and soporifics by inhalation during surgical operations.

He was one of the first to take the surgery of herniorrhaphy and cataract out of the hands of traveling quacks and mountebanks by his radical operations. He insisted upon operating on cancer in the earliest possible stage. (He divided phthisis into two categories: the type where only glandular swelling is present, scrofula, and the type where continuous fever and hemorrhage is evident.) "The last may be fatal within three days."

The "Chirurgia Magna" describes various operations and the instruments needed to perform them properly. The surgeon must be equipped at least with a scissors, speculum, razor, scalpel, needles and a lancet.

He describes five methods of controlling hemorrhage: sutures, ligatures, compression, cautery and tamponade.

Here is Guy de Chauliac's description of the plague which caused the death of millions: "The great mortality appeared at Avignon, January, 1348, when I was in the service of Pope Clement VI. It was of two kinds. The first lasted two months, with continued fever and spitting of blood, and people died of it in three days. The second kind was also with continuous fever, and with swellings in the armpits and groin; and people died in five days. It was so contagious, especially that accompanied by spitting blood, that not only by staying together, but even by looking at one another, people caught it, with the result that men died without attention and were buried without priests. The father did not visit his son, nor the son his father. Charity was dead and hope crushed. I call it great, because it covered the whole world, or lacked little of doing so. . . . And it was so great that it left scarcely a fourth part of the people. . . .

"Many were in doubt about the cause of this great mortality. In some places they thought that the Jews had poisoned the world: and so they killed them. In others, that it was the poor deformed people who were responsible: and they drove them out. In others that it was the nobles; and they feared to go abroad. Finally they reached the point where they kept guards in the cities and villages, permitting the entry of no one who was not well known. And if powders or salves were found on anyone, the owners, for fear that they were poisons, were forced to swallow them..."

The swellings of the armpits and groin that Guy de Chauliac mentions were enlarged glands. A gland so infected is called a bubo—hence the term "bubonic plague." When a person had the bubonic plague, the glands were not only swollen, but also became filled with pus, broke, and made running sores—plague sores.

Guy de Chaluiac, in his brief description of the plague, makes one important statement concerning control of the disease: "Finally they reached the point where they kept guards in the cities and villages, permitting the entry of no one who was not well known." This was the first time that measures of the kind were put into effect—the first use of quarantine. Isolation of the patient for various lengths of time persisted after the epidemic began to subside. Beginning in 1383, travelers of ships suspected of infection were held forty days in the harbor of Marseilles before they were allowed to land, hence the word "quarantine," meaning "forty."

The surgeon, according to Guy de Chauliac, should possess the following qualifications: He should be a man of letters, an expert in his work, intelligent and a man of good habits. He adds, "It is necessary that he especially know anatomy because without anatomy one can do nothing in surgery."

Considering his great influence on surgical progress, it is disappointing to learn that in one respect Guy de Chauliac was a reactionary. He failed to follow the teachings of Henri de Mondeville and Theodoric of Bologna (1205-1295) with regard to the treatment of wounds. He followed the old method of using salves and plasters on wounds and rejected their teaching that it is better if no pus is generated in wounds. In other words his belief in "laudable pus" was almost his only retrogressive theory.

Guy de Chauliac's work passed through many editions. The first was published in Paris in the year 1478. The Latin version was first published in Venice in 1498. A modern edition was published by Nicaise in Paris in 1890.

CHAPTER XVII

MEDIEVAL MEDICINE IN ENGLAND

It is difficult to determine the status of English medicine in the early Middle Ages. The conquest of the British Isles by Claudius (A.D. 43) undoubtedly introduced Roman medical practices in the new colony, and the thirty years of hill fighting unquestionably taught the natives new methods of treating traumatic conditions.

The Saxons who speedily over-ran Britain at the end of the sixth century after the Romans departed, most likely brought along with them from their Germanic homeland the medical lore which they had inherited from early kinsmen. This medical inheritance included prescriptions containing herbs, minerals, and animal substances including various secretions and excretions. A good measure of superstition permeated the whole.[1]

The early healers of Germany were largely women and, according to Tacitus, even the wounded on the battlefield were brought to their mothers and wives for medical attention.

The Angles (of the Northern Kingdom) before they united with the Saxons (of the Southern Kingdom) to form what later became the Anglo-Saxon nation, had their own medical practices. The union of the Angles and the Saxons produced an amalgamation of the medical lores of both nations. To this was added, in the year 597, when Christianity was introduced in England by St. Augustine, the Roman Church medicine as practiced by the monks in the monasteries of Italy. The conversion of England to Christianity took only about ninety years (A.D. 597-686).

Early in the seventh century, when the Angles and the Saxons began to emerge from the cultural lethargy of their ancient peoples, they began to develop a literature of their own. The northern runes, the Beechen tablets and the scratching implements were superseded by the Roman alphabet. The records of the "venerable Bede," the poetry represented by the rugged lines of Beowulf and Cynewulf, the scholarly work of St. Aldhelm, and above all the medical treatise known as the Leechdom of Bald, all illustrate the great cultural change that occurred at that period.

From a letter written to Boniface, the Apostle of Germany, by an English friend, it appears that there was already a medical literature on the British Isles as early as the eighth century. The letter reads: "We have some medical books but the foreign ingredients we find in them are unknown to us and difficult to obtain." The books referred to might have come from Italy or perhaps from Syria where the Greek classics were still read. This would account for the British natives not knowing the ingredients of the prescriptions. It may be inferred from this letter that doctors, known as leeches, existed on the British Isles at this period.

The name "leech" is derived from the Anglo-Saxon "laece" meaning "to heal." The word *dom* means "a law." The word "leech" became applied to a physician because the doctors originally specialized in phlebotomy and used the leech for blood letting. There is no evidence that women occupied the position of leeches as they had done in Germany. The English leeches do not appear to have belonged to the priestly caste as did the Druid healers before them. The last were priests who employed magic arts and other superstitious means in their healing practices.

When the Christian Church became firmly established on the Isles, medicine became sponsored by the ecclesiastics. Gibbon in his "Decline and Fall of the Roman Empire" says that one of the most powerful causes of the spread of Christianity was the miraculous healing powers of the primitive Church . . . Indeed, so acclaimed were the healing powers of the Church that the third century witnessed the rise of a special order of men within the Church whose function was to cast out demons from persons stricken with disease.[2]

That there was some kind of training in the art of medicine available in England in the early Middle Ages may be inferred from the following lines written by an author of that period.

> "Twig runes shalt thou ken
> If thou a leech will be,
> And ken a sore to see;
> On bark shall one then write
> And on branch of wood whose
> limbs to east do lout."

In the Anglo-Saxon work, "Medicinale Anglicum," the expression is frequently met with "as leeches know how," from which it may be inferred that the leeches were professionally trained persons. The early training of the English leech might have been in the monastic infirmaries.

In the seventh century, the darkest of the Dark Ages, England was particularly fortunate, firstly in the appearance of the work "Ecclesiastic History of Bede" which, although its author was primarily interested in religious matters, throws much light on secular matters, and secondly in the arrival in 669 of the monk Theodore of Tarsus. It was Theodore, who later became the Archbishop of Canterbury, who stimulated learning on the British Isles. He, with the assistance of his abbot, Adrian, founded a school of Classic sciences. Due to the activities of Theodore, the Church of England at that period excelled continental Churches both in learning and in cultural developments. Among its great men were Bede, and Alcuin. Both became known for their scholarship. According to the "venerable Bede," students of his own day knew both Greek and Latin as well as their native tongue.[3]

"One of Theodore's pupils," states Bede, "named John of Beverley, Bishop of Hexhaus, was called in to see a young priest who had suffered a concussion of the brain in consequence of a fall from his horse. Through the efforts of this ecclesiastic, the priest regained consciousness." John of Beverley, however, sent for a leech to attend to the priest's injuries. The latter splinted the bones and bandaged the fractured skull.[4]

In the early part of the eighth century (705), a monk named St. Aldhelm included medicine among the essential sciences. The sciences to which reference was made included arithmetic, astronomy, geometry, music, astrology and mechanics.[5]

The status of the leech in the seventh century may be derived from Bede's "Ecclesiastic History." He alludes to ecclesiastics who performed minor operations and phlebotomy. He states that leeches were subordinate to Church healers. Bede mentions the Saxon leech Cynfrid, who attended Setheldryth, the Abbess of Ely, in 579 during her last illness. He lanced a carbuncle on her neck.

The following narrative shows that the ecclesiastics consulted lay physicians on medical matters: A boy who was dumb, came one day to solicit alms from the Bishop St. John of Beverley. The boy had scabs and no hair on his head (perhaps the condition was due to an eruption known as favus which is more or less common among people who live in an unsanitary condition). The Bishop taught the patient how to speak (evidently he was not a mute) but did not attempt to cure the boy's ailment. He called in a professional leech to treat the skin condition and a complete recovery ensued.

We owe to the "venerable Bede" the first description of the plague in England in 664. This epidemic is supposed to have been brought from Ireland where it had raged during the previous year.

Bede is said to have been the author of a work on phlebotomy entitled, "De Minutione Sanguinis Sive de Phlebotomia." In this book he gives the particular days and the time of day most propitious for bleeding. He warns that no bleeding should be performed on certain unlucky days. He states, "Any time by day or night needs we must use phlebotomy in acute diseases and especially in the time from the start of the calends of April to the seventh of June, we have good results from taking away blood because then the blood is undergoing an increase."

The "Saxon Leech Book" mentions the leeches Bald, Oxa and Dun. That the surgery of these leeches was not confined entirely to the use of salves, poultices, plasters, etc., is evident from the following extract: "For hare-lip pound mastic very small, add the white of an egg and mingle as though dost vermilion: cut with a knife with silk, then smear without and within with the salve ere the silk rots. If it draw together arrange it with the hand. Anoint again soon."[6]

After the "venerable Bede" there was a lull in medical progress for a period of 200 years. Medical literature broke its silence in the person of Bald who influenced his friend (perhaps his scribe) named Cild to write the first Anglo-Saxon leech book known as the "Leech Book of Bald" (in Latin "Medicinale Anglicum"). This is the first medical book that was written in the Anglo-Saxon language. Almost all books in Europe at that period were written in the Greek or Latin language.

A few manuscripts of this work remained hidden in Oxford, Cambridge and other English libraries until past the middle of the nineteenth century, when two eminent Anglo-Saxon scholars published it. It was first published in 1864 in the Anglo-Saxon tongue in the "Chronicles and Memorials of Great Britain" by the Master of the Rolls. It was then translated into modern English as part of "Leechdoms, Wort-cunning and Starcraft of Early England,"—a collection of documents for the most part never before printed illustrating the history of science in England before the Norman Conquest. The material for this last work was collected and edited by the Reverend Oswald Cockayne in three octavo volumes which were published in London in 1864-6.

Reverend Oswald Cockayne's collection includes the "Leech Book of Bald" in two books (believed to have been written between 900 and 950 A.D.), the Anglo-Saxon translations from Latin of the "Herbarium" of Apulus Platonici, the "Recipes," a miscellaneous collection of prescriptions, and "Of Schools of Medicine"—a treatise on medical charms and a glossary of the names of plants.[7]

The Anglo-Saxon Leechdoms of the eleventh century, published in the "Rolls" series of medieval chronicles and memorials, are admirably illustrated and exhibit a lion's share of magic and superstition intermingled with a few relics of ancient science which are monastic in character. Similar works, in Latin and other languages, exist in manuscript form in all the great European libraries.

As has been intimated earlier, the principal medical work of Anglo-Saxon origin is "The Leechdom of Bald" known in Latin as "Medicinale Anglicum." "The Leechdom of Bald" occupies 109 manuscript pages and 299 printed pages. It is divided into two books, and 155 chapters, containing very little diagnosis, symptomatology or pathology; it concerns itself primarily with treatment. The diseases for which remedies are prescribed start with the head and proceed down to the feet, after the method first introduced by Alexander of Tralles (sixth century A.D.). The author seems to have been acquainted with the works of Alexander of Tralles, Paul of Aegina and Rhazes.

The first book of "Medicinale Anglicum" begins with a list of the various remedies recommended for affections of the head; next came therapies for ailments of the eyes, ears, throat, parts of the face, teeth, mouth and lips. Coverage then proceeds to affections of the chest (including coughs), the heart, the stomach, the loins, the thighs, the legs, and lastly the feet. The thirtieth chapter concerns itself with chilblains of the feet. After this no regular order is preserved and the remaining chapters contain prescriptions for a great variety of diseases including tumors, smallpox, skin affections, paralysis, fevers, and snakebite.

The second book concerns itself chiefly with internal and abdominal diseases including those associated with the stomach, liver, and spleen, and some miscellaneous prescriptions. It differs considerably from the first book in that it is more learned and includes some recognition of the signs of disease as well as diverse attempts at diagnosis. The second book contains many passages which may be traced to Greek and Latin medical writers.

At the end of the second book are found the following verses:

"Bald habet hunc librum, Cild quem conscribere iussit.
Hic precor assidue cunctis in nomine Christi
Quod nullus tollat hunc librum perfidus a me
Nec vi, nec furto, nec quodam *famine*[8] falso.
Cur? quia nulla mihi tam cara est optima gaza,
Quam cari libri quos Christi gratia comit."

This may be translated thusly:

"Bald is the owner of this book, which he ordered Cild
to write.
Earnestly I pray here all men, in the name of Christ,
That no treacherous person take this book from me,
Neither by force, nor by theft, nor by any false
statement.
Why? Because the richest treasure is not so dear to me
As my dear books, which the grace of Christ attends."[9]

It would seem from this quotation that Bald wanted this book for his own use. Bald himself might have been a physician who asked Cild, who might have been a scribe or a leech, to write this work. The "Medicinale Anglicum," which is undoubtedly of Anglo-Saxon origin, gives evidence that the contemporary leeches were not entirely devoid of learning in Greek and Arabian medicine. As mentioned, the author seems to have been acquainted with the works of Alexander of Tralles, Paul of Aegina, Rhazes and others. The author refers to two leeches named Dun and Oxa.

Bald gives a rough classification of the members and limbs of the body and of the diseases to which they are subject. He enumerates a large list of remedies for various parts of the body as well as for diseases of the special senses. He applies the apt term "flying venom" to epidemics. The term "venomous swelling" probably refers to the bubonic plague. Smallpox is unquestionably referred to.[10]

The following are some pertinent extracts from "Bald's Leechdom":

"Against pockes; very much shall one let blood, and drink a bowlful of melted butter; if they, (the pustules) strike out, one shall dig each with a thorn, and then drop one-year alder-drink in, then they will not be seen." This last instruction, evidently intended to prevent pitting, clearly identifies the disease.

Struma was known to the Anglo-Saxon leeches as "neck ratten," or "purulence in the neck."

Yellow jaundice is termed "the gall disease, from which cometh great evil." It is diagnosed when "the patient's body all becometh bitter, and as yellow as good silk and under the root of his tongue there be swart veins and pernicious, and his urine is yellow." The last observation is interesting as being one of the few instances in Anglo-Saxon leechdoms of good clinical observation and reference to the appearance of the urine.[11]

The drinks or potions against poison are very numerous, and are indicative of the dread of poisoning that existed in Anglo-Saxon times— probably because of the current imperfect knowledge of what was really poisonous.

"Against any poison, boil the netherward part of bishopwort and lupin, and the netherward part of springwort, everthroat, and clote in ale; give to drink frequently."

"If an adder strike a man, wash a black snail in holy water, and give to the sick to drink."

One of the most curious remedies reads as follows:

"If a man eat wolfbane, let him stand upon his head, let someone strike him with many scarifications on the shanks; then the venom departs out through the incisions." The belief in demonic possession is evident in this treatment.

That poisonous snakes were common in the land may be gathered from the many leechdoms (however ineffectual) for the bites of adders and snakes:

"Against a hand-worm: take ship tar, add sulphur and pepper and white salt; mingle them together, smear therewith."

"For hand-worms and 'deaw-worms': take dock or clote, such as would swim, mingle the roots with cream and with salt, let

363

it stand for three nights, and on the fourth day smear therewith the sore places."

"Against a boring-worm: let the man eat new cheese, beebread, and wheaten loaf. Again, burn to ashes a man's head bone or skull, put it on with a pipe."

Another variety of worm mentioned is termed the "ana-worm, which grows in a man." It is referred to as follows:—

"If the worm eat through to the outside and make a hole, take a drop of honey, drop it in the hole, then have broken glass ready ground, shed it on the hole, then as soon as the worm tastes of this, he will die." This description seems to fit Dracunculus medinensis—the Guinea worm.

For devil-sickness, for demonic attacks and for evil eye, the patient is instructed to eat a wolf's flesh, "well dressed, and sodden," and, the leechdom reassures: "The apparitions which ere appeared to him, shall not disquiet him."

"For a man who has the falling-sickness (epilepsy), work to a drink a boar's coillons in wine or water; the drink will heal him."

For the bite of a mad dog, the following curious remedy is suggested:

"Take the worms which are under a mad hound's tongue; snip them away; weave them around about a fig-tree; give them to him that hath been rent; he will soon be whole."

To remove ugly marks from the face, smearing with wolf's blood is recommended, "for it taketh away all the marks."

"For griping," says the leechdom, "let the sick drink hound's blood; it healeth wonderfully."

A curious relic of the ancient mythology of the Gothic races is apparent in the leechdoms connected with the hound.

The popular medical authorities in England during the fourteenth century may be gathered from Chaucer's "Doctour of Phisik":

> "Well knew he the olde Esculapius
> And Deyscorides, and eek Risus (perhaps Ruffus)

Ypocras, Haly and Galyen,
Serapion, Razis and Avycen,
Averrois, Damascien and Constantyn,
Bernard and Gatesden and Gilbertyn."

ANGLO-SAXON SURGERY

Judging from the scattered allusions that are to be found in the manuscripts on surgery, it would appear that surgery was not entirely practiced as a separate calling—notwithstanding the fact that Bede mentions that "other than the physicians were called in to bleed and scarify."

"For broken head: take betony, bruise it and lay it on the head above; then it unites the wound and healeth." Again, for the same: "Take garden cress, that which waxeth of itself, and is not sown, put it in the nose, that the smell and the juice may get to the head."

The use of splints was known to the Anglo-Saxon leeches, and that they employed them in cases of fracture is evidenced from the following:

"If a sinew shrink (that is, when a leg is broken), and after that swell, take a she-goat's turd, mingle with vinegar, smudge it on, soon the sinew healeth . . . Then let him (the patient) duly arrange the bones as well as he can, apply a splint, and it is so much the better the oftener a man bathes with the preparation. If a sinew have pulsation, mugwort beaten and mingled with oil, and laid on, is good. Juice of mugwort mingled with rose oil, smear with that; soon will the quaking be stilled."

For bones that are fractured the following treatment is also recommended:

"If the shanks be broken, take bonewort (generally interpreted as violet or pansy): pound it; pour the white of an egg out; mingle these together for the man whose shanks are broken."

Amputation was performed when gangrene set in:

"If a man have a limb cut off, be it finger, foot, or hand,

if the marrow be out, take sheep's marrow boiled, lay it to the other marrow, bind it very well at night."

As a dressing for wounds, honey appears to have been generally employed:

"For cleansing a wound: take clean honey, warm it at the fire, then put it in a clean vessel; add salt to it; then stir it till it is the thickness of pottage; smear the wound with it; then it cleanseth it."

The antiquity of the use of honey as a dressing for wounds goes back to a very early period, and a knowledge of its antiseptic properties was possessed by the Assyrians many centuries before the Christian era. It was recommended by Hippocrates, and several of the early Greek physicians, in the treatment of wounds.

The Anglo-Saxon leech does not appear to have employed mechanical methods for reducing dislocations. In such cases he applied an ointment.

For a hernia, the following treatment is directed:

"If a mans bowel be out; pound galluc, wring through a cloth into milk warm from the cow, wet thy hands therein, and put back the bowel into the man; sew up with silk; then boil him for nine mornings galluc, that is, comfrey, except need be for a longer time; feed him with fresh hen's flesh."

That surgery had acquired some degree of importance may be gathered from the fact that an operation for opening an abscess of the liver is described in the "Leechdom of Bald."

The actual cautery or blistering rod was extensively used by the Anglo-Saxon leech. This is evident, not only from the references in the leechdoms, but also from contemporary drawings, which show the form of the instrument, and the methods of its employment. It was apparently used in the preliminary treatment of a variety of diseases, from gout to headache.

"If the edges of a wound are too high (excessive accumulations or "proud flesh"), run them round with a hot iron very lightly, so that the skin may whiten."

Bleeding was practiced with the lancet, the cupping-glass or horn, and the scarifier. Thus, for paralysis, blood is directed to be drawn "with a cupping-glass or horn from the sore deaded places."

It is apparent from the historical resume presented that Anglo-Saxon medicine was in a relatively undeveloped state with very little known of anatomy, physiology and methods of diagnosis. Symptoms were treated as diseases and pathology was not known. Anglo-Saxon treatment was of an herbal nature with the herbs gathered at certain hours of the day or night. Therapy was heavily tainted with charms, spells, and magic potions.

The early records of Scotland and Ireland give evidence that the art of medicine in these countries was often transmitted from father to son. The oldest of the family, the chief of the clan and the king were most trustworthy to administer to the sick. When a son succeeded his father in the profession, the prestige of the father at once became his own.

The early Anglo-Saxon medical books specify that only curable cases should be treated. When death seemed imminent or when the patient was in danger of permanent incapacity from illness or accident, practitioners were urged to call in a fellow physician or surgeon to share the responsibility. A great hindrance to the practice of medicine and a deterrent to its study was the fact that the physician or surgeon, when he failed to effect the promised cure, was often heavily fined or even killed. The death sentence was exacted particularly if the patient died under the operation. Medicine and surgery were usually two separate branches. Medicine in the larger cities was often controlled by the Church. There were, however, some lay physicians. Surgery was in the hands of laymen exclusively.

Not before the Norman Conquest in 1066 did medicine become a true profession in England. The Norman kings brought along with them from Normandy learned ecclesiastics some of whom had been trained in the art of medicine at the Universities of Salerno and Paris. The influence of the Norman culture and customs made an indelible impression upon the English people. This was particularly true during the reign of Edward the Confessor who chose Baldwin, a French monk, as his personal physician. Baldwin, being much interested in the medical science, influenced the King to advance medical knowledge in England. The Norman kings were the founders of the higher English schools of learning; the first of which was Oxford University.

UNIVERSITIES OF OXFORD AND CAMBRIDGE

Oxford University, one of the two greatest seats of learning in England, is a collection of colleges under one corporation located on the Thames river fifty-one miles from London. It is the oldest house of learning in England and was originally modelled after the University of Paris. It was founded in the early part of the twelfth century in the town of Oxford near the nunnery of St. Friedeswyde and Oseney Abbey. These institutions appear to have been the nuclei around which the University grew up.

Mr. Rashdall[12] asserts that the University of Oxford had its origin because of the forced expulsion of English students from Paris (1167-1168) during the political disputes between the English and French sovereigns after the Norman Conquest. "There is a striking relation," says Rashdall, "between the sudden rise of Oxford into a 'studium generale' (about 1167) and the issue of an ordinance (by Henry II, during a quarrel with Thomas à Becket over the fact that Phillip the Second was aiding Becket) ordering all clerks possessing revenues in England and being residents in France, to return home and forbidding all clerks in England to cross the channel . . . A very large proportion of the clerks holding English benefices and residing in France consisted of students at the University of Paris. It is certain that many English scholars were forced to leave Paris in accordance with this ordinance." [13]

John of Salisbury (1115-1180) had this expulsion in mind when he remarked: "France, the mildest and most civil of nations, expelled her foreign scholars." [14]

In the year 1257, the Bishop of Lincoln, as diocesan, markedly restricted the liberties of the community. The deputies from Oxford, when proffering their appeal to the King of St. Albans, ventured to speak of Oxford University as a school second only to Paris. Oxford's students at this time numbered about three thousand. However, this enrollment was far from static, and whenever a plague or tumult occurred this led to a temporary dispersion of many of the student body and decrease in its numerical strength.

In the year 1228, a riot broke out among the students of Paris which influenced many students and their masters to come to Oxford. During the reign of Henry the Second, Oxford had a large enrollment. Many students had come from Paris to take courses in Greek and Philosophy. The *"studium generale"* opened in the year 1167 or 1168. By the end of the twelfth century, Oxford was of considerable size.

Rashdall is of the opinion that the number of students at Oxford during its early history never exceeded 3,000 at any one time. Cambridge had a still lower enrollment. The total number of students at Paris and Bologna did not exceed 5,000.[15]

Although Oxford never ranked with Paris, it was highly honored throughout Europe as a center of classical studies. Modern Oxford University gradually developed out of the schools which existed in Oxford as early as the twelfth century.[16]

Theology, for a long period, was considered the "queen of sciences" at Oxford and the seven liberal arts were looked upon as the handmaids of the School of Theology. Medicine was not included in the liberal arts and the medical school did not have a large attendance.

One may assume that lectures in medicine were given at an early date at Oxford, although the regulations of the College founded by Walter de Merton in 1264 contain a prohibition against medical students at the College. The famous schools of Salerno and Montpellier were already in existence at that period, and indeed, a great interest in medicine prevailed among the cultured classes all over Europe. The prohibition in Merton College applied only to students who occupied themselves with medicine only.

The study of medicine at Oxford was, at first, only theoretical. Surgery and bedside instruction were viewed as menial labor not compatible with pure scholarship.

One of the first Merton physicians was John of Gaddeston, to whom reference will be made later in this chapter. John was graduated in about 1309. He may be considered representative of his period.

A great man who was far in advance of his time and one of the first to value direct observation and experimentation as means of obtaining knowledge was Roger Bacon (1215-1294). Yet even he was often empirical with regard to medical treatment. For a certain malady he recommends a prescription consisting of a pearl and various precious stones exposed to the sun for a given period. Robert of Lincoln, to whom reference was made in the chapter on scholasticism, is generally accepted to be the most famous Oxfordian.

Early in the thirteenth century a somewhat progressive tendency became manifest in Oxford and a definite course of study was established for anyone who desired to become a doctor of medicine. Any candidate for a master's degree was required to have a reading knowledge of the "Tegne" of Galen or one of the books of Hippocrates. No special examination was required for an M.A. to become an M.D. When the candidate presented himself for the license to practice medicine, he had to swear that he had read certain books and the nine regent masters and his preceptor were required to testify to his qualification. Five others had to affirm their belief therein.

The University of Cambridge is located in the town and borough of the same name. The first mention of Cambridge University was in connection with the great dispersal which followed the Oxford Suspendium Clericorum of 1209. Cambridge University had its origin in the first half of the thirteenth century. Stimulated by the educational work carried on by the Church of St. Giles, it gradually developed into a regular *"studium generale."* Cambridge as a *"studium generale"* dates at the earliest to 1209.

In the year 1229, Henry III offered an asylum to the dispersed students of Paris promising to assign certain towns in England for their residence. It is possible that one of these designated towns may have been Cambridge. Papal recognition of Cambridge was received in 1233.

In the years 1231 and 1233, certain royal and papal letters afford satisfactory proof that the University of Cambridge was already an organized body with a chancellor at its head. The chancellor was a dignitary appointed by the Bishop of Ely for the express purpose of granting degrees. Students at Cambridge continued to enjoy certain privileges given by the Bishop of Ely until the end of the fifteenth century (after the downfall of scholasticism).

Cambridge remained a third rate university and not a single schoolman can be shown to have taught there until Oxford was rendered open to Wyclif heresy. Following this Cambridge came into its own and it was patronized by orthodox parents.

The first medical lecturer at Oxford was Nicholas Tingewick, a fellow of Balliol College (named after John Balliol). He is mentioned by Edward I as "the physician to whom after God we owe thanks for our recovery from an illness which has lately oppressed us."[17] As intimated, Oxford and Cambridge did not take kindly to teaching surgery. They probably graduated some surgeons but these had to take the entire medical course.

In the prologue of his "Canterbury Tales," the English poet Geoffrey Chaucer presents a picture of the status of medicine of his period. The physician examining the patient had to ascertain whether the nature of the sickness is cold or warm, moist or dry and which of the four humors produced the malady. As soon as he "determined" these factors, the prescription was written and the apothecary was called upon to compound it. As mentioned previously, Chaucer gives a list of authorities to whom the doctor is indebted. This list includes Aesculapius, Dioscorides, Ruffus, Haly, Galen, Serapion, Rhazes, Avicenna, Averroes, Damacien, Constantine, Bernard, Gaddesden and Gilbert.

The esteem in which the University was held by the city authorities may be seen from the agreement made by the City of Oxford with the University. The city, in 1356, formally granted to the Chancellor of the University jurisdiction over the market: "and over all flesh of fish that shall be found to be putrid, unclean, vicious or otherwise unfit . . . on this condition, that the things forfeited be given to the Hospital of St. John." The impropriety of this regulation is obvious. Incidentally, a similar Scottish Act of Parliament (1386) provided that corrupt pork or salmon be forfeited and given to "the poor leper-folk." At Berwick, a similar law added, "If there be no leper-folk, the rotten pork or salmon shall be utterly destroyed." Such "generous" gifts to the poor and downtrodden, may well have been the cause of serious disease in many cases.

The number of students at Cambridge was augmented in 1229-1231 by migrations of students from Paris and Oxford. Cambridge, however, suffered from emigration in the year 1261 and again in 1381 when the strife between the citizens of the town and the students compelled many of the latter to leave the school. On the last date the records of the University were wantonly burned by the townsmen. Throughout the thirteenth century, the University was still a very imperfectly organized institution with no systematic code to govern its member colleges and very defective supervision over the students.

Cambridge University, as Oxford, is composed of separate member colleges. The College of Peterhouse, where medicine was taught, was founded in 1282 by Hugh Balsham who had been elected Bishop of St. John. The students at first received their instruction in the hospital of St. John. Later Peterhouse was established on the principle of Merton College at Oxford. The medical curriculum differed little from that presented at Oxford and Paris. Both Oxford and Cambridge created licentiates in surgery as well as in medicine but only the medical graduates could receive a degree. The Barber-Surgeons of London sent their best scholars to Cambridge and hired able students to lecture to them on surgery and anatomy in order to gain the educational advantages of the University.

The right to license an apothecary student was left to the chancellor who, in turn, appointed some master to act on his behalf. The prospective druggist had to swear to the following oath before he received a license:

"I swear that I will always have in my shop all medicines, species of medicines and confections which concern the art and mystery of an Apothecary, and are necessary for the health of man."

"That I shall be contented once a year (at least) that certain physicians practicing in the University shall visit my shop upon the account of good and bad medicines, in the month of November, or any other time if occasion shall require it, to be adjudged of by the Vice Chancellor, one of the Proctors and the practicing physicians here; and these searchers and tryers of medicines being of the Vice Chancellor's and Proctors' appointment, shall have power to destroy and throw away all bad and unprofitable medicines and drugs."

"That I will sell all things appertaining to my trade at a low and reasonable price, and as sold in other places in England."

"That I will not make up any compound medicines without the presence and advice of some physician admitted to the practice who shall judge those samples fit to be made up into compositions."

"That I will observe these things without fraud or deceit."[18]

The most prominent English physicians of this period were John of Gaddesden, John of Arderne and John of Mireld.

THE THREE JOHNS

JOHN OF GADDESDEN (Johannes Anglicus, 1280-1361)

The successor of Gilbert the Englisman[19] (1250) was John of Gaddesden, a fellow of Merton College, Oxford, and a canon of St. Paul's Cathedral. John was probably the first physician to be appointed to the English court. He refers to his father as possessing a choleric temperament and states that he was fond of fruit and milk. He ascribes the formation of a stone which he removed from a salivary gland of his father to this diet.

When John of Gaddesden attended Oxford, a Master of Arts

had to study medicine for some four years before being admitted to practice as a Doctor of Physik. However, a practical knowledge of medicine was considered entirely unnecessary. This last was in marked contrast to the rigid requirements of contemporary Salerno where practical experience including dissection was a basic requirement.

John of Gaddesden took his degree at Merton College, Oxford, in the early years of the fourteenth century. Having qualified as a Doctor of Physik, he opened his office in London—then a city of about 30,000 population. Besides medicine, he practiced surgery and dentistry. He gave up his general practice when he was formally appointed physician to Edward the Second.

John of Gaddesden became famous when he came out with his book, "Practica Medicina a Capite ad Podem" (1305-1307), commonly known as "Rosa Anglica," because as a rose has five petals, his book has five parts covering fevers, injuries, general hygiene, diet, and materia medica. John was not an overly modest man. He informed his readers that as a rose excels all other flowers so his "Rosa" excels everything previously written on the subject of medicine.

In reality, his "Rosa" contains nothing new. It is a repetition of well known medical works with few original additions. It is replete with superstitious practices. When the young son of Edward II contracted smallpox, John ordered that the prince be swathed in red materials with the floor coverings and window curtains in the room all changed to red.[20] The idea that red cures red, and that red surroundings will cure rashes and reduce fever is an old one. Fortunately for John, his princely patient recovered and John prided himself that the son of Edward II was restored to health by his very original and efficient treatment.

John subscribed to the belief that the "king's touch" cures "king's evil" (scrofula). If his own specific—the drinking of the blood of a dove or weasel—fails to cure the patient of "king's evil," he recommends that the patient be touched by the reigning monarch. He states that he cured a man who had been blind for twenty years with an infusion of fennel and parsley in wine.

John of Gaddesden, as has been intimated, had a great opinion of his book: In the preface, he writes: "I implore those who see this book not to gnaw it with an envious tooth but to read it through humbly for nothing is shown here but what is proved." The word "proved" scarcely tallies with many of the remedies mentioned in the "Rosa Anglica." He was certain that an extract of cuckoo (which bird he believed to get an epileptic attack once a month) mixed with boar bladder and mistletoe is a specific for epilepsy.

He recommends spikenard in treating dropsy and in his own personal practice, was insistent that this medicine be paid for in advance. In treating colic he advises the constant wearing of a seal-skin girdle with a whale bone buckle. John of Gaddesden found a cosmetic gold mine in his prescriptions for perfumes, hair washes and hair dyes. John always prescribed twice as much of any drug for his rich patients as he did for his poor ones.

John advises physicians to demand their fees before commencing the treatment of a case. In addition to his fame as a prescription writer, he also had some reputation as a poet and grammarian.[21]

Regardless of its faults, John of Gaddesden's book, "Rosa Anglica" was well written and was held in great esteem by many of his contemporaries. The "Rosa" went through at least four editions and was popular in Pavia, Augsburg, Venice and Ireland.

Edward Meryon, in his "History of Medicine," states: "He was a type of . . . the fourteenth century and an excellent illustration of the tendency of his age. He glorified in secret practices and was a charlatan of the first order. His remedies too were worthy of being recorded as curiosities in medicine. For loss of memory, he recommended the heart of a nightingale and for scrofula, the king's touch. He had the honesty, however, to confess that if the laity did but know his secret, they would despise him and his art."[22]

The best that can be said of John of Gaddesden's book is that it contains some things that are free from astrological nonsense and that there are some clinical descriptions of a rational nature. His hygienic rules are similar to those of the

"Regimen Salernitatis" of Salerno. John agrees with Avicenna and Galen and quotes them.

Until the appearance of Dr. H. P. Chalmley's book, "John of Gaddesden and the Rosa Medicina" in 1912, John of Gaddesden was almost universally rated as a charlatan. Chalmley, however, evaluates John as follows: "We see therein a man of good education and, as regards his medical education, one who was acquainted with the writings of his predecessors . . . Of anatomy he naturally knew next to nothing; of physiology less."

JOHN OF ARDERNE (1307-1380)

In the reign of Edward III, a surgeon of note appeared in England in the person of John of Arderne (John of Arden, 1307-1380). Born in Arderne the same year that Lanfranchi died, he served under the Dukes of Lancaster in succession at Antwerp, at Algeciras in Spain, and Aquitaine. After twenty years of practicing in Newark, he went to London at the age of 63, (in 1370) where he joined the Guild of Military Surgeons, and where, at the age of seventy, he published his book "De Cura Oculi."

In London, John of Arderne built up a very lucrative practice among the aristocratic and princely families of the great city. He appears to have been on good terms with the physicians of his day—an almost unheard of thing for a surgeon at that period. He refers to himself with pride as, "chirurga inter medicos" (a surgeon among physicians). He looked down upon barbers who practiced surgery.

In contrast with many other medical literary productions, the writings of Arderne are noteworthy because of the richness of his clinical histories and his preference for rational and relatively simple methods of treatment.

In the treatment of intestinal and renal colic, he successfully employed clysters in which a bladder filled with sea water served as a reservoir. Other instillations were recommended by him in bladder and venereal diseases. According to John, "every man should use an enema at least two or three times a year."

John of Arderne was a follower of Lanfranchi, but he always placed his own experience above the dogmatic rulings of surgical authorities. He describes in detail every step of the operations which he presents and he is honest enough to record his failures as well as his successes.

He wrote on the care of the eyes, on bleeding and on sinuses. His only printed work is his treatise on fistula of the anus—a condition that most of his predecessors regarded as incurable. This last is his most important contribution to surgery. This work deals with fistula in general but chiefly with the origin and treatment of fistula *in ano* to which he devoted special attention. In performing his operation, he first put his patient in a lithotomy position following which he incised the outer wall of the fistula and all of its branches. Bleeding was stopped by pressing with sponges wrung out in warm water. The operated area was then powdered, covered with clean dry pads and held in position by a T bandage.

John of Arderne used ligatures to check hemorrhages. He avoided all corrosives in the treatment of wounds. In all operations, he relied upon non-irritating powder and clean dressings for rapid healing.

His method of removing a stone impacted in the urethra is ingenious. He tied ligatures on the shaft of the penis above and below the stone to prevent its slipping. He then made a small incision over the stone and squeezed it out. Following this, he sutured the wound and applied his favorite dressing which consisted of egg white and firmly ground flour. John remarks: "There is no need for alarm in these cases even though the urine escapes from this wound for three or four days after the operation, for the patient will certainly be cured." John's fee for the above operation was 40 pounds, and according to John, his patients paid him cheerfully.

John warned his readers of the danger of mistaking cancer of the rectum for simple ulceration. His differential diagnosis between cancer and ulcer of the rectum is that cancer is painless at first and of stony hardness tending to hinder the passing of feces. Later, it ulcerates and causes pain. Still later there is the desire for frequent defecation and the stools are streaked with blood.

He describes the following essential instruments for rectal operations: a long slender metal probe for examination, a broad silver needle with a curved point and a *"tendiculum"* of wood.

His writings, illustrated with drawings of instruments, exist for the most part in manuscript form only and deal largely although not exclusively with surgery. They exhibit a wide personal experience as well as a good knowledge of the literature. Translations of his works in Old English also exist in manuscript form.

Incidentally, John's fee for the operation for anal fistula is "one hundred mark or fourty pounde, with robez and feez of one hundred shillyns terme of life, by Zere." The minimum fee was "one hundred shillyns." Considering the purchasing power of money, this certainly was a high fee even for the rich. John claims that his patients paid him cheerfully.

In his "Of Ye Manner of Ye Leeche," John advises his colleagues to cultivate modesty, charity and chastity. The leech is advised to abstain from venery and to be particularly careful in his conduct towards the wives, daughters and other women in the house of the patient. "Consider not over-openly with the lady or the daughter or other fair women in great men's houses, nor proffer to kiss them, nor touch their dresses; privately or openly."

John advised that the estimated period of time for cure should be increased over the physician's actual opinion for the benefit of the patient and his family. If the patient became well sooner than the prognostication, the leech should tell him that the quick recovery was due to the fact that he was stronghearted, suffered well and was of good complexion; "for such words makes the patient proud."

His instructions to the surgeon are of high moral tone: He should pray, write or study, "for the study of books is an honor to a leech." Above all he must always be sober, for drunkenness destroys all virtue and brings it to naught: "Drunkenness breaketh whatsoever wisdom teacheth." The surgeon should scorn no one and if another doctor is spoken of, he should answer courteously: "I have nought heard of him but good." He must have clean hands, and well-shapen nails which are neither black nor dirty. He should hear much and speak little for if a patient sees that he keeps other people's secrets, he will naturally put more confidence in him.

"When sick men, forsooth, or any of them beside cometh to the leech to ask help or counsel of him, be he not to them over-stern nor over-homely, but moderate in bearing after the requirements of the persons; to some reverently, to some commonly. For, according to wise men, overmuch homeliness breedeth despising."

John advised the leech to "give no certain answer in any cause, but he see first the sickness and the manner of it; and when he hath seen and assayed it, although to him it seem that the sick may be healed, nevertheless he shall make prognostication to the patient (of) the perils to come if the cure be deferred. And if he see the patient pursue busily the cure, then, after the state of the patient requireth, ask he boldly more or less (fee); but ever be he aware of scanty askings, for over-scarce askings set at nought both the market and the thing."

John warns against telling the patient the exact time of recovery: "If the patients or their friends or servants ask how much time he hopeth to heal it, evermore let the leech promise the double that he supposeth to speed by half; that is, if the leech hope to heal the patient in twenty weeks—that is the common course of curing—add he so many over. For it is better that the term be lengthened than the cure. For prolongation of the cure giveth cause of despairing to the patient, when trust to the leech is most hope of health. And if the patient consider or wonder or ask why he put him so long a time of curing, since that he healed him by the half, answer he that it was for that the patient was strong-hearted, and suffered well sharp things, and that he was of good complexion and had able flesh to heal."

"Have the leech also clean hands and well shapen nails, and cleansed from all blackness and filth. And be he courteous at lords' tables, and displease he not on words or deeds to the guests sitting by; hear he many things but speak he but few . . . And when he shall speak, be the words short, and, as much as he may, fair and reasonable and without swearing. Beware that there be never found double words in his mouth, for if he be found true in his words few or none shall doubt in his deeds. Learn also a young leech good proverbs pertaining to his craft in comforting of patients . . . Also it speedeth that a leech can talk of good tales . . . that may make the patients to laugh, as well as of the Bible as of other tragedies; and any other things which are no trouble, while they make or induce a light heart to the patient or the sick man."

Here he warns against betraying the friends, relatives and servants of the patient: "Discover never the leech unwarily the counsels of his patients, as well of men as of women, nor set not one to another at nought, although he have cause, that he be not guilty of counsel; for if a man see thee conceal well another man's counsel he will trust better in thee. Many things, forsooth, have to be kept by a leech, without these that are said afore, that may not be noted here for over much occupying."

"If the patient insist steadfastly that he be cured, or ask if he may be cured, then say the leech thus: 'I doubt not, if God help us, and thy good patience following, if thou wilt competently make satisfaction to me, as such a cure—not little to be commended—supposing all things to be kept that ought to be kept, and left that ought to be left, as it is said, I shall be able to bring this cure to a loveable end and healthful." [23]

JOHN OF MIRFELD (d. 1407)

The third John of the trio was John of Mirfeld (Johannes de Mirfeld) a scholastic, who was a cleric of the monastery of St. Bartholomew in London. His early history is not known. It is even not certain whether he received his medical education in a recognized medical college or through some form of apprenticeship. It is known, however, that he was closely connected with the St. Bartholomew Hospital—perhaps as a chaplain.

John of Mirfeld is the author of two medical treatises, the "Breviarium Bartholomei Medicina" (1380) and the "Florarium Bartholomei," a theology which also contains one chapter on medicine.

John of Mirfeld's medical books are based on classical and medieval authorities. His "Breviarium" is a resume of contemporary medicine and surgery. He was particularly interested in treatment. There is no theoretical quibbling. In his "Breviarium," he points out the chief symptoms of various ailments which lead to a diagnosis and suggests remedies. Many charms are included. For example, he gives the wording of a charm to be worn by a pregnant woman to facilitate her delivery. He apparently prescribed such charms as a kind of a placebo for he did not believe in their therapeutic worth.

His "Breviarium" is largely derived from Macer Floridus' work, "The Salernitans." The names of the surgeons Roger, Lanfranc, Arnold of Villanova and particularly Gordon, Gilbert Anglicus and John Gaddesden and various Arabic authors are cited. In addition, John's original observations are included.

The "Breviarium Bartholomei Medicina" (1380-1395), is divided into 15 parts. The first two parts deal with fevers. The next five sections cover diseases arranged according to the regions of the body beginning with the head and proceeding down to the toes. Diseases of the head and throat, the chest, the abdomen, the pelvic organs, and the extremities, are included in that order. The eighth part is concerned with abscesses, the ninth with wounds, the tenth with fractures and the eleventh with dislocations. The twelfth, thirteenth and fourteenth parts deal with remedies and particularly purgatives. The last section is devoted to hygiene and phlebotomy. There exists among John of Mirfeld's manuscripts a short treatise on prognosis entitled "Speculum," a chapter of which deals with physicians and their drugs from a dermatological standpoint.

Among John of Mirfeld's prognostic signs are many of a superstitious nature in which he himself might not have believed. For example, if the right eye of a sick man sheds tears, he will die. If the left eye of a woman sheds tears, she will die.

If the sole of a patient is anointed with lard and the lard is then thrown to a dog, if the dog eats it without vomiting the patient will recover; on the other hand, if the dog makes no attempt to eat it or vomits after doing so, the patient will die. These omens are typical of the Anglo-Saxon leechdom prognostics.

John seldom comments on the therapies he prescribes; the only exception to this is the aforementioned charm written on parchment to be worn by pregnant women to assist in delivery. His comment on this is to the effect that, although some men believe in it, he himself has little faith in its use.

The "Breviarium" has some quotations taken from Hippocrates, Galen, Rhazes and Avicenna. The "Anglo-Saxon Leechbook" is also quoted.

John of Mirfeld indicts the quacks and particularly "women who usurp this profession to themselves and abuse it." The surgeon is advised to leave the patient alone if he is in doubt about the outcome of an operation: "for it is safer to leave a man in the hands of his Creator than to put trust in surgery or medicine, concerning which there is any manner of doubt."

John of Mirfeld evidently did not have a good opinion of his contemporaries: "Modern physicians possess three special qualifications and these are to be able to lie in a subtle manner, to show an outward honesty, and to kill with audacity." Perhaps even more crushing is his statement to the effect that few physicians are good Christians.

In the following quotation he shows that medicine and surgery were separated in his day:

"Long ago, unless I mistake, physicians used to practice surgery and medicine, and this, I fear, arises from pride, because physicians disdain to work with their hands, though, indeed, I myself have a suspicion that it is because they do not know how to perform particular operations; this unfortunate usage has led the public to believe that a man cannot know both subjects, but the well informed are aware that he cannot be a good physician who neglects every part of surgery, and, on the other hand, a surgeon is good for nothing who is without knowledge of medicine." [24]

It is apparent that the three Johns, each in his own way, made contributions to the progress of English medicine and surgery. If their beginning was slow, the results of their labors eventually influenced future generations.

Medieval surgery in England was of a minor character and was mostly military surgery performed either by guild surgeons or by barber-surgeons. These two groups became at an early day united into a legal corporation which sometimes included physicians and apothecaries and which always constituted the chief licensing body for surgeons in the various towns.

English surgery during the first half of the Hundred Years' War was by no means on a par with the French. John of Gaunt, the Duke of Bedford, sought to remedy this defect by making available to English surgeons the writings of Guy de Chauliac in the English vernacular. Guy de Chauliac's skill in treating fractures of the skull and wounds of the breast was supreme. His discreet use of sutures and diet for the wounded restored many to health who might otherwise have died on the battlefield. Quaritch, referring to this translation avers that it is "one of the finest English medical manuscripts in existence." The manuscript is a volume of 181 pages, 13x9 inches, beautifully written in double columns.

CHAPTER XVIII

MEDICINE IN MEDIEVAL GERMANY

After the fall of the Western Empire, few traces of organized medical practice remained in the region which later developed into Germany. In the early years of the sixth century, after the Franks conquered most of Europe and took over many Roman institutions, records indicate that physicians were employed at the royal courts, but they did not carry any prestige and were not treated as persons of merit. The last request of Queen Austrichides, who died from the plague was to the effect that her physician be decapitated on her demise. Her wish was promptly fulfilled.

After the conversion of the Germans to Christianity, the Germans, like the Greeks of old who brought the afflicted to the temples for temple sleep, conveyed their sick to the churches for cure. There were few lay physicians and most of these had migrated from Italy and Southern France. Native healing, barring the Church physicians, was largely in the hands of women and wound-healers who attended only to injuries.

Under the rule of Charlemagne, German national unity took a mighty step forward when a long standing struggle ended in 804 A.D. with the submission of the Saxons and the extension of Frankish authority over Bavarians. This brought the German race under a single ruler. The general establishment of the Frankish system of government and the presence of Frankish officials in all the capitals helped to break down tribal and racial barriers. With the conversion of the Saxons to Christianity, the whole German race became Christians. Charlemagne granted land privileges to the prelates and established Bishoprics, monasteries and schools.

In the days of Charlemagne, medicine was largely confined to the monasteries, the most magnificent of which was that of Fulda where a center of learning was established. Charlemagne advocated and sponsored the teaching of medicine in this monastery. The works of the ancient physicians were copied and studied by the monks who at that period were the only learned class. Among their number were various learned medical men including Rhabanus Maurus (778-850 A.D.), Abbot of Fulda, who left a record of the medicine of that period in his work "De Rerum Natura."

In "Indrun" (manifestly a Germanic imitation of the Iliad) we first find the "Heilkunstmeister" Wate, employing roots, salves and powerful herbs in the cure of wounds. He had learned his art from "a rude old woman" (druidess?).

From the earliest times, women seem to have practiced medicine among the Germans and Celts. Medicine was regarded as unworthy of the attention of men. At least in old Germanic writings (as well as in those of Tacitus), medical women alone are mentioned, and it is not until the twelfth century that male physicians are also spoken of. The remedies of these female healers consisted chiefly of charms, runic characters, and natural domestic remedies. Even St. Hildegarde was unacquainted with remedies other than the aboriginal, domestic drugs of the Germans. It was not until the twelfth century that old-Greek medicine and Arabian remedies reached Germany.[1]

Charlemagne (Charles the Great—c. 742-814 Roman Emperor and King of Franks), in his "Capitulare of Diedenhofen" urged that medical herbs should be cultivated around the monasteries. The pupil of Rhabanus Maurus, Walafrid Strabo (807-848), described many herbs and their medicinal actions in a Latin poem entitled "Hortulus," written in the year 827 A.D. In the grounds of the monastery of St. Gallen may be found what can be considered as one of the earliest hospitals. The "house of physicians," the room of the seriously sick patients, and the pharmacy can still be discerned.

Hospitals were usually attached to the larger monasteries. Here not only the sick sought refuge, but also weak and needy pilgrims and travelers. The significance of the monastic hospitals diminished when the cities began to build their own hospitals and staffed them with lay physicians and surgeons.

Leprous patients were sent out of town in leprosariums. Communication was strictly forbidden with such groups. The so-called "municipal hospitals" not only took in the sick, but also the poor and the wayfarers. Insane people were looked upon as either wild animals or disciples of Satan and were treated brutally.

Most hospitals owed their existence to endowments of princes or rich citizens. The hospital physicians received a definite salary from the city treasury. They were required to swear to give their faithful services both to the rich and poor alike and, in case of epidemic, not to flee the city, but remain faithfully on duty.[2]

Pharmacy was a lucrative enterprise in those days and apothecary shops did not have to be established by the municipality. The municipal governments however, regulated the relationships between the physician and the druggist, and often fixed the fees for both. An oath was exacted from the apothecary to the effect that he exercise his trade in an honorable manner. An old statute in Basel forbids an apothecary from treating the sick. Apparently over-the-counter prescribing by druggists was not unknown even in those days.

The German term *"Arzt"* for physician is generally believed to be derived from the Latin "archiater." Eckard, however, is of the opinion, that *Arzt* is derived from *"ars* (art) *medicinalis"* and originally signified one who gathered or prepared herbs for medicinal purposes.

In the early part of the thirteenth century when it became known that some of the clergy were engaging in surgical practice, the Church placed a ban on priests who practiced surgery and as a further development this ban was later extended to include general medicine, thus increasing the need for lay physicians.

The spread of leprosy at that period increased the necessity to train lay physicians at home to combat this dreaded disease. Hitherto, most of the lay physicians who settled in the larger cities had been foreigners. The few native doctors who were trained at Salerno, Montpellier and Bologna acquired positions at the courts of the princes or were employed by the governments of the larger cities upon their return. It was difficult for the small number of lay physicians to cope even partially with the great medical problems of the country.

The bubonic plague of 1348 demonstrated in a most dramatic manner that Germany was in great need of trained physicians at home. There were pitifully few physicians available and the foreign cities stopped admitting German students for fear that they might bring the plague along with them.

"Nothing can be more strikingly illustrative of the cosmopolitanism of the medieval universities," says Rashdall, "than the fact that up to the middle of the fourteenth century Germany possessed no university. Germany was certainly not untouched by the great intellectual movement of the twelfth century, but its two great centers were Paris and Northern Italy."[3]

When the earliest universities arose, Germany was too far behind the rest of Europe in culture and civilization for the spontaneous development of a university, and when the period of artificial foundation arrived, its political dissension was not conducive to such an experiment. German students, therefore, attended all the universities of France and Italy.[4]

The first German university was founded in Prague in 1345 by Charles IV. This king was an ardent friend and patron of all efforts to advance science and art. The university building was known as the Carolinum and was first built in 1348. The studium generale was modeled after the pattern of the University of Paris. For centuries the University of Prague was the scene of many religious discussions. The larger part of the building was occupied by lecture rooms and there were also a library and observatory. This school played a prominent part in the history of Bohemia. The students were mostly Bohemian, Bavarian, Saxon and Polish. At their head was a rector who had to belong to the clergy, be at least 25 years old, of legitimate birth and have lived a blameless life devoid of all sin.[5]

Medicine did not receive much recognition in the beginning, when there were only one or at the most two professors of medicine. Nicolaus de Gevicka, Balthasar de Tusca and Walther are mentioned as famous medical teachers. The first religious quarrel at the close of the fifteenth century caused a decline in medicine. Later the medical school grew in strength. "In no place," said Benesch de Wartinnel (14th century), "did the science receive such careful cultivation as in Prague. Students came thither from England, France, Lombardy, Hungary, Poland and the adjacent countries." It is said that there were in Prague at this time, 30,000 students (perhaps this number includes all enrolled Prague students since the founding of the University).

When once the university movement was started in Germany, it advanced with rapid strides. As in medieval Spain and modern America, the foundation of a university in one State excited the jealousy and ambition of the others.

In 1389, the University of Vienna was founded by members of the Faculty of Paris upon the request of prominent citizens of Vienna. Instruction here was based on the plan of the University of Paris. The first public lecture on anatomy was delivered in Vienna in the year 1404, by Caliazzo de Sophia of Padua. This was the first lecture on anatomy that was delivered beyond the Alps. It took place one hundred years after Italy's first anatomical lecture.

The Provost of the Church of St. Stephen occupied the office of Chancellor. The doctors who had received diplomas there constituted the Medical Faculty and the dean was elected by them. The first teachers of medicine at Vienna were Johann Gallioi of Breslau, Herman Lurch of Nurenberg and Herman von Treysa of Hersen.[6]

The decline of Prague in consequence of the Hussite troubles put Vienna at the head of the German universities. Vienna long resisted the tendency observable in older German universities towards the concentration of power in the hands of an inner circle of senior masters.

Vienna, after the Albertine reorganization, was in the main a university of masters. Yet its constitution permitted the students a larger share in the government of the University than was the case at Paris or Oxford. Whereas the students had no share in legislation, they apparently had a vote in the election of proctors and were eligible to hold office. There was far more magisterial discipline at Vienna than at Bologna or Montpellier, but perhaps rather less than at Paris and Oxford. Marriage was not a bar to graduation although married students are described in the registers in a by no means complimentary manner.

The University of Vienna was followed by that of Heidelberg which was founded by the elector Ruppert in 1386. A bull authorizing its foundation was issued by Pope Urban IV in that year. It was modeled after the University of Paris. Among the medical facilities were an academic hospital, a maternity hospital, a physiological institute and a clinical laboratory. There were also a zoological museum and an observatory. For a long time, the University of Heidelberg was granted state privileges. During the reformation, it became the stronghold of Protestant learning. The "Heidelberg Catechism" was drawn up by famous theologians.

The rector was always taken from the Faculty of Arts, which apparently voted as one body in the general congregation. Few universities of the Middle Ages, not founded by migration from an existing university, could boast so large a membership in the very year after its foundation. By October 1387, 589 persons had been matriculated, including six masters of theology, five doctors, a licentiate of canon law, three doctors of medicine, and thirty-four masters of arts. A year later, the University was nearly emptied by pestilence, quarrels with the town, and the establishment of a rival university at Köln. But Heidelberg regained its equilibrium in the following year and permanently took its place as one of the most important in Germany.

The University, following in the footsteps of its first great teacher, Marsilius (1433-1499), was originally entirely nominalistic. In 1412, we find a prohibition not merely of the "perverse and condemned doctrines" of Wyclif, but of all realistic teaching. After the Council of Constance, however, we find symptoms of the realistic reaction which was everywhere in progress.

Other later universities were Koln founded in 1388, Erfurt established in 1392 and Leipzig opened in 1409.

In Germany, due to the few medical institutions and the limited means, medical education was not very advanced. The teaching in the early universities included the elementary subjects which were taught in the monasteries and cathedrals as well as the subjects that were taught in the community schools.

In Austria, up to the year 1848, two years of philosophy was required before entering medical schools. A similar requirement existed in England.

Emperor Friedrich II decreed that a three year scientific education should precede entrance to medical school. Most academies, before being permitted to present a medical curriculum, were required to present a bachelor of arts degree.[7]

For sometime, it was difficult to get local students to register in these schools because the medical courses were so expensive. The medical teaching staff was very small. There were only two professors: one taught theory and the other the practice of medicine. The designation "professor" came into use during the sixteenth century. There was no department of surgery. This branch of medicine was free for all and was practiced by barbers, old females, clerics and quacks.

The primary qualification for admission to a medical school was the completion of a three year course of study in general education which led to the degree, known as "Artibus." The length of the medical course varied. In Vienna and Leipzig, it was for six years and in Koln, for three years. In Paris, Vienna and Prague, the Master of Medicine claimed the right to determine in what manner the art of medicine should be taught.

The instruction was largely theoretical and consisted of lectures upon ancient medical authorities, Arabic commentators and Italian writers, as well as upon personal medical experience. The works recommended were: the "Aphorisms" and "Prognostics" of Hippocrates, the "Ars Parva" of Galen, the "Liber ad Almansorem" of Rhazes and the "Canon" of Avicenna. In addition there were weekly dialogues by students under the supervision of the professor. In these discussions, students who excelled in dialectic cleverness were considered of the highest caliber. Very little clinical teaching was available. In later years, senior students were permitted to accompany teachers into the sick room.

A textbook entitled "Articella" was popular among German students for several centuries. This work was reprinted several times. The professors' salaries ranged from 35 to 50 dollars per annum, but the physicians' yearly stipends were smaller. In Frankfurt-on-the-Main, there was a municipal physician in 1438 who received a salary consisting of a measure of cloth and ten measures of grain. Later three physicians in the same city received a yearly salary of from ten to 100 gulden each. The first German to receive the degree of Doctor of Medicine was a Salerno graduate. The degree was awarded by Gilles de Corbeil (Petrus Aegidius Corboliensis) of Paris in the twelfth century, who was a pupil in the School of Salerno.

At the graduation ceremony, the candidate was required to defend four theses on Aristotle, Hippocrates, Galen and a modern author and to take an oath. He then received a ring, a wreath of laurel and ivy, a book first closed and then opened, and a kiss—"the kiss of peace"—and the rank of "Doctor in Philosophy and Medicine."

More liberal treatment—even special privilege—was given to physicians with the approach of modern times. They were exempted from taxes and military service and were honored with a special attire consisting of a red coat trimmed with fur borders. The duties of the doctor were regulated by a magistrate.

The municipal physician, from time to time, visited the shops of apothecaries to examine their stocks and see if everything was in order. In those days, the doctor himself took his prescription to the druggist and gave him personal directions as to how to prepare and mix the ingredients in the prescription. If the doctor was summoned on a distant call, he was escorted by a municipal servant.

The statutes of Nuremberg and Silesia of 1350 promulgated by Carl IV prohibited the doctor from preparing remedies and the pharmacist from treating patients.

The statutes of Vienna in the fourteenth century permitted those holding a Baccalaureate degree to practice when accompanied by an instructor or by a practicing physician who was a graduate from the University of Vienna. A doctor who had not been paid by his patient for his professional services was not obliged to attend to the patient if he were called again.

Few original works were written by German physicians in the Middle Ages. The available works were mostly translations of Lanfranc, Saliceto, Guy de Chauliac, etc. The one original work was the "Binderartzner" by the German Ordensritter ("Monastic knight").

There were of course, numerous quacks, hernia specialists, stone cutters (for vesical calculi), cataract couchers and tooth crushers who competed with the physician. In spite of prohibition by the authorities, such illicit practitioners continued in their practice. Driven out from one place they swooped down upon another.[8]

Among the earliest physicians and medical authors of Germany was Petrus Physicus (1292-1378), Bishop of Sarepta. Thomas, as his name was before he became Bishop, practiced in Breslau and in other places of Germany. He wrote upon uroscopy and alchemy, vehemently opposing the latter. He was a staunch advocate of venesection.

Perhaps the most famous physician of that period was Sigismundus Albicus (b. 1347), a student of Prague University who taught at that institution for some three years. His fame as a skilled physician brought him to the attention of King Wensceslas who appointed him court physician and heaped honors upon him.

His writings consist of "Regimen Temporo Pestilentia Medicinale" and "Tractatus de Regimen Hominis." The latter work known in the vernacular as "Vetularius" is a work distinguished by its rationality and independence. All Sigismundus Albicus' works possess marked practical tendencies and sober views. He cites the names of his authorities and frequently mentions Arnold of Villanova whom he particularly admired. While admitting the value of alchemy and metallurgy, he rejects these sciences from the standpoint of medicine. He is of the opinion that the original properties of drugs are interfered with by the process of sublimation. He devotes a chapter to astrology although he is not an advocate of this pseudoscience.

KUNRAT VON MEGENBERG (c. 1309-1374)

Among the famous physicians of the early part of the fourteenth century was Kunrat von Megenberg, the author of "Buch der Natur" (c. 1350). He was a liberal-minded cleric, taught for eight years in Paris and, on his return to Germany, became director of the town-school of Vienna. He later established permanent residence in Regensburg. The "Buch der Natur" is no more than a compilation and frequent reference is made to Aristotle, Hippocrates, Galen and the Arabic authorities. Megenberg's "Book of Nature" follows in its contents the "Liber de Naturis Rerum" of Thomas of Cantimpre (1201-1270), but appears to be based, not upon the original of this work, but upon a Latin translation.

"Regimen Sanitatis" contains various annual and monthly dietetic directions and discusses the influence of the elements upon the temperament of man. This work covers the qualities of various foods and drinks, the proper regulation of sleep, aperients, baths, blood-letting, emetics and clysters. It advises the proper mode of life during plague epidemics and gives directions as to the proper care of the head, brain and eyes. At a later period a symptomatological addendum with short prophylactic and therapeutic recommendations and recipes was added to this work.

BARTOLOMAEUS METLINGER
(middle of the fifteenth century)

One of the most distinguished physicians of his time was Bartolomaeus Metlinger, author of "Ein Regimen wie Man Junge Kinder Halten Sol von Mutterleyb bis zu Siben Jaren, mit Esen, Trinken, Laden und in Allen Kranckheytt die in zu Sten Magen," published in Augsburg in 1473. This little book with the long title is doubtlessly derived from hand-written copies and it quotes Hippocrates ("Aphorisms"), Galen ("Ars Magna" and "Parva"), Rhazes ("Continens"), Avicenna ("Canon"), Averroes ("Colliget"), Constantinus ("Pantegni"), and Avenzoar. It is divided into four chapters, of which the first two deal with the diet and care of children, the third with diseases of children and the fourth with their education.

Chapter I presents general rules of health for the newly-born until they learn to walk and speak, and includes such topics as cleansing the mouth, bathing the new-born, dusting the navel with desiccating powder and other care of the navel, proper sleeping position (with the head elevated), proper methods of lifting, stroking and wrapping the infant and inferences which may be gathered from crying.

Chapter II deals with suckling, choice of wet-nurse, weaning, testing the milk of nurses and proper nourishment of nurses.

Chapter III, following the introductory statement that in the case of a sick nursling the nurse herself must be included in the cure, the following diseases are described: eruptions of the scalp, hydrocephalus, meningitis (?), insomnia, cramp, paralysis, otorrhea, inflammation of the eyes, squint, teething, swellings of the throat, affections of the oral mucous membranes, enlargement of the breasts, disorders of digestion, jaundice, diarrhea, constipation, prolapse of the rectum, worms, colic, umbilical and other types of hernia, urinary calculosis, ulcers of the skin, fevers, erysipelas, measles and chickenpox. In recommending therapeutics, the author relies mainly upon his own personal experience.

Chapter IV presents directions as to how children should be held when learning to walk, and covers their physical and intellectual education up to the seventh year. Eating, drinking, bathing and exercise are discussed and commencement of education is recommended in the sixth year.[9] Wine-drinking is permitted to girls after the twelfth year and boys after the fourteenth year.

Metlinger was an active practitioner in Augsburg.

HEINRICH VON PFOLSPEUNDT (b. 1460)

Heinrich von Pfolspeundt is the author of "Buch der Bundth-Artzeney" which was written in 1460 and published by Haeser and Middeldorpf in 1868. This work deals chiefly with temperance and cleanliness. An important piece of advice is tendered to surgeons who deal with difficult cases which they are not capable of handling. Such surgeons are advised to direct the patient to more experienced masters. Wounds are divided into recent and old (infected) types. According to Pfolspeundt, the former can usually be made to heal only after suppuration which may be facilitated by application of turpentine, oil of roses and wound-plasters spread upon tow or flax and composed of honey, meal and bole. The latter require stimulating, desiccant and caustic remedies, of which a number are enumerated. Pfolspeundt appears to have learned facial plastic surgery from the Italian surgeons.

To arrest hemorrhage, he recommends tampons of cotton or wool impregnated with styptics. He does not even mention ligatures. Among diseases occurring in traumatic wounds are included "Wilde Fever" (erysipelas) and "Gliedwasser" ("watery discharge"—suppuration). He gives clear instructions as to how to suture the scalp. He advocates the use of green silk thread which is left *in situ* for seven days.[10]

The directions concerning extraction of arrows are very minute. Mention is only made once, and then only casually, of shotgun wounds. A most detailed description is given of the treatment of penetrating abdominal wounds (particularly those caused by arrows). Pfolspeundt discusses enlargement of the wound in certain cases and the advisability at times of immediate suture, particularly after the reposition of prolapsed intestines. A ruptured coil of intestines should be removed by section and replaced by a silver cannula. Internal hemorrhage (on account of the dangers incident to clotting) is to be treated by placing the patient in an appropriate position.

Setting of fractures (following reposition of the fragments) is undertaken by means of a "leg-plaster" with appropriate splints of wood, felt and pasteboard. In compound fractures, the seat of the fracture must be left exposed. In fracture of the hip, use is made of a wooden fracture-box to lessen the danger of shortening and mechanical treatment is employed to prevent distortion.

Apart from the above-mentioned diseases, cursory mention is made of diseases of the teeth and mouth, gout, dysentery, thread-worms, dysuria, condylomata and plague buboes.

Noteworthy is the description of a hair-lip operation and directions for employing an anesthetic agent consisting of a narcotic sponge steeped in juice of black poppy, henbane seeds, leaves of mandragora, unripe mulberries, hemlock root, ivy and lactuca seeds.

The great importance of Pfolspeundt's work, however, lies in the fact that it contains the first description of rhinoplasty procedure which hitherto had been carefully guarded as a craft secret. The author, as he admits, learned of this from an Italian who had imparted it to only two other persons.[11]

A very important medieval German work is the "Buch der Wund Artzney" by Hieronymus Brunschwig (Strassburg, 1497). This work, the first in medical literature to deal with the theory and practice of medicine, describes operations and technical procedures.

This book, notable for its illustrations, presents good descriptions of surgical instruments and gives explicit directions to the physician at the bedside and in the pharmacy, to the obstetrician in the delivery room and to the surgeon performing an operation, handling severe fractures and treating all kinds of wounds. This book was reproduced by Klein in 1911 and by Sigerist in 1923.

Among the practicing physicians in medieval Germany were

many Jews. Under Louis the Bald, a Jewish physician named Zedekiah was court physician.

Solomon Pletsch, the city physician of Ratisbon (1394), received an annual stipend of 36 florins and six yards of cloth. He was required to treat the servants of the city council and the sick Jews. His successor, Isaac Friedrich, received only 20 florins. At Basel, one Dr. Jossel held the office of city physician at an annual stipend of 25 silver pounds; Gutleben, his successor, received only 18 pounds. At Wurzburg, Dr. Seligmann (c. 1407) was physician to Bishop John I. The Bishop's successor, John II, permitted a woman named Sarah to practice medicine in the bishopric of Wurzburg. She, with the Jewess Zerlin (c. 1475), who was an oculist at Frankfurt-on-the-Main, were the earliest Jewish women physicians in Germany of whom there is record.

During the ravages of the plague in 1348 and 1349, Jewish physicians were accused of having poisoned the wells. At Strassburg, a Jewish surgeon named Balavignus was executed in 1348 for an alleged crime of this nature.

In 1505, Lorenz of Bibra prohibited Jews from practicing in Wurzburg (this edict was reenacted in 1549). Up to 1517, the physicians who wished to practice in Vienna had to acknowledge under oath their belief in the "immaculate conception."

In 1422, Pope Martin V issued a bull in which he exhorted all Christians to treat the Jews with kindness. He permitted the Jews to practice medicine. However, by the end of the fourteenth and the beginning of the fifteenth centuries, Jewish physicians found the greatest difficulty in practicing medicine. Papal decrees and Church councils (such as at Basel in 1434) restricted them seriously.

Until the fourteenth century, most of the German physicians were educated in Italian or French universities, where they were compelled to go because of the lack of such institutions at home. German physicians generally confined themselves to the practice of medicine and did not engage in surgery. This separation of the medical and surgical arts, which had so marked a cleavage, was also followed in Germany where the occupation of surgery rendered one "disreputable." Such specialization, however, was never the case in Italy, where many eminent physicians and even teachers, did not occupy themselves exclusively with medicine, but also practiced surgery. Where they did not practice surgery personally, they often had assistants who performed the required operations.

The prominent physicians, who at the beginning of the fifteenth century began to belong chiefly to the laity, practiced all the branches of medicine and were called "Physici" ("Buchaerzte" in contrast to the clerical physicians or "Seelenaertze"), "Magistri in Physica," and later, "Doctores Medicinae." To the "Seelenaertze" and to the Church especially credit must be given with regard to the development of the hospital system far beyond anything that had been known in pagan Rome. The early hospitals were partly for the casual sick or poor, but more often still for the aged and infirm. Clement V, in the Ecumenical Council of Vienna (1311), expressed his bitter indignation at the negligence or dishonesty of executors or governors of leperhouses, almshouses or hospitals, who let them go to ruin or embezzled their revenues. The occasional disappearance of these leperhospitals or their conversion to other uses, may have been due mainly to improved conditions of living. The masses of population were perhaps betttter nourished in the fifteenth century.

CHAPTER XIX

MEDICINE IN MEDIEVAL RUSSIA

Properly speaking, the term "medieval" cannot be applied to Russia. Russia had no great early culture and, as a matter of fact, the status of civilization in Russia of antiquity was no better than during the Middle Ages.

All Western superstitions were current in Russia during the medieval period with a large assortment of native hocus pocus in addition. The Russian people believed in magic, sorcery, divination, astrology, the miraculous virtues of various herbs and formulas, the evil effect produced by "lifting the footstep marks" of an enemy, bewitched swords, love philtres, ghosts and vampires. Such factors still play a prominent part in Russian folklore.

Sorcery manifested itself in everyday life. Before a person went to a court of law, he customarily secured a trembling twig from a birch tree and recited the following formula: "As this twig trembles so may my adversary at law and his tongue tremble." When a women felt that she was being neglected by her sweetheart or husband, like as not she would consult a sorceress who would give her a root to place upon a mirror while reciting the words: "As I look into the glass and do not tire of seeing myself so let my loved one never grow tired of seeing me." [1]

As late as in 1598, the Russian people had to take an oath of loyalty to the czar. Each citizen had to pledge that in drinking and wearing clothing he would engage in no evil practice against the monarch. He also had to swear that he would not engage in sorcery nor employ noisome roots to the detriment of the czar and that he would not employ wizards or witches to do harm unto him. He had to promise that he would not efface the czar's footprints with any magical design and that he would not use magic or send any evil to him via the wind. The general public was refused admission to the imperial stables lest some evilly disposed person place noxious herbs or roots in the emperor's saddles, bridles, belts or gloves.

It is recorded that even the most enlightened czar, Boris Godunof, was afraid of malign occult practices. He made all his servants swear never to have recourse to magicians, male or female or to any other means of hurting the czar and czarina or their children and never to cast spells by working magic upon the traces of their feet or their carriage.[2]

The Russian people had more confidence in the concoctions of "wise women" and in the holy water in which a relic had been dipped, than in doctors, whom they generally regarded as not particularly well intentioned. If a doctor did not succeed in curing his patient, he was punished as a malicious magician.

One unfortunate physician, a Jew, was executed publicly by Ivan III for having allowed the czarina to die. Another, a German named Anthony, was accused of causing the death of a Tartar prince. He was delivered to the prince's relatives to be dealt with according to the rule of *lex talionis*. He was promptly stabbed to death. Even at the end of the sixteenth century, when the restrictions against doctors were ameliorated, the medical man was not altogether free from the prejudice of the laity and safe from arbitrary punishment—particularly when he undertook the treatment of a member of the royalty or nobility. The physician was not allowed to see a noble lady's face or expose even the part of the body that was sick or injured. Even her pulse had to be felt through a muslin covering. Yet, the physician was expected to make a correct diagnosis and perform a speedy cure.[3]

A great change took place in Russia at the close of the tenth century when Russia adopted the Greek Catholic Church as the state religion. Nestor (1056-1111), an old monk historian of Kiev, gives an account of how this was brought about: During the siege of Constantinople by Emperor Vladimir (956-1015), that monarch suddenly gave up the attack upon the city when his efforts were on the very threshold of success. Nestor believes that Vladimir, who was a pagan, was impressed with the Greek Catholic Religion and that this siege led him to accept this religion. Others affirm that the prince fell in love with Anna, the sister of Emperor Basil (912-954), and that the latter insisted that he accept her religion for himself and his country. At any rate, the prince, after some hesitation, agreed on accepting the Greek Catholic religion and imposed the Greek Church upon all his subjects.

According to Nestor's version, the conversion of Russia to the Greek Orthodox religion is devoid of any romance with women and developed after the Emperor's sincere search for a true religion for his country. According to Nestor's account, after a prolonged consultation with his boyars, Vladimir sent, in the year 987, envoys to study the religious claims of Mohammedanism, Judaism, and Christianity. The representatives of each of these religions urged Vladimir to enter their faiths and, after due deliberation, he was won over by the enthusiastic accounts given him about the Greek Orthodox Church by his ambassador at Constantinople. The ambassador presented a most attractive picture of the Eastern Service in the Church of St. Sophia at Constantinople.

In his chronicles, Nestor describes the circumstances with which the conversion was associated. While the envoy to the Mussulman Bulgarians of the Volga reported "there is no gladness among them, only sorrow and a great stench; their religion is not a good one" and while the envoy to the Germans saw "no beauty" in their temples, the ambassador to Constantinople reported the splendid full festival ritual of the Orthodox Church. When the envoys witnessed this service, they reported: "We no longer knew whether we were in heaven or on earth and we know not how to tell of it."

Perhaps Nestor's version of the story is right or perhaps Vladimir was more impressed by the offer of Basil to give him his sister Anna in marriage than by the account of his envoys from Constantinople. At any rate, Vladimir was baptised in Kherson in the "Crionae" where also his marriage took place with Anna, the Roman princess. The Greek Church bestowed upon Vladimir the rank of sainthood in appreciation for the conversion of his subjects to the Greek Catholic Church.

The masses of the Russian people were evidently taken by surprise by this act. They were dismayed when the images of Peroun and other gods were cast into the Dnieper River and when they were forced to consult monks instead of their own priests when they were stricken with disease or in time of other trouble.

Evil tongues questioned Vladimir's sainthood. Even the virtuous and learned monk Nestor, whose annals are the chief source of information of the history of the Russian Church, questions his sincerity. He refers to Vladimir as one who encouraged war and sensualities. His true character may be surmised from his behavior towards his own brother and his conduct towards women. It may be recalled that Vladimir was the youngest of the three sons of Sviatoslav, born to a servant at the palace. When the father died, the country was divided among the three sons. To the eldest (Iaropolk) fell the district of Kiev; to the middle one (Oleg) the district of Dievlian and to Vladimir the district of Novogorod. In the civil war that followed after the father's death, Iaropolk slew Oleg and in turn died at the hands of Vladimir. It is emphasized that this last murder was not done to avenge his brother's death, but because Vladimir was lustful for his wife. He also was lustful for the beautiful Rogneda. Later Vladimir demanded her in marriage from her father, the ruler of Polotsk. Rogneda's father objected on the ground that she would not marry the son of a slave. Maddened by this insult, Vladimir laid waste the district of Polotsk, killed Rogneda's father, King Rogvalad, and his two sons and forced Rogneda to marry him. After the triple murder he also compelled his dead brother's wife, a beautiful Greek nun whom Iaropolk had captured in an expedition against Byzantium to marry him. Thus he married the two women by force. One he deprived of her husband (his own brother), the other of her father and two brothers by foul murder. Vladimir also had a Bohemian and Bulgarian wife all of whom bore him sons. This son of a slave was so lost in profligacy that he kept 300 concubines at Vychegorod, 3000 at Vielgorod near Kiev and 200 at Berestof.

It has been said that Vladimir really favored Mohammedanism as a state religion because it permitted polygamy. He did not adopt it, however, because the Moslem faith insists upon circumcision and total abstinence from alcoholic drinks and he did not want to submit to surgery nor give up his wine cellars for any religion. He turned down the Roman Catholic religion because Catholic holy men had to live in celibacy. He accepted the Greek Orthodox Church because it restrained him least.[4]

When Vladimir discovered that he was losing his virility he sent his physician John Simear to Alexandria to consult Alexandrian doctors about his condition. The doctor, however, for reasons which are not hard to discern, refused to return.

A change took place in Russian medicine when Christianity was introduced into Russia (tenth century). Medicine which formerly had been in the hands of the aged, wise women and sorcerers, passed into the province of the priesthood. The previous medical practices of Russia which included so much magic and sorcery were forbidden by the Church.

Vladimir urged everyone to seek medical advice from the monks. He himself, however, employed a lay physician. Of course, in this hypocrisy he was far from unique. Even popes did not trust the monks medically when it concerned their own welfare. Their body physicians were largely lay doctors.

The Kiev-Pichersky Abbey was the first monastery in Russia to practice medicine among the masses. Its founder, Holy Anthony (992-1072), upon returning from the Greek monastery at Athos, settled near Kiev and treated the sick with herbs, roots and leaves. His reputation as a physician spread far and wide, and the Kiev-Pichersky monastery grew up about him.

His pupil, Holy Agapit (1095), who was called the "gratis physician," carried on the work of Holy Anthony, treating the clergy and the laity in the monastery hospital.[5]

As has been intimated, before the days of Vladimir I (980-

1014), the Russians depended on popular medicine which was rich in tradition and folklore. It was based on the instinct of self-preservation and was closely related to their Slavonic religion.

The function of intermediaries between the people and the mysterious powers of nature naturally rested in the hands of those who had gained wisdom through experience and age. The elders of the clan, magicians, wizards, and enchanters were consulted in case of disease. The healers gathered herbs, roots, stones and many other substances to use as remedies.

Medicine in Russia was originally practiced by the *wolkhava* or wolfman who, like the druids of England, and the "wise frauen" of Germany gathered medical herbs to cure the sick and resorted to charms, spells and magic. On a vase of Greek pattern excavated at Koul-Oba there is a representation of a Scythian chieftain having a consultation with a *wolkhava,* a Scythian warrior examining another's teeth and a surgeon bandaging an injured leg. This unique vase epitomizes medieval medicine and surgery in Russia up to the time of the School of Salerno.[6]

Russians of the early Middle Ages ascribed disease to the displeasure of the gods and the malevolence of evil spirits. Attention was paid to the forces that caused disease and sacrifices, incantations and spells were employed. Russian medical folklore, which, incidentally, is still in vogue in rural districts and smaller communities, is of great interest not only to physicians but also to ethnologists and historians.

Kohl relates that Russian villagers seek to protect themselves and their cattle against epidemics by drawing a furrow with a plough right around the village. The plough is dragged by four widows and the ceremony is performed at night; all fires and lights must be extinguished while the plough is making its circuitous course. The villagers believe that no unclean spirit can pass the furrow which has thus been traced. In the village of Dubrowitschi, a puppet is carried before the plough and members of the procession cry out: "Out of the village with the unclean spirit!" At the end of the ceremony, the puppet is torn in pieces and the fragments scattered about.[7] No doubt the demon of the disease is connected with the puppet and is believed to be destroyed with it.

Sometimes, in an Esthonian village, a rumor will spread that the "Evil One" himself has been seen in the place. Instantly the whole village is in an uproar, and the entire population, armed with sticks and scythes, turns out to give chase to the devil. The "Evil One" is generally expelled in the form of a wolf or a cat. Occasionally the villagers brag that they have beaten the devil to death.[8]

The Khirgis of Central Asia, as soon as fever breaks out in their midst, leave the sick behind them in their effort to escape the epidemic.

Among the Georgians, if one of their kinsmen takes sick, the entire family is separated from the patient and an old woman is left with him. Regardless of the motivation of this practice there is no question that from a prophylactic standpoint, those that leave the houses may be spared any communicable disease.

Among the heathen Wotyaks, a Finnish people of Eastern Russia, all the young girls of the village assemble on the last day of the year or on New Year's Day, armed with sticks, the ends of which are split into nine branches. With these they beat every corner of the house and yard while declaring in a loud voice: "We are driving Satan out of the village." Afterwards the sticks are thrown into the river below the village, and as they float down stream, Satan goes with them to the next village, from which he must be driven out in turn. In some villages the expulsion is managed otherwise. The unmarried men receive groats, meat, and brandy from every house in the village and enter every house where there are young unmarried women. They then seize the young women and throw them into the snow while declaring: "May the spirits of disease leave you."

The oldest form of this ceremony is that observed by the Wotyaks of the Kazan Government. First of all a sacrifice is offered to the devil at noon. Then all the men assemble on horseback in the center of the village, and decide—not without much disputation—upon which house they shall begin. They then tether their horses to the paling, and arm themselves with whips, clubs of lime-wood, and bundles of light twigs. The twigs are believed to hold the greatest terror for Satan. Thus armed, they proceed with frightful cries, to beat every corner of the house and yard. They then shut the door and spit at the ejected fiend. Next they mount their horses and ride out of the village, yelling wildly and brandishing their clubs in every direction. Outside of the village they fling away the clubs and spit once more at the devil.[9]

On Good Friday and the two previous days, people in Croatia and Slovakia take rods with them to church, and when the service is over they beat each other "fresh and healthy."[10]

Very little is known of Russian medicine before the tenth century. Skorokhodov in his work, "The History of Medicine," relates that an Arab who came to the Volga district in the tenth century met a tribe of Russians who told him that if one of their number took sick they placed him in a tent out of town and supplied him with bread and water. They kept away from him, and his isolation continued until he either died or got well.[11] This quarantine of the sick was made not because the process of contagion in the modern sense was known but because of the belief that disease is caused by demonic possession and the populace was fearful that demons might pass from the body of the possessed patient to the healthy villagers.[12]

Medieval men visualized demons as substantial entities. He who occupied himself with the practice of casting out evil spirits from the sick was careful to keep his mouth closed while carrying out the exorcism lest the demon might pass from the mouth of the patient to his own. This practice is similar to that of modern physicians when examining the mouth of a patient suspected of contagious disease—although, of course, the rationale behind the practice is very different. It is related that the Khirgis of Central Asia still change their nomadic camping grounds whenever fever breaks out among them. They leave the sick kinsmen behind and flee to escape the terrible fever demon.

Among the medieval Russians, the individual's course of life was entirely conditioned by signs and premonitions. Books of magic and collections of warnings and predictions were passed from father to son and friend to friend. A creaking in the wall or a whistling in the ears foretold a journey. An itching in the palm signified a gift of money. Itching eyes betokened weeping. The croaking of ravens or the crowing of cocks were omens of misfortune.

The people believed in the prognosticating nature of dreams, and framed an elaborate system of reading their significance. They saw portents in the act of sneezing, in the crawling movements of insects, and in every sort of object they came across. It was thought unlucky to meet a monk, a horse whose hair had worn off, or a pig. As early as the twelfth century, we find St. Theodosius censuring those who allowed such occurrences to scare them.[13]

Even among the present day Russian peasantry, the belief in omens and predictions still prevails to an extent without parallel among any other European people. The manifold superstitions of an aged Russian peasant woman are thus set forth in Turgenev's romance, "Fathers and Sons."[14] She was pious and impressionable to a degree; she believed in all kinds of omens, predictions, spells, dreams; she believed in lunatics, in household spirits, forest spirits, unlucky foregatherings, enchantment, popular remedies, Maundy Thursday salt (the salt sprinkled on Maundy Thursday bread ranks as a powerful specific); she believed that the end of the world was at hand, that the buckwheat prospers if the candles are not extinguished at the evening service on Easter Sunday, and that mushrooms cease growing when they have been seen by a human eye, etc.

"Strange as it may seem, they scarcely ever go astray in their predictions. By long-continued observation they have become sensitive to signs which enable them almost unerringly to forecast the weather. Their memories are stored with a mass of all but infallible maxims inherited from the past."[15]

In later medieval Russia, remedies were employed composed of various metals and minerals including copper and iron. Iron was used both internally and externally. Copper, in the form of sulphates and acetates, was used on the skin. Mercury was used externally and internally in syphilis. Gold was employed in cases of scurvy. Great credence was given to the effectiveness of the magnet in curing all sorts of disease and its use was regarded as a favorite means of expelling disease-demons. The magnet was also used by a husband to test his wife's faithfulness. The husband surreptitiously placed a magnet under his wife's pillow at night. If its presence did not disturb her sleep, she was considered true to her husband.

Medieval Russian women were familiar with the use of various devices to keep the uterus in position in case of malposition. Ivanchenco described an operation performed by one women upon another after the patient suffered a sudden violent pain in the abdomen. After an abdominal incision was made, an extra-uterine pregnancy was noted.

Afanasiev reports that to prevent sterility (which was considered by the Russians to be the greatest misfortune) the boiled testicles of a bear were given to the bride and groom. Testicles mixed in wine were regarded as a dependable remedy for sterility even by the *boyars* (nobility) and royalty.

Wounds were treated with various ointments. In some places the wound was washed with the warm urine of a child. Urine was considered as a reliable remedy in a number of diseases. It was applied to burns and skin infections. Abscess was softened by the application of cow manure.

In the year 1551, there was an outbreak of *klikusi* ("the possessed") which greatly disturbed the country and had to be dealt with by the Church Council of Moscow. Those that were affected were principally elderly unmarried women—a group especially liable to hysteria. The victims of this ailment ran about barefoot and unkempt; they shook, they fell, they whirled, they writhed, and, amid such carryings-on, uttered their predictions as to the future. The presence of such women in a city was considered a menace, and the Church Council petitioned the czar to order the inhabitants to expel the lying prophetesses from their midst.

Of somewhat similar character were the prophetic powers

ascribed in Russia to *lunatics*. (The insane fell under the same category as the Roman *monstra*, as is borne out by the Russian terms applied to them: e.g. *jurodivy* derived from *urodu* which means "prodigy" or "monster.") Madmen inspired the Russians with amazement and even with reverential awe. Like the hysterical women just spoken of, their incoherent ravings which seemed to come from another world, were interpreted as conveying supernatural knowledge.

During the reign of Boris Godounof, there lived in Moscow a lunatic of this type who was revered as a saint. Naked and with hair dishevelled, he went about the streets in the coldest weather, uttering prophesies of coming woes. In an awe-inspiring voice he harangued Boris for the murder of his young Czarevitch. The Czar, either afraid of offending the people or else convinced of the man's holiness, did not attempt to interfere with him in the least.[16]

Aside from religious practices, various substances such as herbs, roots, leaves, turpentine, naphtha, arsenic, human blood, human and animal milk, honey, dew drops, sulphur, pitch, hops, (as given in an old manuscript in the Rumjanzew museum), magical amulets made of roots and slips of paper inscribed with magic formulas were employed to combat or prevent disease.

THE RUSSIAN BATH

The steam bath, which probably originated in Russia, was more than a cleansing procedure. One of the most frequently used devices in combating diseases was the vapor bath. This was used for washing away disease as well as for religious purification. Brides were escorted by relatives and friends to the bathhouse a day before and the morning after the nuptial day. Baths, as a rule, were taken on Saturday afternoons and on the eve of the high holidays. After Saturday baths, strong efforts were made to prevent pollution until Sunday morning services.[17]

The bathhouse in Russia served as a gathering place for the peasants of the village. In most instances it was the only public place owned by the community at large, and amidst the relaxing effect produced by the hot steam, they discussed their public and private affairs.

The bathhouse was also the place where the sick were brought in to be cured from colds, rheumatism, arthritis and similar diseases. These were the days when it was believed that the application of external heat was an effective method for withdrawing heat from the body so fever patients were also brought to the bathhouse to be healed.

At the bathhouse, the local healer practiced phlebotomy, and the floors were literally covered with blood. It was customary for every person to be bled at least once a month. Aside from bloodletting by scarification, the local healer was a master in the art of cupping and, where the painful area was extensive, large cups the size of a pot were placed on the back, in some cases, leaving a lifetime scar.

The practice of obstetrics was the function of the village women. The methods used by the midwife to "stretch" the uterus frequently led to disastrous results to the mother and her baby.

The newborn infant was often put through an unnecessary amount of handling. It was steamed with hot broth, shaken with head down to prevent hernia, rubbed with salt, and fed fruit juice and other liquids thought good for the stomach.

The local midwife often brought her patient for actual delivery to the bathhouse because the steam was thought to be effective in stimulating labor pains. It is related that when Czar Fedorowitch suffered from a swelling in the groin (probably hernia), he was taken to the bathhouse where a pint of blood was taken from his veins, following which the swelling subsided. A patient with a hernia was customarily placed on a hot wooden bench and a wet rag was placed on the swelling. A ball of some fiber was then ignited in a cup or pot which was quickly placed over the wet cloth. This method was said to effectively reduce the hernia. Most of these procedures were performed by women healers.[18]

In early times, according to Snegirov, Russian men were accustomed to bathe with women in the same tank. This was forbidden by the decree of Empress Elizabeth in 1743 and again by that of Catherine II in 1783. However, these edicts were never obeyed by the populace at large. It is ironical that these two decrees of modesty should have been issued by two libertines who themselves were so lewd and brazen that their palaces and royal bedrooms were given up to venery and every type of sexual immorality.[19]

The public bathhouse consisted of a large room at one side of which stones were piled up which were heated from below by a furnace. On the other three sides were large wooden benches arranged in progressively higher rows as in an amphitheater. The steam or vapor was produced by pouring water upon the hot stones. While the room was filled with hot steam, the bathers rubbed themselves with brush-like appliances made of twigs or shrubs, and bound tightly together like a broom. After the vapor bath, the bathers immersed themselves in a tank of warm water followed often by a tank of cold water.

Among the northern Finns the *mesarana* or sweat bath was situated in a log hut. The entire family customarily visited the bath at one time.[20]

Mercury was extensively employed in treating syphilis and skin diseases which were frequent among city dwellers. Women attending syphilitic cases often therapeutically licked the diseased eyes of children perhaps imparting lues to their patients.

Gold was used in the treatment of scurvy and was administered in the form of gold-leaf on bread.

Caucasians who use firearms are skilled in treating wounds caused by such weapons. They grease the wound with an ointment containing the plant of echinacea rubrum.

In many places the villagers understood the contagious character of smallpox, leprosy and various fevers and insisted on isolating such cases.

As soon as Christianity was introduced by Vladimir folk-medicine received its greatest challenge. The new Church at once engaged in fierce persecution of the healing sages and wizards. The use of simples became a crime. Equipped with medical experience brought from Byzantium, the clergy undertook the supervision of the medicine of the masses.

Vladimir immediately raised the position of church healers to the rank of ecclesiastics and placed them under the jurisdiction of the bishop. Vladimir's regulations condemned the use of herbs, witchcraft and magic. Magicians were outlawed, persecuted and even burned at the stake. He ordered the opening of hospitals at the monasteries and decreed that hospitals be placed under the supervision of the Church.

When epidemics broke out, he ordered ikons to be placed in the districts where the pestilence prevailed. When this measure failed to ameliorate the situation, a ban forbidding transportation of goods from the stricken area was enforced. Often, contraband goods were burned and with them even the merchant, if he were detected transporting them.

According to the testimony of a Rostow chronicler, Vladimir ordered bread, meat, fish, vegetables, mead [21] and cider be supplied gratis to the sick, needy and disabled. On the basis of previously mentioned information, the reader will unquestionably have grave doubts as to Vladimir's generosity. If history credits him with humane deeds, these were possibly done in atonement for his sins.

There is no evidence that the medicine practiced in the Russian monasteries ever attained the quality of that practiced in Western European cloisters. The Russian monks, by and large were a God fearing people who spent their time in prayer and devotion but had little inclination to read secular books. The Russian monasteries failed to produce a single personality who can be compared to the scholastics of the Western European monasteries. The Russian clerics were not interested in the seven sciences and they apparently did not ever possess any scientific documents. Aside from religious books, there were few works which interested them.

The rise of the universities in Europe was influenced in a large measure by the scholastics who were the first teachers at the universities of Salerno, Paris, and Montpellier. In fact, various European universities actually owe their very existence to the local dignitaries of the Church. The Russian Church did not produce ecclesiastics similar to the scholastics of Western Europe.

The revival of Russian medicine was greatly influenced from without—in spite of the ecclesiastics. The first mention of a doctor was during the reign of Ivan III. A German physician named Anton Nemchin arrived in Moscow in the year 1485. He found favor in the eyes of the Grand Duke for a time, but when he failed to cure the Tartar Prince, Karakech, he was summarily discharged and turned over to the Tartars who took him down to the Moscow River and cut his throat. A similar fate under the same Czar befell a doctor known as Leon the Jew (Leon Zhidovin). He was brought from Venice in 1490 by Andrei Paleolog, the brother of the Grand Duchess and by the Russian ambassador, Palevy, to treat Ivan Ivanowitch, the eldest son of the Grand Duke. The prince appears to have been afflicted with rheumatic fever with rheumatic involvement of his lower extremities. Cardiac complications ensued. He was treated by Leon with various internal remedies and hot applications externally. The treatment was not successful. The young prince died and Leon was imprisoned and executed by decapitation. The living conditions of the Western European doctors must have been pretty bad. Despite the great risk to their life and liberty, some were willing to leave their homes in Western Europe in order to practice in far away Russia. Of course few, if any, knew the fate that had befallen their professional countrymen who had traveled to Russia as "Dead men tell no tales." Of course, not all the foreign physicians that were called to Moscow met with such a tragic fate. Some were well treated and were honored by the royal court.

All the medical men attached to the medieval czarist courts were foreign doctors. The royalty apparently had no confidence in their local physicians. The foreign doctors, as long as their efforts were successful, were favorably treated, but when their royal patients expired, they were severely punished, if not by execution at least by incarceration in dark dank dungeons.

Shortly after Leon the Jew was disposed of, the Russian ambassador, at the request of the Grand Duke, asked Emperor Maximilian I to send him a skillful physician learned in internal diseases and in the methods of treating wounds. In response to this request, the German ambassador, George Delator, in 1518, brought Nicolo Luyev of Lubek with him to Moscow. Luyev, who was a celebrated physician at home, appears to have enjoyed the great favor of the royal family. Perhaps more important than his medical skill was the fact that he knew how to get along with the political and ecclesiastic visitors to the court.

Foreign physicians gradually poured into Moscow from Western countries. In general they received better receptions than were given to the first physicians.

In the twelfth century, many foreign physicians came to Russia. A Syrian doctor named Peter Sirianin attended Prince Nicholas Davydovich of Chernigov. His patient later became his friend and entered a monastery with him in 1106. Sirianin is reported to have taken his patient by the hand whenever he examined him, probably for the purpose of palpating the pulse. Prince Svyatopolk Yaroslavich died after a surgical operation on a swollen gland—an operation which probably had been performed by a foreign doctor. It is known that there were foreign private doctors in Russia during Yaroslavich's time.

The first code of Russian laws, *Russkaya Pravda,* recognized the right of the physician to receive compensation for treating a sick person: "The injured person is to receive three *grivny* and the *lekar* is to be compensated." This additional medical compensation later came to be known as *medicinal.* In general, it may be said that not until Yaroslavich's time did learned doctors appear in Russia and their influence at that period was in large measure due to his daughter's marriage to the French King, Henry I, in 1051.[22]

By the end of the Middle Ages, English physicians were welcome in Russia. The commercial relationship established with England in the year 1553, by the water route through the White Sea, opened Moscow to foreign physicians and artisans. The friendly relationship between the two countries began with the arrival of Richard Chancellor and his staff to Moscow. The relationship continued for three centuries.

The English and Scotch had a prominent part in the introduction and improvement of medicine in Russia.

Under Alexei Mikhailovich, there were eleven doctors, six pharmacists and one head physician. The outstanding doctors were Andrew Engelhardt, who was educated at Leyden and Koenigsberg; Samuel Collins of Cambridge and Oxford; Ivan Osenburg of Koenigsberg University; and the famous doctor, Lavrenti Blumentrost. Doctor Gregory Carbonari went to Moscow in 1689 on the recommendation of Emperor Leopold. In 1690, Jacob Pellarino, noted for his advocacy of smallpox inoculation, entered the service of Russia.

The salaries of medical men in Russia were not stipulated or equitably proportioned. Court doctors received salaries, monetary rewards and presents. One Dr. Sibelist, for example, was given a salary of 250 rubles a year with a food allotment of 50. *Lekars* and pharmacists received from 180 to 360 rubles per annum. Assistants to pharmacists were paid from 100 to 112 rubles per year. Assistant *lekars,* phlebotomists and barbers received from 28 to 30 rubles yearly. Pharmacist students received 36 rubles per year and herbalists eight rubles a year.

During the medieval period in Russia scientific medicine remained inaccessible to the masses, with the sole exception of the army. Dissemination of medical knowledge in Russia was primarily a result of the recognized needs of the army. The first czar to lay a sound and broad foundation for the development of medical practice in the army was young Mikhail Fiodorovich, who sent *lekars* to the regiments. In his calculation of expenses in 1615, it is stipulated that the doctors attached to the army were maintained by the public treasury. In 1616 the regiment doctors were enumerated in the records, and by the end of the seventeenth century, most of the regiments had attending physicians. But the masses, who were burdened with heavy taxes were deprived of satisfactory medical care worthy of the name.

CHAPTER XX

ANATOMY IN THE MIDDLE AGES

The renaissance of the Saracens in the early Middle Ages (seventh century A.D.) brought about a revival of interest in the sciences, mathematics, philosophy and medicine but the "new" learning was based neither on personal experience nor on laboratory evidence. All conclusions were based upon ancient manuscripts which were believed to be infallible. Any contradictions or additions were considered sacrilegious. The science of anatomy, for example, was considered complete and closed with the last word of Galen.

Galen, like most of his predecessors, derived his anatomic knowledge from observations made on apes, dogs, pigs, and various other animals. Man's construction was assumed to be identical with that of animals—which supposition, of course, is very erroneous. The fact is that the internal organs of beasts and cattle differ anatomically from those of humans just as their external aspects vary. For example, for more than a millennium, it was taught that the human sternum or breastbone is divided into sections like that of an ape, that the human uterus has two long horns like that of a dog (the right horn to house male embryos and the left female) and that the human hip bone is spread out like that of an ox.

Up to the sixteenth century, Galen's hold on anatomic knowledge was so strong that when Vesalius demonstrated that the Galenic description of the hip bone was wrong, he apologized for deviating from the master's teaching by stating that man had changed his shape since Galen's time by wearing tight trousers.

A great difficulty with Galen's anatomic concepts was that he often made the structure of the human body fit the erroneous theories of physiology and the religious philosophies of his day. His concept of teleology, for example, assumes that the structure of every part of the functioning body is preconceived and follows a certain intelligent and purposeful plan. "In my view," said Galen, "there is nothing in the body useless or inactive, but all parts are arranged to perform their offices together and have been endowed by the Creator with specific powers."

The fact is, of course, that there are useless organs in man's present economy; as one example may be mentioned the vermiform appendix. Galen believed that there are invisible passages in the walls of the heart that circulate the blood from the left to the right: "We are driven to wonder at the handiwork of the Almighty by means of which the blood sweats from the right into the left ventricle through passages which escape the human vision."

Teleology came to be an actual school of theosophy which explained everything in the human body, and for that matter in all organic life, on the basis of a divine, preconceived, intelligent plan which operates through conscious and purposive causes.

The teachings of this school of theosophy were by no means unanimously accepted even by the Church. St. Augustine, for example, questioned the intelligence of placing the organs of reproduction between the organs of defecation and urination. Among modern scientists, von Helmholtz, possibly the greatest investigator in the field of physiological optics, thought that the construction of the visual organs lacks much in the way of perfection.

For centuries, the concept of teleology had a large following. Isaac D'Israeli relates that because, teleologically speaking, fingers are wisely designed for manipulating objects, the use of forks was denounced for a time by the clergy as an insult to the Creator. When "God in his wisdom has provided man with natural forks (fingers), it is considered impious to substitute them by metallic artificial forks when eating." The same argument was used against the wearing of spectacles. As mentioned in a previous chapter, it is related that Salvinus de Armatus, one of those associated with the invention of spectacles (1290), was censored for his great device. Muschebroek states that the inscription over his grave in the cemetery of Florence reads: "Here lies Salvinus de Armatus of the Armati of Florence, inventor of spectacles. God pardon him his sins."

More time was spent in sophistic discussions, explaining the wisdom of the Creator in the formation of the organs, than in the study of the organs themselves.

Explanations of anatomic structures and functional traits were often advanced on moral rather than on physical grounds. The medievalists were particularly fond of the Platonic explanation that the purpose of the long and tortuous structure of the intestine is to permit the food to remain in the intestinal tract for a long period of time so that the mind may not be disturbed too much in its contemplation by the desire for nutriment.

Religious dogmas even influenced anatomic terminology. The coccyx, for example, was known as the "resurrection bone" because of the belief that this bone would serve as a nucleus from which the body would be restored and resurrected. Jews, Christians and Mohammedans firmly believed in this. A legend is related in the "Midrash" that Emperor Hadrian asked Rabbi Joshua Ben Chananyah to state from what part of the body resurrection would begin. The latter replied, "From the bone *luz* (coccyx, almond bone or nut bone)." To prove his statement he placed this bone in water and it did not soften; in fire and it did not burn; between two millstones and it was not crushed; and between the anvil and the hammer and it was not destroyed.[1] No less an authority than the Arabic philosopher Averroes accepted this legend of the bone "luz" as a fact. In the Middle Ages the coccyx was known in Germany as the *Juden-Knochen* or "Jew bone."

The legend that man has one less rib than woman dates back to the Genesis account of the missing rib of Adam (Genesis 2:21) which persisted until the sixteenth century, when

Vesalius showed it to be erroneous. The spinal column, when found separated from the body, had a mystic import because of its resemblance to a serpent—"the enticer of evil."

Legends concerning the indestructibility of certain parts of the body were abundant among ancient and medieval peoples. Pliny[2] states that the thumb of the right hand of Emperor Pyrrhus was indestructible. Another legend has it that a vertebral bone when found connected to a rib ("sheled")[3] is indestructible. A corpse may be burned by fire or disintegrated by water, but the "sheled" remains undestroyed.

Moral interpretation for the shape and form of organs is given in the Talmud. For example, Providence has designed the fingers to be pointed, the auditory canals to be small and the ear lobes to be soft so as to shut out profane language; the eyelids are fashioned for the purpose of blotting out lewd objects from sight.

At Galen's death (199 A.D.), a school characterized by veneration of the written word and blind belief in authoritative statements came into being. Conclusions were reached purely by sophistical arguments based upon pseudo-Hippocratic writings, corrupted texts of Galen, and disconnected fragments of later anatomists which survived in the Benedictine monasteries. In consequence of this attitude, original anatomic investigations ceased for a period of twelve hundred years.

Lack of interest in anatomy may also be ascribed to the Biblical injunction against any contact with the dead body, the Koranic denunciation of dissection as being unclean and contaminating those who come in contact with a dead body and the belief that the body is of minor importance as compared with the soul and therefore unworthy of intimate study.

To reiterate, although the renaissance of the Arabs in the early Middle Ages (seventh century A.D.) brought on a revival of learning and great interest was displayed in the natural sciences, philosophy, and mathematics, no progress was made in advancing the cause of anatomy. The few modifications in anatomic science were made not on the basis of evidence obtained by dissection, as this was prohibited by the Mohammedan religion, but were conclusions reached from comments and speculations on the text of Galen.

Abd-ul-Latif, the annalist of Egypt, records perhaps the one exception to this statement. This concerns the science of osteology. He informs us that the Moslem doctors did not neglect any opportunity of studying the bones of the human body in cemeteries. He states that he himself once examined a collection of bones and in this manner ascertained that the lower jaw is formed of one piece, that the sacrum, although sometimes composed of several bones, most generally consists of one bone and that Galen was mistaken on these matters.

Medieval Christian Europe was no more advanced in anatomy. The few books found in the monastic libraries were texts of Galen copied by monastic scribes. With each new copy, anatomic knowledge became more corrupt. The "Anatomy of Master Richard" (twelfth century) and the "Anatomy of the Body of Man" are examples of scholastic anatomy. The School of Salerno used Copho's "Anatomy of the Pig" as a text. These textbooks show what may become of science when it is left to ecclesiastics and lay scribes and when ideas such as "the body is of minor importance, unworthy of intimate study" prevail.

Up to the early part of the thirteenth century anatomy was taught almost exclusively according to the text of Galen, which was considered a canon about which there could be no difference of opinion. A turn of events came in 1230 when Frederick II (1194-1250), Roman Emperor and King of Sicily and Jerusalem, issued an edict requiring physicians to study the structure of the human body for one year. There is, however, little indication that this edict was actually carried out.

The credit of being the first country in Europe to revive the study of anatomy goes to Italy. While other European nations were either profoundly ignorant or grossly indifferent of this science so basic to medicine, the Italians made great advances in the science of anatomy, in spite of the great difficulties in opposing the papal edicts that prohibited dissection.

In Italy, autopsies for the purpose of elucidating the cause of death or settling doubts regarding the manner in which death came about and especially for the discovery of poison, were made with increasing frequency in an age when mysterious homicide was common.

From a document dated 1302, it appears that in a fatal case in which poisoning was suspected, two physicians and three surgeons were required to make an autopsy on the corpse.[4] Still earlier, William of Saliceto (1210-1277) presented in his book directions to surgeons for performing dissections.

It is the glory of the University of Bologna that the study of anatomy was advanced in Western Europe early in the thirteenth century. Sarton testifies that anatomy was successfully cultivated as an appendix of surgery if not as a distinct branch of science. The anatomic experts of Bologna, according to the testimony of Guy de Chauliac, were Roger of Palermo (1210), Roland (c. 1250), Jamerius, Bruno of Longoburgo (c. 1252) and Lanfranc.

Ciasca is authority for the statement that the first autopsy in Bologna was made in 1281 on a male cadaver; the first on a female cadaver was made in 1315 by Mondino di Luzzi.[5] Probably dissections for medico-legal purposes were made even earlier. Singer is of the opinion that the first postmortem examinations of the human body may have been to discover the cause of death rather than actual dissections.[6] It is related, however, that the Senate of Venice in 1308 ordered that one cadaver be dissected annually. This ordinance was in direct violation of the prohibition of Boniface VIII in 1300.

That dissection was practiced by surgeons of that period may be inferred from the statement of Thaddeus Alderotti to the effect that he could not with certainty answer a question pertaining to pregnancy because he had not had the means of making anatomies on pregnant women. From this the inference may be drawn that he had dissected other cadavers. One of the earliest medico-legal autopsies recorded was performed in 1302 under the direction of Guilelmo Varignana (born in the 13th century), a pupil of Alderotti, on the body of a certain nobleman named Azzolino who had died under circumstances suggesting poisoning.

MONDINO DI LUZZI (1276-1326)

The first anatomical teacher to struggle with the authority of the Church which prohibited dissection was Mondino di Luzzi, professor of anatomy at the University of Bologna. He aroused the curiosity of the medical profession by his well ordered demonstrations of the different parts of the body. In January 1315, he dissected and demonstrated the parts of two female bodies and, in the course of the following year, he accomplished the same task on the person of a single female cadaver. Acts such as this were done in defiance of the authority of the Church, for a Bull issued in 1301 by Pope Boniface read: "Persons cutting up bodies of the dead and barbarously cooking them in order that their bones be separated from their flesh are by the very act excommunicated." In 1319, criminal prosecution was initiated against a professor and students of Bologna for body snatching.

Mondino was the son of the apothecary Nerino. He was born at Bologna in about 1276. He gave public lectures at the University from 1314 to 1324. He was also interested in civic matters of Bologna and in 1316 he was sent as ambassador to King John the son of Robert of Naples.

His fame, however, is bound up with the art of anatomy and particularly with dissection.[7] His work "Anatomia" is not only a concise treatise on anatomy, but also a manual of dissection. It teaches the students how to study anatomy on the human cadaver. He directs that the incision on the cadaver should begin with a vertical cut in the abdomen followed by a horizontal incision above the umbilicus. (The reason why dissection was to begin with the abdomen was because the viscera tend to decompose quicker than the upper and lower extremities or the head, particularly in warm climates.)

It is said that on certain occasions Mondino did not hesitate to step down from his platform to demonstrate certain anatomic points to his students. This was an unusual occurrence for it was customary that the dissection be done by a barber by means of a razor; the demonstrator who was standing pointed out the different parts in the region that was dissected. The professor himself usually sat on a high platform busy reading the description out of a book of the part dissected. He did not dream of soiling his fingers by touching the body.

Mondino's "Anatomia" as all the books of that period was in the spirit of the Arabian authors or rather that of Galen who was the final authority from whose opinion there was no appeal. Many of his descriptions were influenced by Galen and the Latin translation of Avicenna and Rhazes. He retains in his work most of their nomenclature as for example "Zirbus" for the omentum; "Sipbach" for the peritoneum; "mirach" for the abdominal walls and "eucharus" for the messentary.

It is interesting to note that he found the liver in the cadaver higher than in the living person. He states that the liver has five lobes, the uterus has two "cornus" and that the uterus is enlarged during menstruation, as it is during pregnancy. He suggested the removal of the false ribs when examining the spleen.

Mondino divides the body into three cavities, "ventrae." He first describes the anatomy of the lower (abdominal) cavity, then proceeds to the middle (thoracic) cavity and concludes with the upper cavity which comprises the head, its contents and its appendages. "In the base of the brain," he states, "are two optic nerves" which he thought were the first pair of cranial nerves. The oculomotor he took for second. The fifth nerve he considered to be the third and the ninth to be the seventh. He compares the outline of the choroid plexus to a long red worm. He gives a correct description of the dura mater in describing the cerebral membranes. Mondino considers the upper cavity to contain the animal members, the middle cavity the spiritual members and the lower cavity the natural members. He gives a short description of the location, shape, distribution and texture of the membranes and he mentions the disorders to which they are subject. In the last classification he shows how difficult it was for even a scientific investigator to entirely divorce himself from preconceived notions. In his description of the pleura he distinguishes between true pleurisy, false pleurisy, and pneumonia. The liver and its vessels are minutely if not accurately described. He recognizes the importance of the bile for digestion. The yellow bile is secreted by the gall bladder and the black bile by the spleen; they reach the stomach by imaginary canals. The kidneys are carefully covered. He gives a good description of the pancreas and the pancreatic duct. He points out the pulmonary artery and vein. He describes the infundibulum under the name of "lacuna." The vena cava is referred to as "chilis."

Mondino's coverage of anatomy of the heart shows beyond a doubt that he made observations on human cadavers. His description contains a knowledge of circulation. In the heart three ventricles are described. In the right ventricle one sees two orifices—one directed toward the liver, which is larger because the heart draws through it the blood from the liver, and the other the opening of the *vena arterialis* towards the lung. The left ventricle has two orifices: the *adhorti,* opening with three valves, and the opening of the *arteria venalis* with two valves, through which passes a smoke-like vapor from the lung. The third chamber is described as consisting of various small cavities in the septum, where the blood crossing to the left ventricle may be subtilized.

"It is a remarkable fact which seems to be omitted by all subsequent authors," said F. G. Parsons, "that his description contains the rudiments of the circulation of the blood."[8]

The merit of these distinctions, however, he afterwards destroys by repeating the old assertion that the left ventricle ought to contain spirit or air, which it generates from the blood. For some reason Mondino did not venture to open the skull which practice was so commonplace among anatomists that bodies were frequently stolen to examine the contents of the head, when they could not be obtained otherwise. His osteology of the skull is erroneous. His account of the cerebral tissues, although short, describes the lateral ventricles, with their anterior and posterior *cornua,* and the choroid plexus as a blood-red substance like a long worm. He then speaks of the third or middle ventricle, and one posterior, which seems to correspond with the fourth; and describes the infundibulum under the names of *lacuna* and *emboton.* Notwithstanding the misrepresentation into which this early anatomist was betrayed, his book is valuable, and has been illustrated by the successive commentaries of Alessandro Achillini (1463-1512), Jacopo Berengario da Carpi (1470-1550) and Johann Dryander (1500-1560).

His treatise on anatomy, written in 1316, is the first modern work on the subject. Those who preceded him incorporated their anatomical work in larger treatises on surgery, and do not refer directly to their own anatomical experiences. His work is essentially a practical manual of the subject and he is with justice called "the restorer of anatomy."

Mondino's "Anatomia" is written entirely in the spirit of Galen. He believes with the Pergamon in his concept of teleology as for example, Mondino states that the creator has made the anterior abdominal wall soft without bones in order to stretch sufficiently in the event of flatulence or abdominal dropsy, if perchance this disease should befall one. The uterus possesses seven cells to facilitate the coagulation of the semen and menstrual blood when they meet in that organ. The ovaries secrete a fluid like saliva in order to excite the sexual organs.

His work, however, contains a considerable number of references to actual anatomical procedure. He deals not only with anatomy in our modern sense, but also includes physiology and much discussion of the application of anatomical and physiological principle to medicine and surgery. His book gives a good deal of insight into the scientific knowledge of the day. Thus, it is saying much for Mondino that he took the first and perhaps the greatest step for the advance of anatomy. It was two centuries and more before the next step was taken.

Mondino's "Anatomia" was quickly accepted as a textbook up to the sixteenth century, probably because his descriptions are characterized by discussions and scholastic explanations, intended to allay any doubts that might arise in the reader's mind. To be sure, by modern standards there are many errors in Mondino's work, but considering the scholastic time when it was written, we must not expect any frequent appeal to nature. The fact that he was perhaps the first to demonstrate on the cadaver was by itself a revolutionary step in anatomy. Joseph Hyrtle (b. 1811) points to his superior style in comparison to his predecessors and his contemporaries. It is certain from his book and the notes of his students that he regularly conducted a large number of dissections. It is related that the Duke of Tuscany turned over to students of anatomy the bodies of persons executed for religious and criminal violations. It is probable that Mondino received some of them.

His book should be regarded as the first truly scientific anatomical text, planned as a guide for students of anatomy. He was the first professor to descend from his lofty chair and stand near the cadaver. The oldest edition of his "Anatomia" was printed at Pavia in 1478 and, up to the time of Vesalius, it was the most studied anatomical textbook in the Italian schools.

He died in Bologna in 1326 and was buried in the parochial church of San Vitale d'Agricola where he was placed in a granite tomb. A bas-relief by Boso of Parma pictures him as a master in his chair lecturing to his pupils.

Bertuccio (c. 1347) pupil of Mondino, became professor at Bologna; he was one of the teachers of Guy de Chauliac and Petrus ab Argelata (died 1423).[9]

CHAPTER XXI

THE CHIRURGEON AND THE BARBER SURGEON

The most important surgeon of the Middle Ages was Paul of Aegina (A. D. 650). Of his seven books, the sixth is entirely devoted to operative surgery, and the fourth is largely occupied with surgical diseases. The importance of his work to medieval surgical history is aptly stressed in the following remarks of Francis Adams (1796-1861):[1] "It contains the most complete system of operative surgery which has come down to us from ancient times. Haly Abbas (d. A. D. 994), in the ninth book of his 'Practica' copies almost everything from Paulus. Abulcasim (tenth century A.D.) gives more original matter on surgery than any other Arabian author, and yet, as will be seen from our commentary, he is indebted for whole chapters to Paulus. In the 'Continens' of Rhazes, that precious depository of ancient opinions on medical subjects, if there be any surgical information it is mostly derived from Antyllus, Archigenes and Paul of Aegina.

"As to the other authorities, no one has treated of surgery in a systematical manner; for even Avicenna, who treats so fully of everything else connected with medicine, is defective in his accounts of surgical operations; and the descriptions which he does give of them, almost all are borrowed from our author, Paul of Aegina."[2]

Almost five hundred years elapsed after Paul of Aegina with little or no surgical progress. The famous Arabian physicians did not show any special surgical qualifications. The most noted representatives of the Arabian school, Avicenna (980-1037) and

Averroes (1126-1198), certainly exhibited little surgical interest. Even Rhazes and Avenzoar made no real advances in surgery. They merely copied the surgical works of their predecessors.

The physician of the Middle Ages was an aristocrat. He looked down on practical surgery as base manual labor and he would not soil his lily-white hands in blood. He was entirely satisfied with reading what the ancient masters had to say about anatomy and surgery, but he refused to engage in surgical practice.

As long as surgery was confined to the study of the Graeco-Arabic masters, learned physicians and philosophers were interested in these subjects. But as soon as surgical skill became a practical necessity because of frequent wars, "book physicians" disdained the profession of surgery. The result was that in the Middle Ages, the level of surgery descended to a very low standard. Its practice became monopolized by barbers and bathhouse keepers.

The task of preventing ignorant laymen from practicing surgery was difficult, firstly, because the state needed surgeons on the battlefields and physicians refused to fill this need, and, secondly, because the Church eventually prohibited surgery—especially priestly surgery—on account of its aversion to the shedding of blood. In the year 1215, Innocent III fulminated an anathema against any monk or priest who dared to practice surgery. Thus the barber who had some experience with some minor surgical ills, had little or no competition. He monopolized the art of scalpel-medicine.

Among the Arabs, surgery was never on as high a plane as medicine, largely because of the religious prejudice against mutilation of the body.[3] Male surgeons, moreover, were prohibited by religious custom from examining the female genitalia with the result that gynecology and obstetrics were left entirely to female nurses. Rhazes complained that surgery was entirely in the hands of slaves. Avicenna regarded surgery as an unimportant and separate branch of medicine.

The Arabians were fatalists. They believed in predestination: "What has to be, cannot be changed." If a patient is to die, no operation will change his fate. Even human pain did not move the Arabs to resort to surgery. They accepted with equanimity the suffering that befell them.

Medical surgery was largely connected with the sexual organs and included primarily the procedures of castration, infibulation and circumcision. One of the purposes of castration was to drive out the demon of sexual desire from the system, thus rendering the eunuch eligible for the position of chamberlain. Eunuchs (Eunuch, in Greek, signifies "guard," or "bed keeper") were employed in the harems of the princes and nobles and frequently attained state positions of trust.

The operation of castration was also imposed on foreign captives past puberty, as well as on those of tender age, to prevent intermixture with foreign blood, to cut down the possibility of female infidelity and to afford a means of recognizing slaves by their inability to grow a beard and by their feminine voice. At times castration was merely a religious mutilation to escape sexual desire. This avoidance of sexual sin or temptation was the motive of many cases of emasculation. This form of asceticism appears to have been practiced in early Christian times, its votaries acting on the text of Matthew: "For there are some eunuchs which were so born from their mother's womb, and there are some eunuchs which were made eunuchs by men, and there be eunuchs which have made themselves eunuchs for the kingdom of heaven's sake. He that is able to receive it, let him receive it."[4] Among the self-imposed eunuchs who had the operation performed on themselves were St. Origen and St. Francis.

There were several methods of performing the operation of castration. One surgical procedure included the removal of all the visible genitalia. Another technique involved the removal of the scrotum and the testicles, but not the penis. Resort was only occasionally had to amputation of the penis and distortion of the spermatic vessels.

Hammond (1828-1900) describes an operation by the Indians of New Mexico and Arizona that enabled the subjects to enjoy relationships with women without being able to engender children. Perhaps it is to some such technique that Juvenal refers when he states that eunuchs were held in high esteem by the Roman matrons. Juvenal (100 A.D.) depicts Heliodorus castrating powerful slaves so that their lustful mistresses may use them with impunity: "Matron and maid the sex has turned all whore; to escape abortion they have the Eunuch, but only such as have been gelded at manhood age; all that the navel string could give is present, except the hair, and that is the barbers' loss, not theirs."

The sultans and caliphs considered those eunuchs who had all external evidence of virility removed to be the safest guards over the harems. Owing to the unskilled and septic surgical technique, 75 per cent of those castrated by the most radical method died from this operation; hence those who did not succumb fetched a price three or four times higher than eunuchs who had undergone a less severe operation and had been castrated only for the purpose of slavery. Most of the higher-priced eunuchs were kidnapped or purchased from North Africa in their boyhood. They were castrated when young, taught to take care of harems, and when they reached the age of maturity, were sold to the highest bidders.

The mortality of more conservative castration was no less than 33 per cent. Those who did not succumb to the simple operation brought about $200 each. The great eunuch factories of Egypt were located on Mount Ghebel-Eter. At Abou-Gerghe, a large Coptic monastery existed where unfortunate African children were gathered and emasculated. The Coptic monks from the monastery, trading with Constantinople, Arabia, and all Asia Minor, did a thriving business with much-sought-for and expensive eunuchs. They produced two commercial grades of eunuchs: those who were simply castrated, and those on whom the operation of complete ablation of the sexual organs had been performed. The latter brought from $750 to $1000 per head but only 10 per cent survived this operation.

The crude manner in which the operation was performed and the cruel and ignorant after-treatment were revolting. The helpless and unfortunate prisoner or slave was stretched out on an operating table; his neck was placed in a collar which was fastened to the table; his legs were spread apart and his ankles made fast to iron rings; his arms were held by an assistant. The operator then seized the penis and scrotum and with one sweep of a razor-sharp instrument removed all the appendages. A short bamboo cannula or catheter was then introduced into the urethra, from which it was allowed to project by about two inches. No attention was paid to hemorrhage. The whole wound was simply plastered up with some compound and tightly packed about the hapless subject's body so as to prevent any possibility of movement. Perfect immobility was considered by the monks as the main element required to promote a successful result. It is estimated that 35,000 children were annually sacrificed to produce the Sudanese average quota of 3800 eunuchs per annum.

Emasculation was occasionally performed on young boys to prevent a change in their voices so that they might grow up to take female parts in theater productions or be trained as adult soprano singers.

According to Ernst von Bergmann (1836-1907) the operation of castration for preserving the voices of young boys originated in the Orient. For a time Constantinople became the center of Greek music and the fine soprano solos were sung by eunuchs. Eunuchs were not only prominent singers but also cultivated the art of music. In 1137, Manuel, a famous eunuch singer, established a school of music in Smolensk, Russia. From Constantinople, the custom of employing eunuchs as choristers spread to Italy. Rome became the center of music as it became the center of religion. The eunuchs reached their height in the art of music with the establishment of the Italian opera. There is a dark chapter connected with the rise of eunuch music. The demand for this kind of singer became so great that it offered an opportunity for wicked persons to become enriched by trafficking with children.

Many well-intentioned Italian parents permitted the eunuchizing of their boys for chorister purposes in church services. Their voices, after emasculation, were often developed to perfection. Even after Pope Sixtus (1521-1590) censored this practice and the law of the State prohibited it, it was quietly continued. Pope Leo XIII finally put an end to this shameful practice.

Another operation to restrain sexual indulgence which was not quite as barbarous as emasculation was that of infibulation. The origin of this practice is enveloped in mystery. The operation consisted of the introduction of a metal ring through an opening made in the male at the end of the prepuce, and in the female through both ends of the labia. Both ends of the ring were then joined. Gladiators were infibulated in this manner to restrain them from venery that tended to weaken them. Pliny the Elder (23-79 A.D.) attributed the origin of this operation to a most drastic effort on the part of the masters to prevent their wives from being unfaithful with the virile athletes.

Egyptians punished their prisoners of war by emasculating them. Romans, Spaniards, Britons and Poles punished the crime of rape by excision of the sexual organs. In Nazi-Germany, non-Germans were emasculated to maintain the purity of the Aryan race. Monks were not infreqently muzzled by this process.

In Ethiopia, when a female child was born, its vulva was sutured together, allowing only for the passage of urine. The father was then in a position to guarantee the girl's virginity to the highest bidder. The union of the labia was severed with a sharp knife just before marriage. In some parts of Africa and Asia, married women wore a sort of harness fastened around the body to insure their faithfulness. The contraption is locked by means of a key which is kept in the possession of the husband. Of course, wealthy husbands did not have to resort to this stratagem, as they possessed seraglios and eunuchs to safeguard their interests.

The oldest religious surgery known is that of circumcision. The original purpose of this operation is still veiled in mystery. Voltaire is inclined to believe that circumcision is an outgrowth of ancient phallic worship. He finds confirmation of his view in the passage of Genesis where Jacob asked Joseph to "put thy hand under my thigh." [5] This expression, in the opinion of Voltaire, refers to the phallus. Circumcision among Jews, according to Voltaire, was taken from the older Egyptian religious custom.

Bergmann holds that, originally, circumcision was a method of marking slaves and was a development from an earlier practice of amputation of the organ. Amputation of the phallus was a symbol of disgrace. Thus in battle a conqueror, looking upon the vanquished as unfit to bear the name of man, disarmed him of his manhood by removing his generative organs.[5a]

Arabs practiced circumcision long before the time of Mohammed. According to the Old Testament, Ishmael, the progenitor of the Arabian race, was circumcised at the age of 13. Mohammed himself believed in this religious practice. Pococke refers to a tradition which attributes to the prophet the saying, "Circumcision is an ordinance for men and honorable for women." Arabs, like the Abyssinians, appear to have practiced female circumcision. It is not clear whether the operation was performed on the labia or over the clitoris but M. Murat feels certain that the operation was performed over the clitoris.

In Arabia, the profession of *resectricis nymphrum* or female circumcision was as popular an occupation as that of cock castration or caponizing.[6]

It is related by Abulfeda that when Islam came close to a crushing defeat in the Battle of Ohod, Hamza, the uncle of the prophet, cried out to the Koreish chief of the enemy, "Come on, thou son of a she-circumciser."

HEMOSTASIS

All through the Middle Ages, spider-webs were employed to stop hemorrhage from wounds and after phlebotomy. The flimsy web placed on the bleeding surface speeded coagulation. People of the Arctic regions have used cold objects and snow to check bleeding. In a similar fashion, grandmothers place a large cold iron key on the back of the neck of youngsters to stop nosebleed. In medieval times, after the hemorrhage from an incised wound was stopped, the lips of the wound were occasionally held together with the nippers of a large beetle. The angry creature would immediately plunge its nippers into the wound and lock them, thus holding the edges together. The healer then decapitated the insect leaving the nippers, like modern metallic wound-clips, in place. The nippers were removed when the wound was healed. It is related that the Aztecs of Peru and many natives of Brazil, Venezuela, and Colombia still use beetles to unite the edges of an incised wound.

CANCER OF THE BREAST

Another surgical disease of remote antiquity was cancer of the female breast. Cancer of the breast has always inspired horror. As the name indicates, it was believed to have been produced by a mysterious deadly demon resembling a crab (cancer) that settled in the breast and stubbornly resisted expulsion by all forms of magic and divination.[7] In the Middle Ages, St. Agatha was considered the patron-saint of cancer of the breast. Cancer of the female breast was usually not recognized early because modesty and fear of the surgeon's knife made women keep their tumefaction secret as long as possible.

HERNIA

Another surgical abnormality recognized in the Middle Ages was hernia. Its demonic origin was surely demonstrated by the fact that it could grow in size at a moment's notice and disappear entirely as quickly. It was not until the thirteenth century that Roland of Parma dared to investigate the cause of the "demonic swelling" and to suggest operative interference. An old drawing in a Roland manuscript depicts a surgeon holding a murderous-looking implement in his hands standing over an inverted patient with a female assistant in close attendance.

OBSTETRICAL SURGERY

Obstetrical aid was generally forbidden to women in labor in the Middle Ages. Parturient patients were left to suffer for weeks in cases of abnormal presentations until they died either from complications or exhaustion. No one was allowed to interfere with the fetus' position which Providence had chosen. Literal application of the Old Testament doctrine: "In sorrow thou shalt bring forth children,"[8] was the rule.

The practice of the obstetrical art, up to a century ago, was almost exclusively in the hands of ignorant matrons. Trained physicians, if consulted at all, were only called in case of serious difficulty. So universal was the custom of employing midwives, and so strong the prejudice against men engaging in obstetric practice, that in 1522, Dr. Wartt, of Hamburg, having put on the dress of a woman to attend a case of labor, was burned alive for the offense. A little more than a century later, Dr. Percivall Willoughby, an eminent English physician, assisted his daughter, who was a midwife, in a case of difficult labor. He crawled into the darkened room of the parturient patient on his hands and knees without her knowledge.

CATARACT

The couching operation for cataract was practiced in the Middle Ages. Couching or depression for cataract (*depressio cataractae*) was the only method of operating upon cataract from ancient times throughout the Middle Ages. The procedure was as follows: A needle was passed into the sclera on the outer side of the margin of the cornea and somewhat behind it and was pushed forward until it lay against the upper border of the lens; then the point of the needle was lowered by a sweeping movement and the lens was thus depressed into the vitreous. The moment this was done the pupil became black and the patient regained sight. There were cataract specialists in most municipalities.

During the Middle Ages, "cataract prickers" went from one annual fair to another and operated upon those who were blind with cataract. After the "cataract pricker" received his fee, he traveled on to another place. He did not see his patient again after the operation and this was often most fortunate for him, for the later consequences of the operation were often as sad as the immediate result was brilliant.

URINARY CALCULI

Cutting for stone in the bladder was an operation practiced since the days of antiquity. In medieval times, it was the province of uneducated specialists. The method of removing the stone was as follows: the operator put his finger in the anus and hooked down the stone which could be felt in the bladder, pressing hard against the perineal tissue. He then made an incision on the abdomen over the protrusion with an ordinary razor. The bladder was then opened and the stone extracted with a scoop. What happened to the patient later was not considered particularly important.

The type of surgery practiced in the Middle East at the end of the eleventh century may be seen from the memoirs of the north Syrian Arab poet, Usamah Ibn Munquidh (born 1095 A.D): The Lord of Al Munatirah asked his uncle to send him a physician to treat certain sick persons among his people. His Christian physician named Thabit, after an absence of ten days, returned with the following story: "They brought before me a knight in whose leg an abscess had grown; and a woman afflicted with imbecility. To the knight I applied a small poultice until the abscess opened and became well; and the woman I put on a diet and made her humor wet. Then a Frankish physician came to see the patients and said: 'This man knows nothing about treating you. Which wouldst thou prefer, living with one leg or dying with two?' The knight replied, 'Living with one leg!' The Frankish physician then said, 'Bring me a strong knight and a sharp ax.' Then the physician laid the leg of the patient on a block of wood and bade the knight strike it off with one blow. Since the first chop didn't do the job, he dealt a second blow and the patient died on the spot. The Frankish doctor, having disposed of his first patient, then examined the woman and said: 'This is a woman in whose head there is a devil which has possessed her. Shave off her hair.' Her mental condition took a turn for the worse. The physician then said, 'The devil has penetrated through her head.' He thereupon took a razor, made a deep incision in the scalp and peeled off the skin until the skull was exposed, after which he rubbed it with salt. The woman expired instantly."

The first Arabian surgeon of distinction was Abulkasim (d. 1122) of the Western Caliphate. He was chiefly celebrated for his free use of actual cautery and caustics. He occasionally resorted to trachectomy. He performed a number of operations and some of them appear to be original. His surgical greatness is enhanced by what he refused to operate as well as by the operations he performed. He declined to operate on goitre and refused to meddle with cancer.

Christian Europe was no more progressive with regard to surgery during the five hundred years following the work of Paul of Aegina. There were few surgeons in early medieval Christian Europe. Surgical practice passed into the hands of various religious orders—particularly the Benedictines. When ecclesiastical surgery was forbidden by the council of Tours (1163), surgery passed into the hands of the barbers.

One of the first prominent surgeons in Western Europe after Paul of Aegina was William of Saliceto, who belonged to the school of Bologna. In his "Chyrurgia" (1275) he advocates the use of the knife in many places where actual cautery was used by his predecessors.[9] Even a still greater name in the history of medieval surgery is that of his pupil Lanfranc of Milan, who migrated because of political troubles first to Lyons and then to Paris. Lanfranc distinguished between arterial and venous hemorrhage, and he is said to have used ligatures for the former.[10] Eighteen years before Lanfranc came to Paris, a College of Surgeons was founded there (1279) by Jean Pitard (1238-1315), who had accompanied Louis X to Palestine as his surgeon. The College was under the protection of Saints Cosmas and Damian (A.D. 303), two "practitioners of medicine" who suffered martyrdom in the reign of Diocletian. The College became known as the College de St. Come. After Lanfranc joined the College it attracted many pupils.

One of the most gifted pupils of Lanfranc was Jan Yperman (b. 1280) of Milan and Paris. He later (1308) became famous as a surgeon in his native Ypres.

Yperman was a surgeon of note. He felt that bleeding cannot be satisfactorily arrested with styptics. To assure hemostasis, he recommended ligatures: "Take a triangular needle, thread it with a stout waxed thread and pass it under the artery; tie the two ends of the thread together securely and take care not to pierce the vessel with the needle." As to the use of the cautery to control hemorrhage, he was of the opinion that while it might be successfully employed on large vessels, there is always danger that the scar will fall off and start the bleeding again.

Yperman described a technic of trepanation and recommended a treatment for wounds caused by an arrow. In operating for harelip, after the edges are brought together and the stitches applied, he recommended that the patient should eat through a silver tube until the wound is healed.

Yperman did not discourage "royal touch" in the treatment of "king's evil" (scrofula) but he suggested that curable cases recover without it. Incidentally, Yperman's house and hospital served as a memorial to the surgeon until the First World War when they were destroyed by the Germans.

Contemporary with him in France was Henri de Mondeville famous surgeon of the school of Montpellier, whose teaching is best known through his more famous pupil, Guy de Chauliac. The "Surgery" of the latter bears the date 1363, and marks a great advance in surgical precision, which the revival of anatomy by Mondino made possible.

In England, where for a long time the priests were disposed to unite medicine and surgery, when the separation finally took place, it became more enduring and more sharply defined than elsewhere. Lanfranc in his "Chirurgia Magna," held that it is not possible to be a good physician unless one is at the same time a good surgeon, and vice versa.

Guy de Chauliac, who was both priest and surgeon, dates the separation of surgery from medicine from the time of Abulkasim. In northern Italy the division did not take place until a much later period and came to an end earlier than elsewhere. In Southern Italy, the separation was legally recognized from the thirteenth century onward in the Constitutions of Frederic II. In Venice, in the twelfth century, surgeons were forbidden to administer medicines, even in grave cases, despite the voices heard condemning the separation of medicine and surgery.

French surgery in thirteenth and fourteenth centuries was on a higher plane than elsewhere. Indeed, France produced some of the greatest surgeons of the later Middle Ages. One whose work deserves more attention than it has received is Henri de Mondeville (1260-1320). He was probably born in Normandy and he was a pupil of William of Saliceto. Guy de Chauliac refers to him as a worthy successor of Roger of Palermo (c. 1210). He was a protege of Jean Pitard and was surgeon to King Philip the Fair and Louis X (1304). He brought the new teachings from Bologna to France. He taught medicine at Montpellier and, like his master Saliceto, stressed anatomic knowledge and its importance to students. He was a friend of Bernard de Gordon at whose suggestion and urging he wrote his "Surgery." [11]

Mondeville is justly famous for his advocacy of cleanliness in the treatment of wounds. He was against the use of salves in wounds which was then the common practice. He also taught, like Theodoric of Bologna, that suppuration is not essential to the healing of wounds.

Mondeville divided the medical art into three parts. He called surgery the *"tertium instrumentum medicinae,"* the other two divisions being diet and medicine. His independence of traditional dogma may be inferred from his much quoted epigram in the introduction of his fifth treatise: "God did not exhaust his creative power in making Galen."

His deep sense of medical ethics may be derived from the following paragraph:

"You, Surgeons, if you have operated in the homes of the rich for an adequate sum, and in the homes of the poor for charity, you should fear neither fire, nor rain, nor wind; you have no need of going into religious places nor of making penitential pilgrimages, because by your science you are able to save your souls; ... your recompense is grand in Paradise."

He advised his colleagues against dining with a patient who is in their debt. "Get your dinner at an inn; otherwise he will deduct his hospitality from your fee."

In the introduction to the last part of his work, he wrote: "I cannot live long, being asthmatic, coughing, phthisical, and in consumption."

He stresses the importance of anatomy as the foundation of the surgeon's skill. He places his reliance chiefly on Avicenna.

His conception of the circulation is the common one of the time: The "spiritous fluid" penetrates from an intraventricular cavity into the left ventricle; thence, as "vital blood," it courses through the arteries, which are double-walled to withstand this lively fluid. The veins are single-walled and carry the more sluggish "nutritive blood."

In his chapter on amputation of limbs, Mondeville refers to the ligation of arteries as a recognized procedure, requiring no special discussion. This fact alone gives the lie to the oft repeated claim that Pare is the inventor of arterial ligation.

In the Middle Ages, there developed two kinds of surgeons: the military surgeon who learned his art on the battlefield and was often consulted in difficult cases, and the guild surgeon who remained home during war to take care of the community and to train younger men in the art of surgery. The guild surgeon, as his name implies, belonged to a guild. The sons of members of the guild were permitted to become surgeons in due time and were eventually admitted to the guild. An apprentice had to serve seven years before he was eligible for membership in the guild.

The military surgeons, on account of the frequent wars, remained separated from the guild or civil surgeons. The barber surgeons organized guilds of their own.

The regulations of the military surgeon apprentices were elaborate: Each apprentice had to consult with his master before major operations. Apprentices had to serve six years and then pass an examination.

The methods of warfare at that time were those of the joust or tournament. The lance, the mace and the battle-axe were favorite weapons, and since most of the warriors were mounted and heavily armored, the head of the opponent was the part to be aimed at. Head injuries were, therefore, numerous. A procedure peculiar to military surgery was described by Roger of Palermo (c. 1210): Barbed arrows were removed by inserting an iron or copper tube into the wound, so that it slipped over the barb and permitted the extraction of the arrow. This procedure was recommended only when the barbs were too strong or too deeply placed for the surgeon to flatten with a forceps. If the metal head of a lance or an arrow was very deeply embedded, it was usually left alone. Roger said that in such a case he had seen more harm result from ill-advised attempts at extraction than from the effects of the weapon.

The "Practica Chirurgia" of Roger gives a fine description of herniorrhaphy. It treats at length of wounds of the head and brain, giving the differential diagnosis of injuries of the skull and the indications for trephining. For depressed fractures, he recommends a number of perforations with the trephine and then teaches how to raise the bone without damaging the meninges. Bleeding of the scalp was then controlled, and any loose fragments of bone were removed. The scalp flaps were then pressed together and the wound bound with a linen cloth, which had previously been soaked in white of egg. Thanks to the almost continuous warfare between the Norman overlords of Salerno and their neighbors, Roger had many opportunities of treating fractured skulls and other injuries.

Lesions of the intestine and peritoneum occupy a prominent place in the "Chirurgia." If, after an abdominal wound, a loop of protruding gut became cold, he advises that the abdomen of an animal be opened and superimposed on the wounded part until it warmed up and became soft. Then he recommends the application of a clean sponge soaked in hot water on the parts followed by replacement of the intestine. The wound should then be kept open until the intestine appears normal. Afterward a drain is to be inserted and the wound dressed.

ROGER OF PALERMO (c. 1210)

Roger gives an accurate description of the methods he employed in reducing dislocation. He recommends the use of mercury salts in various skin diseases and refers to the use of seaweed (containing iodine) in the treatment of goiter.

As noted in Chapter XV, "Medicine in Medieval Italy," Roger and his pupil Roland made a grievous mistake in adhering to the Galenic fallacy of "coction" or "laudable pus." His critic, Theodorico Borgognoni (1205-1296) of Lucca, remarked: "For it is not necessary, as Roger and Roland have written and as many of their disciples teach and as all modern surgeons profess, that pus should be generated in the wound. No error can be greater than this. Such a practice is indeed to hinder nature, to prolong the disease and to prevent . . . consolidation of the wound." [12]

This error of Roger was the greatest made by the distinguished surgeon. Even Guy de Chauliac, who reviled Theodorico for criticizing Roger as a copyist and plagiarist, was not able to erase this surgical error.

In England, the first to be referred to as "Magister Chirurgorum" or Master Surgeon was Thomas Stokeley (1392). The Masters of Surgery were not merely Master Surgeons but were actually Masters or Aldermen of the Surgeon's Guild and thus in authority over the members of the guild.

Surgeons proper (Magistri in Chirurgia or Chirurgi Physici) stood next to the physicians in education and rank, as is manifest from the curriculum at Salerno. The practice of medicine was strictly forbidden to them, although this prohibition, as may be easily understood, was often disregarded. These surgeons were not only often excellent operators even in difficult cases, but were also often very capable theorists and authors. Besides, the Magistri in Chirurgia there were also Chirurgi Phlebotomatores (Blood-letting surgeons). France possessed a class of guild surgeons from the middle of the thirteenth century at the earliest. These higher surgeons came from the College of St. Come founded in about 1260 by Pitard. They belonged to the laity, for the Church had forbidden surgery since the twelfth century and with special strictness in the thirteenth. From this period the origin of lay surgeons in France may be dated. Such surgeons either settled in one locality permanently or traveled about from town to town.

Montpellier for a long time ceased to permit doctors the practice of anything but internal medicine and abolished entirely all surgical teaching to medical students. If a surgeon of Paris, ashamed of his position, wanted to obtain a license to practice medicine, he had to swear before a notary never to perform an operation again. In Northern Italy the division of medicine and surgery did not take place until a much later period and came to an earlier end.

Better surgeons appear to have developed in France after the complete establishment of a class of higher surgeons. The surgeons that came from the class of barbers and bathhouse-keepers differed from the regular surgeons not only by the place and manner of their education (i.e., they received no higher education), but also by the extent of their technical knowledge which they acquired hit or miss, by traveling and private study. The "herniotomists" and "lithotomists" were "specialists" among this lower class. They traveled about freely, and were particularly dangerous when, in operating upon cases of reducible indirect inguinal hernia, they laid hands not only on the radix of the hernia, but also on the testicles—a method which was almost the rule until the eighteenth century.

In Italy there existed families of surgeons, in which certain operative procedures like herniotomy, rhinoplasty and various secret "specialties," were handed down from one generation to another.

In England, from an early period, there were surgeons who

were called "bonesetters." Later the profession became divided so that, besides the medical practitioners or leeches there were also "Chirurgeons" (surgeons) and barbers or plaster-spreaders. The Chirurgeons were educated in institutions. The barbers or plaster-spreaders received their training from masters.

In Germany, the lower class of surgeons were represented by the bathhouse-keepers and the barbers, who first made their appearance in the twelfth century and subsequently formed and joined guilds. Until the thirteenth century, this inferior aggregation seems to have been not only the surgical group in Germany, but, in general, the only medical faculty. These bathhouse-keepers and barbers enjoyed a social position comparable to that of the players, fifers and butchers; that is, they practiced a disreputable calling and passed before the law and society as a disreputable group. Probably it was one of these inferior surgeons who, without ceremony, hacked off the foot of Duke Leopold of Austria in 1194, when at a tournament he received a compound fracture of the leg after a fall from his horse.[13]

One wonders when looking at old wood engravings and drawings of surgical operations whether the artist truthfully portrayed the patient as possessing such an unconcerned countenance during surgical procedures. One can readily understand how calmness and equanimity might pervade the patient's countenance at the present time with so many sedatives, hypnotics, and anesthetics at the physician's command, but how indifference could be maintained during surgical procedures, in days gone by, is hard to comprehend. If such indifference did actually exist, perhaps the intense fear of the barber surgeons acted as a psychic sedation, or possibly the patients made themselves insensitive to pain by drunkenness or by the sheer power of concentration.

In antiquity, the Stoics are said to have succeeded in becoming insensitive to pain by "rational repudiation" of pain. It is related that when Pompey visited Poseidonius (a distinguished Stoic who was suffering from an attack of gout), the latter, by concentrating on his distinguished guest, lost all feeling of pain.

In the twelfth century, a monk invented the "potion of oblivion" having soporific and analgesic properties which might have been identical with or similar to that used in Scotland and known as "lethargion." "It is certain, moreover," said Jocelyn, "that many, having drunk the potion of oblivion (which physicians call lethargion), have slept and have never felt when they suffered incision and sometimes burning of the limbs and abrasion even of the vitals, and after awakening from the sleep, have been ignorant of what was done to them." Jocelyn does not indicate, however, its composition but it probably contained opium and hyoscyamus.

While there were many hypnotic drugs in "lethargion," its ingredients seldom became known to the barber surgeons or to physicians in general. It was the property of a few who kept its composition secret. Frequently such soporifics had too strong an effect upon the sick, bringing about an eternal sleep. In consequence thereof, patients were averse to their use, preferring pain, however terrible, rather than taking a chance with a drug that might send them into eternity. Even physicians were prejudiced against these secret hypnotics. As late as the seventeenth century, Guy Patin (1601-1672), a learned physician of the University of Paris, vehemently protested against the barber surgeon, Bailly of Troyes, for putting one of his patients to sleep with an herbal syrup before an operation. Said he, "If Bailly really uses narcotic plants in this way, you had better take him soundly to task. Herbal poisons have worked mischief in more skillful hands than his. See to it that these practices are not allowed, and do not let him go unpunished. The impudent barber should not be able to boast of having done such things with impunity." When the case came before the court, Bailly had to pay a heavy fine and the use of herbal remedies before operation was forbidden to him under heavy penalty.

Narcotics supposed to contain henbane (hyoscyamus niger) and poppy mixed with intoxicating mead were prescribed as sedatives. The "potion of oblivion," mentioned by old Norwegian writers, was supposed to contain herbs of the entire forest. The narcotic qualities of mandragora and poisonous water hemlock (cicuta virosa) were well known.

The first to provide a dependable artificial anesthetic was Joseph Priestley (1773-1804), when he discovered the pain controlling nitrous oxide gas. The next discovery that was destined to revolutionize the art of surgery came a century later. Its honor is shared by two Americans who independently discovered the reliable anesthetic, ether, which has been used with great success all over the world. One of the two given credit as the pioneer in this discovery was a country doctor of Georgia, Crawford Williamson Long (1815-1875); the other was a Boston dentist, William Thomas Green Morton (1819-1875).

BARBER SURGEONS OF THE MIDDLE AGES

Owing to the defective method of preparing young men for the surgical profession, the barber (derived from the Latin "barba," meaning "a beard") of the Middle Ages whose occupation was to shave and to trim hair and beards, became associated with the art of surgery. Thus while the art of medicine, whether it was practiced in the cell of the monastery or in the office of the private physician, has always been considered a learned and scientific profession, surgery separated itself from the bathhouse environment and its practice remained primitive. The achievements made in the surgical field by Hippocrates, Celsus, and Galen were never followed by the surgeon of the Middle Ages.

The barber surgeon, without theoretical knowledge, had little difficulty in associating surgery with his tonsorial occupation. In his shop, he pulled teeth, removed corns, cupped, leeched, administered enemas, opened abscesses, dressed wounds and finally extended his province to major surgical procedures. He operated for stone, reduced dislocations, set fractures and amputated extremities.

During military campaigns, when trained military surgeons were lacking, the care of the wounded and sick on the battlefield was often entrusted to the barber surgeon and even to his assistants. The latter might have been completely untrained persons who volunteered in response to military call. At such times, the care of the wounded on the battlefield was left to a mass of ignorant individuals, called "field barbers."

Until the seventeenth century, surgery was a free-for-all trade; anyone who desired to practice it could do so. In consequence thereof, there developed in addition to the barber surgeon, an army of charlatans who filled the market places and country fairs, presenting themselves as tooth pullers, cataract couchers, and operators for stones. To counteract this chaos and to safeguard their "professional" and economic security, the barber surgeons organized themselves into guilds. In small communities where there were no doctors, the barber attended to the medical needs of the community as well.

In Southern Germany, persons who pull teeth, let blood, remove corns, and administer enemas are still known as *bader* or *dorfbader* ("bath surgeons"). During the days when the baths are not open, these *"Baders"* attend to their patrons in the open fields; hence these barber surgeons are still known in the Germanic countries as *"Feldscherers"* or *"Feldschers"* ("field-haircutters")—a designation first applied in the fourteenth century by the Swiss armies.

Most of the universities that came into existence in Europe during the twelfth and thirteenth centuries had well established faculties in medicine but few were willing to impart a knowledge of surgery. Even years after the Church lost its grasp over the universities, teachers feared to oppose the Church-sanctified teaching that the spilling of blood by surgery is evil.

In the year 1396, the Guild of "Surgeons of the Long Robe," (in contradistinction to the barbers who were known as "surgeons of the short robe") adopted the following regulation: "Masters and bachelors in surgery may take to service no apprentice who is not a clerk-grammarian capable of writing and speaking good Latin." The framers of this rule sincerely believed that the advantage and honor of science depended upon this rubric. They added by way of amplification that "the King and all people of quality take great delight in Latin." Although they admitted that some of the barbers were gifted in their handicraft, they looked upon the barber surgeons as totally uneducated persons who were destitute of basic knowledge and full of cunning. None-the-less in spite of their ignorance of Latin, the barbers due to their increasing surgical skill grew into an increasingly important civic body, so that, in A.D. 1450, the Mayor and Aldermen of London sanctioned a code of laws drawn up for the protection and government of their craft. In 1462, Edward IV granted the barbers a charter of incorporation. The charter was granted to the barbers as a class, referring specifically to ". . . free men of the . . . Barbers of our City of London exercising the Mystery or the Art of Surgery . . .", and goes on to describe their diligent and laborious occupation in tending to wounds, bruises, hurts, and other ailments, and in bleeding and drawing teeth. This charter pointed out a wide field in minor surgery for the barbers, and does not even mention the less dignified activities which for so long had been their province. Shaving, bathing, trimming beards, cutting hair, and delousing are forgotten, and not even a footnote is devoted to the brothel-keeping propensities of the older barbers.

In France, surgery was done almost entirely by proxy. The members of the College de Saint Come were a lordly body of men of superior social standing who charged high fees and wore red robes trimmed with ermine fur as a sign of their nobility. Yet they disdained to soil their hands in manual operations. They absolutely refused to give any didactic instruction to those who did not understand Latin—even if these ignoramuses were the ones who enabled them to receive large fees for the surgical procedures they performed under their guidance.

The faculty of the College of Saint Luc, jealous of the academic strength of the College of Saint Come, eventually gave the barbers special lectures in the French vernacular on condition of their perpetual submission to its authority. These lectures and anatomic discussions were held in secret until the year 1494.

Despite their pledge of submission, the barbers were dissatisfied with the amount of anatomical material provided them and demanded more cadavers for themselves. The result of this agitation was that they were eventually deprived of all the privileges granted to them by King Charles V in the thirteenth century and these included the right to practice bloodletting and perform minor surgical procedures.

The barber surgeons were first styled "barbitonsars" or "barbisarsors," and later were given the more honorable name of "tonsor chirurgici." In 1505 their profession or trade was mentioned in the official register, and was designated as "Chirurgia Tonsuria."

There were two classes of barber surgeons: major and minor. The latter were itinerant vendors of amulets, ointments and antidotes, The major barbers aspired to a higher dignity; they carried scissors, forceps, scalpels, razors, and a variety of ointments with them in open containers. Various of their ointments were allegedly of high repute, such as "the ointment of the Apostles" which was guaranteed to "change the vitality of the tissues" and a yellow ointment which relieved local pain.

During leprosy epidemics, which were a frequent occurrence in those days in France bathhouse-keepers and barbers often assumed the work of the educated physicians who frequently fled from the community in terror. During such times, bathhouse keepers saw an opportunity to make an easy coin and baths were widely acclaimed as the best prophylactic against contracting leprosy.

Although the chirurgeons of the College de Saint Come fled their posts during epidemics, they still claimed as their own the whole field which they had abandoned to their competitors. They even sought legal redress against the unremitting encroachments of the barbers and bathhouse keepers upon their profession.

The unwilling hands of the chirurgeons naturally transferred the practice of surgery to the ready hands of a body of uneducated but ambitious men who were ready to devote their lives to the service and relief of their compatriots. The French barber surgeons served the poor and the lower bourgeoisie, trimmed their beards and wigs, looked after their cupping and bleeding, and attended to their wens, wounds, ulcers, tumors, fractures and dislocations. In fact they performed all surgery with the exception of cataract couching, cutting for stone and hernial operations, which were left to itinerant specialists. The barbers had little use for pride and high stratagems. What they lacked was theoretical education, the ability to read textbooks which were usually in Latin, and proper lectures. The schooling they received from their masters at St. Come did not satisfy them. They looked forward to the day when they could transfer their allegiance to the Faculty of Medicine.

The lot of the barber surgeons in England was better than in France. As early as 1308, they formed a guild which received a charter in 1462, when Edward IV granted the right to practice the craft of surgery. Through the practice of dissection and the attendance of lectures the barber surgeons of England constantly improved their position until finally they were able to organize into a professional surgical guild which subsequently became united with the guild known as the "Barber Company" by act of Henry VIII.

Those achieving the new Barber-Surgeon status did not believe that a mere statutory union of the two guilds would realize for them the ideals for which they had striven. They wanted to raise the cultural status of their profession and they proceeded to organize a course of systematic teaching for all who practiced surgery. Young and well-educated physicians were engaged to teach the anatomy of the normal and the diseased body. Surgery was taught systematically by such learned surgeons as Thomas Vicary (1548), William Clowes (1575) and others. Regulations were drawn up with regard to the supervision and examination of apprentices. At the same time, an effort was made to diminish the number of quacks. The latter effort failed except in the few districts where surgeons were also justices of the peace. One such surgeon was John Halle of Maidstone, who made that district quite uncomfortable for quacks. Anyone who desired to practice medicine or surgery in his district was examined by him.

When the barbers united with the company of surgeons, a law was enacted that barbers should confine themselves to minor operations such as bloodletting and drawing teeth, and that only surgeons should perform major operations. Surgeons were prohibited from "barbery or shaving." In 1745, barbers and surgeons were again separated into distinct corporations.

The barber shop in England was a favorite rendezvous for idle persons. In addition to its attraction as a focus of news, a lute, viol, or some such musical instrument was often used to entertain the waiting customers.

Barber surgeons customarily notified the public when the time for bleeding had arrived by displaying a blood-soaked bandage at their doors. This custom represents the origin of the familiar red-striped barber pole.

One of the Anglo-Saxon medical manuals written in 1480 has this to say about bleeding: "Here teacheth Galen the goud leche of mete and drynke and tume of bledynge to vyse, et cetera ... In ye monthe of Jeniuer vastying whyte wyn hit ys goud to drynk & bloud-letyng forbere thorwe alle thyne, for 7 days ther beeth of grete periole therinne the ferste daye & the 2 daye & the vifthe & the 7 daye & the XVI daye & the XIX daye."

In Paris, during the prescribed season for phlebotomy, barbers often applied for the position of dresser of wounds in the wards of the Hotel Dieu, in Paris. At times they preferred to return to their masters for further practical training and in time of war, they signed up as servants to field-surgeons.

As has been intimated, Paris, the great city of schools and of books, was for a long time a closed citadel to the barber surgeon, for it was open only to those who knew the Latin language. The barber apprentice wanted to read "Le Guidon" in French and William of Saliceto in Italian; he wanted to read the great Lanfranc of Milan as taught at Lyons and at Paris in his native tongue. He resented the fact that his books were written in Latin —a language which was only spoken by the privileged class.

Lyons was first to produce French versions of both Guy de Chauliac and Lanfranc (1480) but these were too costly and quite beyond the reach of a "yellow-beak" (barber surgeon). In 1485 Guy de Chauliac's work appeared in quarto in a cheap, popular French edition under the aforementioned title "Le Guidon" and this was reprinted again by popular demand four years later. The French translator was Nicolas Panis, a Norman surgeon who spent his life in Lyons. Nicolo Prevost's translation of William of Saliceto was also published at Lyons, and these two works became the most popular books read by the barber surgeons.

At the insistence of the barber surgeons, the Faculty of Montpellier, in 1490, arranged instruction in the craft of surgery for the barbers. Griphis, who later became Dean, got himself appointed as first lecturer to this group. For ten years he read and commented upon the text of Guy's "Collectionary of Surgery," reading first in Latin and then rendering the text in the French tongue. John Falco or Falcon, Professor of Messina, who followed the same bilingual method, put forth the substance of his lectures in a book entitled "Les Notabiles Declaratifs." In his prefatory note he states: "I have been happy to prepare, for all surgeons following my ordinary lectures on medicine and who have been reading Guy in the noble town of Montpellier in the year of Grace one thousand five hundred, I have had the pleasure, I repeat, in preparing divers comments upon notable passages in Guy, whereby he may be easily understood, and men may go about the exercise of the aforesaid art without danger or undue peril to the human body." [14]

Louis XII in granting a renewal of the barber surgeon charter, called attention to the danger at Montpellier of too loose a licensing policy. "For many there are here (says the grantor) of ignorant Apothecaries, Surgeons, Barbitonsors and other of that ilk, woefully insufficient and inexpert in medicine who are endeavoring to worm their way into practice—a menace likely to besmirch the fair name and fame of this University." [15] In spite of this admonition the attitude of the Regents of Montpellier was very liberal. System and procedure on the basis of fact began to replace pure theory. Texts and competent lecturers on surgery were provided, and dissections performed. Montpellier was first to avoid purposeless argumentation, endless discussions of "expoundables and insolubles" and wearisome dialectics.

The enlightened policy of Montpellier lured to South France many youngsters who had a natural preference for the University of Paris. The zealots of the Paris Faculty from then on particularly detested Montpellier for in their mind the Regents of Montepellier had wilfully followed a policy of educating a body of poor and ignorant artisans: "It is unthinkable that a sister university should open its doors to inferiorly born, boorish clowns and impart to them the innermost secrets of medicine."

Despite this clamor of disapproval coming out of the North, every quarterly book-fair at Lyons saw something new produced in the mother tongue to supply the needs of the barber-surgeons. The translation of Giovanni de Vigo (1460-1525) by Nicholas Godin of Arras, a military surgeon and a man truly interested in the public welfare, had a great influence on the process of educating and elevating the standards of the barbers.

This book actually vindicated the use of the vernacular and brought down in utter ruin the whole fabric of the dogmatic schools. It appears that some 52 editions of Guy de Chauliac's surgery came off the presses at the end of the fifteenth and beginning of the sixteenth centuries. The run of vernacular translations of Vigo seems to have been endless, for Vigo offered an up-to-date well ordered work, fit to be found in the kit of surgeons attending that greatest of all surgical schools—the school of warfare.

In the medical school at Pavia, the barber surgeons found similar champions. Champier (1472-1579), recently knighted and elected to the Faculty, stood up during a full session of that body and made the proposal of conferring upon the barber of the Duke de Guise the title of Doctor of Surgery. As can be imagined, this aroused the ire of Matthew Curtius, senior Professor of Medicine and caused him to declare: "Champier, we of this University are amazed that you should have brought us all into session to hear you propose the name of a man of no reading and no understanding of the Latin tongue. It seems that you are willing to mock and trick those from whom you yourself have just received vast and unparalleled privileges." To this Champier replied: "Answer we this, brothers and colleagues; suppose Hippocrates the Greek and Avicenna the Arabian were alive and came to Pavia, drawn by the reputation of your University, would you grant the doctoral degree to these wise ones, or would you refuse because they knew no Latin?" "It has been customary in France," he continued, "particularly at Montpellier, in the last twenty-five years, to read Surgery in the Gallican or French language, for as a rule barbers know no Latin. This method has been sponsored by some of our most learned university men, by Griphis a former chancellor, by Dean Falcon, a man of high learning and renown in France, and after him by Dionysius, also a very proficient medical man." The members of the faculty were not stirred by this argument. After the session they angrily let Champier know that such an unspeakable suggestion had never before been brought up at their fair university and that it had better be never brought up again.

An entirely new version of the Surgery of Guy de Chauliac was published by Jean Canappe. He restored Guidon for the barbers and his work went through nine editions. With great ardor, he went about his translation, giving time to the project whenever he could spare it.

With each new preface, Jean Canappe increased his defiance of the privileged and greedy Regents of Medicine and with each new edition his appointment as "reader to the Barbers of Lyons" gathered more respect. Canappe cast his lot with the underprivileged surgeons: "It is for them and in their name," he said, "that I take on the duty of translating from Latin into French. Yes, with a clear unfaltering aim, I am determined to persist in this course from now on, with no intention of satisfying or composing the physicians' querulous outcries against me. For they are the legitimate offspring and heirs of Zoilus, chattering calumniators and detractors."

In a preface to the "Two Books of Simples from Galen," Canappe again makes plain his position: "I have no thought of foisting my French translation upon those who know Greek and Latin: I interpret for others, for those who, though unacquainted with those tongues, follow the profession of surgery and who daily and unremittingly go their rounds curing maladies . . . I make bold to state that I have known many surgeons, unequipped with either Greek or Latin, but tireless in applying their minds to matters germane to their art . . . I would not have you mistake my meaning . . . I am not disparaging those languages, nor calling them hindrances. I would that every student were well versed in them; it would relieve us from this labor of translation."

Help also came to the barbers from unexpected sources: from Fayard of Perigueux, and from the reader in medicine, William Christian of Orleans. They spoke up loudly and clearly in the inferior idiom which all could understand.

But it was Ambroise Pare, who began as a barber-surgeon, who ushered in the period of original surgical contributions in the mother tongue. Pare's first work appeared in 1545. He found critics and tormentors aplenty waiting for him. As he made steady headway against the strong and persistent opposition about him, he continued to hold in dear remembrance the name of Jean Canappe, the first protagonist in the unfolding drama of the rise of the barber-surgeon.[16]

CHAPTER XXII

EPIDEMIC DISEASES IN THE MIDDLE AGES

INTRODUCTION

Having dwelt at some length on the history of medieval medical theories and practices, a discussion of the diseases that prevailed in the Middle Ages will now be covered. It is generally assumed that most physical disorders now prevailing in epidemic form also occurred in the Middle Ages, but many of them, owing to a lack of diagnostic technique, were not recognized. Of the 126 abnormal physical conditions discussed by Paul of Aegina (625-690),[1] he appears to have recognized the contagious character of plague, cholera, phthisis (which had been identified by Hippocrates, Galen and Arataeus), smallpox, trachoma, leprosy and erysipelas. However, he definitely mentions only plague and elephantiasis (lepra) as being epidemic diseases.

Rhazes mentions elephantiasis (lepra), the itch, phthisis, pestilent fever, ophthalmia (trachoma) and malignant pustule (smallpox) as transmittable diseases. Haly Abbas (d. 994) adds measles to the number of contagious diseases stating that measles and smallpox are the most contagious. In the later part of the thirteenth century Bernard de Gordon (1285-1318) enumerates eight contagious diseases: acute fevers (malaria or typhus), phthisis, scabies, erysipelas, epilepsy, anthrax, leprosy and trachoma. He does not mention plague, smallpox, cholera and diphtheria which were prevalent diseases for ages, perhaps because he considered knowledge concerning them to be almost universal. His list includes epilepsy which is not contagious, but which is often familial. Disregarding epilepsy, the total number of contagious diseases known in the thirteenth century was thirteen.

The physicians of the Middle Ages had an idea that certain diseases are contagious but the mechanism of transmission was not understood. The teaching of Hippocrates that disease in general may arise either from the food we eat or the air we breathe generally prevailed all through the Middle Ages and even later. Therefore when a disease seized a large number of different persons of varied ages and sexes at one time, it was considered that it must have taken its origin from the air. This theory was approved by Galen who added that climatic factors also contribute to the outbreak of the malady. Miasmata, given off by water in certain communities, "taint the air and occasion disease."

Haly Abbas (d. 994) attributes the cause of a pestilential state to the nature of the country and the season of the year which cause a change in the atmosphere. Avicenna's account of the cause of epidemic disease, like that of Galen, includes such etiological factors as the humid and warm state of the atmosphere, the stagnant air of caverns, the miasmata of the lakes and the proximity of dead bodies.

The Italian physician, Gentile da Foligno, who flourished during the greatest plague in Europe (1348), mentions astrological causes, corruption of the air due to putrifaction, and the opening of old wells and caverns. Gentile was firm in his belief in contagion when he stated that the plague was brought to Italy by ships trading with the Levant. The dread disease appeared first in Genoa then in Perugia and later in many other cities.

The Moslem poet and physician of the fourteenth century, Ali ibn Khatma al Ansari, said in 1368: "Contagion, according to my long experience, is the result of a direct contact with a person who suffers from a transmutable disease. That person is immediately attacked with the same symptoms. If the first person expectorates blood the second will do so; likewise if he develops a bubo, it will also appear in the other person at the same place, and the second person likewise will transmit the disease to the others." [2]

Avicenna (980-1037) came close to the real cause of bubonic plague in the tenth and eleventh centuries. He observed that before the plague spreads, rats and mice come out of their burrows, stagger about as if drunk and then frequently die. The full meaning of Avicenna's sage observation did not become clear until almost a thousand years after his death.

It is difficult to appraise the moral and religious consequences of the plague. The very fear of contagion often weakened or destroyed family and social ties. Of course, there were men whose faith was tried and even strengthened by the catastrophic test of the epidemics, but others lapsed into pessimism and cynicism. The same trials that hardened the hearts of some men, softened those of others. No generalization can be made.

Whether or not faith was increased or diminished during epidemics, it is certain that superstitions multiplied. The plain people often accepted the plague as a divine punishment in retribution for their sins. The more sophisticated ones wanted a more scientific explanation, and the explanation was frequently astrological. There were also strong tendencies to establish a connection between the calamity of plague and other catastrophes such as volcanic eruptions and earthquakes, and also to relate the epidemic to various mysterious portents such as comets and eclipses.

Relics, images, amulets, talismen, and charms were used both as prophylactics and cures for the plague. Special prayers and incantations were devised. Flagellation was practiced and certain forms of psychosis, such as the dancing mania and witch hunting, were resorted to.

Throughout the entire medieval period it was generally assumed that sorrow and suffering create especially favorable conditions for the rise and spread of disease. The panic prevailing during epidemics was regarded as furthering the spread of disease. Thus the municipal authorities in many cities repeatedly forbade the tolling of the funeral bells, which would otherwise have sounded the entire day.[3]

Terrorized by and in fear of the inexplicable evil, men were driven to seek the guilty ones who had provoked God's wrath.

Numerous individuals openly professed their own sinfulness and formed groups of flagellants who marched from one country to another, lamenting, calling upon the people to repent, and scourging themselves.

As intimated, since epidemics were attributed to the sins of man, a thorough search was made to discover the offenders who were responsible for them. Elders of the Church went from house to house searching for religious irregularities and immoral conduct. The word "moral" signified good sexual behavior. If a man could not satisfactorily explain where he spent his Sundays during Church services, he was thought to be a sinner and the cause of the epidemic. Numerous men and women were disgracefully expelled from the community for minor offenses— real or fancied—as a measure to stop an epidemic. There were scenes of the most despicable brutality as the Church sought to find a scapegoat for the mistaken cause of the highly fatal disease. Hate and racial prejudice were fired to a high pitch. Jews particularly were made victims of the most absurd superstitions. In many German cities Jews were persecuted because they were accused of having poisoned the wells. Such rumors were often spread by the nobility who were indebted to them for advancing large sums of money which they refused to pay back.

THE PLAGUE

While it is true that the frequent epidemics in the Middle Ages brought on an intellectual stagnation, the reverse is equally true: Intellectual stagnation also brought on epidemics. The masses and authorities steadfastly refused to learn anything of the contagious and infectious nature of the pestilences which might have served to prevent or alleviate such scourges in the future. Since the deadly epidemics were generally ascribed to the anger of God for the sins of man, it was deemed futile for mortals to interfere with the will of Providence. While it is true that the epidemics were a result of sin, the primary sin was gross ignorance of the simplest rules of sanitation and hygiene.

Ancient medical writers including Galen (A. D. 131-201) used the term "plague" (which means "a blow") to signify any epidemic disease causing a great mortality. Accordingly, many epidemics recorded in history under the term "plague" do not really refer to the bubonic plague as described in our modern textbooks. The ancient connotation of the term included various contagious and infectious diseases such as smallpox, typhus and typhoid fever.[4] In fact, the so-called plague epidemic of Athens described by Thucydides might have been any one of a number of severe infectious diseases. The same is true of the epidemic which occurred during the reign of Marcus Aurelius (A. D. 164-180) that raged in epidemic form over the whole Roman Empire.

The first description of bubonic plague is contained in a fragment of Rufus of Ephesus (A. D. first century), who lived at the time of Emperor Trajan, which is preserved in the "Collections of Oribasius." Rufus refers to the "pestilential" buboes found chiefly in Libya, Egypt and Syria as being especially fatal. Dioscorides (40-90 A.D.) fully described these buboes in a work on the plague which prevailed in Libya in his time.

It is not until the sixth century of our era during the reign of Emperor Justinian that we first definitely meet with bubonic plague in Europe. This epidemic lasted for fifty years. Procopius (end of the 5th century), the Byzantine historian, who observed the plague with the eye of a physician in Contantinople, gives a graphic description of the process and symptoms of the pestilence. He called it *"pestis inguinaria."* The plague of Justinian, states Procopius, began at Pelusium in Egypt in A.D. 542. It spread over Egypt, and in the same, or the next year passed to Constantinople, where it carried off 10,000 persons in one day. It appeared in Gaul in 546. Here the most severe epidemic was in 565 and this depopulated the country. In 590 it reached Rome and spread over the whole Roman world, beginning in maritime towns and radiating inland.[5]

Whether the numerous pestilences recorded in the seventh century were the plague or other infectious disease cannot now be said with certainty. However, it is probable that the pestilences in England chronicled by Bede (673-735) in the years

664, 672, 679, and 683 might have been this disease, especially since in the year 690 *"pestis inguinaria"* was prevalent in Rome. Gabriele de Mussi narrates how the few who miraculously escaped the pestilence themselves transmitted the contagion to all whom they met.

Old Russian chronicles place the origin of the disease in Cathay (China). This is confirmed to some extent by Chinese records in which it is stated that pestilence and destructive inundations destroyed the enormous number of thirteen million persons. Bubonic plague appears to have passed by way of Armenia into Asia Minor and thence to Egypt and North Africa. Nearly the whole of Europe was gradually overrun by this pestilence.

England was invaded early in the year 1352 and Oxford lost two-thirds of her academic population. The outbreaks of 1361 and 1368, known as the second and third plagues of the reign of Edward III, were doubtlessly of this same disease, although some historians refer to these epidemics as "the black death." Scotland and Ireland did not escape this pestilence.

The "Leech Book of Bald" characterizes the plague that attacked England as "flying venom." In one case the expression "venomous swelling" is used, which has been interpreted as a reference to the buboes of bubonic plague.

The nature of this pestilence has been a matter of much controversy, and some have doubted the diagnosis of bubonic plague. Some of the symptoms enumerated seem to justify the diagnosis of bubonic plague and others seem to adequately differentiate it from Oriental plague. In the latter condition, the pulmonary involvement gives rise to hemoptysis and other symptoms. This lung complication was a marked feature in certain epidemics of plague in India. Guy de Chauliac notes this feature in the earlier epidemic at Avignon, but not in the later.[6]

The most severe epidemics of bubonic plague were those of the fourteenth century which, after circling Europe, devastated the whole of Asia, from China to the Caucasus, as well as Africa. In the single city of Ghaza 22,000 persons died in one month. In the whole East, it is estimated that 23 million persons perished.

The Arabian physicians who give an account of the "Black Death" estimate the number of its victims at two-thirds of the total number of persons living at that time.

From the Crimea, the plague spread after 1347 to Constantinople, Greece and Italy where it arrived in 1348, speedily extending over France, Spain, England, Norway, Denmark and Holstein. It even reached Greenland as well as Iceland in the same year. Both of these northern countries heretofore very populous, were almost depopulated by the ravages of this dread epidemic.

By another route the "Great Death" (which had already in 1348 once visited Germany, coming from France through Alsace) again spread from Carinthia and Vienna in 1349, destroying an estimated million and a quarter human beings. Poland, according to Honiger, with Silesia, Bohemia and eastern France, remained exempt for at least the first three years of the epidemic, but then was ravaged by the disease. Russia, too, in spite of its northern situation and colder climate, was subjected to the destruction of the plague. Even the population of Switzerland, especially of Valais, were thoroughly scourged, so that Luzerne lost 3,000 and Basel 14,000 men. The enormity of the death rate may be inferred from the fact that Strassburg lost 16,000, Danzig 13,000, Vienna 40,000, Schleswig four-fifths of its inhabitants, Paris 50,000 and London 100,000 souls.[7]

The mortality of the first wave of Black Death has been estimated in various parts of Europe at between two-thirds and three-fourths of the total population. In England it was even higher, but some countries were much less severely affected. A. F. Hecker (1713-1811) calculates that one-fourth of the population of Europe, or 25 million persons, perished during the entire series of epidemics.

In the fifteenth century, bubonic plague recurred frequently in nearly all parts of Europe. The epidemic of 1563-1564 in London and other parts of England was very severe, a thousand dying weekly in London. In Paris about this time plague was an everyday occurrence, and some were less afraid of this scourge than of a headache.

GIOVANNI BOCCACCIO (1313-1375)

It is a curious fact that the most graphic descriptions of plague were given by learned laymen, not by physicians. The first to describe it was the great Greek historian, Thucydides (460-339 B. C.). The second was the Roman poet Ovid (43 B. C.-19 A. D.). The third was the Italian author Giovanni Boccaccio (1313-1375), in the introduction to his work "Decameron" published in 1353. His description of the plague of Florence which precedes his stories, is universally acknowledged to be a masterpiece of epic grandeur and vividness. It ranks with the descriptions of similar calamities by Thucydides, Defoe (1659-1731) and Manzoni. Like Daniel Defoe, Boccaccio drew largely on hearsay and his own imagination, it being almost certain that in 1348 he was at Naples and therefore no eye-witness of the scenes he describes. Because of its great medico-historical value, it is appropriate to present his description of the plague in an abbreviated form:

". . . one thousand three hundred and forty-eight, when into the notable city of Florence, fair over every other of Italy, there came the death dealing pestilence, which, through the operation of the heavenly bodies or of our own iniquitous dealings, being sent down upon mankind for our correction by the just wrath of God, had some years before appeared in the parts of the East and after having bereft these later of an innumerable number of inhabitants, extending without cease from one place to another, and now unhappily spread toward the West. And there against no wisdom availing nor human foresight not yet humble supplications, not once but manytimes both in ordered processions and on otherwise made unto God by devout persons —about the coming of Spring of the aforesaid year, it began in horrible and miraculous wise to show forth its dolorous effects, yet not as it had done in the East, where, if any bled at the nose, it was a manifest sign of inevitable death; nay, but in men and women alike there appeared at the beginning of the malady, certain swellings, either on the groin or under the armpits, whereof some waxed of the bigness of a common apple, others like unto an egg, some more and some less, and these the vulgar named plague-boils. From these two parts the aforesaid death-bearing plague-boils proceeded, in brief space, to appear and come indifferently in every part of the body; wherefrom, after awhile, the fashion of the contagion began to change into black or livid blotches, which showed themselves in many first on the arms and on the thighs and (after spread to) every other part of the person, in some large and sparse and in others small and thick sown, and like as the plague-boils had been first (and yet were) a very certain token of coming death, even so were these for every one to whom they came.

"To the cure of these maladies not counsel of physicians nor virtue of any medicine appeared to avail or profit aught; on the contrary—whether it was that the nature of the infection suffered it not or that the ignorance of the physicians (of whom, over and above the men of art, the number, both men and women, who had never had any teaching of medicine, was become exceeding great) availed not to know when it arose and consequently took not due measures thereagainst—not only did few recover thereof, but well nigh died within the third day from the appearance of the aforesaid signs, this sooner and that later, and for the most part without fever or other accident. And this pestilence was the more virulent for that, by communication with those who were sick thereof . . . the mere touching of the clothes or of whatsoever other thing had been touched or used of the sick appeared of itself to communicate the malady to the toucher . . . not only did it pass from man to man, but . . . being touched by an animal foreign to the human species, not only infected this latter with the plague; but in a very brief space of time killed it. Of this mine own eyes (as hath a little before been said), had one day, among others, experience on this wise; to wit, that the rags of a poor man who had died of the plague, being cast out into the public way, two hogs came up to them and having first, after their wont, rooted around among them with their snoots, took them in their mouths and tossed them about their jaws, then, in a little while, after turning round and round, fell down dead upon the rags which they had in an ill hour intermeddled . . .

"The condition of the common people (and belike in great part, of the middle class also) was yet more pitiable to behold, for that these, for the most part retained by hope or poverty in their houses and abiding in their own quarters, sickened by the thousands daily and being altogether unattended and unsuccored died well nigh all without recourse . . . Nor was it only one bier that carried two or three corpses, nor did this happen but once, nay, many might have been counted which contained husband and wife, two or three brothers, father and son or the like . . . there were made throughout the churchyards, after every other part was full, vast trenches, wherein those who came after were laid by the hundred and being heaped up therein by layers, as goods are stored aboard ship, were covered with a little earth, till such time as they reached the top of the trench . . . throughout the scattered villages and in the fields, the poor and miserable husbandmen and their families, without succor of physicians or aid of servitor, died, not like men, but well nigh like beasts, by the ways or in their villages or about the houses, indifferently by day and night . . . they looked for death that very day, studied with all their wit, not to help to maturity the future produce of their cattle and their fields and the fruits of their own past toils, but to consume those which were ready at hand. Thus it came to pass that the oxen, the asses, the sheep, the goats, the swine, the fowls, nay the very dogs, so faithful to mankind, being driven forth to their own houses, went straying at their pleasure about the fields, where the very corn was abandoned, without being cut, much less gathered in . . .

"To leave the country and return to the city, what more can be said save that such and so great was the cruelty of heaven (and in part, peradventure, that of men) that, between March and the following July, what with the virulence of that pestiferous sickness, and the number of sick folk ill tended or forsaken in their need, through the fearfulness of those who were whole, it is believed for certain that upward of an hundred thousand human beings perished within the walls of the city of Florence. . . . How many memorable families, how many ample heritages, how many famous fortunes were seen to remain without lawful heir. How many valiant men, how many fair ladies, how many sprightly youths, whom, not others only but Galen, Hippocrates or Aesculapius themselves, would have judged most hale, breakfasted in the morning with their kinsfolk, comrades and friends and that same night supped with their ancestors in the other world."[8]

Giovanni Boccaccio (1313-1375), the author of this graphic description of the bubonic plague was born in 1313, but the place of his birth is somewhat doubtful. Florence, Paris and Certaldo are all mentioned by various writers as his native city.

At an early age he was apprenticed to an eminent merchant, with whom he remained for six years—a period which Boccaccio felt was entirely wasted. Boccaccio's father yielding to his son's immutable aversion to commerce, permitted him to adopt a course of study of his own choosing. He then went to study with a celebrated professor of canon law.

About the year 1341, by command of his father who in his old age desired the assistance and company of his son, Boccaccio returned to Florence. Nine years later his father died and he was made the guardian of his younger brother, Jacopo. He then entered the service of the Republic and was sent on important missions to the courts of several popes, both in Avignon and Rome.

During the fourteenth century the study of ancient literature was at a low ebb in Italy. Boccaccio relates that when he asked to see the library of the celebrated monastery of Mount Cassino, he was shown into a dusty room without even a door leading to it. He found that many of the priceless manuscripts were irreparably mutilated. His guide told him that the monks were in the habit of tearing leaves from the codices which were either made into psalters for children or amulets for women which sold for four or five *solidi* apiece.

Boccaccio did all in his power to overcome by word and example the barbarous indifference of his age. He bought or copied with his own hand numerous valuable manuscripts. Boccaccio deplored the ignorance of his age. His zealous endeavors to revive the all but forgotten Greek language in Western Europe are well known.

The "Decameron" is a collection of one hundred stories with which a group of people entertained themselves while on a pilgrimage to the grave of St. Thomas à Becket. In the prologue, the various participants are described in a masterly fashion. Among the tales is the story of a rather unscrupulous doctor of medicine who had greatly enriched himself during a plague epidemic. It has been suggested that Boccaccio was actually referring to John of Gaddesden (1280-1361).

The publishing of the "Decameron" in 1353 marks the beginning of the rise of Italian prose. Boccaccio, for the first time, speaks in a new idiom, flexible and tender, and capable of rendering all the shades of feeling, from the coarse laughter of cynicism to the sigh of hopeless love. Boccaccio is considered the "Father of Italian Prose."

In about 1360, Boccaccio retired from the turbulent scenes of Florence to Certaldo. In the following year a Carthusian monk came to him with a posthumous message from another monk of the same order to the effect that if Boccaccio did not at once abandon his godless ways in life and literature his death would shortly ensue followed by eternal damnation. Boccaccio's impressionable nature was deeply moved. In his writings he had constantly attacked with bitter satire the institutions and servants of the Church. Terrified by the approach of death, he sealed his library, abandoned literature, and devoted the remainder of his life to penance and prayer.

The first reaction to the "Black Death" was flight but not everyone could flee. Consequently those who were still well attempted as far as possible to isolate the sick and thus diminish the danger of infection.

Relatives and all who had come into contact with the patient were compelled to remain in isolation. The patient's house door was sealed with brickwork to make certain that the injunction was obeyed. Messengers of the municipal authorities delivered food to such isolated people. During the epidemics crowds were avoided, and festivals and sermons were prohibited. Only processions begging God to cease scourging the city were permitted. Travelers from regions where the plague was raging were forbidden entrance into the city. The dead were lowered through the windows and removed from the city in carts. Burial outside the city was intended to prevent the extension of the epidemic. In every house where a plague patient had died, the doors and windows were kept open for eight to ten days, the rooms were all fumigated, and the clothes as well as the linen of the deceased were burned. Bernabo, Duke of Milan, was the first to introduce a "quarantine" in 1374; yet he was unable to save Milan from the plague of that year. Despite rigorous measures applied, they proved ineffective during the pestilence. The next wave of the epidemic was much milder in Milan than in other Italian cities.

Physicians felt entirely impotent in the face of the plague. Every protective measure appeared to them almost useless. The belief prevailed that one could catch the disease from another without even having the slightest contact with the sick person. Simply looking at the afflicted person exposed one to the greatest danger of infection. If the patient were feverish, he was ordered to keep a sponge soaked in vinegar before his mouth. On the other hand, if the patient were cold, he was supposed to diminish the danger of infection by drinking a concoction of caraway.

The effectiveness of fumigation was regarded with the greatest confidence. Plague patients were advised to light a fire,[9] especially in the evening, and burn rosemary, ambergris, gummastic, and sulphur so that the fumes would purify the air. Bathing was prohibited throughout the duration of the epidemic. Blood-letting was recommended in treating the plague as in all other diseases. It was also believed that people who worked in hospitals and "other foul-smelling places" were protected against infection. The explanation was "that one poison overcomes, and destroys the other." There were people who, in the name of prophylaxis, paid daily visits to particularly evil-smelling places and remained there for hours inhaling the foul odors.

ST. ANTHONY'S FIRE

Among the great epidemics that raged during the Middle Ages in Europe none is more interesting historically than that of St. Anthony's fire. A disease termed *ignis sacer* ("sacred fire") was first mentioned by Celsus who described two clinical varieties. In the first form, the skin is either red or a mottled mixture of redness and paleness and the skin is covered with a great number of small pustules. As the disease spreads, the part first affected either heals or becomes ulcerated from the rupture of the pustules and discharges a humor intermediate between sanies and pus. The breast and sides are mentioned as being the most frequent sites of this disease. This description surely represents shingles (herpes zoster).

The lesions of the second variety are described by Celsus as consisting of superficial ulcerations of the skin. The areas involved are broad and somewhat livid, but unequal, the middle part healing as the periphery spreads: The new areas becoming affected then become swelled and hard, and the color a combination of black and red. This form affects principally old and cachectic persons and especially involves their legs. Perhaps varicose ulcers and erysipelas are covered by the second type.

The treatment of *ignis sacer* consists of various foods and drinks. The ulcers are treated locally by washing them off with hot water. If they spread, hot wine is used. They are then opened with a needle and dressed with astringent applications.[10]

St. Anthony's fire, which first appeared in Europe in the latter part of the tenth century, was first mentioned in the Annals of the Convent of Zanten (c. 857). It proved to be a rapidly fatal disease. It onset was sudden, beginning with a high fever. The limbs, first cold became rapidly burning hot. Blisters quickly developed in the extremities and gangrene rapidly set in. Occasionally the face and genitals suffered the same fate.

St. Anthony's fire was a withering and deforming epidemic disease, striking abruptly like a thunderbolt and quickly leaving behind dead and crippled bodies. Mothers scarcely knew that their children were sick before they were taken from them to be carried to the graveyard. Frequently limbs were lost but the mutilated persons survived. If the viscera were attacked, the outcome was always fatal. The cause of this epidemic has never been ascertained. The French commission appointed in 1776 to study its etiology decided that the cause was some form of plague. The disease, not described before the latter part of the tenth century, occurred in at least six epidemics up to 1129, as described in the chronicles of the times.

According to an eye-witness, the epidemic which prevailed in the year 993 A.D.. (the *"ignis occultus"*—"occult fire") "detached the limbs from the trunk."

According to some accounts, the largest number of survivors of this dread scourge were those who sought aid in the Church of Notre Dame in Paris.

In the year 1129 a Benedictine monk named Michael Feliban stated that Paris and the rest of France was afflicted with the "mal des ardents"—a gangrenous affection that destroyed thousands of lives. The strangest characteristic of this particular epidemic was that debilitated persons, poor people and children were less frequently attacked than members of the healthier and richer classes.

The severe outbreak of the "mal des ardents" in Arras, became surrounded with legendary stories. One is to the effect that the people of Arras, having become terrified by the epidemic in their desperation sought cure from the Virgin Mary. The Virgin appeared to two jongleurs who were carrying a wax candle. Three vases filled with water into which a few drops of the sacred wax had dropped were offered to the sick who filled the church. The legend has it that 143 sufferers who used this therapy were immediately cured but the remaining ones who were not satisfied with the holy water and demanded wine died wretchedly on the spot. The holy candle received the name "joyel" (jewel).[11]

St. Anthony is often represented in art with a fire beside him in the act of protecting and blessing the sick. He is first mentioned with regard to this disease in the Annals of the Convent of Zanten (c. 857). The disease which bears his name occurred in at least six different epidemics up to the year 1129.

Haly Abbas attributes Saint Anthony's fire to a disorder of the black bile. He says: "There are nine kinds of black bile, from each of which humors arise, many diseases such as anthrax, fistula, cancer, lupus, St. Anthony's fire, and the like for which physicians have no sufficient remedies."

THE PLAGUE OF JUSTINIAN

One of the most frightful visitations which has ever befallen mankind bears the name "Plague of Justinian." It raged throughout almost the whole reign of that emperor (527-565) and continued beyond this period, prevailing for 70 years (from 531 to about 600). It ravaged the whole known world and did not spare even the most remote barbarians.

Like the epidemics of ancient times, "the Plague of Justinian" is said to have been attended by harbingers and precursors. Some of these are partially explicable on the basis of famine, inundation and war. Others relate the disease to comets, earthquakes, and solar eclipses. In one case, prior to the epidemic, an earthquake occurred which in a few moments destroyed most of the populous city of Antioch, and, from the resulting conflagration, laid the rest in ashes. It is said that 25,000 persons were buried in the ruins and the flames. In another case it was claimed that a hideous form of camel appeared which was interpreted as a harbinger of the serious plague to ensue.

Frequent "darkening of the sun" and numerous volcanic eruptions were alleged precursors of the epidemics. It is a fact that from the year 438, there raged for a year or more a general famine, which caused countless deaths especially in Italy. Among the Piceni alone, it is estimated that 50,000 peasants perished. Various premonitory markings are said to have appeared upon houses, stones, clothing and even food. The significance of such real or fancied phenomena magnified by religious superstition, was in itself frightful.

After a series of such harbingers and after a destructive conflagration which reduced to ashes the great hospital in that city, there appeared in Constantinople in the year 531 a deadly disease which originally was local. The general plague, as we have seen, originated in lower Egypt twelve years later (542). The "Plague of Justinian," according to eyewitnesses, apparently varied in many respects from the general plague both as to its onset and manifestations, but there are no reliable clinical data concerning it.

TYPHUS FEVER

Typhus fever has prevailed from the days of antiquity, but it was not definitely identified from the other *"morbi contagiosi"* until the later Middle Ages or the beginning of the Renaissance. Adams states that the term "typhus" was used by Hippocrates and that Galen used the word "typhodes" to signify typhus.[12]

The pestilence known as the Plague of Anthony or the Plague of Galen which lasted for sixteen years (164-180 A.D.) is believed to have been typhus. It is this epidemic which, according to some of his inimical contemporaries, prompted Galen to leave Rome. It began in the eastern frontier of the Roman Empire and spread rapidly to the western boundaries. It was introduced into Rome in 160 A.D. by the army which was returning from an expedition to Syria where it had been sent to suppress a revolt, and it spread rapidly.

Typhus fever was known in the Gaelic language as *"buidechar"* and this disease left a deep impression on the Gaelic tradition. Ireland appears to have been especially subjected to this destructive fever. The earliest record available in Ireland is that of the epidemic which occurred in the year 547 A.D. As a countermeasure against this scourge, a hymn was composed.[13] In the seventh century A.D. Kolman composed a hymn entitled "Sende" to save himself from the severe pestilence that raged in Ireland at that period. Gillies believes that "buidechar" was typhus fever which was known in the seventh century as "buidechar fever."[14]

Rhazes (842-926), in the eighth book of the "Continens," describes an eruptive disease which he named "blacciae." The eruption of this sickness is not elevated above the surface of the skin, but is marked by circular red and arid patches.

In the "Leech Book of Bald," typhus fever is known under the name "lent addle." The treatment of this disease is partly medicinal and partly by incantation, as is seen from the following: "A drink against lent addle fever is the herb rams' fall (menyanthes trifoliata), fennel and waybread."

The incantation recommended to go with the medicine is as follows:

"Let a man sing many masses over the worts, souse them with ale and holy water, boil very thoroughly, let the man drink a great cup full, as hot as he may, before the disorder will be on him; say the names of the four gospellers, and a charm, and a prayer, etc. Again, a divine prayer, etc., thine hand vexeth, thine hand vexeth."

Information with respect to typhus fever, according to De Renzi, comes from a chronicler in the convent of La Cava near Salerno, who states that in the month of August, 1083, he saw in the convent a very severe and malignant form of fever with petechiae and parotiditis.

CHAPTER XXIII

TUBERCULOSIS AND OTHER INFECTIOUS DISEASES DURING THE MIDDLE AGES

Tuberculosis has prevailed from the earliest times. The Old Testament perhaps refers to it when it alludes in three places to consumptive diseases (*shapahath*). Among the cardinal symptoms are mentioned extreme wasting of the body and phthisis bulbi. In the Biblical book of "Zechariah" the disease is described as follows: "In this shall be the plague . . . the flesh shall consume away, and the eyes shall consume away in their holes."

As far back as in the days of Hippocrates, tuberculosis was recognized as a disease characterized by the breaking down and destruction of tissues, by cough producing sputum with a putrid odor, and by the production of a discharge containing frothy blood. It most commonly occurs between the ages of 18 and 35.[1]

The name "phthisis," from the Greek word "φθίσις" meaning "wasting away," or "decay," was applied to this malady by Hippocrates. The Father of Medicine considered patients afflicted with this disease as incurable: "Many, and in fact, most of them died; and of those confined to bed I do not know of a single individual who survived for any considerable time. They died more suddenly than is common in such cases . . . Consumption was the most considerable of the diseases which then prevailed, and the only one which proved fatal to many persons. Most of them were affected by these diseases in the following manner: fevers accompanied with rigors, of the continual type, acute, having no complete intermission, but of the form of the semi-tertians, being milder the one day, and the next having an exacerbation, and increasing in violence; constant sweats, but not diffused over the whole body; extremities very cold, and warmed with difficulty; bowels disordered, with bilious, scanty, unmixed, thin, pungent, and frequent defecations. The urine was thin, colorless, unconcocted, or thick, with a deficient sediment, not settling favorably, but casting down a crude and unseasonable sediment. Sputa small, dense, concocted, but brought up rarely and with difficulty; and in those who encountered the most violent symptoms there was no concoction at all, but they continued throughout spitting crude matters. Their fauces, in most of them, were painful from first to last, having redness with inflammation; defluxions thin, small and acrid; they were soon wasted and became worse, having no appetite for any kind of food throughout; no thirst; most persons delirious when near death. So much concerning the phthisical affections."

Speaking of tuberculosis of the spine, Hippocrates states: "And when the gibbosity occurs in youth before the body has attained its full growth, in these cases the body does not usually grow along the spine, but the legs and the arms are fully developed, whilst the parts (about the back) are arrested in their development. And in those cases where the gibbosity is above the diaphragm, the ribs do not usually expand properly in width, but forward, and the chest becomes sharp-pointed and not broad, and they become affected with difficulty of breathing and hoarseness; for the cavities which inspire and expire the breath do not attain their proper capacity. And they are under the necessity of keeping the neck bent forward at the great vertebra, in order that their head may not hang downward; this, therefore, occasions great contraction of the pharynx by its inclination inward; for, even in those who are erect in stature, dyspnea is induced by this bone inclining inward, until it be restored to its place. From this frame of body, such persons appear to have more prominent necks than persons in good health, and they generally have hard and unconcocted tubercules in the lungs, for the gibbosity and the distension are produced mostly by such tubercles, with which the neighboring nerves communicate . . ."[2]

The so-called *"facies hippocratica"* gives a typical picture of the last stage of consumption: "Hollow eyes, sharp nose, sunken temples, tense skin, cold ears, parched and discolored face, livid eyelids, open mouth and blanched lips." This appearance is classical of terminal pulmonary tuberculosis.

Hippocrates had no other diagnostic procedures at his disposal than simple inspection and palpation. He had no stethoscope and no experience in percussion and auscultation. He had no tuberculin, no microscope, no roentgen rays and no cultures to confirm his diagnosis. In spite of all of these handicaps, his diagnoses appear to have been correct, and his therapeutics was far in advance of his time. He advised a young patient suffering from consumption to leave the city and rest in the sunshine, to eat nutritious foods and to imbibe much milk until his flesh returned. He stated the belief that phthisis is caused by small foci of pus.

Of the later ancient medical writers, none surpasses Aretaeus (about 50 A. D.) in his vivid description of tuberculosis. In his book *"De Causis et Signis Morborum"* (The Causes and Diagnosis of Disease), he described with extraordinary accuracy:

". . . the curved nails, shrunken fingers, slender, sharpened nostrils, hollow, glazy eyes, cadaverous look and hue, the waste of muscles and startling prominence of bones, the scapulae standing off like the wings of a bird; the thin, veneer-like frames, the limbs, like pinions, the prominent throats and shallow chests."

He remarked that "moist and cold climates are the haunts of it." Incidentally, Aretaeus was the first to make the following striking observation:

". . . Hemorrhage from the lungs is particularly dangerous, although patients do not despair even when near their end. The insensibility of the lungs to pain appears to me to be the cause of this, for pain is more dreadful than precarious; whereas in the absence of it, even serious illness is unaccompanied by fear of death and is more dangerous than dreadful."[3]

The external signs of habitus phthisicus, which were described in great detail by ancient medical writers, have not changed up to the present time. Indeed, that frail, undersized, emaciated body, with the long, narrow, flat chest, in which the ribs stand out prominently, the chest bone is depressed and the shoulder blades project in the back like two wings, is the classic description still applicable to a large number of patients with tuberculosis.

There is no evidence that Hippocrates suspected contagion or infection to be the cause of these symptoms, although his contemporary, the historian Thucydides, in his "History of the Peloponnesian War," although not discussing consumption, expressed a definite belief in the infectious character of plague and its transmission from one person to another. Describing the Plague of Athens, (see previous chapter) he stated: "Nay, they (physicians) themselves died most of all, inasmuch as they most visited the sick."

Galen believed in aerotherapy for tuberculosis. He ordered his patients to warm climates and to the sunny slopes of Vesuvius. He indicated the infectious character of consumption when he stated that it is a matter of experience that persons who sleep in the same bed with tuberculous patients, as well as those who live long with them or wear their clothes and use their linens, contract tuberculosis.

According to Galen, the phthisical constitution is marked by a narrow and shallow chest, with the scapulae protruding behind like wings; and hence he says chests of this type have been named "alar." He further states that there are two forms of consumption, the one originating in a defluxion from the head, and the other being connected with the rupture of a vessel in the lungs. Galen justly remarks, that, in the ordinary forms of phthisis, delirium is not a common symptom.

In the Middle Ages, tuberculosis of the lymph glands, particularly of the neck, was quite common. The terms "struma" and "scrofula" were applied to this form of tuberculosis. It was also known as "king's evil."

In England, the practice of "king's touch" dates from the reign of Edward the Confessor (died in the year 1056). In the year 1277, Edward I touched five hundred and thirty-three persons in one month. Henry VII reenforced the usual touch by giving each patient an "angel"—a kind of amulet consisting of a gold coin with the figure of St. Michael. The forms of prayer used by James I and Charles I in connection with the "royal touch" are found in contemporary prayer books. The time fixed for healing by touch was usually either Easter or Michaelmas (the 29th of September, the feast of the Archangel Michael). Persons who applied for treatment were examined by physicians and the latter had to testify that the former really suffered from the "evil." That the belief in the efficacy of "king's touch" was well nigh universal may be seen from the records of parish registers, which indicate that many poor persons were given financial assistance to enable them to proceed to London in order to be cured by the touch of the king. From "The Ecclesiastical History of the Venerable Bede" and from the diary of John Evelyn (1620-1700) dated 1660, we have a full description from eye witnesses of the ceremonies connected with the king's touch. The diary of Evelyn reads:

"This day, his Majesty, Charles the Second, came to London, after a sad and long exile . . . being seventeen years. This was also his birthday, and with . . . about twenty thousand horse and footmen, brandishing their swords, and shouting with inexpressible joy, the way strewed with flowers, the bells ringing, the streets hung with tapestry, fountains running with wine . . . Lords and nobles, clad in cloth of silver, gold and velvet; the windows and balconies seated with ladies; trumpets, music and myriads of people . . . so that they were seven hours in passing. I stood on the Strand and beheld it, and blessed God. And all this was done without one drop of blood shed and by the very army which had rebelled against him.

"His majesty began to 'touch' for the 'evil' according to custom, thus: His Majesty sitting in state in the banqueting house, the chirurgeons cause the sick to be brought, or led, up to the throne, where they kneel; the King strokes their faces or cheeks with both hands at once, at which instance a chaplain in his formalities says, 'He put his hands upon them, and he healed them.' This is said to everyone in particular. When they have been all touched, they come up again in the same order, and the other chaplain kneeling, and having angel-gold strung on white ribbon on his arm, delivers them one by one to His Majesty, who puts them about the necks of the touched as they pass, whilst the first chaplain repeats, 'That is the true light who cometh into the world.' Then follows an epistle with liturgy, prayers for the sick, lastly blessings; and then the Lord Chamberlain and the Comptroller of the Household bring a basin, ewer, and towel, for His Majesty to wash."

Another record of testimony is that of Richard Wiseman (1625-1686) a distinguished English surgeon:

"But when the physician upon trial shall find the contumaciousness of the disease, which frequently deluded his best care and industry, he will find reason of acknowledging the goodness of God; who hath dealt so beautifully with this Nation, in giving the kings of it, at least from Edward the Confessor downwards (if not for a longer time), an extraordinary power in the miraculous cure thereof. This our Chronicles have all along testified, and the personal experience of many thousands now living can witness for his Majesty that now reigneth, and his Royal Father and Grandfather. His Majesty that now is having exercised that faculty with wonderful success, not only here but beyond the seas in Flanders, Holland and France itself. The King of this last pretends to a Gift of the same kind, and hath often the good hap to be alone mentioned in Chirurgical Books, as the sole possessor of it, when the French themselves are the authors: yet even they, when they are a little free, will not stick to own the kings of England as partakers with him in that faculty; witness the learned Tagaultius, who in his 'Institutions' takes notice of King Edward's faculty, of doing the same cure, and the continuance of it in his successors. Italy as well as France hath made the like acknowledgments in the Book of Polydore Virgil, who reciting the gift given to Saint Edward the Confessor, doth subjoin these words: *'Quod quidem immortale munus quasi haereditario jure ad posteriores Reges Manavit: nam Reges Angliae etiam nunc tactu, ac quibusdam hymnis, non sine ceremoniis, prius recitatis, strumosos sanant'* ('Which immortal gift hath been derived as it were by an hereditary right to the later Kings; for the Kings of England even now also do cure the struma by touch. &c.')."

Shakespeare alludes to the "king's evil" in Macbeth when Malcolm says:

> "Since my here-remain in England,
> I've seen him do. How he solicits heaven
> Himself knows best; but strangely-visited people,
> All swol'n and ulcerous, pitiful to the eye,
> The mere despair of surgery, he cures
> Hanging a golden stamp about their necks
> Put on with holy prayers; and 'tis spoken,
> To the succeeding Royalty he leaves
> The healing benediction."

In the 15th century the practice of "royal touch" in England grew into a celebrated church ceremony. It found its way into the ritual and became a part of the prayer books. It was removed from the ritual in the year 1790. Of course, the healing of disease by holy men laying their hand upon the victim did not originate in England. We read in the New Testament that, when Jesus was in a certain city, "Behold a man full of leprosy, who seeing Jesus, fell on his face saying, 'Lord! if thou wilt thou canst make me clean,' and Jesus put forth his hand and touched him, saying: 'Thou wilt be then clean,' and immediately the leprosy departed from him."[4]

Pliny stated that Emperor Pyrrhus could cure diseases of the spleen by applying his right thumb on the sick person.[5] Tacitus relates that Vespasian (A. D. 9-79) cured blindness and paralysis by the mere touch of his hand.[6] In France the ceremony of "king's touch" goes back to the year 496 during the coronation of Clovis (466-511).

The practice of curing by apposition of the hand is undoubtedly an outgrowth of the miracle healing of the Anglo-Saxon ecclesiastics and saints. Of course, kings belonged to the circle of holymen. Why one disease like scrofula came to be regarded as especially amenable to cure by "royal touch" is not so apparent.

One day in the year 1684, the crowd seeking relief from "king's evil" by the touch of Charles II was so large that seven of the sick were trampled to death. It is of interest to note here that more people are reported to have died of scrofula during the time of Charles II than at any other period in English history.

CHAPTER XXIV

SMALLPOX DURING THE MIDDLE AGES

Smallpox is another infectious disease which has unquestionably prevailed since deep antiquity. The "pox" of the name is derived from the Anglo-Saxon "pocca" meaning "a pimple." The "small" is to differentiate the smallpox lesion from the "large pox" of syphilis. Similarly, the scientific termination "variola" is derived from the Latin "varus" also meaning "a pimple." Bishop Marius (470 A. D.), of Avenchia was the first to use the term "variola." Notwithstanding the authoritative view of Francis Adams that the Arabs were the first to give an account of smallpox,[1] there is evidence that this scourge was recognized in ancient India and that the goddess Sitala ("she who loves coolness"—a euphemistic expression for the dreaded goddess of smallpox) ruled over this disease. She was also sometimes known as "bisanta Chanli," the crude spring goddess, because the smallpox epidemics mostly prevailed during the spring season.

The Hindus believe that one who is ill with smallpox is actually possessed by the cruel goddess Sitala. The house which the sick person inhabits is therefore held sacred and anyone who enters such premises must take off his shoes and wash his feet as though he was entering a sacred temple. A Brahman will not enter the abode of the smallpox victim at all lest his presence anger the goddess and prove disastrous to the sick person.

It seems that the Vedics were cognizant of the fact that smallpox is contagious for a fire was kept burning continuously on the earthen fireplace and a lamp filled with vegetable oil was kept lit near the patient day and night. To warn the populace that smallpox was in the house, a branch of mistletoe or Indian lilac

(Nulia indica) was fastened on the outside door of the smallpox patient's abode.[2]

In the Anglo-Saxon "Leech Book of Bald," smallpox is simply called "pockes,'" the plural of a word signifying "pustules." On the first appearance of the disease, bleeding was ordered:

"Against pockes; very much shall one let blood, and drink a bowlful of melted butter; if they (the pustules) strike out, one shall dig each with a thorn, and then drop one-year alder-drink in; then they will not be seen."

This last instruction, evidently intended to prevent pitting, clearly identifies the disease. The early descriptions of smallpox were of a superstitious character. In Tibet, for example, when smallpox prevailed, nearly all the inhabitants of the village as yet untouched by the disease tried to prevent the disease from entering the village by placing thorns on the bridge over which the disease had to pass to enter. Those who died of the disease were thrown into the river and carried off by the stream.[3]

Noldeke writes that in one of the war expeditions of Abyssinia against Mecca (c. 550 A.D.), miraculous cures were effected during an epidemic of smallpox that broke out in the invading army.[4]

The early history of smallpox is somewhat obscure, owing to the difficulty of identifying the disease under the names given to it in ancient times. It is asserted that it was named by Gregory of Tours (538-595) when an epidemic form of smallpox struck Arabia, Egypt and southern Europe. There is evidence, however, that it appeared in France in A. D. 567, and according to a manuscript preserved in the University of Leyden, it appeared in Arabia in A. D. 572. The Arabian chronicler, Aaron the Presbyter (c. 622), gave an excellent description of smallpox as it prevailed in his time in his work, "The Pandect." In the tenth century, the Japanese isolated smallpox patients in special houses.

The most accurate and trustworthy medieval account of smallpox is found in the description of Rhazes (860-932),[5] who wrote a treatise on it in A. D. 923. Rhazes distinguished smallpox from measles. His pathology of smallpox is based upon the humoral theory of fermentation.[6] As to the predisposing causes of smallpox, Rhazes mentions a warm temperature. The latter part of autumn and beginning of spring, Rhazes states, are the most prevalent seasons of the year for smallpox.[7]

The symptoms of the disease, according to Rhazes are, ". . . continued fever, pain in the back, itching of the nose, disturbed sleep, and afterwards redness and fulness of the face, pain in the throat, difficulty in breathing, dryness of the mouth, thick spittle, hoarseness, headache, inquietude; and these symptoms are followed by the characteristic eruption of the smallpox or measles; but in the case of the latter there is more anxiety of mind, sick qualms, and heaviness of heart; and in that of the former there is more pain in the back, heat, and inflammation of the whole body, especially in the throat, with a shining redness."

Rhazes then lays down the rules of treatment: He directs to bleed from the arm at the commencement, provided the patient be more than fourteen years old; and by a cupping instrument if he is younger. He forbids, however, the withdrawal of blood after the eruption comes out. He permits light animal foods and acid foods. For drink he recommends water cooled with snow, cold spring water, or some dilute acid draught such as barley-water acidulated with pomegranate juice.[8]

Aaron the Presbyter, one of the authorities whom Rhazes cites, forbids the administration of cold water when the eruption is coming out. The medicines recommended by him are, for the most part, vegetable acids and astringents. The earlier part of his treatment consists of bleeding, cold drinks, and acid draughts. For hastening eruption, when this is deemed desirable, he directs us to wrap up the patient tightly in clothes; to rub his body all over; to keep him in a room which is not too cold; to give him some cold water to drink; to put on a double shirt; and to place near him two small basins of very hot water, one in front of and the other behind him, so that the vapor from them may be diffused all over his body excepting the face. He prudently directs us not to allow the moisture to cool upon the body, but to wipe it off carefully. He condemns the use of furnaces and hot baths as overheating and weakening. He recommends figs as being very effective in promoting the eruption. He recommends various astringent lotions or collyria in treating the eyes. For the care of the throat, he recommends bleeding when there is acute pain, and gargling with cold water, or with astringent decoctions, such as those of acid pomegranate, sumac, and the juice of mulberries. When the pustules on the limbs are large, he directs that they be opened. When there is great pain in the soles, he recommends rubbing them with warm oil or placing the feet in a receptacle of hot water. When the pustules need ripening, he directs the body be fomented with steam arising from a hot decoction of camomile, violets, and the like. When the pustules are too moist, he recommends the prompt application of pounded roses, rice-meal, or millet seed. For removing scabs and eschars, he favors rubbing them with warm oil of sesame, or oil of pistachios. He directs that the larger scars are to be cut off carefully without any application of oil. He points out the difference between distinct and confluent smallpox, and he remarks that the latter is far more dangerous than the former. He also states that when, in measles or smallpox, the eruption is suddenly turned inwardly, it is a fatal symptom. He inculcates the doctrine, time and again, that measles and smallpox are closely allied to each other.

Avicenna's description of smallpox and measles is very similar to that of Rhazes. He confidently pronounces that both diseases are contagious. He states that when smallpox proves fatal, it is usually because of involvement of the throat or ulceration of the bowels. Sometimes, he adds, the disease leads to bloody urine. He agrees with Rhazes that measles is a bilious affection, and he feels that it differs from smallpox only in that in the former the morbific matter is in smaller quantity and does not pass the cuticle. His treatment also is little different from that of Rhazes. At any period during the first four days of smallpox, he approves of venesection, but forbids it afterwards.

The elder Serapion's account of smallpox and measles, as pointed out by Haly Abbas, is very defective. He considers them along with apostemes, and his descriptions of the symptoms are far from accurate. Serapion (802-849) suggests that if these diseases occur during the winter season, the wood of tamarisk be burned beside the patient.

Avenzoar, in his "Treatise on Epidemical Diseases," treats only incidentally of measles and smallpox, for the cure of which he recommends gentle purgatives such as tamarinds, with cooling and acid drinks.[9]

According to Haly Abbas, variola is produced either by external causes, such as a pestilential state of the atmosphere, or from breathing the air of a place which has been tainted with the effluvia from the pustules of persons affected with the disease. It also may arise from an ebullition of the blood when it is loaded with gross humors which nature endeavours to cast outwards.

The early symptoms of smallpox include fever, swelling of the face, itching of the nose, inflammation and redness of the face and other members, heaviness of the head, and roughness of the throat.[10]

With regard to the treatment of variola and rubeola, Haly Abbas recommends venesection during any of the first three days; or, if the patient be a child, he directs the application of a cupping instrument to the back. The patient is then made to drink barley-water in which jujubes and sebesten plums have been boiled; syrup of poppies is to be added if the cough be troublesome or if the pain of the throat be severe. Spoon-meats prepared with spinach, orach, and the like, are also to be given. When the eruption does not come out properly, Haly Abbas recommends a decoction of fennel, lentils and figs to be taken cold.

The patient is to be kept on a scanty diet as in other fevers and his room is to be fumigated with aromatics such as sandalwood, myrtles, and roses. When constipated, the patient is to be given barley-water with manna, prunes, and the like. If diarrhea complicates the case, barley-water with myrtle seeds, gum Arabic, and Cretan earth (chalk?) is to be administered. Haly Abbas forbids purgatives after the seventh day, especially in rubeola, as there is danger of diarrhea or dysentery ensuing, and if these complications should set in, he directs that they be stopped with astringents. He recommends particular attention be paid to the eyes at the commencement of the disease and he directs that they be bathed with an astringent decoction. No animal food is to be allowed until the eruption and heat are gone.[11]

Smallpox under its many and diverse names has always been regarded with horror not only because of its great mortality but because of the loathsome disfigurement of the face which it produces. Men and women and boys and girls of all strata of society were alike attacked by this cruel disease. Smallpox seems to have been introduced into Europe from Asia where it has been recognized from time immemorial as a distinct epidemic affection. Among classic writers, it is likely that variola was mentioned by Galen who discussed it in his works. The Arabian medical sage, Rhazes, has this to say about this matter: "As to any physician who says that the excellent Galen has made no mention of smallpox and was ignorant of this disease, surely he must be one of those who has either never read his works or who has passed over them very cursorily."[12]

Smallpox was brought to Europe by the crusaders from Asia Minor in the thirteenth century. It spread through England in the thirteenth century. Gilbertus Anglicus (d. 1230), an English physician who was chancellor at the University of Montpellier, was first to recognize the disease in Europe as a highly contagious malady. Smallpox terrorized England throughout the sixteenth century.

Before vaccination was introduced, men were anxious to get the disease in a mild form as it was widely observed that this offered immunity against the severe form. In the Orient, a method of direct inoculation was practiced for centuries before reaching Europe. The method of inoculation was not as safe as that of vaccination. In China, smallpox was identified at an early period and the Chinese long practiced inoculation by direct transmission from person to person. Their method consisted of snuffing up in the nose a powdered crust from a smallpox pustule.

The Brahmans practiced inoculation by applying the crust to the skin of the healthy individual. The Persians actually swallowed crusts in their attempt to prevent virulent smallpox attacks. In Europe, before Edward Jenner discovered his method of immunization against smallpox by vaccination, inoculation was practiced by rubbing the clear fluid from the vesicals of a mildly ill smallpox patient into the arm of the one desiring protection.

This form of inoculation met with stubborn resistance in England because it was not altogether safe. On the whole, however, the attack which it produced on the one desiring immunity was mild and the probability of recovery was better than if the disease was acquired by chance during a virulent epidemic.

When in 1721, Lady Mary Wortley Montague, wife of the British Ambassador to Turkey, brought with her from Constantinople the discovery of inoculation against smallpox, it was so strenuously opposed that nothing short of its adoption by the royal family of England brought it into use. A similar resistance was shown when Edward Jenner (1749-1823) introduced his method of vaccination. It was opposed on the familiar ground that since smallpox was a punishment from God, no man had a right to interfere. It was rare to meet a person whose face had not been pitted by smallpox before and immediately after vaccination was discovered.

When the public began to doubt that God desired human beings to be disfigured, for if He wished them to be so, He would have created their faces already impitted, the ecclesiastics found another pretense for opposing vaccination—surely the voluntary introduction of disease into a healthy person is an interference with the will of God. The very year that Jenner published his "Inquiry into the Cause and the Effect of Variola," an antivaccination society was formed in England; its membership consisted largely of religious persons who opposed all scientific innovations. Even physicians denounced Jenner. Among his critics were Doctors Benjamin Mosley and William Browley, who came out with a book opposing vaccination. Their argument was not of a religious nature; they seriously claimed that persons after being inoculated with bovine vaccine assumed various bovine characteristics, such as, for example, growth of hair all over the body. Rumors spread like wildfire that persons who had been vaccinated went about bellowing like bulls. A distracted mother whose daughter had an abundant growth of black hair on her face blamed the bovine vaccine for her whiskers and mustache. Gradually, through the efforts of Jenner and his supporters, the opposition to vaccination weakened and the English people began to realize the advantage of the use of cow pox for vaccination.

Smallpox reached America in the seventeenth century. It was brought over from England to Philadelphia in the year 1661. During the great epidemic in Boston in 1792, out of a population of 18,000 inhabitants more than 8000 acquired the disease. Most of the remaining 10,000 escaped because they already had had the disease and were comparatively immune.[13]

The first physician to practice vaccination in America was Dr. Benjamin Waterhouse (1754-1846 of Harvard) of Boston. In 1802 he vaccinated seven of his children. He later took them to a smallpox hospital and exposed them to smallpox; none of them acquired it.

During the Revolutionary War George Washington ordered the inoculation of all recruits of the Continental Army who had not previously had smallpox. It is said that Washington inoculated himself and that his wife Martha was also so protected. Thomas Jefferson, however, was our first president to be vaccinated and this occurred three years after Jenner discovered his method of vaccination.

CHAPTER XXV

LEPROSY IN THE MIDDLE AGES

Leprosy was a widely spread disease in medieval Europe. The opinion has been widely held that it was brought to Europe from Asia Minor by the Crusaders, but there is considerable evidence that the disease prevailed in Europe in epidemic form long before the Crusades. According to Paul of Aegina, Aëtius, Actuarius, Oribasius, Rhazes and others, leprosy was widely disseminated in the early Middle Ages. The skin lesion of the disease described by these authorities was a circular, uniform, superficial eruption of the skin, like psoriasis, and the Greeks had coined the word *"lepra"* to cover such a condition.

There is, however, nothing in the Greek description of *"lepra"* to suggest in the remotest manner the modern form of leprosy. Indeed, the Greeks, when they referred to true leprosy, used the term elephantiasis.

Some form of leprosy was recognized by the Egyptians as early as 1500 B.C. The Hindus and Chinese for many centuries used chaulmoogra oil for the treatment of leprosy. This drug was introduced into the modern pharmacopoeia by Mourat in the year 1854.

Leprosy has been long prevalent among the Hindus. They distinguished eight different varieties: seven severe forms and one mild form. The Hindus apparently confused leprosy with various other skin diseases.

The Old Testament description of *"zaraat,"* which the Greek version renders "lepra," indicates that this condition included a number[1] of skin affections such as, for example, true leprosy, syphilis and psoriasis.

According to the text of Leviticus[2] the clinical features of leprosy are: (1) bright white spots or patches on the skin, the hair of which is also white; (2) depression of the patches below the level of the skin; (3) the existence of quick raw flesh; and (4) the spreading of the scabs or scales.

An authentic representation of the leprosy of the Middle Ages may be seen in a painting at Munich by Holbein of Augsburg made in the year 1516. St. Elizabeth is pictured giving bread and wine to a group of lepers including a bearded man whose face is covered with large reddish knobs; an old woman whose arm is covered with brown blotches, her leg bandaged with matter oozing through the dressings, her bare knee marked with discolored spots and her white head covered with a plaster; and a young man whose face and neck are spotted with patches of various sizes. Rudolph Virchow, 1821-1902, who made a study of leprosy in the Middle Ages, examined this picture carefully and came to the conclusion that the painter had represented the true eruptions of lepers.[3]

The medieval man viewed the cause of leprosy as a punishment of God inflicted upon those who had transgressed against Him. He examined the Old Testament and noted the case of Miriam, who was inflicted with leprosy because she spoke disrespectfully of her brother Moses;[4] the case of Joab and his family who were punished with *"zaraat"* for the murder of Abner; the case of Ghazi who was smitten because he had provoked the anger of the prophet Elisha;[5] and the case of Uziah who was punished with leprosy because he had usurped the priestly privileges.[6]

Medieval man dreaded leprosy and loathed the person who had so sinned against God as to be inflicted with this disease. A leper was looked upon as a public menace because he was dangerous to the community both physically and morally. Communities hastened to isolate him in order not to be close to a person who had suffered divine wrath.

In the year 583, the Council of Lyons laid down a strict regulation forbidding the free movement of lepers. Lepers were considered to be dead, at least symbolically. A leper could not inherit nor dispose of property except during life. During the tenth century, the son of a leper, if he were born after his parents had entered a leper house, was excluded from all heritage rights by law.

In 786, Charlemagne promulgated a decree ordering lepers to be cared for in special houses. Inhabitants of these leper houses were regarded as legally dead. They eked out a wretched livelihood by being permitted to beg from house to house one day during the week. When a leper was permitted out of doors, he had to wear a distinct garb to identify his disease. This outfit consisted of a black cloak with white patches attached to the breast and a tall hat with a white patch on the front of it. He was obliged to give audible warning of his proximity by sounding a wooden rattle or by ringing a bell. Even if he were in urgent need of provisions or other necessities of life, he was absolutely forbidden from entrance into public places to obtain such supplies. When objects were handed to him, they were attached to the end of a long stick which the leper was obliged to carry. The leper's presence at the door of a house on "begging days" was announced by the blowing of a horn; hence, lepers became known as "horn brattlers." Lepers belonging to rich prominent families were permitted to remain isolated in their own houses.

In Italy lepers were placed in San Lazaro hospital in Rome; hence the Italian leprosarium became known as "Lazarette" (a name which is used synonymously for "hospital" in many countries). In France, the leprosaria became known as *maladeria*. In France, on certain days of the week, the lepers were permitted to leave their isolation and go begging in town.

Before lepers were removed from the community to the leprosaria, men, women, and children gathered to participate in the ceremony which was associated with taking the leper to the leper house. In the presence of a large crowd, the sufferer was wrapped in a shroud, placed in a coffin and taken to the cemetery where he was compelled to step into an open grave. The priest then threw three shovelsful of earth upon him. The leper was then taken to the leprosarium where the priest gave him alms and holy water.

After the eleventh century the gruesome ceremony of the isolation of the leper was modified. Instead of token burial, a solemn mass was read as the community accompanied the accursed individual to his new home outside of the city. The presence of the leper in the leprosarium was symbolized by a white cross. The furnishings of his room were the utmost in wretched simplicity, consisting of an old table, chair and bed. Under the best circumstances, the leper was not expected to live long and after his death his furniture was put to the torch and his property became the possession of the leprosarium.

In Switzerland, the expulsion of the leper passed into the hands of the civil authorities. In England in 1346, Edward III ordered that all lepers be removed from London in a fortnight and that the magistrate should see that they were taken to a distant place from the city.

The leper was not permitted to wash his clothes in the river which was used by the community for washing. No barber was allowed to cut his hair or shave his beard. He was prohibited from entering public churches. Most leprosaria had their own chapels.

The diagnosis of leprosy was not always made by a physician. Frequently it was made by an unfriendly neighbor who quickly spread his discovery to the people of the community. The accused was then examined by a commission consisting of the bishop, several priests and a leper who was regarded as a specialist with regard to knowledge of the disease.

In later days, the authorized commission also included one or more physicians and barbers of the community. If the rumor was decided by the commission to be unfounded, the accused was given a certificate of good health which was posted in a public place.

Occasionally one tried to get rid of a competitor in business or an undesired neighbor by spreading rumors that he was a victim of leprosy. Such accusations ruined many innocent people's lives for it was not easy to eradicate such rumors once they were made public. Later a penalty was placed on those who spread such unfounded malicious rumors.

Occasionally lepers were accused of plotting a world wide conspiracy to make themselves masters of the world. In many places, lepers were suspected of spreading epidemics by poisoning wells and streams, and on the basis of such accusations, large numbers of them were ordered to be burned at the stake and their property confiscated by Phillip the Long.

Until the twelfth century, the final admission of a leper to a leper house was decided by an ecclesiastic. Later, as intimated, a physician was also consulted. In 1456 in Germany, municipal physicians or medical men of the faculty of Cologne attended to such admissions. The number of lepers in Europe in the Middle Ages may be estimated from the number of leprosaria built for them. In the year 1400, France and Germany alone had nearly 10,000 leprosaria. France at one time had at least 20,000 lepers.

One of the best descriptions of leprosy in the Middle Ages was given by the English monk Bartholmeus Anglicus (early thirteenth century) in his encyclopedic work "De Proprietalibus Rerum." He ascribes the causes of leprosy to the ingestion of hot food, the long use of strong peppers and garlic, the eating of corrupt meat—especially that of measled hogs and the bite of venomous worms that decays and corrupts the substance of the humors and of the organs. He divides leprosy into four forms: (1) leonina—that which affects the face; (2) elephantia—that which causes apparent overgrowth; (3) alopecia—that which affects the hair; and (4) that which causes apparent mutilation. He evidently recognized both the nodular and the mutilating forms.[7]

Bartholmeus Anglicus was born in England in the early part of the thirteenth century. He entered a Franciscan monastery. He was not a physician. His encyclopedic work, "De Proprietalibus Rerum" (1230-1240), is a compilation derived from some 150 authors among whom Aristotle plays the chief role. It must be borne in mind that the author had in view nothing more than a compilation and he stresses this both in the preface and in the epilogue. His principal intention was to pave the way for a better understanding of the Scripture in relation to technical subjects. His encyclopedia was very popular for several centuries as may be seen from its repeated translations and editions. It was used for a time as a textbook at the University of Paris, where students rented this work for a definite price. The work is divided into 19 books and treats all subjects. Books four and five cover physiology; book six deals with family life and book seven with medicine. His coverage of medicinal herbs is most informative and interesting. The medical book (book seven) is the one which deals with leprosy. Among other diseases covered are halitosis, colic, dysentery, worm infestations, jaundice, dropsy, insanity and epilepsy. Bartholmeus was aware that leprosy was contagious as well as hereditary.

Bartholmeus' encyclopedia was translated into English by John of Tervisa in 1397-98. The Spanish translation of Vicente is considered a classic in the Spanish language. Other translations are in French and Italian.[8]

Two forms of leprosy are presently recognized: the nodular or tubercular form and the anesthetic, nervous or mutilation form. Generally both forms are present concurrently in one patient. The nodular form begins, as a rule, as round or irregularly shaped spots, commonly of a mahogany or sepia color. These often disappear and are followed by the appearance of nodules. In an advanced stage, the face is covered with firm, livid, nodular, elevations. The nose, lips, and ears are swollen beyond their natural size, the eyelashes and eyebrows are lost, and the eyes are staring. The whole syndrome produces a hideous disfigurement. As the disease progresses, insensibility of the skin and paralysis ensue, and the fingers and toes may rot away.

Leprosy began to decline at the beginning of the fourteenth century, perhaps due to the strict isolation of the patients. In 1871 Hansen announced the discovery of the mycobacterium leprae. It is now generally accepted that this mycobacterium is the etiologic factor producing the disease.

CHAPTER XXVI

DIPHTHERIA DURING THE MIDDLE AGES

Diphtheria is a modern name for an ancient disease which prevailed both in epidemic and endemic forms in the Middle Ages. It was known to Hippocrates and Galen. Hippocrates, in his chapter entitled "On the Prognostics,"[1] describes an affection which has all the earmarks of diphtheria.

"Ulceration of the throat with fever is a serious affection and if any other of the symptoms formerly described as being bad is present, the physician ought to announce that his patient is in danger. Those quincies are most dangerous and most generally prove fatal which make no appearance in the fauces nor in the neck but occasion very great pain and difficulty of breathing. These induce suffocation on the first day, the second day, the third day or the fourth day."

According to Pierre Brettonneau (1778-1862), Aretaeus, the greatest clinician of the Graeco-Roman period (second century A.D.), refers to diphtheria under the title "Ulcero Syriaca." His description of this disease adequately describes pharyngeal diphtheria.

Aretaeus speaks of a pestilential disease with ulceration of the throat marked by white and grey eschars:[2]

"Ulcers occur on the tonsils; some, indeed, of an ordinary nature, mild and innocuous; but others of an unusual kind, pestilential and fatal. Such as are clean, small, superficial, without inflammation and without pain, are mild; but such as are broad, hollow, foul, and covered with a white, livid, or black concretion, are pestilential. Aphtha is the name given to those ulcers. But if the concretion has depth it is an eschar and is so called; but around the eschar there is formed a great redness, inflammation, and pain of the veins, as in carbuncle; and small pustules form, at first few in number, but others coming out, they coalesce, and a broad ulcer is produced. And if the disease spread outwardly to the mouth, and reach the columella (uvula) and divide it asunder, and if it extend to the tongue, the gums, and alveoli, the teeth also become loosened and black; and the inflammation seizes the neck; and these die within a few days from the inflammation, fever, foetid smell, and want of food. But, if it spread through the thorax by the windpipe, it occasions death by suffocation within the space of a day. For the lungs and heart can neither endure such smells, nor ulcerations, nor ichorous discharges, but coughs and dyspnoea supervene.

"The cause of the mischief in the tonsils is the swallowing of the cold, rough, hot, acid and astringent substances; for these parts minister to the chest as to the purposes of voice and respiration; and to the belly, for the conveyance of food; and to the stomach for deglutition. But if this affection occur in the internal parts, namely, the belly, the stomach, or the chest, an ascent of the mischief by eructions takes place to the isthmus faucium, the tonsils, and the parts there; wherefore children, until puberty, especially suffer, for children in particular have large and cold respiration; for there is most heat in them; moreover, they are intemperate in regard to food, having a longing for varied food and cold drink; and they bawl loud both in anger and in sport; and these diseases are familiar to girls until they have their menstrual purgation. The land of Egypt especially engenders it, the air thereof being dry for respiration, and the food diversified, consisting of roots, herbs of many kinds, acrid seeds, and thick drink; namely, the water of the Nile, and the sort of ale prepared from barley. Syria also, and more especially Coelosyria, engenders these diseases, and Syrian ulcers.

"The manner of death is most piteous; pain sharp and hot as from carbuncle; respiration bad, for their breath smells strongly of putrefaction, as they constantly inhale the same again into their chest; they are in so loathsome a state that they cannot endure the smell of themselves; countenance pale or livid; fever acute, thirst as if from fire, and yet they do not desire drink for fear of the pains it would occasion; for they become sick if it compress the tonsils, or if it return by the nostrils; and if they lie down they rise up again as not being able to endure the recumbent position, and if they rise up, they are forced in their distress to lie down again; they mostly walk about erect, for in their inability to obtain relief they flee from rest, as if wishing to dispel one pain by another. Inspiration large, as desiring cold air for the purpose of refrigeration, but expiration small, for the ulceration, as if produced by burning, is inflamed by the heat of the respiration. Hoarseness, loss of speech supervene; and these symptoms hurry on from bad to worse, until suddenly falling to the ground they expire."[3]

Asclepiades says that synanche is a moistening or a flow of moisture to the throat especially to its highest part coming down from the head.

That diphtheria prevailed in the Middle East in the early Middle Ages may be seen from some scattered paragraphs in the Babylonian Talmud. Referring to a disease known as *ascara* (Greek "eschar"), the Talmud states that it is a most fatal disease. If even one case of the disease was discovered in a community, it was required to announce this catastrophe to the community by blowing a horn (*shofar*). In all other infectious diseases the horn was only blown after three cases were discovered. "*Ascara*," says the Talmud, "attacks children at night."[4] *Ascara* is particularly fatal to infants. Adults however are not exempt.[5] The disease begins throughout the entire body but localizes itself in the mouth.[6] The patient dies from suffocation.[7] *Ascara* cannot be cured: "It is like a thorn in a ball of wool which gets more twisted when one tries to unravel it."[8]

Rabbi Eliezer ben Josse states that at one time when he was on board a vessel, he was stricken with *ascara*. The disease was transmitted to the mouth of a sailor who happened to pass near him.[9]

These several scattered passages give in their totality a description of some of the most important symptoms of diphtheria:

Ascara is a fatal disease prevailing largely among children, its place of attack is in the mouth and it is highly contagious and infectious.[10] As a prophylactic measure against *ascara*, Rabbi Yohanan advises the use of lentils. It is interesting to note that lentils were one of the ingredients of a gargle prescribed by Aretaeus and that Hippocrates and Pliny recommended lentils for ulcerative stomatitis.[11]

Caelius Aurelianus gives a graphic description of "synanche": "Synanche, gets its name from its similarity to hanging, for when it is fatal its effect is like that of choking by a hangman's noose, the Greek word for 'hanging' being *'anchone.'* [12]

"We, however, following Soranus' view, apply the term 'synanche' to difficulty in swallowing and acute choking occasioned by a severe inflammation of the throat, or of those parts which are used in swallowing food and drink. In addition to 'difficulty in swallowing' we include 'swift or acute choking' to distinguish this disease from inflammation of the tonsils or of the uvula. For, while it is true that in synanche there is always an inflammation of the tonsils and uvula, it is not true that whenever there is an inflammation of these parts we have a case of synanche. . . . As the disease becomes even more severe, all the parts become inflamed, including the neck and face; there is a flow of thick fluid and saliva; the eyes bulge and are bloodshot; and the blood vessels are distended. And if the disease grows still worse, the tongue hangs out of the mouth, the throat is parched and dry, limbs cold and numb, and pulse rapid and thick. The patient finds it hard to lie, especially on his back or side, and frequently, too, he wants to sit up, his speech is indistinct, confused, and accompanied by pain. And if the disease begins to move toward a fatal conclusion, the face turns blue, the voice is lost, there is a wheezing sound in the throat and chest, any liquid taken in is returned, there is failure of the pulse (Greek *'asphygmia'*); in some cases the patient makes a sound like that of a dog, and in some cases there is foaming at the mouth. Death then inevitably follows." [13]

Caelius Aurelianus approves the use of fomentations, inhalations of steam and applications of hot water or hot sponges to the neck and throat and he recommends cupping of the neck to draw off the inflammation from inside the throat.

Rhazes points out the contagious nature of "synanche" in the following paragraph:

"It happens in a bad form (epidemic) during the spring of certain years. At such times it is best to anticipate the malady by venesection and by extracting blood from the legs with cupping instruments. Some Arabic writers advocate the use of astringents and gargles made of mustard and pepper."

Diphtheria prevailed in Spain in epidemic form six times between 583 and 600. An early description of the disease is found in the Spanish medical literature of the nineteenth century, under the title "Enfermedad del Garrotello"—named after the running noose employed in Spain to strangle criminals. From Spain diphtheria reached Naples where it was described by F. Nola (1620) and others. Marco Aurelio Severino (1580-1656), a well known Italian anatomist of Naples, performed the first operation of tracheotomy in diphtheria in the year 1610 during the epidemic of Naples. The disease was named "diphtherite" in 1826 by Pierre Bretonneau.[14] (1771-1862)

In the sixteenth, seventeenth and eighteenth centuries, epidemics of diphtheria appear to have frequently prevailed in many parts of Europe: particularly in Holland, Spain, Italy, France and England and were described by physicians of these countries under various titles. It is probable that other diseases of a similar nature were also included in their descriptions. No accurate account of this affection was given until Pierre Bretonneau of Tours read his celebrated thesis on the subject before the French Academy of Medicine in 1826.[15] He pointed out that "angina suffocativa," "synanche maligna," "putrid sore throat" and other forms of malignant sore throat are one and the same disease and he gave the name "diphtheria" to this clinical entity.

The exciting cause of diphtheria was identified in 1883 by Klebs and Loeffler. The microorganism causing it became known as the Klebs-Loeffler bacillus.

CHAPTER XXVII

CHOLERA, DYSENTERY AND TRACHOMA IN THE MIDDLE AGES

Cholera (from the Greek *"chole"* meaning *"bile"* and *"rae"* meaning "to flow") was well described by Hippocrates. The Father of Medicine recognized two kinds of cholera: dry and wet.[1] "In dry cholera the belly is distended with wind, there is rumbling in the bowels, pain in the sides and loins, no dejections, but, on the contrary, the bowels are constipated. In such a case you should guard against vomiting, but endeavor to get the bowels opened. As quickly as possible give a clyster of hot water with plenty of oil in it, and having rubbed the patient freely with unguents, put him into hot water, laying him down in the basin, and pouring the hot water upon him by degrees; and if, when heated in the bath, the bowels be moved, he will be freed from the complaints. To a person in such a complaint it will do good if he sleep, and drink a thin, old, and strong wine; and you should give him oil, so that he may settle, and have his bowels moved, then he will be relieved. He must abstain from all other kinds of food; but when the pain remits, give him asses' milk to drink until he is purged. But if the bowels are loose, with bilious discharges, tormina, vomiting, a feeling of suffocation, and gnawing pains, it is best to enjoin repose, and to drink hydromel, and avoid vomiting."[2]

Galen states that cholera is a very acute and severe disease which rapidly depletes the patient and is characterized by violent vomiting, diarrhea and abundant secretion. He states that colic develops shortly after the fever starts. The fever of cholera, like the fever of dysentery, is indicative of dangerous changes going on in the viscera.[3]

The Middle Ages physicians including Paul of Aegina follow Aretaeus who defines cholera to be "a retrograde movement of the matters in the body upon the stomach and intestines, consisting of a discharge upwards and downwards of bile, which if the disease proves fatal, becomes black; and, at the same time, the extremities are cold, with profuse sweats, pulse small and dense, constant straining to vomit, and tenesmus."

Among the symptoms of cholera listed by Aretaeus are spasms and contractions of the muscles in the legs and arms, borborygmus (rumbling of the intestinal flatus), tormina (griping pains in the bowels), and syncope. Cholera, he says, is occasioned by continued indigestion and proves fatal by producing convulsions, suffocation, and retching.

With regard to the treatment of cholera, Aretaeus cautions the physicians not to stop the discharge at first, but to encourage it by the frequent administration of tepid water. When cholera is attended by tormina and coldness of the feet, he advises the application of hot oil of rue to the belly and the rubbing of the legs to restore heat. When the feces are all evacuated, he recommends the administration of cold water to compose the stomach. When concurrent with threadiness and rapidity of the pulse there are profuse sweats and delirium, he advocates the adding of a small quantity of wine to the water. He concludes his remarks on therapy by saying, that, if the symptoms instead of improving, should get worse after this treatment, it is advisable for the physician to give up the case at once.[4]

Alexander of Tralles' concept of cholera differs little from that of Aretaeus. In certain cases, he suggests the use of poppies to sedate insomnolency and wine to support the patient's strength.

Marcellus Empiricus (c. 385) recommends various astringent remedies, both externally and internally. Myrtle-wine, he says, will stop the vomiting of cholera. He also favors the use of opium.

Haly Abbas states that cholera is characterized by a discharge of bile. In mild cases when the strength of the patient continues to be good and the fecal discharge is not immediate, he is of the opinion that vomiting is to be encouraged by giving the patient tepid water with oil of sweet almonds to drink. When there is great prostration of strength and tendency to dehydration, he directs the sprinkling of water on the patient's face, the application of ligatures to his limbs and the rubbing of his feet and legs with a calefacient oil.

Haly Abbas emphasizes that at all costs the diarrhea is not to be rashly stopped unless it becomes excessive, in which case astringents are to be given, such as extracts of roses and pomegranate fruit. He advocates the application of a cupping instrument over the stomach.

Serapion and Rhazes mention an emetic as a remedy for stopping the copious rectal discharge. Rhazes recommends draughts of tepid water, the application of snow over the stomach and ligatures to the extremities and the internal use of wine and astringents. Avicenna's plan of treatment is exactly the same as that of Rhazes. All medieval authorities seem to encourage sleep.

Cholera has been classified into three main varieties: (1) cholera morbus—an acute gastroenteritis with diarrhea, cramps, and vomiting usually caused by improper food. (2) Cholera infantum—a common and often fatal, noncontagious diarrhea of young children prevailing in the summer months. (3) Cholera Asiatica (Cholera Indica or Malignant Cholera). The first two varieties as described by ancient and medieval physicians were not epidemic. Few if any of the European medieval authors list this form of cholera. Among the list of contagious diseases enumerated by Bernard de Gordon in his "Lilium" no mention is made of cholera.[5] This lack of interest in cholera on the part of the European doctors has led various modern authorities to believe that Asiatic cholera was unknown in Europe before the nineteenth century.

The malignant form of cholera is the most fatal type of cholera and has been known by such names as Asiatic cholera, Indian cholera, epidemic cholera, algid (cold) cholera, cholera sicca (death occurs before diarrhea) or fulminating cholera.

India and Bengal are said to have been the native haunts of cholera, whence it spread and swept over large parts of the world. Large epidemics broke out during the Middle Ages in the Middle East, Egypt, and Abyssinia. In Russia an endemic form always exists. A number of outbreaks occurred during the First World War particularly in the Balkans and Mesopotamia.

In India and China, cholera ranks in severity with bubonic plague. Cholera is still one of the most fatal diseases in India. A severe epidemic occurred in India in 1781. The Bengal epidemic of 1823 spread over the whole of Hindustan, reached the Caucasus and the Volga basin and menaced all of Europe.[6] During the year 1934, as many as 287,000 cases were reported in Asia. Out of these, 147,000 died—a mortality of over 50 per cent.

In America epidemics broke out in the years 1826, 1848 and 1870. It appeared early among the settlers of New England. John Huham (1692-1768) gives an excellent description of this disease. Samuel Bard (1742-1821) of New York wrote an excellent essay on the subject.[7]

The cause of cholera, which was ascribed to atmospheric and dietary conditions by ancient and Middle Age physicians, was discovered by Robert Koch in 1883 to be the Vibrio comma (Spirillum cholerae asiaticae).

DYSENTERY

Dysentery (from the Greek "dys" meaning "difficult" and "enteron" meaning "intestine") has prevailed throughout antiquity and the Middle Ages both in endemic and epidemic forms, particularly in the warm climates of the East. It was also known as "bloody flux" because of the bloody stools due to ulceration of the intestines that accompanied severe cases.

Dysentery is still endemic in the Far East. The cause of the disease was attributed to atmospheric changes and digestive disturbances. Hippocrates deals with dysentery in several chapters of his "On Air, Water and Places."[8]

In his aphorisms, Hippocrates states: "Dysentery, if it commences with black bile, is fatal." "If a person is ill of dysentery and substances resembling flesh be discharged from his bowels, this is a fatal symptom." [9]

Galen in his "Commentary on Hippocrates" disagrees with the Father of Medicine on the causes of dysentery but he does not propose any other reasons for its appearance.

The Talmudists viewed dysentery (*"choli meayim"* meaning "intestinal disease") as a most dreaded disease. However, *"choli meayim"* appears to have included many gastrointestinal diseases. The difference in the various types was not in kind but in degree of severity. This classification included even painful tympanites ("tapuach;" Aboth d. R. Nathan, 41a). Rabbi Samuel, the famous Babylonian physician thought that *"choli meayim"* was caused by imprudence of diet and too varied changes in food.[10]

The most fulminating form of *"choli meayim"* is *"burdam,"* signifying a cistern of blood, because of the occasionally bloody stools accompanying the disease. The symptoms of *"burdam"* are severe pain in the abdomen and diarrhea and this condition results in sudden death. "One may die while walking." Visiting such patients was strictly prohibited.[11]

Caelius Aurelianus describes the symptoms of dysentery as follows: The primary sign of the disease is a slimy discharge from the bowels made up of small particles and a thick fluid. At first the fluid is the natural solid matter within the intestines reduced to a liquid state; but later there are various bloody and bilious, and sometimes sanious and feculent discharges with particles of clotted blood. There may also be livid discharges and some containing pieces of flesh adhering to long membranes. The discharges have a heavy odor, and the ulceration is painful; there is also loss of appetite, thirst, and a burning sensation in the inner parts. Other symptoms are sleeplessness and in some cases fever, uneasiness, tossing dullness of the senses, rumbling in the intestines, abdominal distention and gas, difficulty in urination, vomiting, throbbing in the precordial region and cold numbness. The tongue may be moist or very dry and rough and the complexion ashen or bluish. At times there is colliquation of the body. Decomposition of food is accompanied by a burning sensation. There is a continual and unabating desire to empty the bowels and, in connection with that feeling, an irritation throughout all the intestines or in the anus or neighboring parts. There is inflammation either in the small intestines or in the large intestines. "It is hardly possible for the ulceration to be present at one and the same time throughout all the intestines, since death would come first."

Caelius Aurelianus continues: "Now we may infer that the ulceration is in the small intestines if there is a sensation of pain above the umbilicus or beginning at that point (and extending upward), and if the discharges from the bowels are always thin. But if the ulceration is in the large intestines, the sensation of pain is then below the umbilicus, and the discharges from the bowels contain fleshy matter; and, in fact, the feces are frequently compact and solid when only the rectum is affected by the disease, and especially the lower parts of the rectum. That is to say, ulceration of the small intestines prevents the digested food from taking the usual form of fecal matter." [12]

Celsus recommends rest for dysentery patients as motion proves injurious to the ulcers. His medical treatment consists of external cataplasms, washing with warm water in which vervain herbs have been boiled, astringent foods, barley-water decoction of linseed, the yolk of an egg mixed with rose water and tepid water drinks either alone or mixed with strong wine. When the site of the disease is high up in the intestine he advises abdominal section.

Alexander of Tralles points out the importance of attending to the parts of the intestines most affected by ulcerations. His treatment depends upon the exciting cause which is either disorders of the liver which he calls "hepatic dysentery" or derangement of the intestines. In most cases he prescribes gentle drugs and in some cases he approves of bleeding.

Alexander of Tralles states that dysentery may arise primarily or secondarily in the intestines. The clinical course depends on the seat of ulceration. If the upper part of the small intestine is affected, severe abdominal pain is followed after several hours by thin membranous bloody stools. Ulcerations lower down in the small intestine produces early evacuation with a slight admixture of pus. Ulcerations in the large intestine cause pain in the lower abdominal region, tenesmus and curved stools. Rectal ulcerations produce only tenesmus and bloody movements.

In the treatment of dysentery, the degree of diarrhea and the seat of ulceration are to be taken into account. If the ulcers are in the upper part of the intestine, remedies are to be administered by the oral route; if in the lower part, by the anus. Severe diarrhea calls for the administration of demulcent and binding decoctions, astringents, vegetable extracts, opiates, powdered gall pills, arsenic, enemas, astringent fluids, warm poultices, plasters and inunctions.

Aëtius follows Galen's treatment internally. When severe inflammation is present, he advocates the letting of a small quantity of blood from the arms.

Avicenna and Haly Abbas recommend rectal instillations containing arsenic. Rhazes attributes dysentery to debility of the retentive power of the liver and derangement of the bile. In protracted dysentery, he suggests that snow be applied to the abdomen. No other authorities suggest the application of cold in chronic dysentery. Haly Abbas speaks of two forms of dysentery: intestinal and hepatic. For the intestinal type which is characterized by ulceration of the intestines, he recommends clysters. If the ulcers are in the rectum, he suggests tents soaked in a solution of quick lime or arsenic.

Paul of Aegina, who usually selects that which seems to him best of the ancient writers, says: "If blood and ulcerous shreds are mixed with the feces and the patient has griping pains in the bowels, you may be sure that the site of ulceration is in the small intestine and is to be remedied by medicine swallowed by the mouth; but if the feces passed are unmixed with blood it is an infection of the large intestine and will yield rather to clysters." Paul also distinguished between hepatic and intestinal dysentery. Paul gives a large number of drugs. Here are two of his formulas:

℞ Sumac   ʒi
    Gall
    Pomegranate rind, a. a. ʒiv
Signa: Administered ʒi in a tablespoon of urine.

℞ Opium   ʒi
    Sumac   ʒi
    Gall
    Gum
    Acacia, a. a.   ʒii
Signa: administer ʒi diluted in urine.

Paul of Aegina devotes several pages to the materia medica of dysentery.

It is evident that neither the ancient nor the medieval physicians identified dysentery as a special affection and, of course, they were not aware of its true etiology. They realized the gravity of the affection when the attack was in a malignant form.

Medicine had to wait until the year 1874 for Prof. Loesch to discover the pathogenic ameba present in many cases of dysentery; he found this protozoan organism in the feces of a Russian patient suffering from this disease. In 1903 Schaudinn differentiated the pathogenic ameba, Endameba histolytica which is the etiologic agent of amebic dysentery from the harmless ameba commonly found in the intestine of man—Endameba coli.

It should be borne in mind that bacteria and viruses can also cause dysentery, although these forms are usually less virulent than the amebic.

TRACHOMA DURING THE MIDDLE AGES

Trachoma (Ophthalmia Granulosa from the Greek "trachys" meaning "rough") is an infectious disease occurring in endemic form in Egypt and the Middle East. It is one of the most ancient diseases known. One of the oldest medical documents, the Papyrus Ebers (1500 B. C.), describes under the name of "blear eyes" or "dripping eyes" a form of ophthalmia differing from the ordinary form by its profuse purulent discharge and other disturbing eye symptoms. A mixture of equal parts of verdigris and onion was prescribed for this condition.

Aristophanes (c. 448-385 B. C.) refers to trachoma in his "Philus" and other plays. The overcrowdedness and unsanitary conditions of the Athenians during the Peloponnesian War (431-404 B. C.) caused the affection to spread rapidly and increase its virulence.

The Greeks and Romans left no positive description of trachoma so that the very name of the affliction is in doubt. One, however, can hardly agree with the eminent ophthalmologist and historian, J. Hirschberg, in his statement: "Dem Klassischen Altherthum war der Begriff der Agyptischen Ophthalmia ganz fremd" ("To classic antiquity the conception of Egyptian ophthalmia was totally foreign."). Indeed, there is ample evidence to show that trachoma was well known to the physicians of these countries in ancient times.

The Roman oculists, although they left no special name for trachoma, often put the words "ad aspritudo" on the seal of the collyrium intended to cure this disease.

Hippocrates in the third book of his "Natural Diseases," prescribes treatment for a form of ophthalmia. This treatment consists in rubbing the inner surface of the lids with a layer of Milesian wool wound about a spindle-shaped core of hard wood until the blood ceases flowing, and in its place, a thin, water-like liquid appears. Cauterization of the well-rubbed surface completed this often extremely effective procedure. In fact, it is doubtful if any better treatment was developed until the development of modern antibiotics and chemotherapeutic agents. This treatment was closely followed up by the instillation of collyria which contained, as a rule, the peroxide of copper.

Alexandrian ophthalmology, as preserved by Celsus, shows considerable advance in the recognition of trachoma. Celsus gives an excellent description of this disease which he called "aspritudo." The name trachoma was not introduced until three centuries later by Theodore Severus (3rd century). Celsus makes a clear distinction between moist and dry ophthalmia (ophthalmia and xero-ophthalmia).

"Among some people," writes Celsus, "the eyes are never dry; a muco-purulent discharge escapes always from the visual organs and with it is associated a roughness of the lids. Such an affection makes the life of the individual miserable and in some instances the vision is destroyed."[13]

Celsus' treatment for trachoma is essentially that of Hippocrates. He states: "And others are useful too; which are calculated to lessen the roughness of which I am going to speak. This commonly follows an inflammation of the eyes; at times it is more violent, at others more slight. Sometimes, too, a roughness occasions a lippitude, and that again increases the roughness; and in some it is short, in others it continues a long time, and so as to be hardly curable. In this kind of disorder some scrape the thickened hard eye-lids both with a fig-leaf and speculum asperatum, and sometimes with a knife; and turning them up, they rub them every day with medicines. This ought not be practiced, unless in case of a considerable and inveterate roughness; nor even then often. For the same end is better obtained by a suitable regimen and proper medicines. Therefore we shall use exercise and the bath more frequently; and foment the eyelids with plenty of warm water."

Celsus also mentions the "collyrium of Hierax," which, he says "is powerful against a roughness." He approves of escharotics such as cupric sulfate.

The Talmudic doctors recognized trachoma under the term of *"ainei dolphos"* ("dripping eyes"). Those that were affected with this disease were known as *"baalei reathan"* ("men of sight").[14] The chief symptom of the disease is a profuse discharge from the eyes and nose.[15] Some writers, however, believe that *"ziran"*[16] was the Aramaic name for trachoma.[17] It is interesting to note that in the Papyrus Ebers, trachoma is also known as "dripping eyes." The remaining symptoms consisted of the presence of flies on the lids and the escape of saliva from the mouth.

Dr. Mazia of Jerusalem, who treated many patients with severe cases of granular lids, noticed its connection with a "scrofulous diathesis." In children trachoma is frequently accompanied by enlarged and infected tonsils, glandular involvement and the escape of saliva from the mouth.

It appears that the Babylonians were free of trachoma in Talmudic days. Rabbi Yohanan asked, "Why are there no cases of *baalei reathan* in Babylonia?" He gave as the chief reason, "because they bathe in the Euphrates."[18]

Galen has this to say about the treatment of severe trachoma: "In severe cases of trachoma, physicians have, in their perplexity, thought out a singular remedy; namely, having everted the lids, to cleanse them thoroughly, and then to scrape them off without the application of drugs. A few scrape only superficially with a small sharp spoon . . . and afterwards wipe up with a soft sponge that which flows away, and then astringe the lids as far as any roughness remains. Others employ also the superficially rough skins of certain sea-animals in a manner entirely appropriate for this purpose. One of my teachers even prepared an eye-pencil of pumice-stone, and, having everted the lids, rubbed the roughness away from them with this instrument. As a matter of course, a person must pulverize the pumice-stone, and make it into a pencil with tragacanth or gum. When, after the employment of the pencil mentioned, the discharge begins to cease, then we may venture to rub into the lids purifying medicines; but, at first, we should employ only a weak solution, and later, when it is found that the patient bears (the treatment) well, we should gradually strengthen it." Both Galen and later Aëtius favor caustics such as sal ammoniac, calamine and aqua aeria.

In the Middle Ages, the scourge of trachoma was endemic in many Eastern countries. The Byzantine physicians understood the gross pathologic changes in trachoma and recognized granulation as the chief symptom. They also suggested remedies to combat the disease.

The first distinguished physician of the Byzantine Middle Ages was Aëtius of Amida (A.D. 502-575), one of the most exhaustive compilers of Greek medicine. In his "Tetrabiblos," Aëtius gives a most graphic description of trachoma:

"The granules, then, which many also call 'rawnesses,' arise, often, as a result of unskillful treatment, for they appear when physicians make too many instillations. Just as in the case of external injuries, inunction produces proud flesh, in the same way, in the disease which is under discussion, the origin is to be conceived. The disease also arises after chronic, non-acid discharges; for, were they acid, they would destroy the eye before this disease became engrafted on the lids. The affection also arises sometimes without preceding discharge, and without the presence of any obvious cause. And these cases are in no way similar to those arising from discharge; for, in the cases first described (those from catarrh) the everted lids look somewhat raw, granular, and reddened with blood, while, in the cases which arise without discharge, one sees as it were little grains of millet, or small peas, protruding on the inner surface of the lids; and this kind is harder to cure than the others. Furthermore, one should, in these conditions, make the following distinctions: (1) The nappiness is superficial and accompanied by redness. (2) In the granular condition the alteration and prominence are greater; simultaneously with pain and heaviness, both conditions are united with humectation of the eye. (3) The so-called 'fig-formations' show still higher elevations which appear as if notched, and resemble nothing so much as a fig that has burst. (4) The callous formation is an inveterate roughness, or nappiness, and shows the altered parts hardened and calloused —a few physicians try to shave off the asperities, some with the knife, others with fig leaves. But this attempt is very harmful; for, as a rule, in that way the formations are increased and hard scars produced, together with an obstinate discharge, in addition to which the eyes are always irritated by the hard scars which have been added; the granules, in case no ulcer is present on the eye, should be treated in this way: One should, with the remedies for nursing children, already mentioned, when there is no inflammation, evert the lids and anoint them, and massage them for a long time with the head of a sound, for, if one leaves off rubbing too soon, one produces greater roughness and discharge. If the injurious cause continues, stronger medicines must be employed, as for example, the following: cuttle-fish scales, 8 drachms; pumice, 8 drachms; Sinopic red-chalk, ammoniated frankincense, of each 10 drachms; gum, 8 drachms, dissolved in water. By the use of this remedy, you will acquire the greatest reputation; for, immediately after the inunction, a few pieces of the superficial pellicle come away under patting. One should, however, after the use of the remedy as an ointment, cleanse the parts with cold water by means of a sponge.

"Another remedy for old discharge and lid-asperities: cadmium, 16 drachms; annealed copper, 4 drachms; henbane seed, 1 drachm; opium, 2 drachms; myrrh, sweet-broom and gum acacia, of each 4 drachms; gum, 8 drachms; all dry and finely powdered. Rub this up with woman's milk and form collyria. Use it thick as an ointment, after preliminary fomentation.

"A moist trachoma remedy, which is favorably recommended, is roasted copper ore, 3 drachms; saffron, 8 drachms, honey, 9 drachms. Rub up the dry substances with water, and, when the mass has again become dry, add the honey and use.

"The so-called 'Eye-Salve of Theophilus' for fig-like elevations and proud flesh consists of annealed copper, 2 drachms; roasted vitriolic ore, 1 drachm; myrrh, saffron and juice of unripe grapes, of each 1 drachm; Chain wine (or another which is cruder, older and better-smelling), 16 ounces; Attic honey, 10 ounces . . ."

One hundred years later, Paul of Aegina (A.D. 625-690), a native of Constantinople who received his education in Alexandria, in his great "Compendium of Medicine," declares:

"Trachoma is roughness of the inner surface of the eyelid, an intense degree of which has the appearance of clefts, and is called sycosis. When it becomes chronic and callous, it is called tylosis. We must use collyria for it, namely, the one from wine, and that prepared from the two stones; or the eyelid may be rubbed with the bloodstone itself (haematite) and washed with much water. But the collyrium called harmation, with a little of the cycnarius, or the saffron collyrium, answers well with these, and with cases of psorophthalmia without ulceration, when rubbed upon the everted eyelid. But if the callus be hard and do not yield to these things, we must turn the eyelid out and rub it down with pumice-stone, or the shell of the cuttle-fish, or figleaves, or by the surgical instrument called blepharoxyston."[19]

The Arabic physicians of the Middle Ages appear to have readily recognized the disease. Abulkasim gives as the predisposing cause of trachoma, an abnormal condition of the blood (dyscrasia) combined with chronic disease of the conjunctiva.[20]

Sadili of Cairo, a celebrated physician of the latter part of the fourteenth century, complained that the people of Egypt suffered more from ophthalmia than the population of any of the neighboring countries and that it was impossible to get rid of the granulations.[21]

In the year 1488, Rabbi Obadiah of Bertimoro, in a letter to his father in the Italian province of Flori, writes that most of the people of Egypt were stricken with blindness from this scourge.[22]

On the streets of Cairo, one can constantly witness the distressing spectacle of flies literally covering the lids of the poor victims of trachoma and feeding on the secretions. Most pitiful is to see the poor babies, whose little arms are not developed enough to rid themselves of these torturing insects.[23]

The marshy districts of Egypt have always been infested with flies; particularly is this true of the banks of the Nile. Thus, said Isaiah (7:18): "And it shall come to pass in that day, that the Lord shall hiss for the fly that is in the uppermost part of the river of Egypt and for the bee that is in the land of Assyria."

CHAPTER XXVIII

MALARIA DURING THE MIDDLE AGES

Malaria ("bad air") is a new name for a disease which has prevailed since early antiquity. This Italian name was introduced into the English medical literature in 1827 by Macculagh. Prior to this date the disease was variously known as chills and fever, intermittent fever, marsh fever, tertian fever, quartan fever, trench fever, autumnal fever, jungle fever, ague fever, hill fever and fever of the individual country where it occurred.

Malaria throughout ancient and medieval history occurred not only in a mild endemic form but also in a pernicious epidemic form.

The Old Testament refers to malaria as *"kadachas"*[1] a term which is still employed by Jews in Eastern Europe and in Israel. In the Iliad, Homer (1000 B.C.) alluded to malaria in the following lines:

> "And o'er the feebler stars exists its rays
> Terrific glory, for the burning breath
> Taints the red air which fever plagues."

In "The Wasps," the poet and dramatist, Aristophanes, a contemporary of Hippocrates, refers to malarial fever in the following stanza:

> "The agues and fevers that plagued our land;
> That loved the darksome hours of night
> To throttle fathers, and grandsires choke,
> That laid them down on their restless beds
> And against your quiet and peaceful talk."[2]

The scourge of malaria led the Greeks to halt their campaign when they came before the very gates of Troy. When the armies of Hannibal approached the pest-ridden city of Rome ("a vail of Hell"), his losses were "as mist disappearing before the wind."

In the writings of Hippocrates (460-377 B.C.) malaria is considered to be pernicious. In his book, "On Epidemics," Hippocrates left such a graphic description of intermittent fevers that for a period of over two millennia, little of importance was added to it. The following is quoted from the English translation of Hippocrates by Francis Adams:

"During autumn, and at the commencement of winter, there were phthisical complaints; continual fevers; and, in a few cases, ardent; some diurnal, others nocturnal, semitertians, true tertians, quartans, irregular fevers. All the fevers which are described attacked great numbers. The ardent fevers attacked the smallest numbers, and the patients suffered the least from them, for there were no hemorrhages, except a few and then a small amount, nor was there delirium; all the other complaints were slight; in these the crises were regular, in most instances, with the intermittents, in seventeen days; I know no instance of a person dying of causus, nor becoming phrenitic. The tertians were more numerous than the ardent fevers, and attended with more pain; but these all had four periods in regular succession from the first attack, and they had a complete crisis in seven, without a relapse in any instance. The quartans attacked many at first, in the form of regular quartans, but in no few cases a transition from other fevers and diseases into quartans took place; they were protracted, as is wont with them, indeed, more so than usual. Quotidian, nocturnal, and wandering fevers attacked many persons, some of whom continued to keep up, and others were confined to bed. In most instances these fevers were prolonged under the Pleiades and till winter.

"Many persons, and more especially children, had convulsions from the commencement; and they had fever, and the convulsions supervened upon the fevers; in most cases they were protracted, but free from danger, unless in those who were in a deadly state from other complaints. Those fevers which were continual in the main, and with no intermissions, but having exacerbations in the tertian form, there being remissions the one day and exacerbations the next, were the most violent of all those which occurred at the time, and the most protracted, and occurring with the greatest pains, beginning mildly, always on the whole increasing, and being exacerbated, and always turning worse, having small remissions, and after an abatement having more violent paroxysms, and growing worse, for the most part, on the critical days. Rigors, in all cases, took place in an irregular and uncertain manner, very rare and weak in them, but greater in all other fevers; frequent sweats, but most seldom in them, bringing no alleviation, but, on the contrary, doing mischief. Much cold of the extremities in them, and these were warmed with difficulty." [3]

In his book, "Airs, Waters and Places," Hippocrates refers to a form of malaria caused by dwelling near marshy places:

"Such waters then as are marshy, stagnant, and belong to lakes, are necessarily hot in summer, thick, and have a strong smell; since they have no current, but being constantly supplied by rain-water, and the sun heating them, they necessarily want their proper color, are unwholesome and form bile; in winter, they become congealed, cold, and muddy with the snow and ice, so that they are most apt to engender phlegm, and bring on hoarseness; those who drink them have large and obstructed spleens, their bellies are hard, emaciated, and hot; and their shoulders, collar-bones, and faces are emaciated; for their flesh is melted down and taken up by the spleen, and hence they are slender, such persons then are voracious and thirsty; their bellies are very dry both above and below, so that they require the strongest medicines." [4]

Among the ancient Hindus, at the time of the composition of the Atharva-Veda, malaria was known as "the king of diseases." At various times up to two-thirds of the deaths in India have been caused by malarial infection.

In Vedic medicine, malaria was the most dreaded disease. It was predominant in the autumn season and was known as "*takman*" after the demon which is supposed to cause it. There is a long list of hymns in Vedic literature composed for the express purpose of combating the destructive ravages of "*takman.*" The symptoms described are alterations between heat and cold and delirium. Return of the fever either daily or every other day is marked by chills, fever, jaundice, certain eruptions, headache, cough, spasms and itch.[5]

Susruta (A.D. 500) one of the greatest of the Indian medical trio—the others are Charaka (first century) and Waghabota (seventh century)—gives an excellent description of malarial fevers which he actually ascribed to mosquitoes.[6]

Plato (427-347 B.C.) alludes to the various forms of malarial fever ascribing them to imbalances of the four elements. "Continued fever,' he states, "is occasioned by the element of fire, quotidian fever by the element of air, tertian fever by the element of water and quartan fever by the element of earth."[7]

Celsus gives an excellent description of the various forms of malarial fever;

"Fevers are a kind of disease that affect the whole body, and are the most common of all. Of these, one is a quotidian, another a tertian, and a third a quartan. Sometime some fevers also return after a longer period, but that seldom occurs. With regard to the first two, they are both diseases in themselves and a cure for others. (Is this a premonition of modern malarial fever therapy, such as for paresis?)

"But quartan fevers are more simple. They begin commonly with a shuddering; then a heat breaks out; after the paroxysm is over, the patient is well for two days. Then it returns upon the fourth day.

"Of tertians again there are two kinds. One of them both beginning and ending like the quartan; with this difference only, that there is one day's intermission, and it returns upon the third day. The other kind is much more fatal, which indeed returns upon the third day, but of forty-eight hours thirty-six are occupied by the fit (and sometimes either less or more) nor does it entirely cease in the remission; but is only mitigated. This kind most physicians call semitertian.

"But quotidians are various, and different in their appearances. For some of them begin with a heat, others with a coldness, others with a shuddering. I call that a coldness, when the extremities of the limbs are chilled; a shuddering, when the whole body trembles. Again, some end so as to be followed by an interval quite free from indisposition; others so as that although the fever somewhat abates, yet some relics remain, till another paroxysm comes on; and others often remit little or nothing, but continue as they began." [8]

The Roman encyclopedist Marcus Terentius Varro (B.C. 116-27) was the first to advance the theory that fever is caused by minute creatures which dwell in swamps. He described these creatures as being so small that they cannot be seen with the naked eye and he declares that they enter the body with the air through the nose and mouth. In his work *"De re Rustica,"* he bluntly states that precautions must be taken in the neighborhood of swamps because small creatures invisible to the eye fill the atmosphere in marshy localities, and with the air breathed through the nose and mouth, penetrate into the human body, thereby causing dangerous diseases. Columella (first century A.D.) speaks of marshes as breeding mosquitoes.[9]

Fifty years earlier, Titus Lucretius (born about 98 B.C.), agreeing with the Epicurean doctrine of the etiology of disease, presented his theory of how pathogenic seeds or atoms are developed. "Pestilence," he states, "comes either from without, down through the atmosphere in the shape of clouds and mists, or they gather themselves up, and rise out of the earth when it is soaked with water and has contracted a stain, being beaten upon by unseasonable rains and suns." He advises that contact with pestilence be avoided to escape disease.

Cato speaks of black bile and swollen spleen as results of malarial fever.

Celli noted in his work, "Ager Romanus" (1925), that the Etruscans excavated the subterranean tunnels and leveled the hills of Tufa in order to avoid malaria. The Etruscans knew that drainage of the swamps was necessary in order to escape pestilence and they defended themselves by this method. Celli has shown that malaria was a disease of great antiquity and that the early Romans recognized the localities where it predominated and built their towns and houses on elevated places. According to Vitruvius, the district about Rome was considered swampy and thus predisposed the citizens to febrile attacks. They built hydraulic works, drained the swamps and constructed the "clocca maxima." In other words, they did not depend altogether upon the goddess Febris who was invoked in cases of fever.

Julius Caesar is said to have excavated a lake and also planted a forest on the right bank of the Tiber where a swamp had previously existed.

The spread of malaria in the Roman Empire undermined the morale of the agricultural population and drove the peasantry from their farms to the city slums where their physical disease apparently gave way to moral degeneracy.

Pliny the Elder in a number of places refers to quartan and tertian fevers for which he prescribes a number of remedies "recommended by doctors of magic arts." Foremost among such remedies he advocates the wearing of amulets. He adds a long list of magic and folkloristic remedies.

The frequency of malaria among the Romans may be inferred from the satire against the healers by the famous Roman satirist and epigrammist, Martial:

" 'Tis a false report that Tongilius is being consumed by a semi-tertian fever. I know the tricks of the man; he is hungry and thirsty."

"You declaim in a fever, Maron; if you don't know that this is frenzy, you are not sane, friend Maron. You declaim when you are ill, you declaim in a semi-tertian; if otherwise you can't perspire, there is some reason in it. 'Yet it is a great thing.' You are wrong; when fever burns up your vitals 'tis a great thing to hold your tongue, Maron."

"Nothing more scandalous, Maximus, was ever done by Carus than his dying of fever, and it too committed an outrage. The cruel fatal fever should have been at least a quartan! That malady should have been reserved for its own doctor." (Carus was a specialist in quartan fever.) [10]

The Talmud alludes to the various forms of malaria. *"Shimsha bath yoma"* refers to quartan fever.[11] The treatment of malaria in the Talmud is largely folkloristic. The Talmud permits the use of water every hour in the quotidian form of malaria, which was contrary to the teaching of the Methodist School. If the fever is of the tertian or quartan forms, venesection was recommended.[12]

In remittent fever, treatment is more complex for it was evident that the spirit that had entered the body to cause the disease was stubborn and heroic measures were needed.[13]

In the Middle Ages malaria prevailed in an endemic form. Aëtius and Paul of Aegina described its prevalence in various forms along similar lines as did the Greek writers. The Arabian writers Rhazes, Avicenna and Isaac Judeus devoted much attention to fevers. The last authority wrote his *opus magnum* on this subject and he carefully differentiated between the various types of fevers. However, in general, the Arabian writers followed the Greek masters almost verbatim.

Maimonides, in his most bulky work, "Fusul Musa fi't Tibb" ("Medical Aphorisms of Moses"; Hebrew: "Pirkei Moshe"), devotes the entire tenth chapter to fevers describing their etiology (humoral), symptomatology and diagnosis. He follows in the footsteps of Hippocrates and Galen and the subject he deals with, unlike the treatment given by other contemporary writers, is free from superstition and folklore.

The Anglo-Saxon "Leech Book of Bald" prescribes the following remedy for malaria:

"For the *tertia,* or a fever which cometh on a man on the third day, take twigs of this same wort, and fold them up in wool, incense (fumigate) the patient before the time when the fever will be upon him."

The Hippocratic teaching that marshy places are responsible for the fever is reflected in the saying of the famous Babylonian Jewish physician, Mar Samuel (c. third century) who says:

"One that drinks water from (marshy) lakes, creeks and pools takes a chance with his life because *shabriri*, the demon causing blindness, dwells in these waters."[14] He names two kinds of *shabriri*: day *shabriri* (hemeralopia) and night *shabriri* (nyctalopia). Is it possible that the demon *shabriri* was an unintentional premonition of the female anopheles mosquito?

Malaria was associated in the mind of medieval man with all kinds of superstition, being in this factor a close second to epilepsy. The very nature of a malarial paroxysm was enough to frighten, not only the patient, but also the attendants. The sudden onset of chills and fever, the violent tremor of the muscles that shook the patient from head to foot and the final termination in a copious perspiration, conveyed the idea to the primitive mind that a cruel supernatural fiend had entered the patient. Only drastic occult measures could expel such an archdemon. Diseases caused by supernatural forces could hardly be effectively treated by purely physical methods.

During the Middle Ages, Europe was plagued with frequent epidemics of malarial fever as perhaps never before or since. The last great European pandemics were in the years 1659-1669 and 1677-1695.

In order to check new epidemics of this grave disease, varied theories were advanced to explain its cause. Astrologers, as usual, attributed it to comets and astral phenomena, and of course there was nothing one could do to change the course of the stars. There were many, however, who attributed the fever to storms, failure of crops, famine, and other natural phenomena. Clerics placed the etiology at the doors of sinners and a deep religious fervor seized the faithful. Everywhere wailing and lamentation filled the air. Epidemic malaria evoked terror in the hearts of the people which is beyond description.

In Germany and Hungary organizations of "crossbearers" were formed who marched from place to place to investigate and detect the sinners who were responsible for the epidemics. Of course, epidemics do not last forever and after they subsided the faithful ascribed this subsidence to the religious revival.

Inundations were blamed for malarial outbreaks in many

parts of the world. The overflowings of the Nile, the Ganges, the Euphrates, the Volga, the Danube and the Mississippi were frequently followed by some form of malarial fever. Swarms of insects and the poisoning of the wells by Jews were other favorite etiologies.

Physicians, however, were reticent to accept any of these theories as valid. Many doctors favored the Hippocratic concept that marshy districts cause the disease. Just how swamps caused malaria, however, was not explained. The first explanation that really interested the medical profession was the one proposed in 1879 by Edward Klebs (b. 1834) and Tamasi-Crudeli who claimed to have found the true cause of malaria by isolating the bacillus in the mud of the Roman marshes. They described it as a short microorganism which they were able to cultivate in fish gelatine and which reproduced the fever when injected into rabbits. This microorganism, however, did not have the same effect when injected into man.

J. F. Meckel (1781-1833) in 1827, R. Virchow (1821-1902) in 1849, and F. T. von Frerichs (1819-1885) in 1866, noticed microscopic malarial bodies in the blood of patients ill with malarial diseases. None of these scientists, however, recognized the significance of these bodies and their parasitic nature was not suspected until the year 1880.

The tireless efforts of the French army surgeon, Charles Louis Alphonse Laveran, led to the recognition of the true plasmodia of malaria. Dr. Laveran, while doing some research work in Algeria where he was assigned by the French government, discovered on June 18, 1880, the plasmodia of malaria in the mosquito.

In the same year, on November 23, 1880, he announced his discovery to the Academy of Medicine. His discovery was accepted by the medical world several years later. Among the American physicians who corroborated the findings of Laveran were Surgeon General Sternberg, Osler and Welch.

In 1885, Golgi was able to follow the tertian and quartan parasites throughout their entire endogenous cycle of development and he showed that a close relationship existed between certain phases of parasitic growth and the tertian stages of the paroxysm.

The differentiation of tertian, quartan and estivo-autumnal species was accomplished by Grassi and Felleti in the years 1895 to 1898. Sir Roland Ross in 1895 and 1896 demonstrated that certain developmental changes occur in the malarial plasmodia within the stomach of the female anopheles mosquito.

In 1898 and 1899, Italian observers, Grassi, Bastianelli and Bignami proved that the female anopheles mosquitoes transmit malaria by actual experiment upon man and these workers confirmed the developmental changes in the mosquito first observed by Ross.

In 1912, Bass and John first succeeded in cultivating the plasmodia of malaria which were employed as a therapeutic measure in the treatment of paresis.

Most important in the history of malaria was the discovery of cinchona bark and its specific action upon malaria. This discovery was made by the aborigines of Peru. In 1638, when the Countess of Cinchon was stricken with malaria, she was advised by Don Lopez to use the Peruvian bark which had been employed by the natives for many years. Its use resulted in her perfect recovery. The bark was brought to Europe by the Viceroy del Cinchon in the year 1640. The news of the Countess' cure spread all over Western Europe and the Peruvian bark became known as cinchona after the Count Cinchon. The specific curative effect of the bark made it possible to differentiate malarial fever from other febrile affections long before the plasmodia were visualized.

In 1820, quinine was isolated from cinchona bark by **Pelletier** and **Caventou**.

CHAPTER XXIX

SYPHILIS AND OTHER DISEASES DURING THE MIDDLE AGES

There is no other disease in the history of medicine that has aroused so much discussion during the past four hundred years as has syphilis. This long controversy has not developed because of its great mortality, for cancer, tuberculosis, smallpox and cholera have caused even greater mortalities. It has not been engendered because its etiology was shrouded in mystery for the causes of all epidemics were not known until modern times. The real cause of the argument lies in the fact that the sexual nature of the disease was early recognized and false modesty would not permit any country to admit its origin. Europe blamed it on America; America on Europe.

The Italians in whose country the first great epidemic broke out, believing that it was introduced by the soldiers of France, called it *Mal Francesse* or *Morbus Gallicus*. The French, believing that the disease was brought back from Italy by returning soldiers, called it *Mal de Naples,* or Neapolitan Disease. The Germans called it *Franzosen böse Blättern*. In England it was known as France pox. The Poles blamed it on the Germans and called it German sickness, and the Russians named it Polish disease.

John Fernel (1497-1558) who was professor of medicine in Paris and author of "Universa Medicina" (1554) named it Lues Venerea. Always a great mimic and deceiver, syphilis was also known as plague, sacred disease, burning disease of St. Main, the disease of St. Gile, disease of St. Marcellus, St. Anthony's fire, Hell's fire, etc. Ivan Bloch [1] presents a list of several hundred names by which the disease was known. The universal name "syphilis" was finally given by Gerolamo Fracastoro of Verona (1478-1553).

Syphilis prevailed in an endemic form all through the Middle Ages. It reached an epidemic height at the time of the siege of Naples by the French. The movement of troops which accompanied the expedition of Charles VIII contributed to the dissemination of the contagion to a large degree. For a period of two years the epidemic was limited to Italy. Eventually it was spread over all Western Europe as the soldiers returned home.

The outbreak of an epidemic after a war is not rare. The "flu" epidemic in the United States in 1917 and 1918 and its relation to World War I is to the point. Influenza in an endemic form was a usual occurrence before the war but the unhygienic life in the trenches apparently helped develop a virulent form of organism.

The symptoms of the endemic form of syphilis which existed in the Middle Ages were present particularly in fifteenth century Europe, but in addition there were more acute symptoms which eclipsed the classic form. These included high fever, much pain, and psychic disturbances. Symptoms which came to be designated in the Middle Ages as sacred fire or St. Anthony's fire, probably represented a flare-up of the usual endemic form perhaps because of widespread debauchery and general lack of hygienic regulations. "The lesions which we observe at the present time (1850) in syphilis," states Philip Ricord (1799-1889), "resemble the standard pathognomonic lesions of syphilis rather than those of the epidemic of the fifteenth century."

The historians Karl Sudhoff (1853-1938) and Singer are of the opinion that syphilis prevailed in Europe and elsewhere from the days of antiquity. According to Sudhoff, the French march on Naples with its camp followers and its abundance of opportunities for licentiousness stirred up and spread the organism and brought its most virulent manifestations. Sudhoff collected an array of evidence to prove that syphilis existed in France prior to the first recorded epidemic. On the other hand, Ivan Bloch, Pusey, H. V. Williams, Samberg and A. E. Wright (1861-1932) maintained that syphilis was not known in Europe prior to the return of the soldiers of Columbus from America.

It is not within the scope of the present writer to enter into a lengthy discussion on this rather complex subject. He will reproduce some of the evidence available concerning the syphilis of the Middle Ages, and leave it to the reader to judge the matter for himself. After evaluating the facts, the present writer is partial to the opinion of Sudhoff and Singer that Lues Venerea is a disease of great antiquity, but remained unidentified until the fifteenth century.

There is no positive clinical evidence that syphilis has prevailed in antiquity. Now and then one meets with symptoms of a certain disease similar to one of the stages of syphilis. For example, in the "First Book of Samuel"[2] it is recorded that the Philistines who captured the Holy Ark were smitten with *"ophalim"* emerods in their secret place. The word *"ophalim"* technically means "elevation" or "buboes." Again in Deuteronomy[3] *"ophalim"* is mentioned. "The Lord will smite thee with the boil of Egypt and with *'ophalim'* emerods and with the scabs and with the itch whereof thou canst not be healed." In the Assyrian language the word *"ubra"* signifies swelling. According to Jensen, (1902) it should be rendered *"uplu"*—a venereal boil.[4]

Biblical and medical scholars are of the opinion that the "ophalim" (buboes) with which the Philistines were punished in their secret places was syphilis. Evidence that the buboes were of a venereal nature is adduced by Victor Robinson and G. Schickele (1875-1927) from the fact that Moses was angered at the Israelites when they saved the women of the enemy after so many of their number had died from the plague.[5]

The disease of Herod of Judea, as described by Josephus, appears to have been the same malady, and Apion, who is denounced by Josephus, had a similar disease.

In the third chapter of the "Book of Epidemics," Hippocrates (460-376 B.C) tells a story of a young married couple who sought death together because of ulceration of the genitals. Scribonius Largus, a Roman physician of the first century, refers to an unhealthy ulcer of the penis. Others speak of "figs" of the anus and of chancres and corns of the penis.

Galen (130-200 A.D.) of Pergamos describes various types of diseases of the genitalia including phimosis, paraphimosis and buboes.

Celsus, in the sixth book of his "De Medicina," dealing with dermatology, mentions among skin diseases some genital affections such as abscess and phimosis.

As stated, there is no undisputed clinical evidence of syphilis in antiquity. Most of the cases enumerated are merely external manifestations which might be visible during the course of syphilis. The symptoms are far from pathognomonic and might merely represent local conditions which do not involve the system as does syphilis.

There is, however, paleopathological evidence which goes back to prehistoric times. The studies of F. E. Williams (1852-1936) and Deninger on ancient skeletons discovered in America and Europe show that this disease apparently prevailed in pre-Columbian skeletal material.[6] Williams identifies syphilis in three prehistoric skulls from Pecos, New Mexico. Hooton identifies additional prehistoric luetic skulls and long bones from Peru, Mexico, Alabama, Arizona and Ohio. He concludes: "The diagnosis of syphilis on the skulls is as certain as is possible in any dried bones, without clinical history." Deninger diagnoses "adolescent luetic periositis" from long bones found in Illinois mounds, and syphilitic lesions in the facial bones of a skull from Arizona, dating to 1000-1350 A. D.

The problem of prehistoric syphilis has been so thoroughly discussed by Williams and Pales that only a summary is required. In Neolithic France, Parrot, Magitot, Le Baron and Jean Seleme described Neolithic crania with syphilitic lesions *"identiques a celles que produit le craniotabes syphyilitique."*[7] Broca states: "I have found a large number of syphilitic lesions in bones derived from an ancient leper asylum whose cemetery was dug up fifteen years ago" (1860). L. Pales (Paleopathologic and Pathologic Comparatives) found syphilitic bones from Roman, Saxon and Medieval England. In Egypt, Fouquet identified lues of the skulls of Abydos and Kawamil, and Lartet (1801-1871) found luetic skulls in Karnak. On the other hand, Smith (1822-1906) and Jones found no syphilitic bones in 6,000 Nubian skeletons. In the Far East, Adachi reports presumably syphilitic bones from Stone Age Japan and Neolithic Annam.

In the New World, syphilitic bones were identified from prehistoric Peru, Mexico, and North America. The criteria of skeletal diagnosis are found in cranial lenticular exostoses or lesions, premature closure of vault sutures, saber-tibia and tibial hyperostosis, deviations of the palate, and dental malformations, such as erosion, impaction, microdontism, hypercementosis, bifid roots, Carabelli's cusp and hypoplastic enamel. Obviously, the prehistoric syphilis question cannot be settled from skeletal material alone; but neither can prehistoric syphilis be categorically denied.[8]

While such findings cannot be taken as positive evidence, they are of great importance in tending to verify the inconclusive clinical histories presented before.

The facts are that syphilis of the head frequently attacks the nasal bones and the palate. The appearance of cranial syphilis depends upon the degree of the lesion. If the lesion is not severe and not long standing, it is difficult to diagnose; but if the lesion is of a marked nature, the bones are heavy and the external surface may present many elevations possessing a convex surface. Gummata, singly or confluent, may complicate the description of cranial syphilis. Among the skulls found of the Mound Builders in America, bony changes point to syphilis although they might have been produced by other virulent affections such as typhoid fever.[9] Still, without clinical data, one agrees with Krogman that, "The problem of prehistoric syphilis is most controversial." [10]

While there may be some doubt as to the identity of syphilis in ancient times, there can be no doubt that it was identified in the early Middle Ages.

F. Burkart gives a translation of a passage in Vindician's (c. 370) *"De Remediis Expertis,"* which was prepared by the authority on medieval Latin, Philippe Hildebrandt. The passage occurs in the *"De Medicamentis,"* of Marcellus Empiricus of Bordeaux, court physician of Theodocius (A. D. 350) and reads as follows:

"Truly if the venereal poison reaches the parts of the body where it can find a favorable hiding place, the pestilence becomes externally visible. At the same time it hastens back to the point where the brain begins and establishes its nest there. When thereafter it begins to range then the fear must be entertained that it will devastate the skin and penetrate the head and produce all manner of evil in it. It may break through the blood vessels to the ears and cause the man to become deaf, completely destroying the sense of hearing, or it creates maggots in the ears or it favors swelling of the nose or fistulous ulcers about the eyes or damages the teeth and transforms the oral cavity of the patient into an empty stinking hole against which one has to protect himself most. By reason of the extensive destruction of the palate the voice is damaged or paralyzed. The evil may cause destructive changes in the lungs and stomach and may destroy the organs of procreation and the kidneys; or the changes in the humors may begin in the hips and thighs causing the nerves of the legs to twitch, gradually destroying the power of walking. While thus the whole organism becomes saturated with the disease the impression is created that you have killed the patient instead of having treated him, inasmuch as he really passes from life through a violent death."[11]

It seems that Vindician here presents a case of tabes characterized by general paralysis.

In the sixth century, Paul of Aegina, the distinguished physician of the early Byzantine period, writing of warts of the sexual parts, remarks: "If it should happen that an *ulcer of the glans* is situated in the interior of the meatus urinarius," (it is the) *"universal ulcer."* He describes "figs" as "ulcerating, roundish eruptions, slightly indurated, of a reddish color."

In a ninth century manuscript which is found in the "Bibliotheque Nationale," of Paris, there is a passage which testifies to the relation existing between certain morbid growths of the anus and ulcers of the genital organs. The anonymous author claims to have observed at the orifice of the anus, fissures, holes, tumors, vegetations, etc., "and *pustules* of divers sorts, as large as beans, peas or even filberts, and sometimes elevated to such a degree that they seemed to close that orifice.". . . .[12]

The most celebrated physician of the Arabian school, Rhazes, refers to venereal papules, which he calls *"bothor"*; he defines *"bothor"* as an itching followed by a rising (tumor) on the vulva or penis, as a result of coitus.

Mesue, (780-859) Isaac Judeus, (830-940) Avicenna, (980-1037) Avenzoar, (1113-1162) Averroes (1198 and Abulkasim (936-1013) speak of *"bothor,"* apostems, and pustules of the penis and of the vulva. Mesue states that the Persian fire (*ignis Persicus*) was of the nature of chancres (*carbunculorum*) and that the so-called "formica" of the Greeks was an apostem of the skin capable of degenerating into a putrid ulcer (*ulcus putridum*). The terms *"saphati"* or *"asafati,"* of which Avicenna and his successors speak, represented something analogous. Isaac Judeus, after describing apostems of the penis, refers to the "nodes" which arise at the anus as they do at the vulva. Avenzoar speaks of "red pustules" which originate at times upon the glans (*pustulae rubrae in capite virgae*) and which are called, in Arabic, *"alchumbra."* [13]

Among the first physicians in Western Europe who appear to have identified syphilis as a special infectious disease was Guglielmo Saliceto (1210-1260), professor at the University of Verona. In his "Chyrurgia" [14] he speaks of pustules which are white or red, of small pimples large as millet seeds, of erosions and of corruptions which show themselves on the penis and around the prepuce. Such lesions, Saliceto claims, are primarily produced by intercourse with an impure woman or prostitute. He mentions the development of fig-like lesions at the anus and vulva. He recommends ablutions with vinegar-water for those who have had intercourse with an infected woman. Saliceto seems to have recognized the fact that a period of incubation exists between the time of intercourse and the outbreak of the disease or primary lesion.

In chapter 53 he describes crusts and ulcers on the legs for which he advises frictions by means of mercury and saliva. It should be borne in mind that Saliceto wrote in 1270, more than 200 years prior to the siege of Naples.

Petrus Hispanus, (d. 1277) who became pope under the name of John XXI, refers to figs and ulcers of the penis and speaks of the chancre (*cancrum*), which may be found on the penis and other places.

A manuscript of the thirteenth century entitled "Parvus Micrologus," by Ricardus Senior (d. 1252) (known as Richard of Vendom, the Englishman, the Parisian and the Salernitan), contains a passage dealing with venereal ulcerations: "These two organs (i. e. the penis and testicles) become the seat of ulcers after a coitus at the menstrual period, by reason of the acrid humors, which are heated and corrosive, as is abundantly proven by the color of the skin and pustules of bad blood, and also the itching, the stinging, and the burning which is felt."[15]

Lanfranc of Milan in his "Practica,"[16] gives a description of the "fig," of the chancre, and of the ulcer of the penis. The "fig" is an excrescence of a peculiar nature which grows on the prepuce and sometimes on the head of the penis. If it is corrupt, it degenerates into a chancre. Ulcers originate from hot pustules which grow on the penis, or from coitus with a diseased woman or one who recently has had sexual relations with a diseased man attacked with the same infection. The author then advises washing the genital organs after coitus.[17]

The most convincing proof that syphilis prevailed in the Middle Ages is the description of the disease "Persian fire," by Bernard de Gordon (1305). In his "Lilium Medicinae,"[18] the author, referring to diseases of the penis, mentions amongst the causes of ulcers and chancres the fact "of having had relations with a woman whose vagina is diseased, full of sangious matter, of virulence, of flatulence, or of analogous corruptions." Quoting Avicenna, he adds, "Every ulcerating and corrosive pustule may be called Persian fire." Bernard de Gordon refers also to the uncertainty of the physicians of the Middle Ages with regard to the nature and etiology of this disease.

Because of the great interest of Gordon's text, a translation by R. C. Holcomb is appended here:[19]

"Causes: Leprosy is caused either from being introduced in the uterus, or after birth. If arising within the uterus, it is because of conception at the time of menstruation, or because it is the child of a leper, or because a leper shall have had intercourse with a pregnant woman, and in this case the bearing will be leprous, for out of the great corruptions that supervene from such conceptions, leprosy is generated.

"If it should happen after the child has left the uterus, it is because the air is badly corrupted and pestilental, or because of prolonged use of melancholic foods, such as lentils and other legumes, and from such melancholic meats as that of oxes, bears, wild boars, hares and other quadrupeds such as asses and the like. In some regions all such dead animals are consumed. (Different texts list different animals.)

"Leprosy also arises by reason of too much conversation with the leprous, and from coitus with a leprous woman. And it will also break forth in him who lies with a woman who has lain with a leper, the seed of whom remains in her womb. In this circumstance, from coitus with a leper, the woman may not be infected, unless it is continued a long time, because of the dense structure of the womb. But if a healthy man lies with a woman with whom a leper has lain, the leper's semen yet remaining in her womb, he will inevitably become leprous, because the pores of the male organ are loose, and the infection is readily transmitted throughout the whole body. Therefore most extraordinary precaution is to be observed, and if through some opportunity or ill consideration one should lie with such a woman, she should ingeniously expel the seed from the womb, as by dancing, sneezing, bathing and cleansing with clean water and wiping it away. Furthermore, such measures should be taken as far in advance as possible.

"And there are many other means of expelling the semen thus received, to avoid submitting oneself to the risk of carrying the gourd (leper's cup) and clappers, with their everlasting opprobrium.

"Everyone ought guard himself against lying with a leprous woman, for I will cite what happened concerning a certain countess who came leprous to Montpellier, and was under my treatment. A certain bachelor in medicine who was attendant to her, lay with her and she was impregnated, and he was made completely leprous.

"Fortunate then are those who are made cautious through the dangers of others."

"If the word "leprosy," says Holcomb, is changed to the word "syphilis," one has a good picture of chronic syphilis.

That the word "leprosy" was used for venereal disease may be seen from Philip Shepps' "Libra de Lepra." He tells of a carpenter who, having had relations with a leprous woman, was infected with leprosy a short time after. The manner of contamination is that of syphilis as leprosy cannot be communicated in such a manner. According to Dr. Zambaco who carefully studied the nature of leprosy, perfectly healthy men and women may live with their leprous wives and husbands without contracting the disease.

Valescus of Tarentum [20] (1382-1417) gives precise information on the seat and the mode of transmission of venereal ulcer and pustule. The cause must be sought either in traumatism or in contact or in coitus with unhealthy and infected chancrous women. This disease occurs more often in young persons because they more often have relations with women having ulcers on their genital organs.[21]

Theodoric (Theodor of Cervia, c. 1205-1298) refers to the malady as a sort of rottenness that is caused by inflammation of the natural melancholic matter and of the false phlegm. This affection is characterized by a livid, black color, and by large pustules, which are scabby, fetid, not sanious, like rust, almost insensitive, and having a repellent aspect. This disease is seen three times as frequently upon the hips and the tibia as anywhere else.

Roger Bacon (c. 12-14-1292) gives a similar description. The "dead disease," he states, is a sort of rotting *(scabiei genus)*, causing pustules around the legs and shins (*"cirea crura et tibias facit pustulas"*) and which is so-called because the limb attacked by it seems to be struck with gangrene.

John of Gaddesden, like Guglielmo Saliceto and Lanfranc, in his "Rosa Anglica" (Oxford, 1320) regards ulcers of the penis as derived from having coitus with a woman having her menses and he advises washing the sexual organs thoroughly after each suspicious intercourse. He states: "If you wish to preserve your organ from all virus, in case you should have reason to suspect your companion of being infected, wash yourself, as soon as you retire, with cold water to which vinegar has been added, or with urine."

This author, in his *"De Infectione et Concubitus cum Leprosa"* ("Of the Contamination following Intercourse with a Leper"), shows that the term leper was applied by physicians of the fourteenth century to local venereal infection following coitus.

In *"Libellus de Epidemia Quam Vulgo Morbum Gallicum Vocant,"* published in 1497, Leonicenus gives a graphic description of syphilis which he clearly recognizes. He states: "I may dare affirm for certain, that 'lichen' was familiar to the Greeks years before Claudius reigned; because Hippocrates, the most ancient Greek author, . . . especially in the third part of the 'Aphorisms,' in the discussion of summer diseases, makes mention of 'lichen'; so it seems highly probable to me that this disease infested Italy, although perhaps for a long interval of time before Claudius, it was not yet propagated by the Roman Empire to the other nations, and indeed therefore among the Greek physicians frequenting Rome, there were less names for this disease. For this reason while it continued without name, it was poorly understood but after Claudius' reign, with the Greek arts and especially medicine now blooming in the city, naming 'lichen' as well as 'mentagra' made one more illustrious . . . Likewise in a measure this happens in our time, for now a disease of an unusual nature has invaded Italy and many other regions.

"In the beginning pustules are on the private parts, soon on the whole body and frequently located on the face itself besides causing great hideousness as well as a great deal of pain.

Moreover to this disease the physicians of our time do not yet give a name, but it is called by the common name 'French disease,' as if the contagion were imported from France into Italy or because Italy was invaded at the same time both by the disease itself and the armies of the French . . . therefore we may understand briefly the nature of the French disease. This exists not in one kind, but in many types, and we can describe it in this fashion.

"The French disease has pustules, generated from the diverse corruption of the humors, because of too much air and the heat and humidity especially intemperate, at first on the privates, then the rest of the body and commonly accompanied with great pain. Why do they attack the private parts first, then the rest of the body? . . . the noxious humor which nature makes more feeble, which nevertheless is able to come to the surface, also settles in the nerves of the joints, and there it produces great pain. . . . Hippocrates suggests the first type, when in another aphorism he enumerates lichen, leprosy and ulcerous pustules among the diseases of spring, many of which according to the same Hippocrates are shared with summer. Now the second when phymata, which are properly tubercles, arise in the glandular parts (as Paul as well as Galen knew) and soon cause pain of the joints. . . . For this reason it is thought in the French disease, it produces at one time the same material and pustules and it is believed to excite pain in the joints, and as far as this is concerned it is believed it may belong not to two diseases, but to one alone, of which pain is a symptom.

"For those, who themselves have no pustules on the external surface, nevertheless can have similar abscesses on the inside, with sometimes (as they say) a greater pain. Certainly many physicians have discovered this to be so in certain dead persons, whom the French disease infected while living, their diseases investigated, thanks to dissections. . . . This I hold regarding the nature of the French disease and the causes of the disease itself. Even if I believe firmly, that the French disease under another name was common to the ancients, and that I should have described a simple type, yet it would not have been possible for me for the multiplex nature of the disease itself demands explanation.

"Finally it is seen that Hippocrates had regarded in his teaching of viruses that a similar epidemic happening in his time was from a similar cause and described completely various types of ulcers as well as tumors. Because if anything is supposed to be known by Hippocrates himself he would attempt to define better the French disease." [22]

NICOLO LENICENO (1428-1524)

Nicolo Leoniceno was born in Lonigo and studied at Vicenzia (a neighboring city) and at the University of Padua where he occupied for a time the position of Professor. He also taught at the University of Bologna.

Leoniceno was a great Greek scholar. He translated Hippocrates and Galen into Latin. He was a great admirer of Hippocrates and quotes him repeatedly in his medical writings. He praises the scholarship of Rhazes but in general he had no high opinion of the Arabian physicians and especially of Avicenna whom he criticizes frequently. He finally settled in Ferrara (1464) where he served as professor for sixty years and where he died in 1524. Leoniceno is discussed more fully later.

The "Blasphemy Edict" of King Maximilian to which was attached a paragraph referring to syphilis (*"Grosse Blattern"*) was promulgated on August 7, 1495. This document indicates that syphilis was widely disseminated in Europe at that time, and that it therefore could hardly have been imported by the returning soldiers of Charles VIII as at that date the army was still in Italy.

Johannes Widmann (1440-1524), a physician of Tubingen, Württemberg, shows that the word "saphata" or "asphati" ("leprosy"), as employed by the Arabian physicians, applies to syphilis which prevailed 37 years before the siege of Naples. He himself had seen such cases long before the siege. He states that pestilential disease manifests itself by fevers, chancres, ulcers, measles, variolous eruptions, cutaneous affections such as the pustules of "formica" or those of "asphati" which is also called French disease, which disease has spread itself from country to country with most grave symptoms from the year 1457 up to the current time.

A similar description of venereal ulceration is that presented by Richard Vendom an English physician, alchemist and anatomist who is better known as Ricardus Anglicus or Richard of Wendover (d. 1252). From 1222 to 1224 he was physician to Pope Gregory X. After 1241 he removed to Paris. When he returned to London he was appointed Canon of St. Paul. He was the author of many works, largely based on Greek and Arabic sources and particularly on the translation of Ibn Sinai by Gerard of Cremona (1114-1187).

G. B. Silvaticus (1550-1621) states that the *bothor* of the Arabians was an excrescence of flesh or a pustule. He, as well as Theodoric (1205-1298) described *formica* as a small projecting pustule.

Edgood quotes from a translation of a Persian work on syphilis by Hakim Imad-el Mahmud ibn Mascud ibn Mahmud, written in Harat (1511) and comes to the conclusion that syphilis has always existed in Europe in a sporadic and mild form but that its virulence became exacerbated with the return of Columbus' sailors from America.[23]

CAUSES OF SYPHILIS

Before the true cause of syphilis was disclosed, many theories concerning its etiology were presented. It was thought to be due to a disturbance of the yellow bile. It was ascribed to contaminated air, bad food and drinking water and other unhealthy living conditions. Inundations and earthquakes were blamed for polluting the air and water, destroying the pastures, causing famine and inflicting syphilitic disease. Astrologists ascribed lues to the conjunction of the planets Saturn and Mars as well as to eclipses of the sun and moon.

Roger Bacon attributes the etiology of syphilis to unnatural debauchery which, in the western Middle Ages, was allegedly very prevalent. Emperor Maximilian of Austria ascribed the *bösen Blattern* to the use of the Lord's name in vain.

Leoniceno of Lombardy, referred to previously, states that syphilis is caused by the action of telluric miasmata which he declares "is caused by divine wrath as the theologians believe, by the influence of the stars as the astrologists declare or by certain unseasonableness of the air as physicians think." He himself is inclined to the last opinion, for inundations were commonplace at that period in all parts of Europe.

CHAPTER XXX

DIABETES DURING THE MIDDLE AGES

The term diabetes derived from the Greek "dia" ("through") and "betes" ("to go") is an euphemistic expression for the frequent urination so characteristic of both diabetes mellitus and diabetes insipidus. Diabetes was known as a clinical entity to the ancients. The Papyrus Ebers (c. 1500 B.C.) indicates that the ancient Egyptians had a number of remedies to combat the passing of too much urine (polyuria).

The early Greeks apparently missed diabetes and the Hippocratics did not mention it. The later Greek writers, however, including Aretaeus, Celsus and Galen described this syndrome. According to Caelius Aurelianus, Apollonius of Memphis (230 B.C.) coined the name "diabetes."[1] Celsus is also credited with having named this pathologic condition "diabetes." Neither the Egyptians nor the Greeks, however, differentiated between diabetes mellitus and insipidus and their descriptions tend to adequately describe only the latter condition. Aretaeus gave the best description of diabetes insipidus.

Hindu physicians, on the other hand, far back in antiquity, seem to have recognized diabetes mellitus for they observed that flies and insects fed on the urine of certain patients. The Ayur Veda refers to the sweet taste of the urine of certain diseases.[2] A document discovered about 200 years ago shows that Susruta (c. 1000 A.D.), considered to be the Father of Indian surgery, was familiar with the clinical picture of the disease and with the sweet taste of diabetic urine. In India diabetes mellitus is still a highly prevalent disease.

Caelius Aurelianus quotes Apollonius of Memphis to the effect that the latter thought diabetes to be a form of dropsy: "One form of dropsy is marked by retention of fluid, and another by an inability to retain, so that whatever the patient drinks is immediately discharged as if it is passed through a pipe." And he declares, in agreement with most physicians, that the type of dropsy which involves retention appears in the three different forms. But Demetrius of Apamea (276 B.C.) more properly distinguishes diabetes from dropsy. The disease in which any fluid that is drunk is immediately discharged as urine . . . he calls . . . diabetes.[3]

Paul of Aegina defines diabetes as "a rapid passage of the drink out of the body. Since the liquid is voided by the urine as fast as it is drunk, this disease is attended by immoderate thirst. Therefore the affection has been called 'dypsacus,' because it is occasioned by a weakness of the retentive faculty of the kidneys . . . and deprives the whole body of its moisture." To counteract the bodily dehydration, Paul advises various kinds of wines and foods to help make up for the loss of liquid in the body. He recommends pot-herbs, endives, lettuce, rock-fishes, the juice of knotgrass and elecampane in dark colored wine and decoctions of dates and myrtle. He advises the application of cataplasms to the hypochondrium, and over the kidneys. These are to be prepared from vinegar, rose oil, the leaves of various vines and navel-wort. He advocates the promotion of sweat and vomitus and warns against the use of all diuretics. He does not object to venesection in these cases.[4]

The Arabian writers, Rhazes (865-925) and Avicenna (980-1037), probably received their knowledge of diabetes from the Arabian translation of Susruta Samhita made at the end of the eighth century.[5]

As previously stated, Aretaeus was the first to graphically describe the clinical history of diabetes insipidus:

"Diabetes is a wonderful affection, not very frequent among men, being a melting down of the flesh and limbs into urine. Its cause is of a cold and humid nature, as in dropsy. The course is the common one, namely, the kidneys and the bladder; for the patients never stop making water, but the flow is incessant, as if from the opening of aqueducts. The nature of the disease, then, is chronic, and it takes a long period to form; but the patient is short-lived, if the constitution of the disease be completely established; for the melting is rapid, the death speedy."

His description of the symptoms of diabetes insipidus is very striking: "a fiery thirst, a never-ending desire to make water, a parched skin and a dry mouth." Diabetes, according to Aretaeus, is a species of dropsy in which the water is shunted to the urinary organs instead of to the peritoneum as in ordinary dropsy. With diabetes, life becomes disgusting and painful, the thirst unquenchable, and the drinking excessive. More urine is passed than water imbibed and one cannot stop such patients either from drinking or making water. If for a time they abstain from drinking, their mouths become even more parched and their bodies dry; the viscera become scorched. They are affected with nausea, restlessness, and a burning thirst and at a not distant term they expire.

"If the disease be fully established, it is strongly marked; but if it be merely coming on, the patients have the mouth parched, saliva white, frothy, as if from thirst (for the thirst is not yet confirmed), weight in the hypochondriac region. A sensation of heat or cold from the stomach to the bladder marks, as it were, the advent of the approaching disease; they now make a little more water than usual, and there is thirst, but it is not yet great...

"But if it increase still more, the heat is small indeed, but pungent, and seated in the intestines; the abdomen, shrivelled, veins protuberant, general emaciation, when the quality of urine and the thirst have already increased; and when, at the same time, the sensation appears at the extremity of the member, the patients immediately make water. Hence, the disease appears to me to have got the name 'diabetes.' The fluid does not remain in the body, but uses the man's body as a ladder, whereby to leave it. They stand out for a certain time, though not very long, for they pass urine with pain, and the emaciation is dreadful; nor does any great portion of the drink get into the system, and many parts of the flesh pass out along with the urine." [6]

Galen states that he only recollected having met with two cases of diabetes. He maintains that its effect on the urinary organs is analogous to that of dysentery on the bowels. He is decidedly of the opinion that the kidneys are primarily affected and not the stomach, as some of his predecessors had supposed. He explains his views on the nature of the disease with great precision.

Aëtius has given a full account of diabetes insipidus. Upon the authority of Archigenes of Apama (45-117 A.D.), he recommends at the commencement of the disease, bleeding and diuretics, the latter being given to clear away the vitiated urine from the kidneys. If the disease be of long standing, he advocates the use of both of these measures. He also recommends a cooling diet, and diluted wine, internally and cooling applications to the pubes and loins. In certain cases, he advocates the use of narcotics such as opium and mandragora.

J. Actuarius (c. 1257) recommends purgatives to relieve the strain on the kidneys and he advocates the use of astringent and refrigerant remedies in general.

A full and accurate account on the subject of diabetes is presented by Avicenna. In certain cases, he favors venesection at the commencement of the disease. The remedies in which he seems to place the greatest reliance are emetics and sudorifics which he gives with the intention of altering the determination of the fluids to the kidneys. He particularly directs the patient to avoid taking all diuretic foods and drugs and to engage in exercise on horseback and to employ moderate friction. In the later stages of the disease, he favors the use of tepid baths with fragrant wine.

Haly Abbas presents, with his usual precision, the theory of Galen and other Greek authorities, namely, that the disease is occasioned by a preternatural increase of the attractive faculty of the kidneys, arising from excessive heat within the viscus. Agreeable with this theory of the etiology of the disease, his remedies are refrigerants and astringents. According to Rhazes, the affection is connected with preternatural heat of the kidneys and debility of their retentive faculty. He says it resembles dysentery of the intestine.[7]

Among the physicians of the Renaissance concerned with diabetes may be mentioned Cardona (1501-1576 A.D.) who studied the urine of diabetics and found that the volume of fluid passing from their bodies through the kidneys, was more than the volume of fluid taken in.

As previously intimated, the Hindus early discovered diabetes mellitus as a distinct medical entity. The works of Susruta having been lost for centuries, diabetes mellitus had to wait until 1574 to be rediscovered as a distinct disease. The first European physician in modern times to note the character of the urine in diabetes was Thomas Willis (1622-1675).

Willis ascribes the cause of diabetes to a humoral change in the blood brought about by immoderate drinking of cider, beer and sharp wine as well as various psychologic factors. He relates the case of a patient who drank Rhinish wine immoderately for twenty days, contracted an incurable diabetes and died within a month.

According to Willis, the symptoms of diabetes are thirst, dry throat and fever and he states that in this condition, the heart and lungs "are provoked into a more rapid motion." The sweetness of the urine is due to a chemical change: "If salts that are of a divers nature both fixed and volatile be mixed with an acid thing the acrimony of either is diminished or lost; therefore we need not wonder that the urine of those laboring with diabetes is not salty."

According to Willis, those that are sick with diabetes pass more urine than they take in by drink, and by taking liquid food. He also states that diabetes is an affection of the blood rather than of the kidneys.

The process of changing the blood into fluid "is apt to be dangerous." The serous fluid passes out of the body and "provokes a huge thirst." . . . "The humors that are within the solid parts are sucked up from the blood; hence it is that those laboring with this disease are exceedingly thirsty and quickly grow lean." . . . "I am led to believe that the watery particles cannot be constrained by the more thick, but that they quickly slide from their embraces, with sulphurous sweetness, but being very much loosed so that very many parts separate the one from the other, it scarce or never can be restored . . ."

According to Willis, it seems probable that the sweetness of the diabetic urine is produced by the union of saline spicules. As to treatment, "Its cause lies so deeply hid and hath its origin so deeply remote that it is most hard to draw proportions for curing." He recommends astringents as remedies.[8]

John Rollo, the greatest authority on diabetes mellitus of his period (1798) was first to notice the existence of an excess of sugar in the blood of diabetic patients.

About the fifth decade of the last century, Claude Bernard (1813-1878) advanced the idea that the presence of sugar in the normal blood is produced by glycogenolysis from the glycogen stored in the liver. In 1848, L. Traube (1818-1876) noted that when carbohydrates are eliminated from their food, the sugar in the urine of diabetic patients tends to disappear but promptly reappears when carbohydrates are again added to the diet.

The findings of Mehring and Minkowski in 1889 to the effect that diabetes mellitus can be artificially produced in dogs and certain other animals by removal of the pancreas, enabled Banting and Best in 1921 to isolate the hormonal secretion of insulin from the Islets of Langerhans of the pancreas and this greatly advanced the knowledge of diabetes mellitus and its treatment. Oral hypoglycemic agents such as Orinase and Diabinese are just now coming into vogue.

CHAPTER XXXI

EPIDEMIC PSYCHOSES DURING THE MIDDLE AGES

INTRODUCTION

The visitation of one plague after another gave the exhausted medieval population scarcely any time to get back to normal life and any semblance of sound reasoning. The people lost faith in physical remedies which brought them no relief and turned to religion for help. Emphasis should be placed on the fact that the type of religion to which they turned was not that to which people turn in normal times. The bitterness of their lives drove them to seek vulgar and base religious superstitions and the greater the catastrophes to which they were subjected, the deeper the abyss into which their base superstitious practices sank. At times actual maniacal outbreaks became the order of the day.

Aside from religious mania, other forms of functional nervous disorders were prevalent. The strangest of these affected large groups of people and followed the footsteps of the great epidemics. At such times, pent-up emotions exploded among the survivors of the great epidemic scourges and manifested themselves in various forms of mania. What a modern psychiatrist would term "manic depressive psychoses" or "manic exhilarating psychoses" became widespread. Wild delusions and fantastic mental aberrations prevailed on all sides.[1]

Caelius Aurelianus gives a graphic description of many forms of mania and particularly the form characterized by "impairment of reason resulting from a bodily disease or indisposition." He states that when a mania lays hold on the mind, "it manifests itself now in anger, now in merriment, now in sadness and now as some relate in an overpowering fear of things which are quite harmless." Caelius describes many forms of monomania. He declares that some suffer impairment of all the senses and some are affected by various other forms of aberrations. He cites the case of one victim of mania who pictured himself as a sparrow and another who thought he was a cock. Others were deluded into thinking they were a god, an orator, a tragic actor and a comic actor. One, who was sure that he was an infant, cried like a baby and begged to be carried in the arms. Caelius Aurelianus thus gives us a picture of the forms of mania prevailing in the early Middle Ages.[2]

The last form of nervous disorder known as monomania not infrequently attacked the inmates of the convents. Don Calimet tells of nuns in a German convent who imagined themselves transformed into cats and went around mewing continuously. Patients troubled with monomania frequently have an urge to imitate the sounds of animals. This condition, according to Freud, is caused by isolation and suppression of natural inclinations. It is a variety of mania particularly prevalent among religious groups practicing celibacy. Suppression of normal sexual functions tends to exaggerate and pervert normal sexual instinct and often leads to illusions, optical aberrations and other types of mental disorders.

Freud[3] has called attention to the fact that our ideas, thoughts, emotions and experiences are naturally grouped in our minds into certain complexes, each of which is somewhat independent of the rest and yet influences the others. For example, all the thoughts and feelings connected with one's religious education or with one's political affiliations or with one's family life may be termed the religious complex or the political complex or the family complex. Every one of these complexes, even when not apparently within the field of attention, has an influence upon the subject within the field of attention and tends to modify any resulting conclusion which would follow from the consideration of that subject. One may be wholly unaware that the fact of such a complex is determining the thought or the conclusion arrived at; yet the complex nevertheless has its continuous and permanent effect. We express this by saying that a person is "unconsciously biased" in his thought. The mind, then, never acts freely, but is always influenced by these underlying complexes to a greater or lesser extent. The more fundamental and primitive the complex affecting it, the more dominating will be the effect of that complex upon the mental activity.

According to Freud, the most fundamental of all complexes is the sexual complex, which, he believes, originates very early in infancy and maintains its dominating influence throughout life. He holds that all love, even the love of the child for its parent, is primarily sexual in origin. It is the tendency, however, of general education to repress the discussion of this sexual complex. Many ideas connected with it are unpleasant, mortifying or shameful, and the tendency of training is to combat its expression. For Freud, sexual abuse or sexual trauma exists in everyone at an early age. The constant effort to ignore or to repress these disagreeable and shameful experiences connected with the sexual complex produces a state of mental perturbation and this in turn causes a very morbid stress of mind, attended by unpleasant emotions. The group of ideas constantly being pushed into the background is detached from the conscious life by an effort attended by emotion, but the emotion is one of anxiety to conceal the sexual complex, or of fear lest it be discovered, or of shame at its existence, and hence any thought which suggests the sexual complex tends to awaken the emotions connected with it.

If the repression is eventually successful, the complex after a time no longer consciously influences the course of thought. It is not thereby obliterated from the mind but remains in the domain of the subconscious. From the subconscious, Freud imagines that there is a constant tendency for the complex to emerge and hence the process of repression is kept up all the time by an act of the mind which he calls "censure." Such an act is attended by more or less emotion and hence the individual may be constantly under an emotional strain. This emotion may then be transferred from the unconscious train of thought to some conscious train of thought, lending an emotional character to some mental act that otherwise would be without emotion. Freud thus explains the existence of morbid fears; that is, the existence of fear connected with some act which normally would go on without fear. If this complex energy with its emotion is diverted into a physical channel, Freud terms the process "conversion" and believes that it is the basis for many hysterical physical symptoms, such as spasms, convulsions, paralysis and anaesthetic areas. He holds that every case of hysteria is the result of some preceding psychic trauma and that such a trauma may be produced by any experience which produces the emotions of fear, anxiety or shame. In his opinion, such experiences are always in the sexual sphere.

Perhaps the earliest work to indicate that man possesses a subconscious state of mind is found in the Old Testament. There are many instances in the Old Testament describing things that lead to such a conclusion. Take for example "which saw the vision of the almighty falling into a trance, but having his eyes open."[4] Dreams[5] and the story of King Saul who was troubled with the evil spirit[6] and expressions such as the "Thought of the Spirit," memory, perception, (daath, machshava, hashaga, habanah).[7]

The Old Testament probably did not know the cause for the change of spirit as given by Freud, but was acquainted with the subconscious condition.

There is a vast amount of historical facts which indicate that almost since the dawn of civilization man has had an understanding that mind activity outside of our waking consciousness does truly exist. There are a great many written words describing such things as double personality, automatic behavior and unreality of feelings, that allow us the understanding that an unconscious process was established long before the advent of Freud.

The earliest work to indicate that activities of our outside of waking consciousness do exist, may be found in the *Upanishads.*[8]

The Upanishads set forth quite clearly the "four states of self." They are:

1. The waking state *jagarita-sthana*: equivalent to the "conscious." In this state, man accepts the universe as he finds it. Perception, volition, and memory are preserved.

2. The dreaming state *svapna-sthana*: the "subconscious." Here the self loses contact with reality, and the soul fashions its own world in the imagery of its dreams.

3. The deep-sleep state *susupta-sthana*: a deeper level of the subconscious approaching complete unconsciousness. This is a state of bliss in which there is no contact with reality, no desire, no dreams.

4. The fourth state *caturtha, turiva, turya:* the "super- (or supra-) conscious." "According to Vedanta, it is in this state that Seers get flashes of Great Truths in the form of vague apprehensions, which are afterwards elaborated in the jagrat state of waking consciousness."

The same might be said about the three souls of Plato (427-347 B.C.),[9] which are treated in a similar way in the New Testament—spirit, psyche, flesh, equivalent to super-ego, ego, and id, and the sense of which was first clearly set forth in the *Katha Upanishad.*

"10. Higher than the senses are the objects of sense.
Higher than the objects of sense is the mind (manas);
And higher than the mind is the intellect (buddhi)
Higher than the intellect is the Great Self (Atman).

"11. Higher than the Great Self is the Unmanifest (Avyakta).
Higher than the Unmanifest is the Person
Higher than the Person there is nothing at all.
That is the goal. That is the highest course." [10]

Plato in *The Republic* states as follows: "Of pleasures and desires that are not necessary, some seem to be contrary to law, —which indeed seem engendered in all men: though owing to the correction of the laws, and of improved desires aided by reason, they either forsake men altogether, or are less numerous and feeble, while in others they are more powerful and more numerous. Will you inform me what these are? said he. Such, said I, as are excited in sleep, when the rest of the soul—which is rational, mild, and its governing principle, is asleep, and when that part which is savage and rude, being sated with food and drink, frisks about, drives away sleep, and seeks to go and accomplish its practices;—in such an one, you know, it dares to do everything, because it is loosed and disengaged from all modesty and prudence; for, it pleases, it scruples not at the embraces, even of a mother, or any one else, whether gods, men, or beasts; nor to commit murder, nor abstain from any sort of meat,—and in one word, it is wanting neither in folly nor shamelessness." [11]

Aristotle (384-322) in the *De Memoria et Reminiscentia*, sets forth his theories of memory, association, and mental activity outside of consciousness of which the subject was unaware. Extracts from this work are so clear as to require but little explanation: The process of movement (sensory stimulation) involved in the act of perception stamps in, as it were, a sort of impression of the percept, just as persons do who make an impression with a seal.

Rhazes (864-925 A.D.) the great Arab physician was an astute psychologist, and drew from Plato when writing of the soul and emotions. In his *Spiritual Physick,* Rhazes applied the Platonic idea of suppression of the passions in order to maintain the health of the body.

During the Dark Ages, nothing is found to illustrate the subject with which we are concerned. Toward the end of the fifteenth century, two great names in medicine strike our attention; apparently both of them had an understanding of the mental processes outside of awareness. They were Paracelsus (1493-1541) and Juan Luis Vives (1492-1540). Paracelsus was of the opinion that mental illness was due to unhealthy changes in the spiritus vitae, and rejected the prevalent demonological concept of mental illness, which in itself was no mean accomplishment for his time, since everybody believed that people became mentally ill from inhabitation of the body by demons or spirits. He offered the name "chorea lascive" for St. Vitus' dance, and suggested the sexual nature of hysteria. He formulated the theory that imaginative ideas, elaborated from seeing or hearing something, were the cause of hysteria: "their sight and hearing are so strong that unconsciously they have fantasies about what they have seen or heard." Vives[12] had clearly seen the importance of psychological associations and recognized the emotional content that many associations carried with them. He described in *De Anima et Vita* (1538) how ideas could be registered without our conscious knowledge and could later be discovered by association.[13]

As epilepsy was considered a form of mania that prevailed in epidemic form and at a period of life when one becomes conscious of the sexual instinct, it will be treated here among other forms of mania caused by the same condition.

MENTAL EPIDEMICS
EPILEPSY

Epilepsy (derived from the Greek "*epi*" meaning "upon" and "*lepsy*" meaning "to seize") is a term applied to a nervous disorder, characterized by a sudden loss of consciousness and a fall attended with a convulsive seizure. Epilepsy was well known in ancient times and was regarded as a special affliction[14] dispensed by the gods. Hence the ancient names "morbus sacra" and "morbus divus." It was also termed "morbus Herculeus," after Hercules, who was supposed to have been an epileptic.

In the Old Testament Balaam is the personage described in the following: "The saying of him who heareth the words of God, who seeth the vision of the almighty, Fallen down yet with opened eyes."[15] This description covers the two essential symptoms of epilepsy.

Hippocrates refutes the concept that epilepsy is a sacred disease. "To me it appears that such affections are just as much divine as all others are, that one disease is neither more divine nor more human than another but all are alike divine for each has its own nature." Hippocrates ascribes epilepsy to a cold phlegm secreted in the brain and causing coagulative obstruction while passing down through the blood vessels. He remarks that inferior animals such as goats are subject to this complaint and that in such cases, water is occasionally found in their brain.

Aretaeus divides epilepsy into acute and chronic forms. In the acute form, he advises bleeding, clysters and emetics and he recommends copper given with cardamum. In chronic cases he suggests opening a vein or artery in the head or even "boring the bone" down to the diploe, and applying the actual cautery to it. As a test of epilepsy he recommends the use of the "agate" stone, the smell of which is said to be diagnostic in that it brings on an immediate attack. He approves of general bleeding if the disease is accompanied with plethora.

Celsus evidently thought that epilepsy is created by an impoverished blood condition and he recommended the blood of a slain gladiator as being of curative value in treating epilepsy. "If these devices do not suffice," Celsus declares, "let the epileptic's head be shaved, then anoint it with oil, adding vinegar, niter and salt water over this." The purpose of such therapy was to stimulate the circulation in the head.

Caelius Aurelianus has this to say of epilepsy: "It is known as 'sacred disease' either because it is thought to be sent by a divine power or because it is centered in the head which in the judgement of many philosophers is the sacred abode of that part of the soul which originates in the body, or because of the great power of the disease, for people generally call what is powerful 'sacred.' " [16]

He goes on to say that the contributory causes are drinking too much wine, indigestion, compression of the brain and fright. The whole nervous system is affected by epilepsy and especially the brain. He approves of venesection after the first attack unless the stomach is overloaded with crudities. If the headache is severe he is in favor of applying leeches to the painful spot. He does not approve of the use of heat to the head and sinapisms to the other parts of the body. He recommends applying eschartics to the head. He is contemptuous of such favorite treatments as the application of a bull's blood or that of a man recently killed. He is against the use of chalybeates, hellebore and scammony.

Haly Abbas states that epileptic convulsions come either periodically or irregularly. Such seizures arise from the brain directly or from a sympathetic reaction within the stomach or other parts of the body. According to this authority, epilepsy is due to a morbid humor collected in the ventricles of the brain or from cerebral compression produced by a fracture. He takes note of the aura and the reaction of the patient's mouth.

Like Hippocrates, he holds that if epilepsy occurs before puberty it is not difficult to cure, but cases originating in adult life are very hard to cure. He advises the application of cupping instruments to the neck and drastic purgatives in persistent cases. If the seizures emanate from the stomach, he recommends emetics, and drastic purgatives such as black hellebore and colocynth. In infant epilepsy, he directs that both the infant and the wet nurse be placed on special diets.

Epilepsy has always been associated with superstition. Alsaharadius, although treating other diseases in a rational fashion, states that he possessed positive proof that epileptics are truly possessed by demons. He recommends the use of amulets to be worn both for prophylaxis and cure.

The Hindus attributed epilepsy to demonic possession. In the Vedic writings, mystic exorcism is generally recognized as the best cure.

Leo Africanus states that the common people term epilepsy "the demoniac disease" or "the lunacy disease," the latter term originating from the belief that it is caused by the action of the Moon.

Even such a judicious and original thinker as Alexander of Tralles (sixth century A.D.) expresses confidence in the use of amulets, at least for their psychological effect.[17] Internally he recommended the use of purgatives and emetics. Venesection was recommended by some Arab authorities.

Paul of Aegina, who flourished at the start of the Middle Ages, gives the causes of epilepsy as (1) humoral, (2) gastric disturbances, and (3) secondary to pathology in other parts of the body, such as when a cold aura ascends to the brain either from the legs or from the fingers or when the condition proceeds from the uterus during pregnancy in which latter case cure usually follows delivery (eclampsia?).

Aëtius regards epilepsy as profoundly influenced by being oversexed, and he advises extirpation of the testes as an infallible cure for epilepsy in males. This opinion is in advance of his time and affords a premonition of the Freudian explanation of neurotic and hysterical convulsions in young people.

An unusual form of epidemic psychosis which combined the symptoms of epilepsy and mania prevailed in the Middle Ages. Bernard de Gordon includes epilepsy among the eight contagious diseases of the Middle Ages. The others are: bubonic plague, tuberculosis, scabies, erysipelas, anthrax, trachoma and leprosy.

Von Storchs quotes Arnold of Villanova (1235-1311 A.D.) as saying: "I hold that epilepsy is an occlusion of the chief ventricles of the brain, with loss of sensation and motion; or, epilepsy is a noncontinuous spasm of the whole body. This disease takes rise from different causes, such as superfluous foods and drinks, poisons, the bites of mad dogs or reptiles, and from poisoned and pestiferous air. When the pores are constricted, superfluities are retained and natural heat is lessened, there follows a filling up of the chief ventricles of the brain. These are the three causes which principally induce epilepsy." [18]

To treat epilepsy, Arnold recommends the flesh of birds (except those living in the marshes), and the flesh of yearling lambs, swine, and goats flavored with strong-smelling wine. Fish which live in rivers are only suitable if cooked dry on hot coals. The epileptic was permitted to eat spinach, parsley, fennel, asparagus, and well baked wheat bread. He might drink yellow wine and white wine of good odor. Other therapeutic measures prescribed by Arnold consist of mineral baths at midnight, purges, and cauterizations, a course of treatment almost as distressing to the epileptic as the seizures themselves. Foods to be avoided by the epileptic, according to Arnold, are cabbage, lentils, beans, brains of animals, and celery. Celery should especially be avoided because of its tendency to induce epilepsy.[19]

From the time of Edward the Confessor (reigned 1042-1066) to that of Queen Anne (reigned 1702-1714), epilepsy was considered only second to scrofula as being curable by royal touch.

Epilepsy was treated in England [20] by the wearing of cramp rings. Cramp rings were often made of silver employed for the communion service. Many were made of coffin nails. The legend is that Edward the Confessor, while dedicating a church to St. John the Evangelist, gave his ring to a beggar who asked for alms. The beggar was later revealed to be St. John himself. According to Crawford this legend explains the synonym of epilepsy, *morbus sacer*. According to the tale, the ring was returned to Edward and endowed with miraculous powers. Although it was buried with him in 1066, it was later exhumed and employed to endow other numerous cramp rings with virtue.

In France the wearing of an emerald ring was looked upon as a protection against "the falling sickness." It also "can fortify the memory, and resist the forces of carnal lust."

According to an Erfurt Codex unearthed in Germany by Sudhoff, the following treatment was recommended: "For epilepsy, take holy water and pour it into the right hand and then say: 'I pour you out in the name of our Lord Jesus Christ born in Bethlehem.' Then pour it over the patient's face and say: 'I pour this over you in the name of our Lord Jesus Christ who was tortured in Jerusalem.'"[21]

Another cure for epilepsy is cited by Frazer: "If a man drops on the ground with falling sickness, you need only whisper in his right ear, 'Gaspard fert myrrhem thus melchoir Balthazar aurum,' and he will get up at once. But to make the cure completely you will knock three nails into the earth on the precise spot where he fell; each nail must be exactly the size of his little finger, and as you knock it you must utter the sufferer's name."[22]

Trephining of the skull was practiced in the early Middle

Ages among some people as a sure cure for epilepsy not because it was thought that the disease was due to a growth or a morbid humor pressing on the vital centers of the brain but for the purpose of effecting an exit for the evil spirit causing the epileptic attack.

That epilepsy was still not divorced from superstition in the seventeenth century is seen from the following formula: "Against the falling sickness, take a jay, pull off her feathers, and pull out her guts; fill her belly full of cummin seeds, then dry her in an oven until she be converted into a mummy (possibly a substitute for the expensive Egyptian *mumia* employed during this period). A dram of her, being beaten into a powder, seeds, and all, is an excellent remedy for the falling sickness, being taken in any convenient liquor every morning."

A so-called "proven-cure" for epilepsy was the following formula: "Take a bone from the heart of a stag, seeds of wild rue, a peony and the hoofs of the forefeet of an ass; pulverize them, and snuff up in the nose one ounce of the powder every morning." A postscript, "In a short time this will cure the epileptic," is added. Another recommended formula: "Take one half a dram of a wolf's gall, with one grain of musk, and place it in the nostrils of the epileptic at the beginning of the month; it helps greatly."

"A wonderful electuary against epilepsy," is vouched for by the author of the following prescription: "Take of the leaves of rue, of the seed of hemlock, of the dung of doves, of polypody, of mistletoe, of castor, of black hellebore, of aloes, of epitheme, of asafetida, of each two drams; of turpeth, of lapis lazuli, of the pulp of colocynth, of mastic, of spikenard, of the root of the peony, of agaric, of each one dram. Grind them all to fine powder; mix with oil of sweet almond; make into the form of an electuary; prepare with a syrup of sugar and dried rue; every morning give the patient one or two drams of it, because it is wonderful and approved." [23]

At the present time the fantastic idea of demonic possession is difficult to condone, but anyone who has observed the symptoms of epilepsy may realize how natural it was in the infancy of medicine to accept demonic possession as an etiologic factor of epilepsy. The sudden onset, the staring eyes, the strange gestures, the fall, the froth-covered mouth, the frantic and beastly voice, the jerking of the body and the twitching of the muscles, surely suggested to those to whom the natural order of things was not known that such an episode was the work of a malicious fiend.

In epilepsy, the demonic seizure was so sudden and mysterious that quick measures had to be taken to inspire fear in the demon so that he would leave the body of the epileptic instantly. In this case, water from the skull of a suicide was poured down the patient's throat so that the demon would have a quick taste of the dregs of destruction. The demon would then surely know to make hasty exit before destruction overtook him.[24]

Some of the great historical personages of ancient and modern times are said to have been epileptics such as, for example, the Persian King Cambyses (521-621), Julius Caesar (100-44 B.C.), Mohammed (570-632), Dante (1265-1321), Mortier (1622-1673), Napoleon (1786-1812) and, in more modern times, A. C. Swinburne (1837-1909) and J. Swift (1667-1745). Indeed, the great Italian criminologist and psychiatrist, Cesare Lombroso (1836-1909), maintained that epileptiform neurosis is a factor closely related to genius.

MANIA

The Latin term *"mania"* has its origin in the myth that a possessed person is dominated by the goddess Mania. In the Middle Ages, madmen whose hallucinations took the form of religious fervor, were often regarded with veneration, but those whose ravings were blasphemous or obscene, were supposed to be possessed by demons. Treatment for possession was exorcism by the priest. If this measure failed, the blame was placed on the madman's obstinacy, and he was treated cruelly, chained, whipped and starved into submission.[25]

Some of the medieval methods of dislodging demons from the body of the sick had such a terrifying effect on the patient that he forgot all about his ailment. He was shown corpses, coffins, skulls, gallows, and graveyards. The method for casting out the demon causing ague (malaria), for example, was the application of chips of gallows upon which a criminal had recently been hanged, to the patient's body. This had a double purpose: firstly, to warn the demon that he might be punished with the extreme penalty; and secondly, to make the patient forget his pain. Malaria, it must be remembered, is a disease characterized by the sudden onset of fever and convulsive chills that shake the body from head to foot, terminating in a copious perspiration. Because of the nature of the disease, the primitive mind conceived it to be the work of a cruel supernatural fiend against whom drastic action was necessary if it was to be dislodged. Since the gallows was the extreme penalty for offenders of the law, the demon who stealthily entered the person's body needs must tremble at the thought that he too will suffer the supreme penalty if he refuses to depart at once.

INSANITY

Next to epilepsy, insanity was regarded as a supernatural disease, and accordingly, it called for heroic and fantastic treatment. Throughout the Middle Ages, imbeciles and insane persons were considered possessed by a frenzied avenging diabolic demon, which called for the intervention of a special saint, as, for example, St. Avertin. In mild cases of insanity, plaintive prayers or the imposition of the hands of a holy man were deemed sufficient to effect a cure. When medicinal measures were resorted to, the ingredients were many, and most disgusting to swallow.[26]

In Anglo-Saxon times insanity was treated "first by working herbs into clear ale; seven masses were then said over the preparation while adding garlic and holy water: the mixture was drunk out of a church bell."

Superficially it appears difficult to condone the fantastic theories of the ancient and medieval peoples and particularly their revolting remedies for epilepsy and mania. But, if one takes into consideration the status of medicine in general in those days, he will find an excuse for their indulgence in medical superstition. Ignorant of the very rudiments of science, our forebears endeavored to obtain an understanding of life guided by their special senses and intuitive powers. The appearance and behavior of one suffering from an illness, in which he no longer expresses his customary thoughts and no longer speaks with his familiar voice, suggested that some strange being had entered that person. Anyone who has observed the symptoms of epilepsy can realize how natural it was, in the infancy of medicine, to accept demonic possession as the etiologic factor of epilepsy.

Evil spirits were held responsible for all ills. If one suffered from a choking sensation, a demon was said to be strangling him. If a person was troubled with pruritus around the genital organs, he was accused of cohabitation with a she-demon. If one had a cancerous growth on his lip he was guilty of having conspired with a devil. When one lost his hearing or speech, he had a deaf or dumb evil spirit in him.

In the Middle Ages lunatics whose delusions were of a religious nature were treated with veneration, but those of a raving and obscene character were suspected of being possessed by the devil and were taken to an exorcist to have the evil spirit expelled. If the fiend refused to leave, the demented person was blamed. He was brutally whipped, starved, chained, and placed in a dungeon until brought under control. If all these tortures did not induce the devil to depart from the body, the demented person was burned at the stake. Lunatics, until the days of Philippe Pinel (1755-1826) were looked upon as human beasts deserving of no sympathy.

As late as in the eighteenth century, "witch towers" were constructed for witches and the raving insane and "fool towers" for peaceful and religious maniacs. Occasionally the insane were on public exhibition and admission was charged to curious visitors for the privilege of watching these unfortunate beings. Vienna has its "lunatic towers" and London its Bedlam. The treatment of the insane in days goneby is a shameful blot on the history of civilization.

CHAPTER XXXII

THE DANCING MANIA AND OTHER EMOTIONAL DISORDERS

The most extraordinary mass emotional disturbance of the Middle Ages prevailed during the fourteenth century. It was known as the dancing mania. The participation in rhythmical dances as a form of religious exultation is as old as religion itself. It is a primitive expression of fervor and devotion. David ". . . danced with all his might before the Lord," at the solemn procession of the Ark at Kirjath Jearim.[1] Rhythmic thanksgiving accompanied by music was popular among the Athenians. Sophocles led the choir in the dancing at the celebration of the victory of Salamis. Among the Abyssinian Christians, dancing still forms a prominent part of worship. In the seventeenth century it was the function of the senior canon to lead a dance through the streets of Luxemburg to the shrine of St. Willibrod, in St. Peter's Church and the Hasidic dances among the eastern Jews in the synagogue on certain calendar days are an important part of the ritual.

However, the medieval dancing mania had no relation to religion. The men and women who participated in the wild dances did not know why they danced. The epidemics of dancing mania were the aftermath of periods of great physical and mental duress and afforded release from the long pent-up emotions of people who had suffered to the limits of human endurance. Dancing mania may be considered to be the strangest emotional disorder that has ever affected large groups of human beings.

The dancing mania began in Italy and spread to all parts of Europe. The dancers are described as wild hordes of individuals with fixed and staring eyes and with the muscles of their faces and limbs twitching. For hours or even days they jumped, screamed and foamed from the mouth until they fell exhausted. Often the participants had convulsions and abdominal distention.

Dancing began in the year 1374 or about twenty years after the fearful epidemic of Black Death. From Italy it spread to Aachen (Aix-la Chapelle), Prussia, and one morning, without warning, the streets were filled with men and women who joined hands, formed circles and seemingly lost all control over their actions. They danced together, ceaselessly, for hours or days, and in wild delirium, the dancers collapsed and fell to the ground exhausted, groaning and sighing as if in the agonies of death. When recuperated, they swathed themselves tightly with cloth around their waists and resumed their convulsive movements. They contorted their bodies, writhing, screaming and jumping in a mad frenzy. One by one they fell from exhaustion, but as they fell, others of the town took their places. These wild dancers seemed insensible to external impressions. They apparently neither saw nor heard.

Of course, the contagion of the dancing mania was a mass mental contagion spread by suggestion from the dancers to the onlookers. The dancing attacks were often followed by epileptiform convulsions. The victims fell to the ground, fainting and laboring for breath. They foamed from the mouth and suddenly sprang up to dance again. Many later claimed that they had seen the walls of heaven split open and that Jesus and the Virgin Mother Mary had appeared before them. Others fancied that they had been immersed in streams of blood and that this had prompted them to leap so high while dancing.

To quote J. F. C. Hecker (1795-1850),[2] "a convulsion infuriated the human frame . . . entire communities of people would join hands, dance, scream and shake for hours . . . music appeared to be the sole means of combating this strange epidemic . . . loud, shrill, tunes played on trumpets and fifes excited the dancers; soft calm, harmonies, graduated from fast to slow, and high to low proved efficacious as a cure."

"Where the disease was fully developed," says Hecker, "the

attacks were ushered in with epileptiform seizures. The afflicted fell to the ground unconscious, foaming from the mouth and struggling for breath, but after a time of rest, they got up and began dancing with still greater impetus and renewed vigor. This mental disorder varied in its course in accordance with individual physical endurance, the locality of the epidemic and other circumstances. Eye witnesses made no notation as to the variations of the malady. They noted only the chief characteristics of the disease." [3]

Hecker declares that in the seventeenth century, the tarantella in Italy reached its climax not only among the natives but also among foreigners, regardless of nationality, color, or creed. Negroes, Gypsies, Spaniards and Albanians were attacked with the dancing malady. There was no cure for the madness. It is said that ninety-year-old persons, at the first sound of the tarantella, threw away their canes and crutches and joined the dancers.

Contemporaries speak of this strange phenomenon as "the mental epidemic." It found ready victims among people suffering from nervous disorders, but even mentally healthy people unquestionably were so afflicted. The tarantella, then, was primarily a mass mental disorder of a "contagious" character which especially affected those whose minds had been unbalanced by their mental or physical condition or spiritual views. A common physical symptom which followed these spasmodic ravings was a sort of tympanites ... a kind of psychosomatic colonic gaseous distention of the abdomen due to spasms of the colonic valves. Thumping on the affected parts was said to ameliorate the distention and swathing relieved the pain.[4]

After a few months, the disease spread from Aachen to the neighboring cities of the Netherlands and thence to many Belgian cities, towns and villages. From all over, people flocked to see them. Some were merely curious and were not affected by contact with the dancers; others, more susceptible to impression, quickly joined the raving dancers. In Metz, the number of dancers reached eleven hundred and in Cologne five hundred. In Erfurt, in the year 1237, more than one hundred children were attacked by the dance mania. Those that didn't collapse, jumped and danced all the way down to Arnstadt. Some of the children died and it is stated that some remained with permanent contractions of the muscles of the limbs and body. On the Mosel bridge at Utrecht, in 1278, two hundred were attacked with the dance mania. They danced so hard on the bridge that the structure gave way and many drowned.[5]

Strassburg was visited by the dancing plague in 1418. It is said that in this city, the dancing mania reached its highest peak. The hordes affected could be seen, day or night, dancing madly to the accompanying music. A Strassburg chronicle dating from 1418, contains the following verse.

> "Viel Hundert fingen zu Strassburg an
> Zu Tanzen und sprungen, Frau und Mann,
> Am offnen Market, Gassen und Strassen
> Tag und Nacht ihrer nicht viel assen.
> Bis ihn das Wuthen wieder gelag.
> St. Viets Tanz war genannt die Plag." [6]

Strassburg was the first city where a concerted effort was made to treat the dancing maniacs and to prevent spread of the epidemic. The city authorities isolated the victims under the supervision of skilled persons who prevented them from coming in contact with the normal population.

Suspecting that their affliction was due to demonic possession, some of the victims were taken by priests to the shrine of St. Vitus to be cured. As is the case with hysterical persons, they were often influenced by suggestion. The priest did his best in the presence of the figure of St. Vitus to pacify these extremely nervous and overexcited persons through exorcism and other spiritual measures and, not infrequently, the habitual contractions of their muscles and the purposeless movements of their bodies, ceased temporarily or even permanently. The abatement of the symptoms was ascribed to the miraculous work of Saint Vitus. Hence, the condition became known as St. Vitus' dance, a name still applied to a nervous disease among children characterized by choreiform movements and known as Huntington's chorea, or Sydenham's chorea.

Judging from the large number of paintings on canvas, ivory miniatures, frescos, and tapestries, the dancing hysteria that prevailed in the Middle Ages must have been of enormous proportions. The victims of St. Vitus' dance were splendidly depicted by the Flemish School. The Italian masters of the Renaissance portrayed the demoniacs and the Spanish artists painted the ecstatics. In the convent of Grotta Ferrata, there is a fresco by Dominico Zampieri (1581-1641), "The Miracle of St. Vitus," which depicts a young girl suffering from contractures of the back, arms, and hands while dancing.

In Italy as well as in Germany, the dancing maniacs were often readily affected by colors. Some intensified their fury while others diminished it. The colors varied from country to country.

There is no doubt that, wherever it occurred, the epidemic was subconsciously intensified by ill-balanced people and consciously by evil persons, minstrels and impostors who found personal or monetary profit from these orgies.[7] Young girls were the worst sufferers.

TARANTELLA

Thanks to Athanasius Kircher (1599-1680), one musical number played for the dancing maniacs has survived. This piece is known as the tarantella a most lively bit of Italian folk music, which derived its name from the tarantula (a large venomous spider prevalent in Apulia, Italy). The mad dance was attributed to the bite of a tarantula. It was believed that it was the venom of this spider that made the dancers twist, squirm and dance, and that lively music was the best remedy for those who were so bitten. The tarantella was played on woodwind instruments.

When one was attacked by the dancing mania, the village musicians were called instead of the doctors. The musicians customarily played the flute, oboe, and turkish drum.

Incidentally, Athanasius Kircher, (1599-1680) who preserved the music of the tarantella, was a Jesuit professor of philosophy, mathematics and oriental languages at the "Collegeo Romano." He was also first to call attention to Egyptian hieroglyphics. His opus magnum, "Magnes Siva de Artes Magnetica," was published in 1654.

At the end of the fifteenth century and at the beginning of the sixteenth century, severe spider epidemics were common in Italy. Those that did not die from the venom of the spiders were often left with poor sight or poor hearing. Some victims of spider bite lost their speech apparently out of fear of contracting the dreaded dancing mania; many became desperate and melancholic. The Italians have always been great lovers of music. Some merely tried to drown their depression by playing the flute. Others thought that the music had a direct effect on the venom of the spider or scorpion and, as a natural sequel to this thought, there followed the belief that music was the natural remedy for those bitten by the Apulian spider.

As late as in 1695, the illustrious Dalmatian physician, Giorgio Baglivi (1668-1707), a Baconian experimentalist who has been likened to Sydenham, wrote a treatise "De Anatome Morsu et Effectibus Tarantulae," in which he analyzed the disease ascribed to the tarantula. This physician concluded that dancing and music were the best remedies. Baglivi was less than 40 when he died.[8]

Alexander ab Alexandro states that he saw, in a village of Italy, a young man who was very ill from a tarantula bite. The patient kept continuously twitching the muscles of his limbs and body and engaged in wild and uncontrollable dancing when the music was playing, but as soon as the music stopped, he fell exhausted and unconscious. He rose as if by magic as soon as the music began to play and regained consciousness. This remarkable phenomenon convinced everyone that the venom of the tarantula becomes harmless when dancing, because dancing scatters the venom throughout the body and eliminates it through the skin. The little poison that was left in the blood vessels was expelled via the music.

In France there were those who believed that the effect of the music cure on tarantula poisoning was only temporary. Epidemics tended to recur during the summer months.

It is related that an Italian Capuchin friar named Tarenta

became affected with the dancing mania and the Cardinal Cajetano was summoned to visit the cleric. As soon as Tarenta looked at the cardinal in his red robe, he ceased dancing, but he continued to suffer from twitching of the muscles. Fear and respect of this high dignitary of the Church caused the friar to stop dancing, but he became depressed and fainted. When the Cardinal presented him with the purple hat, he pressed it to his breast, began dancing again and was much revived.

The fact that in mental institutions dancing mania is only met with among individual patients and that mass dancing is extremely rare at the present time shows that the dancing mania of the Middle Ages started as a religious fantasy and gradually drew to its banners the weak minded, the hysterical and various epileptic persons.

The problem as to whether music has any curative effect on physical abnormalities has never been fully settled. Herbert Spencer (1820-1903), when he evaluates the virtues of music, was unable to concede any further therapeutic virtues to it than its action as a psychologic stimulus. Ancient and medieval physicians had much less doubt about its remedial values. It is recorded that Aesculapius himself used the trumpet to cure sciatica. He claimed that the continuous trumpet sound made the fibers of the nerve palpitate and the pain vanish. He also treated disorders of the ear by the same means. He applied soothing potions to wounds received on the battlefield and, at the same time furthered healing with "soft enchanting strains."

The Greeks understood the relation of mind and body; melody and rhythm were employed when the soul lost its harmony. They believed there is a close relationship between the health of the soul and health of the body. Apollo was both the god of health and music.

Music was used by Homer to combat anger, fear, worry, and fatigue and for promoting health-giving emotions.

Pythagoras said that health and all mental and physical emotions depend upon harmony and if certain prescribed music was made part of the daily living it would have a general beneficial effect on health.

Caelius Aurelianus cites the brother of Philiston (c. 370) in book XXII of his work "On Remedies"[9] to the effect that a certain person would play his instrument over the affected parts and that this would start up a throbbing and palpitation which would banish the pain and bring relief, and that some hold that it was Pythagoras who discovered this kind of treatment.[10] But, in the opinion of Soranus, anyone who believes that a severe disease can be banished by music and song is a victim of a silly delusion.[11]

In the Middle Ages, music was employed by priests to expel evil spirits from the bodies of the sick. Inspirational religious music has been used to stimulate religious ecstasy and to promote religious frenzy. There has been a custom among certain peoples of singing to the sick.

As late as in 1874, "the Shakers," a sect of dancers who worshipped God to the accompaniment of violent movements and dances, was founded by one Mrs. Girling in Lymington, England. When they were banned by the authorities, 135 of them danced on the public streets unceasingly for a day and a night in violation of the law.

It is probable that patients suffering from certain nervous conditions are susceptible to music. For instance, in the depressive phase of manic-depression, one may be cheered and his mood elevated by suitable music. In the overwrought, hypermanic phase, one may be calmed and slowed down. This applies also, to a relatively lesser degree, when the patient is not psychotic but is suffering from a more or less severe emotional disturbance. However, it is very doubtful if any organic or febrile disease may be benefited by any kind of music. It should be mentioned here that the use of ultrasonic waves as a form of physical therapy is presently undergoing extensive investigation.

FLAGELLATION (GEILERN)

Flagellation was another form of psychosis prevailing during the plague epidemics of the Middle Ages. Voluntary flagellation as a form of exalted devotion has been practiced by almost all religions since deep antiquity. Herodotus states[12] that it was the custom of the ancient Egyptians to beat themselves during the annual festival in honor of the god Isis.[13] Plutarch (A. D. 46-120) relates that in Sparta children were flogged before the altar of Artemis Orthia until their blood flowed.[14]

On the Greek Peloponnesian peninsula, women were flogged in the temple of Dionysius. At the Roman Lupercalia women were flogged by the priests to avert sterility. This rite was believed to insure fertility and easy delivery.

In the early Middle Ages, ritual flagellation was ordered by the Beth Din[14a] as punishment for transgression. Symbolic flagellation, as a penance, is still practiced in the synagogue among orthodox Jews of the East before the Day of Atonement. Christians of the Middle Ages employed flagellation as a means of punishment. Parents and school masters commonly flagellated the children and students and even bishops did not hesitate to use this ritual on offending priests and monks.

In the eleventh century, self-flagellation was practiced in the monasteries of the West as a penance. The early Franciscans flagellated themselves with much vigor. The Flagellants eventually organized themselves into fraternities. Flagellation came into special prominence in the eleventh century through the practice of the monks, Dominicans, and especially of Locartus (1060) and Peter Damiane, Cardinal of Ostia (1072). The latter advocated the substitution of self-flagellation for the reading of penitential Psalms.

Bodily punishment probably originated from the idea that the body was a separate entity and especially subject to sin, for corrupting the heavenly soul. In the monasteries, priests castigated themselves to suppress the cravings of their flesh, although this practice sometimes excited rather than diminished them. Flagellation was frequently prescribed for penitents in which case the priest administered the castigation.

The mental shock sustained during the frequent epidemics of plague, wars and famine in the thirteenth and fourteenth centuries brought about the spread of flagellation in European countries as a means of penance. It spread rapidly as far as the Rhine provinces and across Germany into Bohemia from northern Italy.

In 1260, attacked by religious frenzy, whole communities set out to either scourge themselves or to suffer themselves to be whipped by their associates, until their bodies were full of bloody stripes, so that their very appearance excited compassion. These penitents continually sang hymns of penitence and their expeditions commonly lasted thirty-three and a half days. Their sanctifying procedures took place at first in the churches, later, in the daytime before the walls of the city and in the open fields, and finally at night. The flagellants marched into Italy carrying leather scourging thongs which they liberally applied to their limbs with such violence that blood gushed from their wounds.

The outbreaks of the flagellation epidemics coincided with the outbreaks of the plague epidemics until 1349. The plague added fuel to the heated zeal of the flagellants.

To quote Hecker,[15] "An awful sense of contrition seized the faithful everywhere; they resolved to forsake their evil ways, and seek reconciliation with their maker and to revert to self-chastisement due for their former sins."

They appeared in great numbers. Hundreds and even thousands gathered to watch the spectacles. At first the flagellants were divided as to sexes. Gradually they roved about in mixed armies. Cooper states, "These flagellants roamed about half naked with only a hat with a red cross on their heads and a mask over their faces. They scourged themselves by day, and at night the half lewd assembled.[16] Thus gross immorality developed out of religious insanity, with manifest results, with regards to the female participants."

In Germany and Hungary, flagellant organizations known as "Cross Bearers" were formed, the members of which marched from place to place in large numbers. They were robed in somber garments with red crosses on their breasts, back, and cap. Their eyes fixed to the ground and torches in their hands, they entered the cities singing and chanting psalms. They attracted great numbers to their ranks, including priests and nobles. Men and women dropped their work to welcome them and to enlist in their forces. When they entered the city of Strassburg (1349), the church bells tolled and almost the entire community paid homage to the brotherhood, citizens joining their forces by the thousands.

The upheavals of the fourteenth century, especially the earthquakes, and the Black Death, which had spread over the greater part of Europe, gave impetus to the flagellants. The flagellants added to the religious strife in Germany which was already in a bad state because of the struggle between the papacy and Louis of Bavaria. In the spring of 1349, bands of flagellants spread their propaganda in the south of Germany. Each band was under the command of a leader, and assisted by two lieutenants. Obedience to the leader was enjoined upon every member upon entering the brotherhood. The leaders read a letter which they said had fallen from heaven, and which threatened the earth with terrible punishments if men refused to adopt the mode of penance taught by the flagellants. Some of the masters used their spiritual power to drive out demons and even claimed to raise the dead.

On several occasions, the flagellant brotherhoods incited the populations of the towns through which they passed against the Jews, and also against the monks who opposed their propaganda. Many towns shut their gates upon them but, in spite of such discouragement, their organizations spread from Poland to the Rhine, and penetrated as far as Holland and Flanders.

Whosoever was desirous of joining a brotherhood, was bound to remain in for thirty-four days. If married, he was obliged to have the sanction of his wife and to give the assurance that he was reconciled to all men. Penance was performed twice every day, in the morning and in the evening. When the members arrived at the place of flagellation, they stripped the upper part of their bodies and took off their shoes, keeping on only a linen dress reaching from the waist to the ankles. They then laid down in a large circle in different positions, according to the nature of their crime—the adulterer with his face to the ground, the perjurer on one side holding up three fingers, the murderer on his back. They were then castigated by the master, who ordered them to arise in the words of a prescribed form, usually after they had lain on the ground for as long a time as it would take to say five paternosters.

All flagellants were then chastized by their own hand or by the hand of the Master with a three-tailed scourging whip, while chanting psalms and uttering loud supplications to avert the plague. The frosts of winter did not lessen their zeal.

All sorts of sins were confessed, enemies were reconciled, vanities and follies were renounced, and men prepared themselves as for a new spiritual stage of life. Salimbene (1221-1288) writes in his chronicle:[17] "The flagellants came through this world, all men both small and great, noble knights, and men of the people, scourged themselves naked in processions through the cities with the bishop and men of religion at their head; and peace was made in many places; and then restored what they had unlawfully taken away and they confessed their sin so earnestly that the priests had scarce leisure to eat; in their mouths sounded the word of God and not of man and their voices were as the voices of a multitude."

Penitents turned to the master flagellants for confession. For a time the flagellants gained more credit than the priests. Some of the masters determined to form a lasting league against the Church. This prompted the withdrawal of the sympathy shown them by several cardinals who condemned the sect as constituting a menace to the priesthood. On the 20th of October, 1349, Pope Clement published a bull commanding the bishops and inquisitors to stamp out the growing heresy, and in pursuance of the pope's orders, numbers of the flagellants perished at the stake, or in the cells of the inquisitors and at the hands of the episcopal justices. In 1389, the leader of a flagellant band in Italy called the "Bianchi" was burned, by order of the pope, and his followers dispersed.[18]

The processions of the "Brotherhood of the Cross," as they were known, undoubtedly promoted the spreading of the plague instead of diminishing it as they hoped, by flagellating themselves. They transmitted the plague germ from town to town, and infused a new poison into the already despondent minds of the people. Some cool-headed observers undoubtedly noticed this fact and the flagellation mania gradually passed out of the picture.

THE CRUSADES

The people of the Middle Ages never thought of themselves as free-born citizens, who could come and go at will and shape their fate according to their ability or energy or luck. Heretics, heroes, rich, poor, beggar and thief accepted their lot as an ordinance and asked no questions. Poverty was considered by the Almighty a blessing. The Lord blessed the serf to remain a slave so that he might bestow upon him an immortal soul and live and die as a good Christian. This world he was assured was merely a temporary abode; the world hereafter-in-Heaven might be a paradise of wonderful delights or a Hell of brimstone and suffering—depending upon his behavior. To acquire the blissful life in Heaven he was enjoined to devote the greater part of his time preparing for it.

No one dared to question the wisdom of the religious teachers that the cause of their afflictions was their sin.

Those who possessed civic or religious power looked upon "progress" as a very undesirable innovation of the "Evil One" that had to be discouraged and as they happened to occupy the seats of the mighty, it was easy for them to enforce their will upon the ignorant serf and the illiterate knight. Here and there a few brave souls ventured forth into the forbidden region of science, but they fared badly and were considered lucky when they escaped with their lives or a jail sentence of twenty years.

When an epidemic of a malignant disease broke out and communities were swept away by the cruel epidemic, the grief of seeing all that was dear to them carried away by the fearful disease, was not sufficient. They also lived in dread of the final hour of the gruesome day of Judgment for their sins. The fear for the future filled their souls with humility and piety. They turned their backs upon a world which was filled with fear, suffering and disease and sought to atone for their sinful behavior. Being totally ignorant, they readily accepted any suggestion offered by religious authority. In the year 1095 at the council of Clermont in France to consider the cause of the epidemic disease and other catastrophes, the Pope rose and emphatically declared that the terrible horrors which inflicted Christian peoples were due to the ungodly action of the infidels (Turks). He gave a glowing description of the land which ever since Moses had been overflowing with milk and honey, and he exhorted the knights of France and the peoples of Europe to leave their wives and children and deliver Palestine from the hands of the Turks. The Pope's speech was interrupted by cries "God will it" which came to be the slogan of the crusaders in the campaign that followed.[19]

In obedience to the urgent request of the head of the Church, the farmer threw away his plow and the builder his ax. They left their homes, their families and took the nearest route to Jerusalem. This religious mania had a catastrophic consequence.

In 1096, five divisions of "knights" were marching from France and England along the Rhine. They were headed by Peter the Hermit of France, barefooted, clad in rough garments and bearing on his shoulder a huge cross. He rode on an ass. His fiery zeal and eloquence added to his army thousands of impoverished men who left their families to join the brave and "holy" army known later as "the Knights Templars."

These armies were hastily organized; a division of 20,000 under Walter the Penniless and one of 40,000 under Peter the Hermit were cut to pieces when they reached Bulgaria, and their survivors were utterly annihilated by the Turks at Nicaea. Another army of 15,000 Germans who followed them were slaughtered in Hungary.

The most horrible consequences followed the crusade known as "Children's Pilgrimages" (Kinderfahrten). Boys and maidens, all of them under age, immature and deluded, set out from France with the purpose of taking possession of the Holy Sepulchre. Thirty thousand of them, headed by a peasant-boy named

Stephen, set out from France for the Holy Land by way of Marseilles. A like army of German children, 20,000 strong, led by a boy named Nicholas, crossed the Alps by a more easterly route, touching the sea at Brindisi. Those of France were taken on board ships by slave traders at Marseilles on the promise that they would be taken to the Holy Land but they were brought to the slave markets of Egypt where they were sold as slaves. None of the German children reached Italy.

None attained the object of the expedition; few only returned to their homes. Many, after the loss of discipline which had been at all times very loose, strayed about aimlessly in the greatest misery. Many of the girls, scarcely having reached the age of puberty, became pregnant to add to their woes.

We speak of First, Second and Third Crusades. To be more exact, the Crusades were one continuous process. For a period of two hundred years, scarcely a year passed in which new bands did not come to the Holy Land. There was the disastrous Crusade of 1100-1101, the Venetian Crusade of 1123-1124; the Crusade of Henry II in 1172, and that of Edward I in 1271-1272. Crusades appear to have been dignified by numbers when they followed some crushing disaster—as for example—the loss of Edessa in 1144, or the fall of Jerusalem in 1187.

The First Crusade consisted of a wild mob of penniless bankrupts, and fugitives from justice following the half crazed Peter the Hermit and Walter the Penniless. They began the campaign against the infidels by murdering all Jews whom they met on their way. They got as far as Hungary. The armies of Fulcher and Gottschalk were destroyed by the Hungarians in just revenge for their excesses. Two other divisions, however, reached Constantinople in safety. The first of these, under Walter the Penniless, passed through Hungary in May, and reached Constantinople, where it halted to wait for Peter the Hermit. The second, led by Peter himself, passed safely through Hungary, but suffered severely in Bulgaria. He reached Constantinople with sadly diminished numbers. These two divisions in spite of good treatment by Alexius committed excesses against the Greeks. They united and crossed the Bosphorus in August, Peter himself remaining in Constantinople. Those who were successful in crossing the Bosphorus perished at the hand of the Seljuks.

In the following years, when crusading assumed a political aspect the inspired Templars waded into streams of blood up to their ankles not only in their fight against their natural foes the Islamic tribes, but against all that came in their way. Such epidemics of religious frenzy include the orgies devoted to the burning of Jews, "Judenbrands," especially in the years 1348-1350.

Among the Crusaders were many "God fearing" knights who joined in a wild "Judenhetze" in a town on the Rhine, during which some 10,000 Jews perished as the first fruit of the crusading zeal.

The crusaders first would murder all the women and children of a captured city and then they would devoutly march to a holy spot with their hands gory with the blood of innocent victims and pray that a merciful heaven forgive them their sins. But the next day, they would once more butcher a camp of Saracen enemies without a spark of mercy in their hearts.

But the crusades instead of checking the deadly epidemics as Peter the Hermit had assured, merely intensified them. The marching armies transported along with them various diseases from one place to another. To cope with the situation of caring for the diseased and wounded it became necessary to establish religious orders such as the "Knights Hospitalers" and "Teutonic Knights," and hospitals were established in the Holy Land and at home. Hospitals had to be built to accommodate the many diseased and crippled crusaders. In France alone there were 2,000 lazarettos (after Lazarus) and more than 200 hospitals were constructed in England. The buildings were rather primitive. Patients with various diseases mingled together.

Aside from religious motives there were as stated above other motives on the part of the masses to attract them to the Crusades. Famine and pestilence at home drove them to emigrate hopefully to the golden East. In 1094, there was pestilence all the way down from Flanders to Bohemia; in 1095 there was famine in Lorraine, and the stream of emigration that set them towards the East was like the modern rush towards a newly discovered goldfield.

Under the stress of the repeated plagues, emigration became increasingly frequent and in 1064, it assumed large proportions. Streams of humanity from many directions set out to wander about. Groups joined forces and included heterogeneous elements such as escaped prisoners, tramps, bankrupts, paupers and fugitive monks. They were penniless and supported themselves by plundering the countryside if food was not offered them. To others wandering was looked upon as a penance and chastisement for the sins that caused ravaging pestilence. It was considered by the Church as a kind of self-affliction, like fasting and flagellation.

The Crusade idea particularly appealed to the Normans who were a people of sojourners. It appealed to the old Norse instinct for wandering—an instinct which found a natural outlet in the expedition to Jerusalem. Finally, the idea appealed to the kings who desired to gain fresh territory.

The six armies under Godfrey of Bouillon, Robert, Duke of Normandy and Tancred the hero of the crusades, numbering 600,000 men subdued the Turks for a period of 50 years. In 1187 Saladin recaptured Jerusalem from the crusaders with terrible bloodshed on both sides. The efforts of Philippe Auguste, King of France, and Richard the Lionhearted, King of England, stemmed the onslaught only for a period of twenty-one months.

The crusaders contributed a good deal of suffering at home. In addition to the physical ills there was a general lack of occupations for those who were fortunate enough to return home. This is particularly true with respect to women who outnumbered men seven to one. The unexampled indolence explains the foundation of cloisters for "converted widows" and "maidens" as well as the religious orders of "Daughters of Magdalen" and "Penitential Sisters." The latter order was recruited from "the fallen." Besides there were "itinerant wives and maidens"—a female association which at fairs and at religious councils and on similar festive occasions sacrificed themselves at request upon the altar of love or as "schohne Frauen" acted as housekeepers to the clergy. There were 1400 of them at the council of

Constance. The clergy employed these "itinerant wives" as domestics and house-keepers and "not of course as pleasure."

Finally there arose at this time from common street prostitution the somewhat more respectable brothel system. The inmates of these houses of iniquity chose their regular female superintendents. They were subject to the magistrate or more frequently to the Bishop and formed often for the clergy a favorite field for missionary labor and a fine source of income as they were taxed one-tenth of their receipts.

Regulated prostitution was maintained to a great degree by the laxity of morals so highly developed in the preceding barbarous ages but debased by the excesses of the crusading "nobles."

In London there were eighteen of these houses under the jurisdiction of the bishop of Winchester. In Nordlingen the authorities found it necessary to recommend to the reverend clergy that they should pursue their search for converts in the brothels rather by day than by night. How very widespread evils of this kind must have been is shown by the fact that such houses were considered at this time, institutions of prophylaxis and were deemed just as indispensable as ordinary inns. In England the institution of brothels under episcopal supervision seems to have been in its prime, and to have been very carefully regulated. These houses had special names, such as "The Crane," and "The Boar's Head."

The brothels of London were situated on the Bankside, and Southwark, and were visited weekly by the sheriff's officers. They were privileged by patent and regulated by statute from the reign of Henry II (1162) until the last year of Henry VIII (1547), when they were formally suppressed. The statutes of 1162, confirmed by an act of Parliament, the following paragraphs:

1. "No host or hostess shall suffer a maiden to go out and come in at pleasure.
2. No such maiden shall be provided by the host with board and lodging out of the house.
3. The maiden shall pay for her apartment not more than fourteen pence per week.
4. On holidays no one shall be permitted to enter the house.

5. No maiden shall be forcibly detained in the house.
6. No host shall receive a female from ecclesiastical institutions, nor shall he receive a married woman.
7. No maiden shall receive pay from a man unless she has passed the whole night until morning with him.
8. No host shall keep a maiden who has the dangerous burning disease; nor shall he sell bread, meat or other victuals." [20]

In 1129 it was forbidden to grant licenses to the "Focariae" in London. As late as 1321 an English cardinal purchased a brothel in London as an investment for sacerdotal funds! In France the barbers quite generally kept houses of assignation.[21] Brothels were generally established over rooms occupied by students of law and medicine. In 1179 an archbishop of Mayence, a man of extraordinary erudition for his day, was charged with supporting such a retinue of prostitutes that their maintenance entailed heavier expense upon his diocese than the charges of royal representation. In 1190 the Danish peasantry joined the priesthood in opposing an ordinance of the bishops, which exacted the expulsion of concubines from religious houses, on the ground that the execution of the ordinance would endanger seriously the chastity of their own wives and daughters. In 1291 the Knights Templar are said to have supported no less than 13,000 prostitutes. It must not be forgotten that the episcopal supervision of the question of prostitution was designed to regulate what was then regarded as a necessary evil, and that the facts mentioned were abuses of an institution designed for beneficent purposes.

CHAPTER XXXIII

THE RENAISSANCE OF MEDICINE

Historic epochs seldom have sharp lines of demarcation. They do not begin nor end abruptly. This especially is true of the period known as the Renaissance (rebirth) roughly estimated from the middle of the fifteenth century to the end of the sixteenth century; a period of about 150 years. The term Renaissance applies especially to the revival begun in Italy in the fourteenth century and gradually spread to other countries. Petrarch and the early humanists of the fourteenth century may be regarded as the precursors of the Renaissance. The revival of letters and art was greatly stimulated by the arrival in Italy (1453) of Byzantine scholars who, fleeing from Turkey after the taking of Constantinople by the Turks, brought the literature of the ancient Greeks into Italy.

The fall of the Eastern Empire caused a scattering of Greek scholars. Many of the exiles were great teachers, well read in Greek and Latin classics; they were in possession of genuine manuscripts which they rescued from the ruins of Constantinople. The search for manuscripts became a fashionable pursuit, so that the monastic and cathedral libraries were literally ransacked. Manuscript dealers exerted all their resources to procure copies of Greek writings which had remained hidden in the east for centuries or had been scattered when Constantinople fell.

One of these bibliophiles was Thomas da Sarzana (born c. 1400) who later became Pope Nicholas V, founder of the Vatican library and discoverer of the original Celsus manuscript in the Church of Ambrosius. From this manuscript, the Epitome of Hippocratic medicine was discovered, and it proved much different from the dog-Latin text long in vogue. The "De re Medicina" of Celsus was one of the first medical books to be printed.

The Italian Renaissance was at its height at the end of the fifteenth and early sixteenth centuries as is evident from the lives and works of Lorenzo de Medici, Michelangelo, Leonardo da Vinci, Raphael, Niccolo Machiavelli (1469-1527), Angelo Ambrogini Politian (1454-1494), Ariosto Lodovico (1474-1533), Aldus Manutius (1450-1515), Tiziano Vecellio (1477-1576), and others.

The Renaissance was aided everywhere by the spirit of discovery and exploration of the fifteenth century. It was the age which saw the discovery of Copernicus, the invention of printing, the discovery of America, and other breathtaking discoveries. In England the revival of learning was fostered by Erasmus, John Colet (1467-1519), William Grocyn (1466-1514), Thomas More (1478-1535), and others. In France there was a brilliant artistic and literary development under Louis XII (1498-1515) and Francis I (1515-1547).[1]

The Renaissance of learning really began with the opening of the universities and particularly from the time when the scholastic grip of thought was loosened by the influence of Roger Bacon, Duns Scotus, and William Occam. The Franciscan imprisoning of Roger Bacon for venturing to examine what God had meant to keep secret; the escape of Occam from a papal prison to the protection of Louis of Bavaria, and the philosophy of Duns Scotus, indicated the beginning of the spirit of revolt against ecclesiastic authority. Dante (1265-1321) evidently initiated the movement of modern thinking though he did not lead the revival as a separate movement in this evolution.

The Renaissance was noted by no light-heartedness but rather by a severe spirit which brought not peace but the sword, such as the *autos-da-fé* of Seville and Madrid, the flames of Giordano Bruno (1548-1600), Etienne Dolet (1509-1546) and Paleario Aonio (1500-1570), the dungeon of Campanella Tomasco (1568-1639), the seclusion of Galileo, the massacre of St. Bartholomew, and the brutal death of the Huguenot scholar of Paris, Petrus Ramus, who was shot for opposing Aristotelian doctrine.

A half a century later the Italian poet Francis Petrarch (1304-1374), the great reviver of learning in medieval Europe, unlike the scholastic thinkers of his time, tried to restore a taste for good classical Latin in place of the dog-Latin of the schoolmen and to recover the true spirit of thought with absolute liberty of reason. Petrarch first opened a new method in scholarship and revealed what he denotes as humanism. In his teaching he makes it clear that the work for humanism consisted mainly of a just perception of the dignity of man as a rational, volitional and sentient being. It involves a varied recognition of the goodness of man and nature. Petrarch may be regarded as the rediscoverer of literature; but for him the revival of learning might have been indefinitely delayed.

Petrarch, who lives in the memory of most people nowadays chiefly as a great Italian poet, owed his fame among his contemporaries, rather to the fact that he was a kind of living representative of antiquity, that he endeavored by his voluminous historical and philosophical writings not to supplant but to make known the works of the ancients, and wrote letters that, as treatises on matters of antiquarian interest, obtained a reputation which was natural enough in an age without handbooks. Petrarch himself trusted and hoped that his Latin writings would bring him fame with his contemporaries and with posterity. He thought so little of his Italian poems that, as he often remarked, he would gladly have destroyed them if he could have succeeded thereby in blotting them out from the memory of men.

Influenced by the writing of Petrarch, Giovanni Boccaccio (1313-1375), while still young, began to read the classic authors. Petrarch, with whom he came in personal relationship, may be considered the moulder of his thoughts in literature and philosophy.

A great impetus towards the revival of learning was the invention of the printing press in the middle of the fifteenth century by Johann Gutenberg (1397-1468). It enabled scholars to reproduce classical works, to displace the corrupted texts that had accumulated throughout the centuries of medieval stagnation. Printed critical texts of Hippocrates and Galen soon displaced the old manuscripts that passed through a linguistic "transmigration" from Greek to Syrian, from Syrian to Persian, from Persian to Arabic, from Arabic to Hebrew and finally into a corrupted Latin. By the time the last copyist and commentator were finished, the contents of the text had so changed that it was difficult to say what Galen and other classical writers had really said.

In the latter part of the fifteenth century there was a great advance in Greek scholarship. Original manuscripts were discovered, more accurate translations of Greek were made and printed copies of the improved translation appeared, which contributed to the progress and the knowledge of science and philosophy. The great printers of the Renaissance were Sack of Mainz, and Adolph of Nassau (in 1462) and the first book printed in Italy was the text of Lactantius (1465). The Florentine press was set up in 1471, and later the printing-houses of the Aldi and Giunti in Venice, Stephanus and Colinaeus in Paris, Herbst (Oporinus) and Froben in Basel, Wynkyn de Worde and Wyer in London, Plantin at Antwerp, Elzevir in Leyden, vied with one another in the issue of stately folios and beautiful texts.[2]

But the greatest change in the scientific outlook of the universe was the discovery of Nicholas Copernicus (Nicolaus Kopperingk, 1473-1543), mathematician and astronomer, born of a Polish father and German mother who Latinized his name to Copernicus. His discovery that the earth was not flat and that it is not at rest, but that it is revolving daily on its axis and yearly around the sun, fell like a bombshell upon all medieval Europe. It violated the basic dogma of medieval scholasticism and it required great originality of mind to resist all arguments against it. Both Christian factions joined the chorus of denouncing Copernicus and his discovery. "The fools," said Luther (1483-1546) "want to upset the whole science of astronomy, but the Holy Scripture shows Joshua commanded the sun to tarry."[3]

But even fifty years later Galileo did not dare to teach the Copernican hypothesis, which he was to demonstrate with his telescope, because in dethroning the earth from its central position in the universe he contradicted the Ptolemaic system approved by the Church, and finally he was tried and punished for asserting that the earth really moves.

The reawakening of learning not only restored the classics, it also encouraged theological criticism. But it is a mistake to think that the revolt of Martin Luther (1483-1546) against the Roman Catholic Church was merely an innerchurch polemic. When Luther made his first appearance in Germany he scarcely referred to religion. He spoke almost exclusively of the social, financial, educational and moral problems of his day. It would be difficult to distinguish the German movement of the Reformation and the Italian movement of the Renaissance in their original form. Both had a common starting point in the reaction against long dominant ideas.

That the religious element of the Reformation has been greatly overestimated can hardly be questioned. One of the most distinguished students of church history has ventured to say that the motives both remote and proximate which led to Lutheran revolt were largely secular rather than spiritual.

Both the Renaissance and humanism had been anticipated a century before in England when Geoffery Chaucer (1343-1400) gave an early foretaste of Renaissance and humanism, but before it affected the bulk of the English people. It had already permeated Italy and France. Of greater value than the humanistic interest in ancient language was the spirit of free inquiry and the impulse towards the study of everything that "humane letters" gave to Europe after centuries of medievalism.

The humanists paved the way for the revival of science, and widened the mental horizon which made it possible for science to advance. Without them it would have been most difficult for the scientific mind to throw off the intellectual fetters of theological preoccupation.

HUMANISM

Humanism, is a term especially applied to a movement which in the fifteenth century broke through the medieval tradition of scholastic theology and philosophy in Western Europe and devoted itself to the rediscovery and direct study of ancient classics. This movement of its very nature arose as a revolt against ecclesiastical authority and is the parent of all modern development whether intellectual or scientific. Humanism is a genetic form for classics and it means literally, humane literature, which consists of Greek and Latin classics.

As the competitor of the culture of the Middle Ages, which was essentially clerical and was fostered by the church, there appeared a new civilization built on the foundations of classical antiquity. According to Poggio[4] only such persons could say they had lived, who had learned and read books in Latin or translated Greek into Latin.

The humanistic movement began in Italy with Francesco Fileffo (1398-1481), who was born in 1398 at Tolentino in the Province of Macerata. He studied grammar, rhetoric, and Latin Literature at Padua, where he was later appointed professor at the early age of eighteen. In 1417 he received an invitation to teach eloquence and moral philosophy at Venice. Here he remained two years, forming connections with the Venetian nobility. After being admitted as a citizen of Venice by public decree he was appointed secretary to the Baily (Bailo, or Consul-General) of Constantinople.

Equipped with Greek learning and a large supply of Greek books he returned to his native country after an absence of seven and a half years. It is related that he had mastered the whole literature of the ancients in both classic languages, could wield the Greek of Homer and of Xenophon and the Latin prose of Cicero, the verse of Horace and of Virgil with equal versatility. He was recognized as the most universal scholar of his age. In 1427 he was called to Venice to occupy the chair of eloquence but, owing to the plague that was ravaging the city, the nobles had taken flight to their country houses and there was no one to attend his lectures. He therefore accepted an offer as professor of eloquence and moral philosophy in Bologna (1428). He died at Florence at the age of 83.

Another prominent humanist was Guarino da Verona (1370-1460). He studied Latin under Giovanni de Ravenna and while still a lad of 18 years he traveled to Constantinople to learn Greek. After an absence of five years he returned to Venice, and began to lecture to crowded audiences. Like all humanists of that time, he seems to have preferred temporary to permanent engagements—passing from Venice to Verona, from Trent to Padua, from Bologna to Florence, and everywhere acquiring that substantial reputation as a teacher and scholar.

Guarino, like his friend Vittorino da Feltre (1387-1476), was celebrated for his method of teaching, for the exact order of his discipline. Students flocked from all cities of Italy to his lecture room. In this way he labored for many years, maintaining his great reputation as a teacher, and filling the universities of Italy with pupils. He was one of the few humanists whose moral character won equal respect with his learning. He died at the age of eighty-nine.[5]

Among the very first to combine science with humanism in Germany was Johann Muller (1436-1476) of Königsberg, Prussia, who studied under teachers of the new learning in Italy. He translated into Latin the astronomic works of Ptolemy (the "Almagest" and perhaps also his "Optics") and other Greek writers and founded an observatory at Nurnberg where he invented a weight driven clock. He also suggested improvements in teaching practical astronomy.

Perhaps the most prominent figure among the Northern European humanists was Desiderius Erasmus (1467-1536), a Dutch scholar and theologian of Amsterdam. Humanism to him was the means of combating the chief evil of his day which consisted of monastic illiteracy, scholastic pedantry and low moral standing. He battled against artificially interpreted texts, rendered by scholastics and theologians, and tried to explain what the Bible really meant. His revolutionary spirit could no longer be content with monastic life. He resigned from priesthood and traveled through many educational centers of Europe. During this time he mastered the Greek language. In London he wrote his witty satire, "In Everyone's Land" (1528), which has been widely read. Some of his sayings are "My heart is Catholic but my stomach is Lutheran," "The Yoke of Christ would be sweet if petty human institutions had not added to the burden," "Would that people let Christ rule through the command of His word and not try to build their tyranny with human decrees." Long before Luther's name was heard of, he was a strong critic of the Catholic Church. The current motto was "Erasmus laid an egg and Luther hatched it."

The poet Hermelaus Barbarus (1453-1493), was one of the leaders of humanism. He made a careful translation of Aristotle, taught Greek in public and gathered about him the most illustrious scientists of the end of the fifteenth century. He became a doctor at Padua in 1477. He held many public offices, in 1486 he was Venetian ambassador to Emperor Frederick and in 1489 he was ambassador to Innocent VIII, who created him cardinal and patriarch of Aquilea. He was crowned as a poet at the age of fourteen by Frederick III. He died in 1493 before the age of forty, leaving an enormous amount of learned works which exhibit great knowledge of Greek and ancient literature.

The most read humanist who exerted considerable influence on the medical literature of the fifteenth century was the Latinist Georgio Valla (1406-1447), a promoter of a more scientific form of language. In his work he attempted to purify the text of Pliny that had been corrupted by the copyist of the Arabian translators. He wrote a commentary on Dioscorides.

John Hall (c. 1565) was a physician who protested against both *Chyrurgerie* and *Physyke* and tells of a typical mountebank, "one Valentyne":

> "When anye came to him wyth urines . . . he made
> them believe, that onlye by feling the weight
> therof, he would tell them of theyr diseases
> in their bodies, or wythout: And otherwhile

made them believe, that he went to aske counsel of the devil, by going a little asyde, and mumblying to him selfe, and then comming agayne, would tell them all and more to."

THOMAS LINACRE (1461-1524)

In the course of the Renaissance a school of medical humanists arose whose object was to turn their eyes from medieval medicine and to direct their attention to the fountain heads of learning, to the new version of Hippocrates and Galen. Among the first medical humanists was Thomas Linacre, who performed an everlasting service to English medicine by his excellent translation of Hippocrates, Galen and Aristotle from Greek into Latin. The accuracy of these translations was generally praised by contemporaries and the elegant style made the Greek masters accessible to all readers of Latin.

He was practically the founder of the College of Physicians in London and was its first president. He established leadership in Greek medicine in Oxford and Cambridge and in the College of Physicians (1518) in London, and placed valuable estates in the hands of trustees for their maintenance. Erasmus eulogizing his Latin style remarks "Galen spoke better Latin in the version of Linacre than he had before spoken Greek, and even Aristotle displayed a grace which he hardly attained in his native tongue." Erasmus praises Linacre also for his fine critical judgment. He was regarded as a master of Greek, not only in language but also in philosophical and scientific works. The chief cause why Linacre has not left more original literary memorials as Erasmus said was his habit of acute accuracy.

Very little is known of Linacre's parentage. He was probably born in Canterbury where he received his early education at the Cathedral School then under the direction of William Tilly of Selling who was at that time Prior of Canterbury. Probably from this teacher Linacre received his first incentive to classical studies. He entered Oxford in 1480. He accompanied Selling to Italy where the latter was sent by Henry VIIII as an envoy to the Vatican. Linacre took the degree of M. D. with great distinction at Padua and for some time Linacre was instructor at Florence. Inspired with the learning and imbued with the spirit of the Italian Renaissance he formed a circle of scholars when he returned to Oxford. Among them were the humanists John Calet, William Gracyn, and William Latimer; who were greatly eulogized by Erasmus.

On the accession of Henry VIII, he was appointed the king's physician. Among his patients in London may be mentioned Cardinal Wolsey. Aside from his grammatical and linguistic works he translated a number of Galen's medical writings,[6] *De Sanitate Trienda* (Paris, 1517), *Methodus Medendi* (Paris, 1519), *De Temperamentis* (Cambridge, 1521), *De Naturabilus Facultatibus* (London, 1523), *Symptomatum Differentiis, et Causes* (London, 1524), *De Pulsum Usu,* (London, without date). His fine moral qualities are summed up in the epitaph of John Caius: *Fraudes dolosque mir perosus fidus amicis omnibus juxta carus.* (Thoroughly detesting frauds and cheats, faithful to all friends, dear one near at hand.)

NICOLO LEONICENO (1428-1524)

Another distinguished medical humanist was the profound Greek and Latin scholar, Nicolo Leoniceno of Italy. His fame began with his elegant translation of the "Aphorisms" of Hippocrates into Latin, for whom he expressed great admiration in his medical writings. In his later years while professor at Ferrara he started on an accurate translation of Galen into Latin; it is not known how far he proceeded in his work. He was a great critic of the Arabic versions of Hippocratic and Galenic works. He was especially hostile towards Avicenna's teaching but he expressed great reverence for Rhazes.

His contribution to science lies chiefly in the task of correcting the botanical errors contained in the *Natural History of Pliny*. This labor put him to much undeserved trouble and to a stream of invectives on the part of the timid and credulous scholars of his day who believed that Pliny was infallible. It required courage at that time to question the authority of Pliny.

There were before Leoniceno critical commentators of Pliny but their criticism was only aimed at the orthography and grammar. Leoniceno, however, questioned the veracity of the statements of Pliny himself, who was regarded as unimpeachable. Even his friend Palasiano Colucio fired abuses at him for questioning the accuracy of Pliny.

Leoniceno paved the way for the botanical science later developed in Germany by such distinguished investigators as Mattheolus (1501-1577), Cordus (1515-1544), and others. Without tearing down the old notions and fantastic ideas in which botany was enveloped materia medica could not progress.

Leoniceno's classical treatise on syphilis has already been discussed in the chapter dealing with this subject.

Nicolo Leoniceno was born in the Italian town of Loniga near Vicenza. He received his education in Padua where he graduated in medicine. As was the custom in those days, he embarked on a journey when he received the doctorate. He traveled all over Europe, residing in England for a time. When he returned to Italy he was appointed professor at his alma mater—the University of Padua, where he remained for a few years. His fame as a physician, and scholar of Greek and Latin, spread all over Italy and he was soon called to the University of Bologna to occupy the chair of professor of medicine. In 1464 he finally was called to the University of Ferrara where he occupied the professorship for sixty years. He died at the advanced age of 96 years.

FRANCOIS RABELAIS (c. 1490-1553)

The most prominent humanist in France was Francois Rabelais. He was born at Chinon on the Vienne in the province of Touraine. His birth, parentage, youth and education depend upon tradition. His father was either an apothecary or a tavern-keeper. He had four brothers and no sisters. Tradition takes him either to the University of Angers or to the convent school of La Baumette. The next stage in his career is the monastery of Fontenay le Comte, where he was holding a position of recorder of deeds for the community. There he pursued the study of letters, and especially of Greek. The letters of the well-known Greek scholar Budaeus show that an attempt was made by the heads of the convent or the Benedictine order to check his scholarly zeal but it failed.

On or before 1530, he abandoned his Benedictine garb for that of a secular priest. He entered the faculty of medicine at Montpellier on the 16th of September of that year and in a remarkably short interval, he received the degree of bachelor. Early in 1531 he lectured publicly on Galen and Hippocrates. In 1532 he had moved from Montpellier to Lyons. At this time Lyons was the headquarters of an unusually enlightened society, and indirectly it is clear that Rabelais became intimate with this society.

Here he plunged into manifold work, literary and professional. He was appointed physician to the Hotel Dieu, with a salary of forty livres per annum, and lectured on anatomy with demonstrations on human subjects. In the year 1532 he edited for Sebastian Gryphius, the medical *Epistles* of Giovanni Manardi (1462-1536), the "Aphorisms" of Hippocrates, the *Ars Parva* of Galen, and an edition of two supposed Latin documents. At this time probably appeared the beginnings of his work "Pantagruel" which was to make Rabelais immortal.

The earliest known edition of *Pantagruel* is of 1533; of *Gargantua*, 1535. The first was condemned as an obscene book by Calvin in a letter dated 1533. In the spring of 1535 the authorities of the Lyons hospital, considering that Rabelais had twice absented himself without leave, elected Pierre de Castel in his place. Existing documents, however, do not seem to infer that any blame was found against his professional work. The permanent appointment of his successor was definitely postponed in case he should return. In 1537 he took his doctor's degree at Montpellier and soon he was appointed lecturer on the Greek text of Hippocrates and the following year he made a public anatomical demonstration.

He passed nearly the whole of 1546 and part of 1547 at Metz. He was town physician at a salary of 120 livres in Lorraine. He died on the 9th of April, 1553.

MEDICAL REFORMERS

It was the medical humanists who largely effected the liberation of medicine from the domination of Galen and Avicenna as they began to study Hippocrates and other Greek texts in the original and with open mind. Yet, before the average medical mind could be permeated with the experimental method of study, it was necessary to clear the atmosphere of the rubbish that had accumulated during the centuries of medical stagnation, and particularly to rid medicine of the antiquated notions pertaining to anatomy and physiology. Physiological knowledge was not on a par with anatomical progress because physiology was not fortunate enough to produce a Vesalius, a Fallopius, a Pare, a Gersdorff, a Clowes or a Bartisch, and without a clear knowledge of physiology, progress in pathology was well nigh impossible. This explains why it took longer for the physician to throw off the yoke of tradition than the surgeon. The lack of scientific knowledge bound medical practice to superstition, to the belief in amulets, and to reliance on herb decoctions, astrology, and uroscopy.

The medical writers of the day made constant reference to the great Arabian authorities on medicine and gave all credit to the foundation of medical science to Galen, a second-century Greek, who was aware of Christianity but doubted its validity. The old proverb, "Wherever there are three physicians, there are two atheists," was widespread during this period. Medicine was associated with black magic, secret charms, incantations, and strange remedies.

The Galenists were under the suspicion of impiety from the start, while fuel was added to the flame by the circulation of the writings of Paracelsus, an early and violent advocate of chemical remedies. The Paracelsans attacked the Galenists for defending a heathenish philosophy going back to Aristotle, and at the same time their own orthodoxy was being challenged because their chemical preparations suggested sorcery. The public's confidence in medical men was severely shaken by the charges and countercharges hurled back and forth.

Progress in medicine was greatly helped by the invention of the printing press which enabled writers to publish their experiences and the establishment of many universities in Europe which adopted critical and unbiased methods in their courses of study and refused to accept medieval medical tradition as theological dogmas. The Reformation (1517) brought independent views into the open, promoted the growth of vernacular literature and rejected the idea that anything not written in classical Latin is unworthy of reading. These factors added to the impetus created by the discovery of America, materially aided the revival of medical science.

CHAPTER XXXIV

MEDICAL REFORMERS

PIERRE BRISSOT (1478-1522)

The first to break the ties with the Arabo-Galenic medicine was Pierre Brissot. At the present time when phlebotomy as a therapeutic measure has almost entirely disappeared from our textbooks it is hard to conceive how such a trifling matter could bring about a revolution against a system of medicine that was rooted in the minds of physicians for over a millennium but strange as it may seem histories of great revolutions and reform movements often start from what appear later to be insignificant matters.

Brissot had long been a staunch follower of the Hippocratic method of bleeding by which a large amount of blood is taken at the beginning of the disease (e. g. pleurisy and pneumonia) from an area near the diseased part. The later Greek and the Arabian writers contended that, at the onset of an inflammation, blood should be taken at a distant area as far as possible from the site of the pathology and in small quantities taken slowly, drop by drop. These latter writers asserted that considerable bleeding in the vicinity of the diseased part could only increase congestion in the inflamed part and further weaken it. Abstraction of blood from the diseased part was known as *revulsion* and removal of blood away from the diseased part was known as *derivation*.

In the severe epidemic of pneumonia in Paris in 1514, Brissot's method of bleeding proved to be more effective and he became known as a "medical reformer," second only to Paracelsus. He attracted to his views such eminent physicians as Villemore and Helin (1516), members of the Paris Faculty, and many distinguished teachers of other lands such as Giovanni Manardi (1464-1536), Jerome Cardan (1501-1576), Andreas Vesalius (1514-1564), Emilo Campalogo (c. 1589), Ambroice Pare, Guido Guidi (d. 1569), Giovanni Battista and Da Monte (1498-1551). Among his adversaries were equally eminent personalities such as Thomas Erastus (1523-1583), Gunther von Andernach (a foe of Paracelsus), Vittore Trincavella (1496-1548), and Amatus Lusitanus (1511-1568).

The opposition to the *revulsion* method was so strong that the French Parliament actually prohibited this method. Charles V of Portugal, where Brissot came to agitate in favor of the Hippocratic method, condemned it at the instigation of Brissot's enemies who claimed that his method was "just as bad as the Lutheran heresy." In spite of the fact that Brissot met with success during an epidemic in Evora, his enemies in Portugal, led by the court physician named Lusitanius Dionysius, published a criticism of Brissot's method, to which the latter replied in his "Apologetica Deceptatio."[1] Fortunately for Brissot, one of the emperor's relatives had recently died of pleurisy in spite of the Arabian method of bleeding. This incident perhaps saved the burning of many medical heretics, for burning heretics was common in those days in Spain and Portugal.

The large number of those who were pro and con furnishes sufficient evidence of the profound seriousness of this controversy. It divided the physicians of Western Europe into two camps. The most distinguished physicians took part in the controversy, especially the Roman physicians, who, as late as the beginning of the twentieth century, were still not completely agreed on the proper method of venesection.[2] The matter was afterwards brought before the University of Salamanca and was decided in favor of Brissot.

The significance of this agitation turned into a much deeper inquiry, namely, whether or not the authority of Galen and his Arabian followers should be upheld.

JEAN FRANCOIS FERNEL (1497-1558)

Jean Francois Fernel or Joannes Fernelius was born at Clearmont, France, in the Diocese of Amiens. He received his early education in his native town. He afterwards attended the College of Sainte Barbe, Paris, where he studied philosophy. In 1519 he received the degree master of arts and shortly after he entered the medical school. He graduated from medical school in 1530. While he was still a medical student he experimented on the exact measurement of a degree of the meridian, as is recorded in his work *Cosmotheoria* (1528).

From 1534 he gave himself up entirely to medicine. His extraordinary general erudition, his skill and the success with which he sought to revive the study of the old Greek physicians, gained him a reputation, and ultimately the office of physician to the court.

Fernel quickly achieved fame in his medical practice. It was said that no patient however poor was refused treatment by him. He gained the friendship of Catherine de Medici who believed that his skill helped her become fertile. She paid him a fee of C. 10,000 at the birth of her first child and the same fee at that of each of her succeeding children.

Fernel died in despair a few months after the death of his wife.

Fernel did much to shake off the yoke of medievalism. In his work *Universa Medicina* (1554), he presents a case history of a seven-year-old girl, pointing to the fact that he recognized the condition now known as appendicitis with perforation. Here is a part of his description:

A girl of seven afflicted with diarrhoea, passed for many days from the bowels a white, putrid and foul material, with no pain. The grandmother was tired of this daily flowing and to stop it took counsel with some other old women. In this case a quince as large as one's hand was secured and the patient devoured it, with the result that the stools were suppressed so that during the day and the following night nothing was passed. But with violent, most severe pains and cramps in the belly she swelled up until the swelling suddenly became putrid. A physician came who, suspecting the true state of affairs, tried first injections of mild clysters and then more severe ones to dislodge the noxious stinking material from the intestines and to ease the pain with fomentations; but in vain. Indeed with increasingly severe pains, repeated loss of consciousness and moreover with vomiting of a fecal liquid she died miserably in two days. On opening the body the caecum intestinum (appendix?) was narrowed and constricted; also the quince was found adherent to the inside and stopping up the lumen, so that it absolutely could not pass through any other way: whence it happened that this acrid and corrupt material prevented from passing; the obstacle overflowing opened up itself an unusual route into the abdominal cavity, by a necrosis and perforation a little above the obstructed place; from whence in the gut just as by the outlet and the passage escaping it filled up the abdomen to its entire capacity. Hence the suffering of most severe pains, hence distention, hence loss of consciousness, the most cruel death following shortly the appearance of foul vomiting. The history will be of value to those who in an excessive flow of abundant and toxic fluid from whatsoever the cause, hasten intemperately to stop and subdue it to the greatest misfortune of the patient.[3]

PARACELSUS (1493-1541)

Perhaps the greatest reformer of Renaissance medicine was Philippus Theophrastus Aurealus Paracelsus Bambas von Hohenheim, a younger contemporary of the French reformer Brissot. He was regarded by some as a dangerous heretic worthy of the stake, and by others as "the Martin Luther of medicine." His verbal violence eventually brought him bodily harm. He was hostile to the academies and tradition. His violent attacks on tradition were perhaps justified in a country like Germany where traditions were so profoundly rooted.

In compensation for his lack of reverence toward tradition and historical personalities, he gained the confidence of the masses with whom he came in contact medically and from whom he drew his strength. At the bedside of the sick he was a clinician in the true sense of the word. For the benefit of the patient, he utilized the observations that he had made during his travels and the histories that he had obtained from the workmen, peasants, and merchants with whom he had more in common than with the masters and philosophers.

He exhibited the true temperament of the practical physician in that he learned more from his daily contact with the patient than from books. It was his habit to gather with his pupils about the bedsides of patients rather than in the lecture rooms of universities. The secret of his success, as stated, was his appeal to the common people, lecturing and writing in their own German language, not in Latin, as was customary for the erudite physicians and university professors of his period.

Paracelsus was one of the first to break away from the orthodox schools of Galen and Avicenna. He truly applied to medical problems the same independence which Luther employed with regard to religion and Galileo with respect to astronomy. He used his own observations and experiences. "The human mind," he says, "knows nothing of the nature of things from the inward meditations. . . . That which his eyes see and his hands touch, that is his teacher." "Science is a search for God in his creation and medicine is God's gift to man."

Medicines are created by God. However, He does not prepare them completely. The active principles are hidden in the slag. It is for the therapist to remove the active principles from the slag. All things have been created in *prima materia* and it remained for *Vulcanus* to convert them into the *ultima materia* through the art of alchemy. This is the art of separating the useful from the useless.[4]

Nature is sufficient for the cure of most diseases; the medical art has only to intervene when the internal physician, the man himself, is tired or incapable. Then some remedy has to be introduced which should be antagonistic to the disease process. His chemistry taught men to experiment and not to rely blindly upon authority; this is a cornerstone in the development of independent thought.

Paracelsus taught that all matter is composed of salt, sulphur, and mercury. Salt, the solid, is indestructible by fire; mercury, the fluid, is vaporized but unchanged by fire; and sulphur is both changed and destroyed by fire. These alchemistic elements were contained in the *Mysterium Magnum* which Paracelsus and Basil Valentine (c. 1450) regarded as the component parts of all metal. Theophrastus holds that it is the component part also of organic substances and is contained in the Archaeus (active principle).

"Doctors, I advise you to use alchemy in preparing *magnolia, wysteria, arcana,* and to separate the pure from the impurities so that you may obtain a perfect medicine. God did not choose to give us the medicines prepared. He wants us to cook them ourselves." [5]

Out of that *Mysterium* flowed, and from various combinations of the three bodies above mentioned, originated, the four common elements; air, water, earth, as representatives of the earthy material, and fire, as the celestial element. Each of these has an archaeus or active principle, which, in contrast to dead matter, possesses a creative, formative power of its own. From the union of the elements originating within that triad, and arising organically, all material objects and all beings take their origin.

While attempting to apply chemistry to medicine Paracelsus made a number of chemical discoveries. Under "sulphur" he describes a substance *extract of vitriol* which has the ear marks of ether. "The substance," he says, "has an agreeable taste" even chickens will eat it, whereupon they sleep for a moderately long time and reawaken without having been injured.[6]

Incidentally, it was Valerius Cordus (1515-1544) who gives a clear description of the preparation of ether by the action of oil of vitriol (or sulphuric acid). Paracelsus' description of the extract of vitriol shows that he passed from alchemy to chemistry. Among the vegetable preparations, he introduced the tincture of opium still bearing the name *laudanum* which he

599

gave it. He also introduced antimony, a mineral remedy which gave rise to controversy in France.

The followers of Paracelsus were distinguished from the Galenic school by the use which they made of chemical drugs in medical practices. They discovered a number of drugs which proved to be of value. Theophrastus introduced mineral baths, and was one of the first to analyze them. He made opium (*laudanum*), mercury, lead, sulphur, iron, arsenic, copper sulphate, and potasium sulphate (called the *specificum purgans Paracelsi*), as a part of the pharmacopoeia, and regarded zinc as an elementary substance. He distinguished alum from ferrous sulphate, and demonstrated the iron content of water by means of gallic acid.[7] He recommended new forms of medical preparations such as extract and tinctures.

"He had pills which he called laudanum and which had the form of mice excrements, but he used them only in cases of extreme emergency. He boasted that with these pills he could wake up the dead, and indeed he proved that patients who seemed to be dead suddenly arose."

He divided syphilis into local and general, primary and secondary. He refers to its inheritance, its manifold forms, and its influence upon the course of other diseases. He employed internally a great number of mercurial preparations, prepared after alchemistic formulae, and discarded the popular abuse or regimen during the treatment. He erroneously regarded gonorrhea as an initial stage of syphilis, but was correct in ascribing its causation to coitus.[8]

He held the union of divided parts is accomplished by means of a "natural balsam or animal mummy," separated from the body within wounds. To protect the latter is the task of the physician: "Every surgeon should understand that it is not he who heals, but the balsam within the body is that which heals," and "thou art a good surgeon, in that thou offerest to nature defence and protection in the wounded part."

Paracelsus' surgical studies, particularly concerning the treatment of wounds, reveal an intimate knowledge of the subject. He held strongly to the cleanliness of wounds, in direct opposition to the custom of that day: "I have often seen the ignorance of you surgeons, while the wounds fairly stank and poured forth a foul pus, like a stinking old hole in elephantiasis, which suited you!" He recommended further spare diet and regulation of drink and was sufficiently acquainted too with the accidental complications of wounds.

In fractures he opposed the barbarous efforts and methods for the reduction of the broken bone, and laid stress upon the fact that nature could accomplish repair in these injuries also, without any aid. In other places, however, he recommended bandaging the fractures twice a day.

He denies the importance of the knowledge of anatomy in medicine. "You will learn nothing from the anatomy of the dead; it fails to show the true nature, its working, its essence, quality, being, and power. All that is essential to know is not dead. The true anatomy has never been dealt with. It is that of the living body, not of the dead one. If you want to anatomize health and disease, you need a living body."

The operative side of surgery, however, was not in his line. He ascribes high value to "local" anatomy in surgery. Lithotomy alone he permitted, but otherwise prohibited entirely all cutting, burning and stitching by the "torturing idiots" as he called them. On the other hand his treatment of wounds shows rich experience in military surgery.

In curing ulcers he almost did miracles in cases which had been given up by others. He never forbade the patients food or drink. On the contrary, he drank with them all night and, as he said, cured them with their stomachs full. He used precipitate powder with theriacum or mithridatum or cherry juice, made into pills to purge.

PHYSIOLOGY

The physiology of Theophrastus recognizes the *archaeus* as the active and life-giving agent in man whose location is in the stomach. The archaeus separates the material useful for nutrition from the waste substances; the "essence," from the useless (the "poison"). The archaeus thus becomes the "alchemist of the body." Moreover it is the spirit of life, the *astral body*—the "essence" in the body. The "poison" is excreted by two routes—all excrements are "poisons". Each part of the body attracts, extracts and assimilates what is appropriate for it since all possess their own special archaeus. Digestion is a kind of putrefaction, by which, on the one hand, it assimilates the nutritive slime, on the other hand, it renders possible the formation of the excrement. Health is recognized by the regular action of this archaeus. The archaeus presides also over generation.

The semen is a secretion from the *liquor vitae,* from the general fluids of the body, which secretion is effected by the exciting influence of the woman upon the fancy of the man, and takes place only momentarily during coitus. It is the quintessence of the fluids, which is being derived from each member of the body and is therefore in a condition to reproduce each member.[9] The woman supplies no semen, the uterus is merely the soil on which the male semen flows and is deposited; the nutrition of the embryo is derived from the breast which in some unknown way reaches the uterus. The uterus attracts the semen as a magnet attracts iron.

PATHOLOGY

In a similar way he sets himself in opposition to Galen with regard to the general pathological conceptions of health and disease. Health, according to Theophrastus consists in the due proportion of "sulphur, salt, and mercury" in the body, together with the correct action of the archaeus: disease is the opposite of this. "Therefore, the physician should know that all diseases lie in these three substances, and not in the four elements." The so-called fundamental humors are only results and expressions of disease.

SYMPTOMATOLOGY

His symptoms and diagnosis are bound up with the ancient ideas of microcosm and astrology. The pulse reveals to him the temperature of the body. He finds seven kinds of pulses, conforming to the seven planets. The pulse of the sun lies beneath the heart; two pulses in the neck belong to Venus and Mars; two in the feet to Jupiter and Saturn; those of the temples to the moon and to Mercury. The physician must know the planets of the microcosm, the meridian line, etc., before he can determine the vital actions of the body and can cure diseases.

"No belief was as popular in the sixteenth century as astrology, among intellectuals as well as the masses. Paracelsus would not give an enema or bleed a patient when the moon was in the wrong constellation.[10] In prescribing charms and amulets he consulted the Zodiac; and he attributed the bad 'humor' of a patient to a harmful exudation of his planet. At the same time, his criticism of astrology was outspoken."

> "The stars determine nothing, incline nothing,
> suggest nothing; we are as free from them as
> they are from us." [11]

> "The stars and all the firmament cannot affect
> our body, nor our color, beauty and gestures,
> nor our virtues and vices. . . . The course of
> Saturnus can neither prolong nor shorten man's
> life." [12]

"If a disease is in the body all the sound organs must fight against it; not one, but all. Nature notes this fact." "Nature is the physician, not you!" If she refuses, then first begins the office of the physician—the "external physician"— to support the *archaeus*—the "internal" physician—so that he may gain victory. He insists that the first and last duty of medicine is that of healing. In one of his outbursts of anger he cries out: "If God will not help, so help me the devil!"

Theophrastus assumes that a remedy exists for every disease. He considers no disease incurable. "If thou lovest thy neighbor, thou must not say there is nothing which can help thee; but thou must say I help thee!" One should be willing to cure not only with opposing remedies, like the Ancients, but also with similar remedies, not only *contraria contrariis*, but also *similia similibus*.

To know the nature of man and how to deal with it, the physician should study, not anatomy, which Paracelsus utterly rejected, but all parts of external nature. Life is a perpetual germinative process controlled by the indwelling spirit or *archaeus* and diseases are not natural but spiritual. Besides the various remedies the physician must know above all their relations to celestial things (macrocosm) and to the organs, since the stars impress their "signature" upon all drugs. This he said is recognized by the form, color, etc., as woman is by her breasts. Therefore, the testiculate orchis-root indicates its use in diseases of the testicle; the black spot on the flower of the euphrasia points to the pupil of the eye; the color of the lizard, to unhealthy ulcers; gold, which, according to the mystic assumption, harmonizes with the heart, indicates its employment in diseases of the heart, etc. "For where there is a new disease, there is also its remedy." The special duty of the physician consists, according to Theophrastus, in finding for each disease its special remedy, the specificum and arcanum.[13] *Arcana*—a word corresponding partly to what we now call specific remedies, he applied to a mysterious connection between the remedy and the "essence" of the disease. Elixir is the "hidden power which preserves" and is like a balm; which "can change us, bring about transmutations, can renovate and restore us." "Arcanum," is that "immaterial talent" of substances which embodies their "virtue," and is the effective principle of a remedy. In the *Arch-wisdom*, he still called "arcanum" any hidden virtue. Later, he used it for medicines specifically. Arcana bore often a physical resemblance to certain parts of the body; from which rose the famous doctrine of *signatures*, or signs indicating the virtues and uses of natural objects, which was afterwards developed into great complexity.[14]

The doctrine of *signature* is probably the earliest therapeutic system in the history of medicine. It was based on the belief that the Creator stamped all objects medically beneficial to mankind, and on the assumption that there is a connection of every part of the human body (the microcosm) with a corresponding part in the world of Nature.[15]

Nicholas Culpepper (1652), a well-known therapeutist of his day, wrote: "If a bean be parted in two, the skin being taken away, and laid upon the place where the Leeche hath been set that bleedeth too much, it stayeth the bleedings—The Huskes boiled in water to the consumption of a third part thereof stayeth a Lax and the Ashes of the Huskes made upper with Hogg's gress helpeth the old Pains, contusions and wounds of the sinews, the skiatica and the Gout. Beans eaten are extremely windy mete, but if after the Dutch fashion when they are half boiled you huske them and then seive them, they are wholesome food." [16]

We shall now survey the life and personality of Paracelsus who was born in 1493 in Einsiedeln near Zurich, Switzerland, the son of Wilhelm von Hohenheim, who had a hard struggle to make a subsistence as a physician. His mother was superintendent of the hospital at Einsiedeln, a post she relinquished upon her marriage. He was named Theophrastus after the botanist who had been a pupil of Aristotle. The name "Paracelsus" was probably one of his own making, and was meant to denote his superiority to Celsus.[17]

His father, his first teacher, took pains to instruct him in all the learning of the time, especially in medicine. At the age of sixteen he entered the University of Basel, but probably soon abandoned the studies pursued there. He next went to Wurzburg, where he took up chemical research. The belief in the stone of the philosophers so characteristic of the notions of that time was too remote a possibility to gratify the fiery spirit of Paracelsus. He left school and started for the mines in Tirol. The sort of knowledge he got there pleased him much more. He saw all the mechanical difficulties that had to be overcome in mining; he learned the physicial properties of minerals,

605

ores and metals; he got a notion of mineral waters; he was an eyewitness of the accidents which befell the miners, and studied the diseases which attacked them; he was convinced that positive knowledge of nature was not in schools and universities, but only by going to nature herself, and to those who were constantly engaged with her. He attached no value to mere scholarship; scholastic disputations he utterly ignored and despised—and especially the discussions on medical topics, which turned more upon theories and definitions, than upon actual practice. After spending time at Tirol he went wandering over a great part of Europe to learn all that he could. In the book of nature, he affirmed, is that which the physician must read, and to do so he must walk over the leaves. The humors and passions and diseases of different nations are different, and the physician must go among the nations if he will be master of his art; the more he knows of other nations, the better he will understand his own. He argued that he knew what his predecessors were ignorant of, because he had been taught in no human school. "Whence have I all my secrets, out of what writers and authors? Ask rather how the beasts have learned their arts. If nature can instruct irrational animals, can it not much more men?"

Although Paracelsus was not properly educated in medicine, he possessed an ingenious medical instinct. Through his extensive travels and his liberation from the narrowing and rigid education of the schools of his time, he was better fitted for the work of a reformer than were the literati of the profession, who followed slavishly the paths of Galen and the Arabs. "The physician should be a traveler . . . ," said Paracelsus, "Does not traveling supply more information than sitting by the fireside? He who wishes to investigate nature thoroughly must tread her books (evidently referring to Galen and the Arabs) with his feet. The first schoolmaster of medicine is the corpus and the material of nature. What is it to enter medicine by the right door? Is it through Avicenna, Galen, Mesue, Rhazes, etc., or through the light of nature? This is the right door, the light of nature!" In the Basel program he styles himself "Doctor of both Medicine and Surgery."[18]

That Paracelsus really believed that he conceived a great new medical system may be seen in the following: "That I here in this work introduce a new *Theoricum,* also *Physicum,* together with new Concepts which heretofore have never been held, nor understood by the philosophers, astronomers, nor physicians, comes to pass for the reasons which I shall now relate to you: One reason, for instance, which is sufficiently proven, viz: that the old *Theorici* described the *Rationes* and *Causae Morborum* wrongly and inaccurately and thus introduced such error, and so confirmed this error, that it was held and considered just and incontrovertible. And it is so deeply rooted and so tended and preserved, that no one may any more seek an alternative, or the same is deemed an error. This I wish to make known to you, for I am bound to judge such a thing as great foolishness: since heaven is forever learning and creating *Ingenia,* new *Inventiones,* new *Artes,* new *Aegritudines* in the light of nature, should not these also be valid? Of what avail is the rain that fell a thousand years ago? That which falls at present avails. Of what avail to the present year is the sun's course of a thousand years ago?" [19]

His boastful manifesto aroused opposition from his antagonists as well as from his admirers. Here are some of his egotistic utterances:

"Follow me, not I you, follow ye me, follow me Avicenna, Galen, Rhazes, Montagnana, Mesue, and ye others. Follow me, not I you! ye of Paris, Montpellier, ye of Suabia, ye of Meissen, ye of Cologne, ye of Vienna and the banks of the Danube and the Rhine, ye islands of the sea, Italy, Dalmatia, Sarmatia, Athens, ye Greeks, ye Arabs, ye Israelites, not one of you shall remain in the remotest corner upon whom the dogs shall not void their urine! I shall be the monarch, mine the monarchy! How does this please you, Caeophrastus? This dung must ye eat! And ye Calefactores, ye shall become chimney-sweeps. What will ye think when the sect of Theophrastus triumphs?" [20]

"Very few physicians have exact knowledge of disease and the causes but my books are not like those of other physicians copying Hippocrates and Galen. I have composed them on the basis of experiments which are the greatest masters of everything, and with indefatigable labor. If any of you feel the desire to penetrate the divine secrets of medicine and feel like acquiring the medical art in the shortest time come to me at Basel and you will find much more than I can promise you with my words." Another of his vitriolic outbursts was "All the universities have less experience than my beard. The down on my neck is more learned than my antagonists. You must follow my footsteps. I shall not go in yours. Not one of your professors will find a cover so well hidden that the dogs will come and lift them by the legs and defile them. I shall become a monarch, mine will be the monarchy which I shall rule to make you gird up your loins." [21]

This self-assertion and self-exaltation was not conducive to making friends. His writings in the German language made him unpopular among the learned. His alchemistic and astrological practices had so condemned him among the apothecaries that he was compelled to wander from place to place.

He then settled in Strassburg where his fame as a skillful physician reached Basel. In the last city there was a prosperous printer by the name of Frobinus who suffered with a severe malady of his foot, which his attending physician advised him to amputate. Frobinus decided that before submitting to the operation he would consult the doctor from Strassburg, who fortunately cured Frobinus from his malady without resorting to surgery. This opened up Frobinus' printing press for Paracelsus' manuscript and secured for him the position of municipal physician as well as lecturer at the University at Basel, Switzerland. The lectures were in German, not Latin as was customary. They were expositions of his own experiences, of his own views on pharmacology and medicine and his own methods of curing. He gathered many pupils about him. Some of them were driven chiefly by a desire for lucre and only utilized those parts of his teachings that furthered a charlatanism cloaked in glittering formulas. While at the University of Basel, in a fit of temper he is said to have expressed his antagonism to medical tradition by publicly burning the text of Galen and Avicenna.

The truth of Paracelsus' doctrines was apparently confirmed

by his success in curing or mitigating diseases for which the regular physicians who used all kinds of "shot gun" prescriptions, and loathsome drugs, could do nothing. For a few years his reputation and practice increased to a surprising extent but his attacks on traditional medicine made his stay at the University impossible. His enemies watched for slips and failures; they maintained that he had no medical degree, and insisted that he should give proof of his qualifications. Moreover, his pharmaceutical system did not harmonize with the commercial arrangements of the apothecaries, and he did not use their drugs like the Galenists. The growing jealousy and enmity culminated in a dispute with Canon Cornelius von Lichtenfels, who, having called in Paracelsus after other physicians had given up his case, refused to pay the fee he had promised in the event of cure; and, as the judges sided with the Canon, Paracelsus had no alternative but to tell them his opinion of the whole case and of their notions of justice. His friends advised him to leave Basel at once to escape the punishment for the attacks he made on the authorities. He departed in such haste that he carried nothing with him. Then he began his wandering life, the course of which can be traced by the dates of his various writings. In this way he spent some dozen years, till 1541, when he was invited by Archbishop Ernst to settle at Salzburg, under his protection, where he died on the 24th of September.

The opposition of his practices long outlived Paracelsus himself. The greatest outcry against him has been directed against his new prescriptions. The use of inorganic, particularly metallic, elements in internal remedies was attacked as unnatural and poisonous for more than a century and the argument found one of its most acute expressions in the famous fight of the Paris faculty about antimony. He has been accused of using poison; this accusation was largely aimed at the chemical aspect of his medical system. Paracelsus was adamant in his contention that the physician must be a chemist, and supported the contention on the ground that all things are poisonous if taken without respect to their proper dosage. He accused his opponents of not knowing the proper dosage. The enemies of Paracelsus conducted against him a violent campaign full of abuse and grave accusations, especially in Germany and in Basel.

Regardless of his violent temper and his egoism he occupies an important place in the history of medicine. He is a personality about whom most opposite opinions have been expressed. Two centuries after his demise Dr. J. G. Zimmerman could write of him that "he lived like a pig, looked like a coachman and took most pleasure in the company of the loosest and lowest mob . . ." and that "all his writings seem to have been written during intoxication."[22] He possessed one might say, a double personality, a mixture of concise ideas with distorted conceptions—natural as well as supernatural, a mixture of mathematics, astrology and magic. It is difficult to form an opinion of him as, for example, of Galileo and Luther, the other pioneers of the Renaissance. He had an independent spirit but unlike the calm and considerate scholars of his time he advanced medicine by wandering from place to place, picking quarrels, and browbeating his listeners into accepting his views.

In France many medical men rallied to his defence; Jacques Gohory professor in Paris, published in 1567 a summary of the philosophy and medicine of Paracelsus, and Joseph du Chesne (Quercetanus), 1521-1609, wrote an introduction to Paracelsian "antimony," in France.

The best-known Paracelsists in Germany were Adam von Bodenstein (d. 1576), Michael Schutz, Michael Doring (d. 1644), of Giessen, and Gunther von Andernach (1806-1871). In England, Robert Fludd (1574-1637), of pulse timing and early vaccinating fame. In Italy, Peter Soerensen (Severinus, 1540-1602) who published a letter in defence of Paracelsus (Florence, 1570) and later exploited his views in a book, *Idea Medicina Philosophicae*.

His enemies asserted that he died in a low tavern in consequence of a drunken debauch of some days' duration. Others maintain that he was thrown down a steep place by some emissaries either of the physicians or of the apothecaries, both of whom he had during his life most grievously harassed. According to Sudhoff, he died of cancer at the age of 48. He was buried in the churchyard of St. Sebastian, but in 1752 his bones were removed to the porch of the church, and a monument of reddish-white marble was erected in his memory.

How the character of Theophrastus was judged in unprejudiced circles of his own day, may be inferred unequivocally from his epitaph, even if we make some little allowance for the "De mortuis nil nisi bene" principle. The epitaph read as follows: "Here lies Philippus Paracelsus, the famous Doctor Medicinae, who, by his wonderful art, cured bad wounds, lepra, gout, dropsy and other incurable diseases, and to his own honor divided his possessions among the poor."

Paracelsus is said to have composed more than 300 treatises written in German; some of them were later translated into Latin dealing with various phases of medicine and surgery. Among them are his *Chirurgia Magna* (1536), *De gradibus Basel* (1568), his manual *The Use of Mercurals in Syphilis* (1553). About fifteen works and editions have since been published. B. Aeschner rendered his work into modern German in 1920. In English, we may mention *Four Treatises* by *Theophrastus von Hohenheim*.[23] The most exhaustive study of Paracelsus was made by Karl Sudhoff.

JEAN BAPTISTA VAN HELMONT (1577-1644)

A most interesting figure of Renaissance medicine was the erstwhile Capuchin friar and later the founder of the Iatrochemical school, Jean Baptista Van Helmont. Like his master Paracelsus he believed that each part of the human body is governed by a special archaeus or spirit and that the physiological process of the entire body is controlled by a chemical force, a ferment of a special nature which he named "gas." Van Helmont recognized different kinds of aeroform substances which are absorbed by the various archaei to perform the bodily functions under the supreme control of the soul, which is lodged in the stomach. The sensitive soul and the immortal mind, investing the body with superior and inferior archaei, enabled

Van Helmont to make use of the strictest mechanical conception of the body now attributed to the brain and the nervous system. He denied the existence of a sensitive soul in animals and plants. Van Helmont understood that there are gases distinct in kind from atmospheric air.

He claimed to have discovered CO_2 (1641) our carbon dioxide which he called "sylvestre" gas. He resorted to urinalysis, of several 24-hour specimens, but drew no deductions from the test. Van Helmont introduced a complicated system of supernatural agencies like the *archaei* of Paracelsus, which preside over and direct the affairs of the body. He added a central *archaeus* controlling a number of subsidiary *archaei* which move through the ferments. Diseases are primarily caused by some infection of the *archaeus,* and remedies act by bringing it back to normal. In addition to the *archaeus,* which he described as "aura vitalis seminum, vitae directrix," Van Helmont had other governing agencies resembling the *archaeus.* He taught that there is the sensitive soul which is the husk or shell of the immortal mind. When the body perishes the immortal mind can no longer remain in the body.

For the physiology of the gastro-intestinal tract he relied on the authority of Hippocrates. He created six ferments for his six types of digestion. He regarded nature as derived from divine power, which is represented in man by a vital body force, *archaeus insitus,* and an *archaeus influus,* the divine force which regulated physical and mental phenomena in man. Every modification of the *archaeus* produced by the *idea morbosa* results in disease, every alteration of the regulating germ has as a secondary consequence the alteration of matter.

Disease, according to the new concept of Van Helmont, is an actual entity existing as an invisible principle endowed with various properties. This is not an opposition of two forces or a diathesis resulting from the struggle of contraries or an imbalance of the humors. The products of disease are seminal generations, so that they depend on the seeds that are reproduced.[24]

In general the physiologic speculations of Van Helmont's thought, in some respects ingenious, can be dismissed as unconstructive, with no advantage over those which he attacked. His explanations of different *archaei,* of which the supreme *archaeus* governs fecundity explained nothing. Van Helmont deserves, however, an important place in the history of medicine for throwing a brighter light on the chemical path which was previously begun by Paracelsus.

He explicitly denied that fire is an element. He also maintained that earth is not one because it can be reduced to water. He believed that air and water are the two primitive elements. That plants, are composed of water he sought to show by the experiment of planting a willow weighing 5 lbs. in 200 lbs. of dry soil and allowing it to grow for five years; at the end of that time it had become a tree weighing 169 lbs. and since it had received nothing but water and the soil weighed practically the same as at the beginning, he argued that the increased weight of wood, bark, and roots had been formed from water alone.

Chemical principles guided him in the choice of medicines viz., undue acidity of the digestive juices was to be corrected by alkalies and *vice versa;* he was thus a forerunner of the iatrochemical school, and he enhanced the art of medicine by applying chemical methods in its preparation.

Van Helmont was born at Brussels in 1577.[25] He was educated at Louvain and for some time he was a Capuchin friar and after changing from one science to another, turned to medicine, in which he took his doctor's degree in 1599. A few years he spent in traveling through Switzerland, Italy, France and England. He settled in 1609 at Vilvorde, near Brussels, where he occupied himself with chemical experiments and medical practice. Van Helmont was a disciple of Paracelsus, swaying between science and mysticism. A mystic with strong leanings toward the supernatural, an alchemist who believed that with a small piece of the philosopher's stone he had transmuted 2,000 times as much mercury into gold.

The philosopher's stone known as the "quintessence" was not only supposed to transmute the base metals into gold, make precious stones, but also confer perfect health and length of days. It was described by those who chanced to see it, as of a reddish luster. Paracelsus likened it to a ruby; Van Helmont to saffron with the luster of glass.

His life reflects a picture of his period vibrating between doubt and faith, between spiritual revolt and acts of contrition. He was denounced to the inquisitors by his enemies for daring to speak against dogmatic religious conceptions. He steadfastly adhered to the chemical theories of Paracelsus whom he surpassed in the depth of observation and scientific knowledge.[26]

JOHANNES LANGE (1485-1565)

One of the opponents of the Arabs in Germany was Johannes Lange of Lowenberg, Silesia, a friend of Melanchthon (1497-1560), and Casper Peucer (1525-1562). In his "Epistolae Medicinales" he combated the practice of uroscopy and advocated Greek semiology. Uroscopy was based upon Galenic doctrine that the natural forces of a person can be determined from the condition of the urine as the spiritual forces may be learned from the pulse.[27]

Here is in brief his well known description of chloriasis: "There are many illnesses in the catalogue of diseases, lacking a name but not a treatment. Nor has this disease a proper name, as much as it is peculiar to virgins, might indeed be called virgineus, which it is the custom of the matrons of Brabant to call white fever, or pale face and the fever of love: since every lover becomes pale, and this color is proper for a lover, although a fever very rarely is present. But this disease frequently attacks virgins, when now mature they pass from youth to virility. For at this time, by nature, the menstrual blood flows from the liver to the small spaces and veins of the womb: which when from the narrow mouths, which are not yet distended, also obstructed by thick and crude humors, and finally the thickness of the blood, cannot escape: then carried backwards through the vena cava and the large arteries flows to the heart, liver, diaphragm and veins of the diaphragm: also a good part is distributed to the head, and grave accidents appear in the viscera, dyspnoea, a tremulous throbbing of the heart, inflation of the liver, nausea of the stomach, cardalgia: not rarely epilepsy with loss of senses, and delirium.

"Finally, whether your daughter ill with this affection ought to marry, and what should be the treatment of it I therefore say, I instruct virgins afflicted with this disease, that as soon as possible they live with men and copulate, if they conceive they recover, if indeed they be not attacked by this disease in puberty, then it attacks a little later unless they have been married." [28]

John Lange was born in 1485 in Lowenberg, Silesia. He studied at the University of Leipsic, from where he received his master's degree in 1514. Then he went to the University of Ferrara where he studied under the distinguished teacher Nicolo Leoniceno. He received his medical degree from the University of Pisa in 1522.

Upon his return he served as physician to four Electors for a period of forty years. He accompanied the Electors on two occasions when their armies marched against the Turks under Suleiman. He died in Heidelberg in 1565 at the age of eighty.[29]

CHAPTER XXXV

THE REVIVAL OF ANATOMY

Along with the revival of learning there came the renaissance of the arts. We have referred to Michelangelo, Leonardo da Vinci and Raphael who began to study the human form carefully. It was realized that to represent the human form accurately a knowledge of anatomy and especially of the bones and muscles was needed. The artists, therefore, began to dissect human cadavers.

LEONARDO DA VINCI (1452-1519)

Leonardo da Vinci's accurate anatomic drawings were made from actual dissections carried out by the painter himself. His observant eye accurately noted the effects of hardening of the arteries on the peripheral vessels.

"And you who say that it is better to see the dissection than such drawings, you would speak well if it were possible to see all these things which are demonstrated in such drawings in a single specimen, in which you with all your genius will not see and will not obtain knowledge except of a few veins. For, I have true and full knowledge from dissecting more than ten human bodies, destroying all other organs, consuming with the very minutest particles all the flesh which surrounded these veins, without making them bloody except with insensible sanguinification of the capillary veins. One body did not suffice for so long a time, so that it was necessary to proceed by degrees with so many bodies that the complete knowledge might be fulfilled, which I twice repeated in order to see the differences."[1]

A review of the anatomical work of Leonardo da Vinci shows that he was interested in anatomy in all its branches. Leonardo was the first to present exact reproduction of the uterus which up to his time had been described as a vessel with rigid walls. He accurately described the fetal membranes. He studied myology with the same gusto as osteology and carefully examined the embryos of animals before occupying himself with the study of the human fetus *in utero*. He dissected the brain and concerned himself intensively with those mechanical and hydraulic problems that he had studied in his youth. The physiology of cardiac action was studied by him in a long series of experiments on the cadaver. The cardiac valves and their functions were subjected to a most careful examination. Injection of liquid wax into bovine hearts facilitated the study of the ventricles. Leonardo da Vinci was the first who, with impartial judgement, completely freed himself from Galenic traditions.

Leonardo was the first successfully to attack the problem of the anatomy of the human eye, and his account of the internal ear shows that he fully appreciated the structure of the malleus and the incus.[2]

According to the memoirs of the Cardinal of Aragon, Leonardo dissected thirty bodies of men and women of various ages, ten of which were employed for the study of the veins only. His anatomical technique may be regarded as excellent, for he injected the veins and the body cavities with liquid wax and made serial sections. His most admirable feature, however, was his faithful and exact reproduction of anatomical subjects made with an accuracy and exquisite artistic sense that has never been surpassed. From anatomy the next step is physiology, and here, too, Leonardo is found to be far in advance of his age. He described how the blood makes and remakes continually the whole body of man, bringing material to the parts and carrying off the waste products, as a furnace is fed and the ashes removed. He studied the muscles of the heart and made drawings of the valves which seem to show a knowledge of their functions. He compared the flow of the blood with the circulation of water from the hills to the rivers and the sea; from the sea to the clouds and back to the hills as rain. It seems that Leonardo understood the general principle of the circulation of the blood a hundred years or more before it was rediscovered and Harvey gave the knowledge to the world. His art led him to another scientific problem—the structure and mode of action of the eye. He made a model of the optical parts, and showed how an image was formed on the retina. He ignored the view still held by his contemporaries that the eye throws out rays which touch the object it wishes to examine.[3] Leonardo was one of the greatest living experimental scientists of all ages as may be seen from his writings. The following aphorisms of his reflect his contribution:

"Practical work without science is like a pilot of a ship without compass or rudder. Practical work must be based on a good theory."

"There is no certainty where mathematics is not involved or which cannot be considered mathematically."

"An experiment is the repetition of a natural process designed to discover the laws of relations presented by science."

"An experiment is never fallacious, only our interpretation of it may be wrong."

"No action in nature is without cause. If you understand the cause you need no experiments."[4]

Leonardo da Vinci was the son of a Florentine lawyer, born out of wedlock of a mother of humble station. The place of his birth was Vinci in the Florentine territory near Empoli. Leonardo's mother was named Catarina. Her relations with Ser Piero da Vinci seem to have come to an end almost immediately upon the birth of their son. Piero was married four times and had nine sons and two daughters by his last two wives. From the first he acknowledged that he was the father of Leonardo and he brought him up in his own house in Florence. In that city, Ser Piero followed his profession with success and acted as legal counsel to many of the best families of the city. Leonardo's great promise soon made itself manifest. An inexhaustible fountain of intellectual energy and curiosity lay hidden beneath his amiable exterior. Among the many pursuits to which the young Leonardo set his hand, his favorites were music, drawing and modeling. He received his first training in the studio of Lorenzo di Credi (1470-1477). Among his contemporaries with whom he formed special ties of friendship were the painters Sandro Botticelli and Pietro Perugino. By 1472 he was already enrolled in the painters' guild of Florence.[5]

Leonardo was not one of those artists of the Renaissance who sought to revive the ancient glories of art. He did not seek to imitate ancient models. He drew from first hand experience directly from life with a precision and subtle accuracy which no draughtsman before his time ever equaled. He was the first painter to recognize that the effects of light and shade are among the most significant and attractive features concerned with the appearance of objects.

Leonardo da Vinci was magnetically attracted to all odd formations. Strangely shaped hills and rocks, rare plants and animals, unusual faces and figures of men, quizzical smiles and expressions—some beautiful, others grotesque—far-fetched objects and curiosities, were things he loved to study, record and remember. Mere appearances did not satisfy him; he tried to probe their hidden laws and causes.[6]

ALESSANDRO ACHILLINI OF BOLOGNA (1463-1512)

Toward the end of the fifteenth century anatomical studies advanced all over Italy and especially at Padua where anatomy was pursued with intensity.

Achillini of Bologna, the pupil and commentator of Mondino, appears to have been the most distinguished of his disciples. He was the first to describe two of the auditory ossicles: the malleus and the incus. In 1503, he showed that the tarsus consists of seven bones. In neuroanatomy he rediscovered that band of white substance under the callosum, extending from the fimbria to the corpora mammilleria, known as the fornix and the funnel-shaped extension of the third ventricle extending through the hypothalamus to the end in the pituitary body known as the infundibulum. He was the first to observe the course of the cerebral cavities into the inferior cornua. He was the first to recognize the function of the first pair of cranial nerves. His gastrointestinal anatomy included a description of the orifices of the bile ducts, later more completely described by Thomas Warton (1610-1673). He described the ileocecal valve and his discussion of the duodenum, jejunum, ileum and colon shows that he was better acquainted with the site and distribution of these intestinal components than any of his predecessors or contemporaries. Achillini of Bologna had the conviction of firsthand knowledge so necessary to correct some of the errors of Galen.

ANTONIO BENIVIENI (c. 1440-1502)

Contemporaneous with Achillini were Antonio Benivieni an able Florentine surgeon who performed autopsies to determine the cause of death and to explain puzzling symptoms, and Alexander Benedetti (c. 1460-1525), a teacher of anatomy at Padua who avidly stressed the necessity for dissections even beyond the custom then in force of allowing the schools to dissect only the cadavers of legally executed criminals. Benedetti had an anatomical theater constructed at Padua, in which, after 1490, public demonstrations were held. This was later eclipsed by Fabricius' superb anatomical presentations in his magnificent structure.

Matthew de Gradibue, a native of Gradi, a town near Milan, distinguished himself by composing a series of treatises on the anatomy of various parts of the human body (1480). He was the first to describe the ovaries of the human female properly, thus anticipating Nicolas Steno or Stensen (1638-1687).

Another contemporary of Achillini was the anatomist, Gabriello de Zerbis (1465-1505) who flourished at Verona. He assumed the title of *"Medicus Theoricus"* and derived his information from actual dissection of human subjects. He rendered the best description of the olfactory nerves up to his time.

GIACOMO BERENGARIO DA CARPI (1470-1550)

Among the great Italian anatomists of the sixteenth century was Giacomo Berengario da Carpi who was professor at Bologna from 1502-1522. In the field of anatomic study he was a patient and gifted investigator; to him we owe the first descriptions of the sphenoid sinuses, a careful description of the tympanum, of the thymus, of the vermiform appendix, and of the ventricles of the brain. His book *De Fractura Galvariae sive Cranii* was published in Bologna in 1518. His celebrated "Commentary on the Anatomy of Mondino" contained twenty-one tables of drawings of muscles, blood vessels and genital organs. It was printed in Venice in 1521. In his *Isagogae* (1523), Berengario paid careful attention to the anatomy of the heart.

He is the first to undertake a systematic view of the several textures of which the human body is composed. He treats successively of the anatomical characters and proprieties of fat, of membrane in general (Panniculus), of flesh, of nerve, of fibre (filum), of ligament, of sinew or tendon, and of muscle in general. He rectifies the mistake of Mondino as to the olfactory or first pair of nerves, gives a good account of the optic and other nerves. Berengario is the first observer who indicated the principal divisions of the carotid arteries. He possessed an accurate knowledge of the position and shape of the ventricles, which he named the anterior, the middle and the posterior. He was also a celebrated surgeon.

GIOVANNI BATISTA CANANO (1515-1579)

A contemporary of Vesalius was Giovanni Batista Canano of Ferrara. Canano hailed from a distinguished medical family. He developed into an anatomist while young. His home contained a library and a dissection room. He discovered the muscle known as palmaris brevis and valves of the veins. The last he communicated to Vesalius. He was trained by Marcantonio della Torre the associate of Leonardo da Vinci, whom he succeeded.

The new professor Canano published *Muscularum Humani Corporis Picturata Dissectio* in Ferrara, 1541. (Dissection of the Muscles of the Bones of the Body with twenty-seven drawings by Girolamo da Cappi.) Canano's descriptive material, which is brief, clear and authoritative was the first printed book in which each muscle was figured separately; the relationship of the muscles to the bones was indicated. Never had twenty leaves given so much information. He had prepared a large treatise on anatomy but his "liber primus" was the only manuscript published: Only eleven copies are now extant, he suppressed even this first installment. (Streeter suggests "It is logical to suppose that when the great work of Vesalius appeared Canano realized that it was futile for him to attempt to equal this stupendous achievement). Despite the praise of Amatus Lusitanus and Fallopius, Canano disappeared from the anatomical arena, as soon as Vesalius became known.

ANDREA CESALPINUS (1519-1603)

Cesalpino of Aarazo, maintained the analogy between the pulmonary artery and aorta and the pulmonary veins and veins in general. Cesalpino observed the swelling of veins below ligatures and inferred from it a refluent motion of blood in these vessels.

The concept of circulation is indicated roughly by Cesalpino's attacks on Galen's concept regarding the liver as the center of the movement of the blood by showing that the vena cava is of a larger size near the heart than the liver. "The orifices of the heart are made by nature in such a way that the blood enters at the right ventricle of the heart by the vena cava from which the exit from the heart opens into the lungs. From the lungs there is an entrance at the left ventricle, from which in its turn opens the orifice of the aorta. Certain membranes placed at the opening of the vessels prevent the blood from returning so that the movement is constant from the *vena cava* through the heart and through the lungs to the aorta."[7] He was regarded by the Italians as a discoverer of the circulation of the blood before Harvey (1571-98). The physiologist, P. Flourens (1794-1867),[8] who investigated the function of the individual parts of the brain remarked: "The concepts of Cesalpino of general circulation could not have been better conceived nor more concisely defined." It is Cesalpino who first used the term "circulation of the blood" (in 1559). Strange as it may seem, Cesalpino believed that frogs might be generated from mud with the help of the sun and even suggested a similar origin of the aboriginal American. He still believed that organic and psychic life is governed by a principle called *anima*. He also adhered to the ancient concept of the human microcosm.

Andrea Cesalpinus was professor of medicine at Pisa before he was called to Rome by Clement III to be his personal physician. He was also Director of the Botanical Garden at Pisa. Clement III gave him the professorship of medicine at the Sapienza. His philosophic system crowned him with the name of "the Pope of Philosophers." He was an encyclopedist in his learning. Besides anatomy and physiology he was devoted to botany, biology, zoology and mineralogy. He came near to grasping the mechanical theory of human physiology (he only lacked convincing experiments). As Director of the Botanical Garden, which had been founded there in 1543, he collected plants from all over Europe and classified some 100 plants into fifteen classes. His "De Plantis" was published in Florence, 1483. He was honored by the Italians with statues and other monuments. He was called by Linacre "Primus Verus Systematicus" (the first true systematizer in botany).

Although dissections were carried on for over 200 years prior to Vesalius, comparatively little progress was made in anatomy. In Bologna the professor of anatomy only was permitted to give lectures on practical anatomy whenever he wished, while to the other professors it was allowed only at stated times. In spite of the improvement in the conditions of anatomical instruction, it was still considered a special attraction for a university, and still more for a professor or a physician, to possess an entire skeleton. The price of a skeleton in that day was very high.

The task of procuring cadavers in Bologna rested upon the students and competition for suitable subjects was so keen that heated arguments and fist fights often ensued. It was finally ordered that no doctor or pupil would be permitted to acquire a body without a license from the rector. A suit was instituted in 1318 against a professor and some of his pupils in Bologna for disinterring a buried body in order to dissect it.

According to the earlier statutes of Bologna, only doctors, surgeons and students had the right to attend an "anatomy," and then only after the beginning of their third year of study.

A total of twenty students were permitted to witness the dissection of the cadaver of a man and thirty of the cadaver of a woman. At first, two dissections were held a year, one on a man, one on a woman.

By 1521, as many as 500 students and citizens at a time attended public dissections. At times the payment of a fee was prerequisite to seeing the dissections. The dissection was usually done either by a surgeon or barber. The physician, who customarily thought himself too dignified to employ a scalpel or touch the body, supervised the dissection from the rostrum.

Because of the warm climate in Italy, dissections were held only in winter. "Anatomies" were performed in private or public, in lecture halls or in the open air before groups of medical men. In the fifteenth century special buildings were constructed for this purpose and public dissections usually lasted for three or four days. The cadaver was either placed on a table or fixed upright to a wooden cross.

Generally speaking, the contributions of France, England and Germany to anatomy were small and not comparable to those of Italy. The Italian dissectors were greatly stimulated by the painters and sculptors who exhibited a keen interest in human anatomy.[9]

Before and after each special dissection religious ceremonies in many places were considered necessary. In order that those who came into contact with the corpse might not become "disreputable," the corpse was first made "reputable," the professor beginning the proceedings by reading a decree to that effect from the lord of the land or the magistracy and then, by order of the Senate or the medical faculty, stamping upon its breast the seal of the university. In the second half of the century public anatomical theaters were established. Paris and Montpellier got one in 1551. Such a theater was built by Fabricius ab Aquapendente in Padua (the most popular and famous medical institution of the sixteenth century) at his own expense in 1549. Basel had an anatomical theater in 1588.

Among the able anatomists of this period was Jacques Dubois Sylvius (1478). Despite his fanatic adherence to Galenism, he made contributions to anatomy. The names jugular, subclavian, renal, popliteal and other blood vessels were given by Sylvius. He also named many muscles. The sylvian aquaduct is first mentioned in his book "Isagogue" (Venice, 1536), and the sylvian fissure is well known.

The greatest credit for the development of anatomy was due to the Renaissance artists and sculptors, for their efforts toward perfect representation of the human body. The first great anatomist whose work was illustrated with figures drawn accurately, in all details, was Vesalius.

ANDREAS VESALIUS (1514-1564)

While there was undoubtedly a great passion among the Italians for the independence of science, there were few who dared to question the veracity of Galen's anatomy. Michael Angelo Biondo (Blondus, 1497-1565), a prominent surgeon of his day declared "It is more honorable to err with Galen than to be right with others." "Beyond Galen thou shalt not go" was the motto.

At the medical schools of Paris and Lorraine anatomy was taught by two ardent Galenists, Gunther von Andernach a learned humanist of whom Vesalius said he never used a knife except at the table, and the other Jacques Dubois Sylvius, the head of the University of Paris faculty.

The first anatomist who had the courage to maintain that Galen's anatomical conclusions were based on the study of animals and not on the dissection of human cadavers was Andreas Vesalius. His has been the task of writing the first real anatomical textbook based on direct observation of the human cadaver.

He disagreed with his immediate predecessors, Mondino and Berengario da Carpi, whose knowledge of anatomy had been limited by acknowledging the supreme authority of Galen and his Arabian commentators. Vesalius acknowledges no authority beyond what his eyes could see and his mind perceive. Galen he said "was cheated by his monkeys in the manifold divergence of the human body from that of monkeys. He hardly noticed anything different except in the fingers and the bend at the knee."

At the age of 25, Vesalius occupied the position of anatomy at Padua where, for three centuries the Pergamene had the last word on the subject. Padua now became the center of anatomic studies; students from all over Europe flocked to that university.

It is not know how he succeeded in gaining the confidence of the senate for he had no difficulty in receiving permission to get bodies needed for his lectures.

Vesalius was appointed professor of surgery in Padua on condition that he lecture on anatomy and perform surgical operations. In those days the professor of anatomy occupied also the chair of surgery. He lectured on tumors and fractures. More than 500 students, physicians and distinguished laymen crowded his lectures which began in 1537. The dissection course lasted sometimes three weeks, including morning and evening sessions. When there was not a sufficient number of cadavers at his disposal, he dissected dogs and monkeys.

Vesalius was aided in his investigations by the liberal Venetian republic which showed the greatest measure of freedom to teachers. Students were admitted to the school of Padua regardless of religion, race, or nationality.

His method of teaching was to summarize the opinions of others especially Galen and then proceed to dissection without reference to the text. He once drew a plan of the veins which proved to be so pleasing to all the physicians and students that they urged him to supply a description of the arteries and the nerves.

Vesalius' career is the most romantic in the annals of medicine. After five years experience in Padua, in the year 1538, he published his *Tabulae Anatomicae Sex* and five years after (1543) appeared his monumental work *De Humani Corporis Fabrica Libri Septem*, works which marked an epoch in breaking with the past and overthrowing Galenic tradition. The last work with the engravings of Stephan Calcar was published at Basel about the same time as his *Epitome*. This publication raised a tempest among the timid members of the profession; even Sylvius, his master, turned against him with coarse abuse, while his own pupil, Realdus Columbus, cast discredit and derision at him. A controversy also arose with the publication of the *Fabrica*. The first attack came from Paris and from his own teacher, Jacques Dubois Sylvius (1478-1555), who called upon his pupil to renounce his heretical utterances and to confess his mistakes and his sin in departing from the footsteps of Galen. But when Vesalius replied that he had nothing to retract, and that he insisted upon the truth of his statements, the attack of his old teacher Sylvius became acrimonious and personal, who declared he was not "Vesalius" but *Vaesanus*: a madman and a two-legged ass. He eventually went so far as to ask Charles V, at whose court Vesalius was appointed physician, that "Vesalius be punished and in every way restrained lest, by his pestilent breath, he poison all of Europe."

Vesalius had the support of most of his pupils who admired him as a scholar and teacher. Vesalius complained that while his enemies attacked him, many of his critics in France, Germany, Spain and England tried to copy his work under their own name and in a changed form.

In three years he had revolutionized the methods then in vogue. He had accomplished the change not in an abrupt manner but in an orderly way. He rectified errors and added much to the stock of anatomical knowledge possessed by his contemporaries. His great and engaging personality made dissection not only possible but also respectable.[10]

Vesalius soon recognized that the system of teaching anatomy was wrong; "The detestable procedure now in vogue is that one man has to carry out the dissection of the human body while another gives a description of the parts. The lecturers are perched up aloft in a pulpit like jackdaws and with a notable air of disdain. They drone out information about facts they never approached at first hand but which they merely commit to memory from the books of others or of which they have descriptions before their eyes; the dissectors are so ignorant that they are unable to explain the dissections to the onlookers and botch what ought to be exhibited in accordance with the instruction of the physician who never applies his hand to the dissection and steers the ship of the manual, as the saying goes. Thus, everything is wrongly taught, days are wasted in absurd questions and in confusion; less is offered to the student than a butcher in his stall could teach the doctor."

At last he was persecuted by the authorities who checked his future scientific activities. In a fit of indignation, he burned his manuscripts, left Padua and accepted the post of court physician to Emperor Charles V.

Vesalius was scarcely twenty-nine years of age when he completed his monumental *Tabulae Anatomicae*. He himself supervised the engravings which were made directly from the cadavers. In his "Tabulae Anatomicae" Vesalius gives an accurate description of the *venaazycos* and the *ductus venosis*. He points out Galen's error of the existence of pores in the septum of the heart ventricles. "I do not see how a small amount of blood could pass from the right ventricle to the left through the septum." He described the sphenoid bone, the division of the sternum and sacrum, the structure of the pylorus, the omentum, the mediastinum, the pleura and particularly the brain. He points out errors in Galen's description of the liver, bile-ducts and uterus. In other words, Vesalius introduced a new and rational conception of human anatomy no longer hampered by tradition and religious fancies.

The *Tabulae Anatomicae Sex* (six anatomical plates) closes with a chapter on vivisection, where he takes issue with Galen who is of the opinion that when the thorax is open, life is impossible. Vesalius shows that artificial respiration may prolong life for an indefinite time.

To be sure some of his anatomic teachings needed revision, as for example: "The crystaline lens is situated in the center of the eye." That there are seven ocular muscles and that the vena cava originated from the liver, etc. But generally speaking it is the greatest anatomic work ever written.

Andreas Vesalius was born at Brussels where his father immigrated from Wessel on the Rhine. He hailed from a family of physicians. His father was a pharmacist, who was somehow connected with Charles V. Young Andreas received his early education in Louvain and Montpellier. From Montpellier he went to the University of Paris where he studied under Guido Guidi (d. 1569) and Sylvius; the latter a strong follower of Galen. His fame as anatomist spread while he was a student at Paris. He received a call from the University of Padua as instructor of anatomy.

In the nine years (1537-1546) he taught at Padua, he manifested a great gift for originality and independence in the field of anatomy. Indeed, Harvey's discovery of circulation might have been impossible if it had not been for Vesalius' correct anatomical descriptions of the circulatory apparatus.

Vesalius left Padua abruptly out of fear for the authorities of the church who disapproved of his outspokenness. That he acted wisely by leaving Padua is shown by the fate suffered by another anatomist for being outspoken. His younger contemporary, Michael Servetus (1509-1553) of Villanova, Spain, was burned at the stake by the order of John Calvin for similar offenses against church dogmas. He was disgusted with the controversy over his work and particularly hurt by the hostility of his teachers. In 1544 when only thirty years of age he decided to resign his professorship. He burned his medical books and some of his unpublished manuscripts.

With the resigning of his position of the University of Padua, his interest in anatomy had come to an end. He received the appointment of court physician to Charles V and in 1556 when the monarch died he was continued in the same position by Phillip II at Madrid, where he married and for some years he lived a quiet life.

In 1563 Vesalius started out on a pilgrimage to the Holy Land, perhaps as a pretext for getting away from his tiresome surroundings, or as others would have it, he went to the Holy Land as a penance for an accidental human venesection. Be this as it may, he never returned to Europe, for on his way back (1564) to Padua, where he was invited to reoccupy his old chair of anatomy which was vacated by the death of Fallopius, he contracted an obscure malady and died on the island of Zante.[11]

The fabric of the human body of "Fabrica" which was written in Latin in 1543 and was never translated, once and for all disposed of the belief that the Galenic anatomic doctrine was infallible. There he laid the foundation of the entire gross human anatomy.

The *Tabulae Anatomicae Sex* is not only of interest to the student of anatomy but also to the Semitic philologist: the author has included a Hebrew anatomic terminology in his "Tabulae Anatomicae" taken first from the Hebrew Bible where the names of such organs are found; next from the Mishna and he also employed the nomenclature used by the Hebrew translator of the "Canon" of Avicenna.

It is known that the Hebrew terms of both works of Vesalius (the *Tabulae Anatomicae* published in 1538, and his great anatomic work *De Humani Corporis Fabrica Libri Septem* commonly known as *Fabrica,* published in 1543) were prepared with the assistance of Hebrew friends of the great anatomist. The Hebrew terms in the *Fabrica* were the work of Lazarus de Frigeis and those in the "Tabulae" of another friend whose name is not given. Lazarus adopted to a large extent the names of the bones found in the printed Hebrew translation of the "Canon" by Israel ben Joseph.

The "Hebrew friend," responsible for the scientific terms of the bones in "Tabulae Anatomicae" followed different sources. His vocabulary is very different from that of Lazarus in the *Fabrica*; it contains several non-technical Arabic words, probably "of the current medical jargon of the Italian medical doctors of the time."

"The Semitic words quoted by Vesalius in the *Tabulae Anatomicae* are representative of contemporary oral usage of obscure sources: Arabic, Hebrew, and Romance." The Hebrew anatomical terms reveal the peculiar character of medieval Hebrew, consisting frequently of idioms used by people who spoke many languages, "yet there is always one generally recognized source of a purely scientific usage, namely the works of the classical writers of antiquity"; i.e., the Bible, Mishna (Oholoth 1.8), Talmud and later Hebrew writers, from whose sources the authors endeavored to trace the anatomic terms of the bones in the *Tabulae*.

Asaph Judaeus' anatomical terminology, which is tinctured with many Rabbinical words, appears to have been known to the translators of the "Canon" of Avicenna as it was to Donol in *Sefer ha-Yakar*. The translators of the "Canon," Nathan ha-Meathi, Zerahiah Graciano (13th century) and Joshua Lorci (14th century) used many talmudic terms in their works and there are indications that in the *Tabulae Anatomicae,* the friend of Vesalius drew on the Talmud for the names of teeth and bones.

The *Fabrica* published in June 1543, is a superb example of the typography of his friend Oporinus (Herbst) of Basel, sumptuously illustrated by Titian's pupil, Johan von Calcar. The splendid wood-cuts, representing majestic skeletons and flayed figures, dwarfing a background of landscape, set the fashion for over a century, and were copied or imitated by a long line of anatomic illustrators.[12]

Singer ranks the *Fabrica* (workings) of the human body as "The first great positive achievement of science itself in modern times." It ranks with another work that appeared in the same year; the treatise of Nicholas Copernicus "On the Revolution of the Celestial Spheres." The work of Copernicus removed the earth from the center of the universe. That of Vesalius revealed the real structure of man's body. But the work of Copernicus is one of close and subtle reasoning, still claiming many medieval elements and is hardly a great exposition of what we call "experimental method." The works of Vesalius far more nearly resemble a modern scientific monograph than does the treatise of Copernicus.[13]

MICHAEL SERVETUS (MIGUEL SERVETO, 1511-1553)

The anatomic seeds planted by Vesalius have struck root and brought about a rich harvest. From Vesalius descended a dynasty of important teachers who carried on the Vesalius tradition. Uninterrupted progress in anatomy continued despite the fact that the anatomic teaching of Galen still occupied an important place at the universities for some years after the death of Vesalius.

The most able anatomical successor after Vesalius was Servetus who went beyond the teaching of his predecessors with regard to the heart. He taught that the septum between the chambers was not perforated and he rejected the hypothesis that the blood passes through the septum of the heart which indicates that he had grasped the true features of pulmonary circulation namely the passage of the blood from the right side of the heart to the lungs and back to the left side of the heart. Servetus' only obscure point in his theory of lesser circulation (pulmonary circulation) is that the blood returning from the lungs to the heart to the pulmonary veins contains *pneuma* (air) and blood.

Michael Servetus distinguished himself from boyhood by his literary accomplishments. His early training was for the ministry but as medicine was the function of the church he became interested in the writings of Galen. In his book *Christianismi Restituto* where he gives his celebrated description of the lesser circulation (*Christianismi Restituto,* 1546, page 169), the following passage occurred:

"The vital spirit has its origin in the left ventricle of the heart, the lungs especially helping toward its perfection; it is a thin spirit, elaborated by the powers of heat, of a yellow (light) color, of a fiery potence so that it is, as it were, a vapor shining out of the blood, containing the substance of water, of air, and of fire. It is generated through the intermingling, which is effected in the lungs, of inspired air with the elaborated subtle blood communicated from the right ventricle to the left. That communication does not, however, as is generally believed, take place through the median wall (septum) of the heart; but by a single orifice, the subtle blood is driven by a long passage through the lungs. It is prepared by the lungs, is rendered yellow (light), and passes from the artery-like vein. In the vein-like artery it is mixed with the inspired air, and by the expiration is cleansed from its fumes. And so at length, a complete mixture, fit to become the vital spirit, is drawn in by the left ventricles through the diastole."

Michael Servetus was born in 1511 at Tudela in Navarre, his father being Hernando Villanueva, a notary of good family in Aragon. His surname is given by himself as *Serveto* in his early works. Later he Latinized it to "Servetus." Of his education we only know that his father sent him to study law at Toulouse, where he first became acquainted with the Bible (1528).

He was promoted in 1530 to be confessor to Charles V. At Bologna he witnessed the coronation of Charles in February 1530. The spectacle of the adoration of the pope at Bologna impressed him strongly in an anti-papal direction.

He attracted considerable attention by his first publication, *De Trinitatis erroribus* (1531, printed by John Setzer at Hagenau). It is a crude, but original and earnest work and shows a wide range of reading very remarkable in so young a man.

We next find him at Lyons (1535) editing scientific works for the Trechsel firm, adopting the *Villanovanus* surname, which he constantly used till the year of his death. He studied medicine under Johann Gunther, Jacques Dubois and Jean Fernel. In Paris (1536) Servetus succeeded Vesalius as assistant to Gunther, who extols his general culture and notes his skill in dissection. In June 1538 he writes from Louvain (where Servetus enrolled as a university student on the 14th day of December 1537 as

Michael Villanova) to his father and explains his removal from Paris, early in September, in consequence of the death (8th August) of his master, says he is studying theology and Hebrew, and proposes to return to Paris when peace is proclaimed. After this he practiced medicine for a short time at Avignon, for a longer period at Charlieu, where he contemplated marriage, but was deterred by a physical impediment. In September 1540 he entered for further study in the medical school at Montpellier.

Among those who attended his Paris lectures was Pierre Paulmier, since 1528 archbishop of Vienna. Paulmier now invited Servetus to Vienna as his confidential physician, where he earned a livelihood for twelve years (1541-1553) by his practice, and also renewed editorial work for the Lyons publishers, in which he constantly displayed his passion for original discovery in all departments. Outwardly he was a conforming Catholic; privately he pursued his theological speculations.

In 1536, Calvin met Servetus, in Paris and as he himself says proposed to set him right on theological points.

In 1546, he opened a correspondence with Calvin, forwarding the manuscript of a revision of his theological tracts and expressing a wish to visit Geneva. Calvin says he replied, *plus durement que ma coustume ne porte* (more severely than my custom calls for). Evidently Servetus had warning that if he went to Geneva it was at his own peril. Writing to Able (in or about 1547) he complains that Calvin would not return his manuscript. However, an edition of 1000 copies was secretly printed at Vienna by Balthasar Arnollet.

On the 26th of February, a secret letter wherein was published Servetus' denial of the tripersonality of the Godhead, the eternity of the Son, along with his anabaptism, was discovered which made him abhorrent to Catholics and Protestants alike. Calvin furnished samples of Servetus's handwriting, expressly to secure his Christocentric scheme of the universe. The inquisitor general at Lyons took up the case on the 12th of March; Servetus was interrogated on the 16th of March, arrested on the 4th of April, and examined on the two following days. His defence was that, in correspondence with Calvin, he had assumed that the offensive expression was only for purposes of discussion. At A. M. on the 7th of April he escaped from his prison, evidently by connivance. He took the road for Spain, but turned back in fear of arrest. His own account is that he never left France.

On Saturday the 12th of August he rode into Louyset, a village on the French side of Geneva. He walked into Geneva, where he attended afternoon service, was recognized at church and was immediately arrested. The process against him lasted from the 14th of August to the 26th of October, when sentence was passed and carried out next day at Chapel (Oct. 27th, 1553). Servetus' martyrdom for science was soon recognized by the civilized world.

In 1876 a statue of Servetus was erected by Don Pedro Gonsalez de Velasco in front of his Instituto Antropologico at Madrid; in 1903 an expiatory block was erected at Champel; in 1907 a statue was erected in Paris, another was prepared (1910) for erection at Vienna.[14]

REALDO COLOMBO OF CREMONA (c. 1516-1559)

The successor of Vesalius at Padua was his pupil, Realdo Colombo of Cremona, known as Columbus. The latter was a classmate of Fallopius but unlike his famous colleague (Columbus), was a bitter opponent of Vesalius.

Columbus claims that he had examined a thousand cadavers. Columbus is accused by some of his contemporaries with plagiarizing his facts from Servetus who was burned at the stake six years before. His book *De re Anatomica* was published in 1559. He used the title engraving for his book from his master's frontispiece, the "Fabrica." Harvey quoted Colombo without attributing to him his full importance.[15]

Columbus distinguished himself by rectifying and improving the anatomy of the mouth and by giving a correct description of the shapes and cavities of the heart, an account of the pulmonary arteries, the aorta and their valves and tracing the course of the blood from the right to the left side of the heart and for giving the first good account of the larynx. To him belongs the credit of stating that the arteria venosa carried blood, not air.

BARTOLOMEO EUSTACCHIUS (1524-1574)

Another critic of Vesalius was Bartolomeo Eustacchius famous for the discovery of the tube that bears his name. He discovered the thoracic duct, the suprarenal bodies and the abducens nerve. He also gave a correct description of the origin of the optic nerve, the cochlea, the pulmonary veins, the muscles of the throat and neck, the adrenal glands, the uterus and advanced the study of comparative anatomy and of the finer structure of the teeth. In spite of his being a Galenist in his teaching his original discoveries show that he was often an enthusiastic adherent of the new school. His *Tabulae Anatomicae* was published by Lancisi in 1714, long after his death. His plates are accurately executed and are the first medical illustrations on copper.

GABRIELLO FALLOPPIO (FALLOPIUS) (1523-1562)

The chief pupil of Vesalius was Fallopius, who carried on the work of the master. He was without doubt the most illustrious of the Italian anatomists of the sixteenth century. He was born at Modena where he became a canon of the cathedral. He studied medicine at Ferrara and after a European tour became teacher of anatomy in that city. He removed thence to Pisa (1548) where he occupied the position of superintendent of the new botanical garden. He died at Padua on the ninth of October, 1562, at the age of 40. His treatise *Observationes Anatomicae* appeared one year before he died (Venice, 1561).

A collection of his works under the title *Opera Genuina Omnia* appeared in Venice (1548) in Frankfort (1600) and again at Venice (1606). He was the most independent anatomist having the boldness to attack Galen even more than did his master Vesalius. Fallopius discovered and described the chorda tympany, the semi-circular canal, the sphenoid sinus, the stylo-mastoid canal, the ovaries, fallopian tubes, the circular fold of the small intestine known as the valves of Kerchring, the Poupart ligament and the glossopharyngeal nerves. He gave a correct account of the generative organs in men and women. He describes the clitoris and named the vagina and placenta, as well as the arteria profunda of the penis. He gave a splendid account of the ocular muscles and the lachrymal passages.[16] According to Daremberg, "Fallopius was a genius, while Vesalius was only a scientist." Some writers stress the importance of his discoveries and place him on an equal footing with Vesalius.[17] In his polemic with his master as to the course of the cerebral arteries, the impartial critics agreed with Fallopius that it arose from the sinus.[18] It is difficult to estimate the comparative greatness of this man. In any case he may be regarded as the shining light between Vesalius and Malpighi.

GEROLAMO FABRICIO DE ACQUAPENDENTE (1537-1619)

A pupil of Fallopius was the famous scholar and physician, Gerolamo Fabricio De Acquapendente. The last part of his name refers to the town of his birth. He, like his teacher Fallopius, strove to render anatomical knowledge more precise by repeated dissection. Fabricio was the teacher of Harvey at Padua and doubtlessly influenced the latter's interest as to the true function of the valves. He was equally a physiologist and a surgeon. He investigated the formation of the foetus, the structure of the esophagus, stomach and intestines and the peculiarities of the eye, ear, and larynx. His anatomic fame rests, however, on his discovery of the membrane of the folds which he named valves in the interior of the veins. Several of these folds had been observed before by Sylvius and Vesalius. Fabricio may be regarded as the last of that illustrious school of anatomic teachers of Italy. The discoveries which each made and the errors which their successive labors rectified tended to give anatomy the character of an accurate science and paved the way for physiological discoveries such as the circulation of blood. Though obscurely conjectured by Aristotle, Nemesius, Mondino and Berenger and partially taught by Servetus, Columbus, Andrea Caesalpinus and Fabricio, it was nevertheless reserved for William Harvey fully and satisfactorily to demonstrate.

JULIUS CAESAR ARANZIO (1530-1589)

One of the most distinguished anatomic researchers was Julius Caesar Aranzio anatomical professor for thirty-two years in the University of Bologna. Aranzio was the first to show that the muscles of the eye do not, as was falsely imagined, arise from the *dura mater* but from the margin of the optic hole. He also corroborated the views of Columbus regarding the course which the blood follows in passing from the right to the left side of the heart. Aranzio described distinctly the inferior cornua of the ventricles of the cerebrum, recognized the objects by which they are distinguished, and gave them the name by which they are still known (*hippocampus*); his account is more minute than that of the authors of the subsequent century. He speaks at large of the choroid plexus, and gives a particular description of the fourth ventricle, under the name of *cistern of the cerebellum,* as a discovery of his own.[19]

GIOVANNI FILIPPO INGRASSIAS (1510-1580)

Ingrassias was a learned osteologist who corrected many errors of Galen in his commentary on the Greek anatomist. He gave the first account of the sphenoid and ethmoid bones, and description of the third bone of the tympanum called *stapes* though this also was claimed by Eustacchius and Fallopius.

FELIX PLATTER (PLATERUS PLATTER 1536-1614)

Another distinguished anatomist was Felix Platter the son of Thomas Platter of Switzerland; he was a zealous and careful observer. He received his education at the University of Montpellier. After graduation he returned to his home city where he became professor of anatomy at the University of Basel for forty years and ordinary physician of the Margrave of Baden. Johann Chiari (1817-1854) credits him with having dissected more than three hundred bodies in a period of fifty years. He was among the early systematic nosologists, dividing diseases into three classes: (1) disturbance of function, which includes diseases of the mind, the senses and motion, (2) pains (Febrile diseases) and diseases of the fluids, (3) defects of formation and secretion. He reported cases of stones beneath the tongue, overgrowth, *Gigantism,* enlarged thymus, intestinal parasites, cystic liver and kidney. His *Praxis Medica* (1602-1608) gives a modern attempt to classify diseases.

AMATUS LUSITANIUS (1511-1561)

Amatus was a Portuguese physician who studied medicine in Salamanca and was driven by the Jewish persecution to Antwerp. He later became professor of medicine at Ferrara. He is chiefly known for his work *Curationun Medicinalium Centuria Septum* (Venice, 1563) which contains much valuable information on medicine, especially along the lines of symptomatology, diagnosis and treatment; Vesalius' observations on the location of entrance of the azygos vein into the vena cava and Vesalius' choice of the right arm for bleeding in pneumonia. Amatus describes the discovery of the valve at the orifice of the azygos vein. His interest is entirely centered on its bearing upon the controversy concerning phlebotomy.

Amatus writes as follows: "Wherefore it is evident that Vesalius' entire argument was wrong, for the azygos vein does not return the blood which it receives from the vena cava; on the contrary, it is so constructed at the orifice where it joins the vena cava, that there is a definite valve here, which holds back the blood (haurio) that flows in; then it is closed so that the blood which was received cannot freely pass and is released from the vena azygos in the same manner as in the case of the urinary bladder or in the orifices of the vessels of the heart. That this is a fact beyond doubt we have proved in the dissection of bodies. For if you place a tube in the upper part of the vena cava and blow downward, both the vena cava and the azygos will be inflated and will rise up, bulging. But if you blow air into the lower part of the azygos, the vena cava will not be inflated; it is not possible for the air to escape on account of the valve or operculum mentioned; whence it is clear that if air cannot pass out of the azygos into the vena cava it is all the more certain that blood, much thicker than air, cannot flow through. These doctrines have been made known by us and cannot be doubted for we have given the proof a thousand (!) times in the year 1547; in Ferrara we made dissections of twelve human bodies and of animals and in all it happened just as described before a large gathering of learned men, and on the same occasion Canano, the admirable anatomist likewise observed this." [20]

Here was a remarkable error made by Amatus in his interpretation of the function of the valve as holding back the flow of blood from the azygos vein into the vena cava; all the more astounding because the experimental method he applies was so appropriate!

CHAPTER XXXVI

THE RENAISSANCE OF PHYSIOLOGY

Anatomy is to physiology what geography is to history. It is impossible to obtain a knowledge of the bodily functions carried on by the organs without first knowing the structure of the organs, for the organs are the instruments which perform the functions.

The lack of physiological knowledge during the Middle Ages was not due to a lack of interest in the subject. On the contrary, ever since man became conscious of himself he has been eager to understand the secret of his own existence. What is the force within him that causes the movement of his limbs? What makes him think, will, love, hate, see and hear? What takes place in his system that subjects him to sickness and afflicts him with physical sufferings? Meager knowledge of physical structure and the consequent lack of rational explanation obliged man to localize in himself a spiritual entity or soul that governs the mechanism of his body.

The first attempt to explain man's vital phenomena on a natural basis was the doctrine of *pneuma* proposed by the followers of Hippocrates. This concept first found clear expression in the medical system of Galen, according to which the origin of all vital phenomena was a very fine aerial substance, the *pneuma*, which was supposed to be in the atmosphere. The *pneuma* was inhaled into the lungs and thence spread through the arteries to all parts of the body; whence the name "arteries" or air vessels. This doctrine, which was transferred to the Middle Ages together with the Galenic system, while not entirely natural or materialistic, was at least rational.

The translators of Galen into Arabic, Hebrew and Latin, however, rendered the word *pneuma* as the equivalent of the Latin *spiritus;* thus the concept of *pneuma* lost its original meaning. Galen intended to convey by the term *pneuma* the entrance into the body of a material substance from the air that had to be renewed constantly through respiration; and not a fixed entity blown into the body at the time of birth or conception. The *spiritus animalis* of the Middle Ages developed into a mystical power, a disembodied supernatural entity that controls all the phenomena of life.

The blood was assumed to remain stagnant in the veins, being transmitted at birth or conception from parents to progeny and inherent in the clan or race from the very origin of the racial stock. This concept has been the cause of blood feuds and wars among clans, tribes and nations and still remains the basis of strife between peoples of various nationalities. The racial theory revived by Hitler in Germany is reminiscent of the primitive and fantastic idea that the blood of a people is inherited from the very first progenitor of that people, or race, and that the blood of certain peoples contains higher spiritual powers than that of neighboring peoples. The conclusion was drawn that the blood of the mythological Roman heroes still flows in the veins of the modern Italians, and that the mythical blood of Wotan still circulates in the blood vessels of the twentieth century Nazis.

Expressions such as "racial blood," "tribal blood," "family blood," "royal blood," "cold blood," "hot blood," or "half" or "full blood," which convey the idea that there are different kinds of blood in the human race, originate in the ancient blood superstition. The expression "blue blood" was coined by the nobles of Castile (Spain), who claimed to be free from all admixture with the supposedly darker blood of the Moors and Jews.[1]

The discovery that the blood continually circulates throughout the body and keeps renewing itself all the time not only destroyed the very basis of all such antiquated concepts but revolutionized the science of physiology from its very foundations. It introduced a definite mechanical conception into discussions concerning the inner workings of the human economy.

The internal functions of the blood have been compared by physiologists with the external functions of the air and food supply. "It is absolutely essential to the life of every part of the body that it should be in such relation with a current of blood that matters can pass freely from the blood to it, and from it to the blood, by transudation through the walls of the vessels in which the blood is contained." Thus it was disclosed that the blood is literally the vehicle of life throughout the organism, and this function is discharged by means of its constant circulation from the left lower cavity of the heart through the arteries, arterioles and capillaries and thence back through the venues and veins to the right upper cavity of the heart. The nourishment of the blood itself is derived by absorption from the food which enters the intestines. The venous blood is changed into arterial blood by the absorption of oxygen through the lungs, the lesser or pulmonary circulation being maintained from the right lower cavity of the heart to its left upper cavity.

The pulmonary circulation was described by Servetus in 1546, and, probably independently by Realdus Columbus in 1559. Caesalpinus recognized that the flow of blood to the tissues takes place in the arteries and the arteries alone, and that the return of the blood from the tissues takes place in the veins and not via the arteries. Fabricius described the valves of the veins in 1574. His pupil, William Harvey, was the first to demonstrate the circulation of this blood. The essential feature of Harvey's new view was that the blood passing through the body was the same blood, coursing again and again through the body, passing from arteries to veins in the tissues, and from veins to arteries in the lungs and heart, all the time undergoing changes in the substance and pores of the tissues. Thus, the long-established doctrine of the *pneuma* or *spiritus* was discredited, and the modern science of physiology established.

The chief cause that retarded the progress of physiology prior to the anatomical advances of Andrea Vesalius and his school was the lack of knowledge of practical human anatomy. To attempt to learn the mechanisms of man without knowing the instruments by which they are performed is like trying to explain the cycle of diurnal revolution without knowing the springs, gears and wheels which set it in motion. As a matter of fact, prior to Vesalius and his school of anatomists even the rudiments of the mechanisms of the bodily organs were not understood.

The physiologist not only had to study the bones, muscles, ligaments, tendons, nerves and blood vessels, but he had to wait until the character and the function of the nervous system and the circulatory fluids had been explained. The advances made during the fifteenth and sixteenth centuries in chemistry and botany further stimulated an interest in physiology.

Servetus' line of reasoning remained dormant for nearly three-quarters of a century until William Harvey of Kent, England, revived it prior to any publication of Servetus' original work. Harvey's description of the circulation of the blood was both precise and complete except for the fact that Harvey did not see the capillary channels by which the blood passes from the arteries to the veins. This gap in the picture was elucidated thirty years later by Marcello Malpighi (1628-1694),[2] who described the capillary circulation four years after Harvey died. Until the capillary system was identified by Malpighi, it was thought that the arteries delivered the blood directly into the tissues and that the veins collected it directly from them.[3]

The monumental discovery of the circulation of the blood was soon supplemented by the discovery of the lacteals and lymphatic vessels.

The contributions of Malpighi to physiology, histology and embryology were numerous. With painstaking care, he focused his microscope on even the minutest parts of the animal system. Malpighi also investigated the structures and physiology of insects and plants. He demonstrated the basic histology of the skin, spleen and liver. Some of the bodily structures still bear his name. After Malpighi observed the capillary current in the lizard, his younger contemporary Anton van Loeuwenhoek (1632-1723) made similar observations on various larvae, frogs, eels, etc., with his improved microscope. Loeuwenhoek was able to study the red and white corpuscles more thoroughly than Malpighi had done and his microscope was a modification and improvement of that of Galileo.

SANTRIO SANTRO (1561-1635)

The most representative of the medical school of physiology was Santrio Santro of Carpodistria d'Istria, Professor at Padua. He was the first who attempted to give a physical explanation to all vital phenomena by means of weighing, measuring and calculating. He is, therefore, considered the leading representative of the iatro-physical school. The food put in the stomach was compared by this school to the fuel put in a furnace. The processes of digestion and absorption were compared to the burning of the fuel and the bodily heat that was generated was likened to the heat of the furnace. Such heat was necessary to the comfort and life of the occupants of the house. The combustion of the fuel and its transformation into the elements of water, gases and solids found its counterpart in the elimination of the food as urine, faeces and gases. This school also noted that the heat generated by the body is directly proportional to the amount of ingested food just as the amount of heat given off by a furnace depends on the quantity of fuel consumed.

Digestion was considered to be essentially a mechanical trituration, and the absorption of the chyle was explained as due to the pressure arising from the action of the intestinal movements upon the comminuted food. In a similar way the bodily secretions were referred to the resistance created by the corners, curves and angles of the vascular system, and to the difference or similarity of the specific weights of the secreting parts and the secreted materials. Respiration was presumed to be entirely dependent upon the mechanics of the motions of the thorax, warmth upon the friction of the blood-corpuscles, sensation upon the vibrations of the nerves, the action of the heart upon the mechanism of the cardiac pump, the circulation upon the laws of motion of fluids in tubes and locomotion upon the action of the muscle-tendon-bone levers. Health accordingly requires only the undisturbed performance of the physical and mechanical processes in the body.

The osseous system was considered to be the foundation of the animal machine; it supports all parts of the body. The muscular actions of the body were explained on the principle of two opposing forces: the "flexors" and "extensors." The power of a muscle grows in proportion to the resistance with which it meets. Since the extensor muscles are generally weaker than the flexors, the most natural position is the state of flexing.

Santro is the author of *Ars Statica Medicina* which was published in Venice in 1614. This work had a large circulation and stimulated others to employ experimental methods as a basis of their investigations.

Santro introduced an apparatus for comparing the rate of pulse beats. He contrived a bathing apparatus for bed-ridden invalids and devised many surgical instruments. He recorded the seasons of the years when diseases are most prevalent. He noted the climate, the bodily temperature (the time of the onset of the disease,) the urine, the faeces, etc. His investigations continued for thirty years.

He investigated the changes in the human body by weighing himself in a scale and proved it loses weight by mere exposure, which he attributed to imperceptible respiration.[4] By this experiment he laid the foundation of the modern study of metabolism.

The school of iatrophysics investigated the pulse by means of a kind of a pulsometer and the temperature by a modification of Galileo's thermometer. One of his most striking calculations is that the "insensible" sweat in twenty-four hours amounts to 1½ kilograms. This closely agrees with present calculations made with precision instruments.

The important role which perspiration plays in the human economy was also stressed by the iatro-chemists who sought to vindicate their exaggerated sweat cures. The iatro-chemists claimed that chemistry—not physics—is the basis of all physiological action.

GALILEO GALILEI (1564-1642)

Galileo, the founder of modern physics, was born at Pisa and died at Arcetri, near Florence. It is easy to recall Galileo's position in time, if we remember that he was born on the day of Michelangelo's death and that he died in the year of Newton's birth. In his early years he was attracted towards a religious life but his father, Vincenzo, who desired that young Galileo should apply himself to medicine, withdrew him from the care of the monks and matriculated him in the year 1581 at the medical school of the University of Pisa under the celebrated physician, anatomist and botanist, Andrea Cesalpino. There a brilliant career awaited him, not only in medicine but also in mathematics and mechanics, literature, eloquence, music and art. From 1592 to 1610 he held the chair of mathematics in the University of Padua. The remainder of his life was mostly spent in Florence.

While in popular estimation Galileo is ranked as a great astronomical discoverer, and rightly so, his chief service to science is the establishment of modern dynamics. To him we owe the statement that nature always behaves in the same way in the same circumstances. To him we owe also the idea which underlies the first two of Newton's laws of motion. He first enunciated the correct laws of falling bodies, showing that, if we neglect the resistance of the air, the path of a projectile must be an *ellipse*.

Galileo did not invent the telescope, as is often asserted; but he used this instrument with great skill to discover spots on the sun. He measured its rotation period, discovered four of the satellites of Jupiter, observed the phases of Mercury and Venus and found the elongated form of Saturn which Huygens later showed to be due to the planet's rings. But no astronomical service of Galileo can outrank that which he did in establishing the Copernican system by showing the mechanical principles upon which the solar system is constructed.

In 1616 he was warned by the Inquisition not to "hold, teach or defend" the Copernican system, and agreed to obey this advice. Nevertheless, in 1632, he published his "Dialogue concerning the Two Great Systems of the Universe."

Galileo was practically the first who laid the foundation of the science of mechanics as applying to the human body. His researches in that field had shown the way of looking at the objects of nature in a new light. From Galileo scientists learned to measure size, shape, quantity and motion, the "primary qualities," and express knowledge in that measured form.[5]

There was a third medical sect known as the Vitalists, who were of the opinion that a vital force (which is neither physical, nor chemical) is responsible for bodily functions. The members of the three sects attempted to explain all bodily activities on the basis of their favorite science only. For a time these sects actually retarded the progress of physiology, for it is impossible to explain all the phenomena of the human body by a single science. As a matter of fact, even the union of all these sciences cannot account for all bodily phenomena. Whereas the facts obtained from natural philosophy, chemistry, mechanics and geometry are applicable to the solution of many great problems of the vital economy, it cannot be too often repeated that he alone can hope to reach valid and comprehensive conclusions, who in the application of the laws of natural philosophy to living bodies, will take into account all the powers inherent in organized nature.

RENÉ DESCARTES (1596-1650)

The most distinguished disciple of Santro was the philosopher, René Descartes. His *De Homine* (1662) is the first modern textbook on physiology, although he laid his foundation on theoretical grounds. His attempts proved a sound beginning for the science of physiology. The stress he laid on the nervous system and its power of coordinating the various bodily activities, was the strongest point of his teaching.

Descartes' idea that all the activities of the organism are forms of motion that can be submitted to precise physical and mathematical examination, was the very basis of iatrophysical medicine. His observations on chemical phenomena that take place in the organism justify the veneration that the iatrochemical school had for the great French philosopher whom they considered as their master.

The tendency of Descartes' school was to explain the functions of the body on physical, and especially on mechanical principles. The movements of bones and muscles were referred to the theory of levers; the process of digestion was regarded as a process of trituration; nutrition and secretion were considered to be dependent upon the tension of the vessels, etc. The influence of his theories on practical medicine was not great for although he attracted many physicians among his students, most of them refrained from hastily applying his mechanical principles to their daily practice.

In the science of physics he included chemistry and biology, and reduced these branches to problems of mechanism. He believed that his mechanistic theories afforded an explanation of every phenomenon of organic life, especially in animals and man. The organism he regarded as a machine, constructed from the particles of the seed, which in obeying the laws of motion arranged themselves in the particular animal shape in which we see them. The finer particles of the blood, which become extremely rarified during circulation, pass off in two directions; one portion, and the less important in the theory, to the organs of generation, the other portion to the cavities of the brain. From the brain these are conveyed through the body by means of the water of a spring to act upon the mechanical appliances in an artificial fountain. The nerves conduct the animal spirits to act upon the muscles, and also convey the impressions of the organs of the brain.

The Aristotelian idea that man and animals alike possess vegetative and sensitive souls was ruthlessly swept away by Descartes; only one soul, the rational, remains, and that is restricted to man. Reason and thought, the essential qualities of the soul, do not belong to brutes; there is an impassable gulf between man and the lower animals. The only sure sign of reason is the power of language, i.e., of giving expression to general ideas; and language in that sense is found only in man. The cries of animals are touched in a certain way, the wheels and springs concealed in the interior perform their work; there is no consciousness or feeling. "They see as we do when our mind is distracted and keenly applied elsewhere; the images of outward objects paint themselves on the retina, and possibly even the impressions made in the optic nerves determine our limbs to different movements, but we feel nothing of it all, and move as if we were automata."

But while all the organic processes in man go on mechanically, and although by reflex action he may repel attack unconsciously, still the first affirmation of the system was that man was essentially a thinking being. Of course a unity of nature is impossible between mind and body so described. You cannot in the actual man cut soul and body asunder; they interpenetrate in every member. But there is one point in the human frame—a point midway in the brain, single and free, which may in a special sense be called the seat of the mind. This is the so-called cnarion, or pineal gland, where in a minimized point the mind on one hand and the vital spirits on the other meet and communicate. In that gland the mystery of creation is concentrated; thought meets extension and directs it; extension moves towards thought and is perceived. Two clear and distinct ideas, it seems, produce an absolute mystery.

Among Descartes' prominent pupils were Nicolaus Stensen (Steno, 1638-1686), William Cole (1635-1716), Lorenzo Bellini (1643-1704), Giorgio Baglivi (1669-1707), Archibald Pitcairne (1653-1713), a Scottish physician who was professor at Leiden, and perhaps the most distinguished of all, Giovanni Alfonso Borelli (1608-1679).

René Descartes was born at La Haye, in Touraine. Joachim Descartes, his father maintained a lofty rank in French society. He had three children, a son who afterwards succeeded his father in parliament, a daughter who married M. du Crevis, and René.

From 1604 to 1612 René studied at the school of La Fleche,

which Henry IV had lately founded and endowed for the Jesuits. René required exceptional privileges; his feeble health excused him from morning duties. At a tender age he began to distrust the authority of his teachers and tradition. At sixteen he went home to his father, who was now settled at Rennes, and had married again. Here he made the acquaintance of Claude Mydorge, one of the foremost mathematicians of France and Father Mersenne, of the order of Minim friars. The withdrawal of Mersenne in 1614 to a post in the provinces was the signal for Descartes to abandon social life and shut himself up for nearly two years in a secluded house on the Faubourg St. Germain.

French politics were at that time characterized by violence and intrigue to such an extent that Paris was no fit place for a student. Moreover, conditions in France offered but little attraction for honorable military service. Accordingly, in May 1617, Descartes set out for the Netherlands and took service in the army of Prince Maurice of Orange.

Descartes returned to Paris in June 1625, in the quarter where he sought seclusion before. By this time he had ceased to devote himself to pure mathematics, and, in the company with his friend Mersenne and Mydorge, was deeply interested in the theory of the refraction of light, and in the practical work of grinding glasses suitable for optical instruments. But all the while he was engaged with reflections on the nature of man, of the soul and of God.[6]

GIOVANNI ALFONSO BORELLI (1608-1679)

Stirred by the success of Galileo, Borelli (a pupil of Galileo and a teacher of Malpighi) like Santro and Descartes, gave mathematical expression to the workings of the human body, particularly to that branch of physiology that treats of muscular movements. He explained these movements on mechanical principles. Borelli estimated the power of a muscle by its weight. The flexor muscles, being stronger than the extensors of the same articulations must occasion a more extensive motion of the limbs and determine them towards a state of flexion.

Borelli applied the laws of mechanics to all physical phenomena. He regarded the human organism as a machine. The circulation, respiration and digestion are mechanical facts which function according to physical laws. He pointed out the importance of the intercostal muscles and the diaphragm in respiration. His neurogenic theory of the heartbeat attributes the heart action to the action of the nerve juice on the heart through its various nerves.

Borelli occupies a leading position in mechanistic physiology and his effect on the mechanical orientation of medicine is one to which modern medicine owes much. According to Borelli, the immediate instruments by means of which the soul brings about movement are muscles, which receive the motive force by way of the nerves. He distinguished muscles of various forms and structures. He maintained that one could correlate the individual action of muscle fibres and voluntary action.[7]

Borelli denied the old theory that fever originates in excessive action of the heart-muscle due to irritation of the latter by an acid nervous-fluid. "There is no such thing as corruption of the blood" . . . a stoppage of the organs of secretion is rather to be assumed. The periodicity of fever he explained by this last mentioned device. In his therapeutics, Borelli considered invisible perspiration most effective in combating fever. His pupil, Lorenzo Bellini (1643-1704), of Florence, who, at the early age of nineteen became a professor in Pisa and subsequently occupied a similar position in his native city, referred both fever and inflammation to a retarded motion of the blood occasioned by its thickening and by the friction of the blood corpuscles—a theory also promulgated by the Bolognese professor Giacomo de Sandris (about 1696).

Borelli was born at Naples on the 28th of January 1608. He was appointed professor of mathematics at Messina in 1649 and at Pisa in 1656. In 1667 he returned to Messina, but in 1674 was obliged to retire to Rome, where he lived under the protection of Christina, Queen of Sweden. He died on the 31st of December 1679. His best-known work is the aforementioned "De Motu Animalium" (Rome, 1680-1681) in which he sought to explain the movements of the animal body on mechanical principles. He ranks as a founder of the iatrophysical school.

Giorgio Baglivi (1669-1707) was a pupil of Malpighi, and a fellow student of Borelli. A man of universal education, he became professor at Rome. He divided diseases into those of the blood and those of the vital spirit. In theory he embraced the mechanical principles so fully that he compared the lungs to a pair of bellows, the heart and vessels to waterworks and their pipes, the teeth to scissors and the stomach to a flask; but in therapeutics he was a follower of Hippocrates.

Baglivi is the author of the maxims: "He who diagnoses well cures well." "Reasonable thought and observation are the chief roots of medicine; observation, however, is the thread by which the conclusions of the physician must be guided." "Very frequently the result does not correspond to the expectations of the physicians, although these were founded, indeed, upon reason and experience—because of numerous unexpected encounters with both external and internal conditions, environmental factors or the carelessness and faults of the patient and of the physician in prescribing and deciding those things required for the cure. Medicine is not a production of human reason, but a daughter of time, originating in long experience. The simple polish of academies or the visiting of libraries, wealth in books which continue unread, to shine in all the journals—all these do not contribute the least to the comfort of the sick."

Another contemporary of Borelli was Domenico Guglielmini (1655-1710) of Bologna, Professor at Padua. He assumed "fermentation of ethereal and saline particles" to be the cause of fever and he uses the laws of hydraulics and the diameter of the mouths of the vessels, in order to explain the processes which take place in the sound and the diseased body. He was half an iatro-chemist and half an iatro-mechanist.

Finally between the years 1598 and 1600, a young Englishman, William Harvey, pursuing his anatomical studies at Padua under Fabricius, learned from that anatomist the existence of the valves in the veins of the extremities, and undertook to ascertain the use of these valves by experimental inquiry. It is uncertain whether he derived from the writings of Caesalpinus the fact observed by that author of the tumescence of a vein below a ligature. He was aware of the lesser circulation as taught by Servetus and Columbus. Combining the facts already known, he, by a series of well-executed experiments, demonstrated clearly the existence, not only of the pulmonary, but also of the general circulation from the left side of the heart by the aorta and its subdivisions, to the veins and thence to the right side of the heart. This memorable truth was first announced in the year 1619.

WILLIAM HARVEY (1578-1657)

William Harvey was the eldest son of Thomas Harvey, a prosperous Kentish yeoman, and was born at Folkestone on the 1st of April 1578. After passing through the grammar school of Canterbury he became a pensioner of Caius College, Cambridge. At nineteen he took his B.A. degree and soon after he went to study at Padua under H. Fabricius and Julius Casserius. At the age of twenty-four Harvey became doctor of medicine. He settled in London and in 1609 obtained the post of physician at St. Bartholemew's hospital.

In 1616 he began his course of lectures, and first brought forward his views upon the movements of the heart and blood. In 1618 he was appointed physician extraordinary to James I, and on the next vacancy physician in ordinary to his successor. In 1628, the year of the publication of the *Exercitatio anatomica de motu cordis et sanguinis,* he was elected treasurer of the College of Physicians.

The work on which he had been chiefly engaged at Oxford, and indeed since the publication of his treatise on the circulation in 1628, was an investigation into the recondite but deeply interesting subject of generation. Charles I had been an enlightened patron of Harvey's studies, had put the royal deer parks at Windsor and Hampton Court at his disposal, and had watched his demonstration of the growth of the chick with no less interest than the movements of the living heart. Harvey had now collected a large number of observations. He had now reached his seventy-third year. His theory of the circulation which had been opposed and defended, was now generally accepted by the most eminent anatomists both in his own country and abroad. He was known and honored throughout Europe, and his own college (Caius) voted a statue in his honor (1652). In 1654 he was elected to the highest post in his profession, that of president of the college; but the following day he met the assembled fellows, and, declining the honor for himself on account of the infirmities of age, recommended the re-election of the late president Dr. Francis Prujean (1593-1666). He accepted, however, the office of consiliarius, which he again held in the two following years.

He had furnished the library with books, and filled the museum with "simples and rarities," as well as with specimens of instruments used in the surgical and obstetric branches of medicine. At last he determined to give to his beloved college his paternal estate at Burmarsh in Kent. His wife had died some years before, his brothers were wealthy men, and he was childless, so that he was defrauding no heir.

Harvey, like his contemporary and great successor Thomas Sydenham, was long afflicted with gout, but he preserved his activity of mind to an advanced age. In his eightieth year, on the 3rd of June 1657, he was attacked by paralysis, and though deprived of speech was able to send for his nephews and distribute his watch, ring, and other personal trinkets among them. He died the same evening, "the palsy giving him an easy passport," and was buried with great honor in his brother Eliab's vault at Hempstead in Essex. In 1883 the lead coffin containing his remains was enclosed in a marble sarcophagus and moved to the Harvey chapel within the church.[8]

The epoch-making discovery of Harvey seemed to have resulted in the overthrow of the Galenic tradition. This now came under the influence of Descartes and Locke who represented the materialistic element of the medical profession and of Leibnitz who was the master of the spiritual philosophies of medicine. John Locke (1632-1704) in early years was a student of physics and chemistry. He turned to medicine at the age of forty-two. Locke followed the school of reasoning of Descartes and founded the school of Empiricism in England where he was in controversy with Leibnitz. He discussed with Leibnitz the views on nature and medicine which each held. The philosophic differences are shown in the short exchange of ideas alleged to have passed between them in his chief book "Essay concerning human understanding" (1670).

CHAPTER XXXVII

THE NEW BIRTH OF PHARMACOLOGY

The revival of learning covered all branches of medical science and particularly pharmacology. It brought about a careful study of plants, minerals and metals, and their medical qualities and consequently it produced a notable advance in therapeutics—a subject that was badly deteriorated. The medical substances used in the treatment of disease by the Arabians had grown to be burdensome. They were too numerous and too difficult to compound, multitudes of drugs being used in one prescription.

Among the first in the sixteenth century to free pharmacology from the Arabian bonds was the Portuguese physician, Amatus Lusitanus (1511-1562). He reviewed the works of Dioscorides, removed all the useless clutter gathered by the Arabian commentators on the works of the "Father of Botany" and on materia medica, and added a large number of drugs which he himself had discovered. Amatus collected the result of his studies and made a careful study of the earlier works on botany and materia medica, from Dioscorides and Pliny to his own day, in his work, *In Dioscorides Anazarbei Dei Materia Medica* (Venice, 1553). His work *Herbarum Vivae Icones* (published by Brunfels, 1530-36) is particularly noted for its botanic illustrations. He pointed out many errors on the part of contemporary writers, among whom was the Italian pharmacologist, Mattioli, a recognized authority on Dioscorides. The criticism of Amatus on Mattioli occasioned quite a stir among students of botany and materia medica even exceeding that of the controversy caused by Brissot by his attack on the Hippocratic method of phlebotomy. This polemic contributed in no small measure to the revival of interest in pharmacology.

In the present case the attack was more one-sided. The rejoinder from Mattioli was bitter and rather on personal grounds. Mattioli refers to Amatus, his critic, as a calumniator. He devotes one hundred pages to attack Amatus. Mattioli calls Amatus "Amathus Lusitanus" (which in Greek signifies ignorant). He heaps upon him violent invective, abuse and calumny. He charges him with heresy and apostasy and calls him a Marano and a Jew. Here is a paragraph in his work which refers to Amatus:[1]

"I am satisfied if I have destroyed all your calumnies; if I have also vindicated myself in your judgement I shall be very happy. I, however, know that you are stubborn and remain so . . . you will receive the definite and just verdict for your peculiar ignorance; you have most perfidiously turned away from God the Eternal . . . you are not only a burden and an object of disgust to yourself alone but to all others. . . . Therefore, Amathus, desist from your calumnies and cease to be futile I beg you . . ." Amatus' references to Mattioli on the other hand were dignified and befitting a scholar. In the very dedication of his work Amatus refers to him as "a great scholar who has recently published Dioscorides in the Italian language, embellished with commentaries."

Mattioli also contradicted other famous botanists, viz. Fuchs, Manardus, Brassavola, Ruelius and Gesner. Haller said of Mattioli "His reputation would be much better had his spirit been less arrogant and less contemptuous of other deserving men."

In considering the intensity of Mattioli's polemics one must consider the temper of the period. The most striking example of unjustified attacks are those which Vesalius suffered after the publication of the *Fabrica*. The first came from his own university of Padua and his pupil Realdus Columbus, the second from his teacher, Sylvius, the distinguished professor of surgery at Paris, who wrote of Vesalius as "vasanus, the madman whose pestilential breath poisons Europe!" Nor were the enemies of Vesalius satisfied with such published calumny, but they "reached out to malign him to the Emperor and caused Vesalius in desperation to destroy a part of his unpublished manuscripts." At a time when such were the amenities of leading scholars, the outrage upon Amatus becomes easier to comprehend. The fury of Mattioli's outburst against Amatus should not take away from Amatus the value of his contribution to pharmacology.

PIETRO ANDREA MATTIOLI (1501-1577)

Mattioli of Siena was a student at Padua, Siena, Perugia, and Rome. At Trent he became the friend of Bishop Bernardus Clesius. Because of his efficient work in a severe epidemic at Goricia, his fame spread rapidly. He was among the first in Italy who sought to liberate pharmacology from Arabian traditions. His work may be regarded as an encyclopedia of Renaissance Pharmacology.

Mattioli's commentary on Dioscorides (Venice, 1554) may be regarded the best work on pharmacology of this period. He studied hundreds of plants, examined them, sorted them and described them. The illustrations of his work are the best that had been produced up to his time in Italy. His book on Dioscorides served as a textbook on the subject for two centuries. He died of the plague in Trent in 1577.

Germany produced five herbalists and pharmacologists during the Renaissance, Fuchs, Cordus, Gesner, Brunfels and Bocke. Of these Leonard Fuchs and Brunfels are the most important.

LEONARD FUCHS (1504-1566)

Fuchs is best known for his *De Historia Stirpium* (Basel 1542) where he gives a full glossary of technical terms used; it is the first document of its kind in general literature. The plant illustrations are of a high level seeking to express the individual character of each species. At the end of the book are the portraits of the three artists who contributed to the beauty of the work. His work passed through a number of editions. Fuchs was professor of philosophy and medicine at Tübingen for thirty-one years, and was the most violent opponent of the Arabians.

OTTO BRUNFELS (1465-1534)

Otto Brunfel's *Herbarium* was published in Strassburg in 1530. The book is known especially for its beautifully drawn pictures.

An outstanding work was the *Herbarium Vivae Icones* (Strassburg, 1530-36) which contains one hundred thirty-five original woodcuts of plants. It was a work that outweighed the popular Horti of the fifteenth century. The *Kreutter Buch* by Jerome Bocke (1498-1544) appeared in Strassburg (1539) and gives a fine and exact description of the plants.

VALERIUS CORDUS OF ERFURTH (CARDI, 1515-1544)

Another distinguished pharmacologist was Cordus. He described some five hundred new species of plants. His commentary on Dioscorides was published by Gesner, posthumously (Strassburg, 1561). Cordus was the discoverer of sulphuric ether (1540). He is also the pubilsher of the first adequate pharmacopoeia, the *Dispensatorium* (Nuremberg 1535). His pharmacopoeia was the model of similar works often published at cities such as Basel, Antwerp, Augsburg, and Cologne. In his short life, of twenty-nine years, he left a permanent mark on history.

CONRAD GESNER (1516-1565)

Gesner referred to above, was known as the "German Pliny" because of his attainments in botany, zoology, physiology, medicine and surgery. Gesner who was a conspicuous figure in the Renaissance period was the son of a poor Swiss furrier. He received his medical degree in Basel in 1541 and after practicing medicine in many European cities he was appointed professor of natural history in Zurich (1551). He was ennobled in 1545. He wrote a Latin, Greek, and Hebrew catalogue of all kinds of writers. He made gynecology into a special branch of medical science. The medical part of his writing was unfortunately never completed. Gesner's *Historia Plantarium* (Paris, 1541) is a handbook on botany which he describes in alphabetical order. He edited and published the works of Valerius Cordus in 1561. His faculty of remembering names was extraordinary. It was Cuvier who called him the German Pliny on account of his attainments in botany, zoology, bibliography and in general erudition. He is credited with the authorship of thirty-nine works.

The most interesting chapter in fifteenth century medical literature is furnished by the herbals which made their appearance in the fifteenth century. They were intended for the instruction of monks in the monasteries and began to be printed at the end of the fifteenth century not as scientific books but as popular works for the laity on the curative virtues of plants.

The earliest printed herbal was that of Pseudo-Apuleius of the fifth century, in Rome by J. P. Lignanime in 1489.

Peter Schoeffer, Gutenberg's pupil, published the first of the herbal series which was reprinted in Germany, France, Holland and Italy in the fifteenth century. Those herbals were frequently reprinted. The Herbal of Apuleius was beautifully illustrated.

The herbals are valuable documents for the pictures they give for the medicines of the time, and for valuable observations. These herbals not only describe medical plants but also medical stones. They also mention the examination of urine and constitute veritable encyclopedias of medicine.

Among the first pharmacopoeias in Germany was that of Nurmberg, published by Valerius Cordus in 1535 (or 1546); the pharmacopoeia of Cologne, 1565; that of Bonn, 1475; and the pharmacopoeia of Bergamo, 1580.

Military pharmacy, too, made genuine progress in the sixteenth century. The sixteenth century, finally, may lay claim to a herbal with plates which made its way into Russia as early as 1534.

Visiting of bathing resorts, in accordance with the prescription of physicians (a proceeding customary as early as the fifteenth century), began to become more and more frequent in the sixteenth century.[2]

Of course the greatest contributor to materia medica of the Renaissance was Paracelsus. During his time pharmacy shops acquired the greatest importance and pharmacology was enlarged by a great number of mineral and metallic remedies. Paracelsus was the first to give mercury internally.

Although Paracelsus displayed insolence and vanity in the most extravagant degree, he rendered important services to pharmacology. He broke down the despotism of the schools and sects of his time, and introduced some valuable and powerful remedies. "His example and teachings excited the envy of some, the emulation of others, and the industry of all." He wandered from place to place, generally intoxicated, seldom changing his clothes, or even going to bed. But he taught fragments of truth which the world could not appreciate till the discoveries of four centuries later corroborated their merits.

The discovery of America speedily exercised its influence upon pharmacology. Among the newly introduced vegetable remedies should be mentioned the guaiac wood (1508) celebrated in verse by Ulrich von Hutten in 1517; China root (1525); sarsaparilla (1530). In the Augsburg pharmacopoeia nearly seven hundred herbs were specified.

During the Renaissance the universities developed botanical gardens on the campuses. One of the statutes of the medical faculties of Frankfurt on the Oder (1588) was that: "The Dean of the Medical Faculty, after having made a requisition upon the doctors specially and individually, shall twice each year summon the graduates and scholars together, in the spring, to visit the meadows, mountains and valleys, in order to acquire information of herbs and their properties. To these gatherings the apothecaries shall be invited. In the autumn the object of these excursions shall be to gain a knowledge of the roots of importance in medicine. The scholars shall provide the usual banquet." These botanical excursions, which existed also among the Arabians and were, indeed, adopted from them, terminated with great enjoyments.

The preparations of drugs were increased by essences, quintessences, specifics, tinctures, arcana, extracts, etc., enriched by the use of mineral waters. In comparison with the pharmacy of earlier times, the new pharmaceutical science was somewhat simplified; yet under the head of "simple" remedies (a name used at this period in contradistinction to the endless composite remedies) some very complex mixtures were still included. The pharmacopoeia of the year 1564 classified its remedies in the following order: From the vegetable kindom: such as leaves, flowers, fruits, juices, woods, and barks. Substances from the animal kingdom: fat, marrow, bones and hair. Substances from the mineral kingdom: such as mineral oil, bitumen, pitch and water containing mineral salts; from metals, stones, gems and earths. Substances from the kingdom of the sea: coral, salt, pearls, shellfish, etc.

Pharmacy shops acquired great importance in the Renaissance and evoked works of art as pharmacy jars. The celebrated potters of Italy fashioned jars especially for the pharmacies of the royalty and nobility.

In contrast to Germany, the French Parliament forbade the use of antimony as a medicine and the faculty of Paris not only prohibited the use of chemical remedies but would not even allow the mention of them in the examinations.

The addition of metallic substances in the pharmacopoeia caused much controversy and bitterness among the followers of Galen who opposed all metallic remedies. The controversy over antimony which arose at the close of the sixteenth century had exceeded in intensity the quarrel led against Brissot over phlebotomy, or that against Vesalius over his innovations on Galenic anatomy, or the fight of Mattioli against Amatus on the subject of botany and materia medica.

The antimony quarrel prompted the faculty of the Paris University which was against the use of antimony formally to place Theodore Turquet de Mayerne (1573-1655), the famous Swiss physician, and the leading exponent of bedside study of disease, and all those who favored its use, under a ban (1603). The ban reads—"All physicians who practice medicine anywhere are admonished to banish from themselves and their threshold the said Turquet and all similar monsters of mankind and monstrosities of opinion and to remain true to Galen." A certain physician by the name of Bresnier was banished from the faculty until he repented and swore not to use antimony in 1609. (This ban was not removed until 1660).

The use of antimony as a remedy at the outbreak of fevers was recommended by Basil Valentine (c. 1415) (the discoverer of antimony) and Johann Tollat Von Wochenberg (c. 1450), who under the pseudonym of "the Mystic," wrote a book entitled *Triumphal Chariot of Antimony*, recommending to physicians the use of this powerful emetic compound in fevers.

The name antimony according to tradition signifies anti-monk. It is related that an alchemist who happened to live in the vicinity of a monastery, had mixed this metal in the feed of his hogs and discovered that the hogs grew fat from the mixture. He suggested that the monks take antimony, "this being a metal there could be no objections to use even on fast days." The metal, however, had the opposite effect on them, for many of them died. In consequence thereof it was decided that antimony may be wholesome for hogs but it is injurious to monks and the metallic drug was named anti-monk or antimony in French.

Strange as it may seem there was no restriction on the use of mercury. Mercury was used as an inunction in the treatment of leprosy from the earliest times. The Arabs used such inunctions in treating infestations of lice: probably syphilitic manifestations. The so-called "saracenic ointment" contained 9% of mercury. Physicians used weaker doses of mercury but the quacks administered massive doses. Although the first results with mercury were often encouraging, soon stomatitis, debility and other signs of mercurial poisoning often set in. The patient was often literally smeared from head to foot with the semi-fluid mercurial mixture. Those entrusted with the application of the ointment were called "greasers of pox." After the application, the patient was taken to a sweat bath and given cooling drinks with a base of wild cherry. It is said that the baths were so hot that some patients frequently were found dead from the heat of the chamber.

In spite of all these innovations the apothecary shop still retained many nostrums such as for example the mumia, the unicorn and the bezoar stones. Mumia was probably the most monstrous remedy that ever entered the pharmacopoeia. Visitors to Egyptian relics at museums, who stand marveling at the workmanship of the bivalvular coffins of the Egyptian mummies and of the skill of the ancient embalmers and artisans, would hardly believe that the remains of the Egyptians, embalmed over thirty centuries ago, have been widely used as a remedy against miasma, insect bites, and other diseases. According to Johannes Wiedman (1440-1542), powdered mumia derived from dried mummies was one of the most valued remedies on the shelves of Austrian apothecary shops. Pomet, a medical writer of the seventeenth century, relates that the demand for mumia in his day was so great that it was impossible to supply it, and as a result, medical charlatans grew rich selling fake mumia. Medical textbooks as late as two centuries ago dwell upon the specific qualities of mumia in many diseases; they describe the scope of its efficacy and the methods of its administration. The use of mumia was possibly due to the fact that nothing was known of the contents of these bivalvular trunks. Perhaps the medical virtue in mumia, if there was any, was due to the fact that the Egyptian embalmers used, in the process of embalming, the water of the Dead Sea, which contains such chemicals as asphalt and bituminous substances.

Even Ambroise Pare, who greatly advanced operative technique and who invented many surgical instruments, showed strange credulity for a time with regard to mumia. He considered it an efficient remedy for internal use, in cases of pains, bruises, and sprains. Whatever objection he had to mumia was not because he questioned its effectiveness but because he doubted its genuineness. He thought that it was obtained from recently executed criminals whose bodies were stolen, dried in an oven, and covered with pitch. While in surgery Pare was thoroughly rational, in medicine he was empirical. He employed medical agents said to be of value and seldom questioned their efficacy. He frequently paid high prices for remedies claimed by others to possess medical virtues in order that he might use them for the benefit of the poor. He acquired in this way the poppy salve for which he claimed great merits in the treatment of wounds. The salve was compounded by mixing poppies, earthworms, and Venetian turpentine with the bodies of newborn whelps boiled in oil of lilies.[3]

The "superspecific" medical mystery of the unicorn horn was never solved. It continued to be widely acclaimed by healers as a most potent remedy in many internal diseases. This fabulous horn, to which medical virtue was attributed, was exhibited in churches in all parts of Europe. The most extraordinary beliefs were entertained with regard to the medicinal influence of the unicorn; the horn was regarded with invincible faith as a specific against all kinds of poisons.

The horn, mounted on gold, was brought out at banquet tables, to touch the dishes and vessels of wine, in order to assure their purity. A seventeenth century physician testified that "If this horn is mixed with angelica root, it makes a fine preparation to expel venom and to provoke sweat." Many a quack waxed rich by selling feigned unicorn horns for a fabulous price. Stags' and rhinoceros' horns were employed therapeutically as a substitute. Travelers in China report to this day that doctors of outlying districts prescribe ground-up horn of rhinoceros, either made in the form of a bolus the size of a walnut which cannot be swallowed unless thoroughly masticated, or in the form of an infusion or decoction administered in tremendous doses.

A specimen of unicorn in Dresden was valued at that time at 75,000 dollars and Venetian merchants in vain offered 30,000 sequins for a piece of unicorn in Germany.[4]

Ambroise Pare doubted the existence of such an animal as the unicorn whose horn was believed to be of great value as an antidote for all sorts of poisons. He thought that the remedy was counterfeited from the horns of domestic animals and that it was worthless.

His aversion to these remedies brought him in opposition with the entire Paris faculty against which Pare had to defend himself. He was bitterly attacked by M. Grangier, dean of the Paris Medical School. The latter argued that the value of the horn was obvious because the king had rejected an offer of 120,000 crowns for one at Saint Dennis.

Another medicament in which the physicians in Pare's time had great confidence was the bezoar stone. The bezoar stone was believed to be formed in the eye of a deer bitten by a snake. In reality it is but a calcareous mass partly mineral and partly organic found in the digestive tracts of herbivorous animals and was used as a general antitoxic agent. Avenzoar, the famous Arabic Jewish physician, called by his contemporaries "The wise and illustrious," was a great believer in the bezoar stone. He was first to write of its therapeutic value.[5] This stone was so highly thought of that it was incorporated in the first issues of the London Pharmacopoeia. There were two varieties, the oriental bezoar and the occidental bezoar. The former was given in doses of from four to sixteen grains; the latter in doses of sixteen to thirty grains. The bezoar stones were also carried in gold or silver cases as amulets. During the plague they were rented out by the day, much the same as radium is at the present time. An eastern nabob gave Queen Elizabeth a large bezoar stone which she highly treasured. Arabs sold spurious bezoars to Europeans for fabulous prices. In one instance it is known that a large bezoar stone was given in exchange for a feudal castle. Oliver Wendell Holmes (1800-1894) in his *Medical Essays*, relates that Governor John Winthrop sent to East India for a bezoar stone. Governor Endicott sent him one which he had obtained from a certain Mr. Humphrey, with the remark, "I hope it is genuine, for they cheat infamously in the matter of this concretion." King Charles IX possessed a valuable bezoar stone, one that he prized highly.

The bezoar stones lost much of their medical prestige when Pare found them to be of no value. Pare, who questioned the value of the stone medically suggested that they try the stone on a condemned criminal given poison. The King, eager to test the merits of the stone, was told that there was a poor cook who had stolen two silver plates from his master and who in accordance with the pitiless custom of the time, was to be hanged and strangled. The King told the provost that he wished to experiment with a stone which they said was good against all poisons, and to ask the cook if he would take a certain poison, and that they would at once give him an antidote; to which the cook willingly agreed, saying that he liked much better to die of poison in the prison than to be strangled in view of the people.

The prisoner was given the poison and the bezoar. He died seven hours later. The stone was returned to the King. He is said to have thrown it in the fire.[6]

It is apparent that Pare, like Vesalius and Paracelsus, used experimental methods to test the value of drugs. They were experimenting on the merits of many traditional medicaments that had no therapeutic value and which would never have been used if physicians had carried the spirit of independent observation to their practice.

The introduction of chemistry by Paracelsus and Von Helmont as a factor in pharmacy stimulated the Iatro-chemical school of medicine which played an important part in the seventeenth century in Holland and Germany. The founder of the school was Francois Sylvius (1614-1672), professor of medicine in Leiden, who studied the works of Van Helmont, founded the school of iatro-chemists and combined chemistry with medicine. He held that health depended on the fluids of the body, acid or alkaline which by union with each other produced a milder and neutral substance; a doctrine which was adopted in chemistry as well as in medicine. Sylvius' theory is of great historical importance as it is the first general theory of chemistry not based on the phenomena of flame, the fundamental ideas of which are still of use in science. It led Nicolas Lemery (1697) and P. J. Macquer (1718-1784) to distinguish clearly between acids and alkalies (or bases). The recognition of the opposite qualities in different bodies and their tendencies to unite sometimes with violence, suggested the idea of chemical attraction or affinity. The formation in this manner of neutral compounds led to the conclusion that every salt was formed by the union of an acid and a base. This foreshadowed the classification of chemical compounds in a series of types; a theory which proved stimulating in the organic chemistry of the nineteenth century.

As stated, Sylvius paid much attention to the study of salts and attained the idea of chemical affinity, an important contribution to the chemical advance of his day. He accepted the borderlines of the mechanical advance of biology such as circulation of the blood and the mechanics of muscular motion. He sought to interpret other activities in chemical terms. His popularity as a teacher gave his views wide currency. All forms of vital activity were expressed in terms of acid and alkali and fermentation. The latter process was assumed to be of a chemical order. His school added much to the knowledge of physiological processes. The discovery that the blood moves through the body in a circle, while it made an end to many of his concepts, revolutionized the science of physiology. It introduced mechanical force in human physiology, notably in the studies of gastric fluids such as saliva, gastric juice and the secretion of the pancreas.

CHAPTER XXXVIII

THE PROGRESS OF SURGERY

In the chapter dealing with medieval surgery it was noted that owing to the lack of interest in practical surgery on the part of the chirurgeons, and the consequent disrepute into which surgery had fallen in England, chirurgeons were prompted to associate themselves more and more with the "bachelor company" or barber surgeons who became very strong. The incorporation of the two companies into a union was recognized by an act of Parliament on July 12, 1512.[1] The barber surgeons thus were fighting their way up both professionally and socially. Toward the middle of the sixteenth century they were recognized officially by the city of London as important craftsmen deserving the protection of their rights to practice surgery in the city of London. Twelve years later (1567) by an act of Edward IV a charter of incorporation was granted them "to exercise the mystery of the art of surgery," pointing out a large field of minor surgery which they were permitted to do. Whether it was due to the rapid growth of the barber surgeons professionally or to a lack of energy on the part of the chirurgeons, the fact is that in the latter half of the fifteenth century the chirurgeons dropped their superiority complex of practicing surgery by proxy. They realized that a powerful competitor was gradually growing up in their midst.

In France the famous faculty of Paris had to procure an indulgence from the Holy Father in 1505 to practice surgery. They admitted barber surgeons into their midst, and instructed them in human anatomy in the French tongue and gave them the honorary title of "Tonsores Chirurgici" (Barber Surgeons) in return for which they were required to promise to employ no internal remedies and always to consult a fellow of the faculty.

It was not until towards the end of the sixteenth century that the barbers began to receive an education in the College of St. Come and the Hotel Dieu. A few, especially the powerful surgeons-in-ordinary, were possessed of large influence. Their pay, however, amounted annually to only 100 francs except that of the "First Royal Surgeon," who also treated the venereal diseases of their majesties.

Other reasons for the development of surgical art during the Renaissance were the advance of anatomy at a time when most anatomists occupied also the chairs of surgery and the continuous wars demanded the services of able surgeons in the army.

AMBROISE PARE (1517-1590)

One of the most prominent barber surgeons of France was Ambroise Pare who had obtained anatomical knowledge and adapted it to the use of the army.

Pare left for Paris early to learn the surgical art. He secured a position as a surgical orderly in the famous Hotel Dieu, the largest hospital in Paris, where he worked for three years. His earliest opportunities were in military surgery. It was during the Campaign in Northern Italy (1536-1545) during the reign of Francis I in Piedmont. Instead of treating gunshot wounds with hot oil, according to the practice of the day, he had the temerity to trust a simple bandage; and from that beginning he proceeded to many other developments of rational surgery. Surgeons had taught that wounds made by fire were poisoned. It was therefore necessary that they should be cauterized. This was done simply by holding the edges of the wound widely apart, and pouring into it a mixture of oil of elders, boiling hot. Each surgeon had hot irons, hot pitch, or hot oil for cauterizing severed bloodvessels, wedges of wood with which to keep the wound open, metal spoons for ladling the boiling oil or pitch and rough dressings.

Field surgeons did not realize that wounds would heal well if treated gently and dressed with some simple mixture, whatever the nature of that mixture.

In 1545, he published at Paris a treatise on the care of battle wounds. The same year he began to attend the lectures of Vesalius, the Paris teacher of anatomy, to whom he became prosector; and his next book was *"Breve Collection de l'administration Anatomique, etc."* (1550). His most memorable service was to get the use of the ligature for large arteries generally adopted, a method of controlling hemorrhage which made amputation on a large scale possible for the first time.

It should be remembered that no less a surgeon than Guy de Chauliac was against performing amputations, because of the hazardous bleeding. He asserted that it was better to let a limb drop by sphacellation than to amputate. He compressed the limb with pitch plasters to force its decay.

The method of stopping bleeding by ligation was not new. In the Middle Ages Roger and Roland and Johan Yperman used ligatures, and so did many lesser surgeons. But despite the fact that ligatures were known, surgeons were never enthusiastic about undertaking larger amputations. The results of amputation were uniformly disastrous, because the stump of the limb was always soaked in scalding oil or roasted with a red-hot iron or treated with styptics of rabbit's fur and aloes and the like.

Pare realized that it was these things which injured the flesh and set up a high fever in the patient, and not the operation itself which was at fault. He experimented with the forgotten ligatures, and, after tying the vessels at the point of amputation, he applied one of his simple dressings instead of rabbit's fur. Each advance that Pare made was in the direction of a rational simplicity and reasonable cleanliness.

Just as he had revived and popularized the use of the ligature and the "turning" of unborn children within their mothers' wombs, Pare also maintained that a deepseated abscess need not be opened every day; if it was opened once and a drainage tube inserted, it would remain open till all the pus was evacuated and healing began. His insistence on cleanliness was shown by the way he ordered new, or at least freshly-washed, bandages to cover the original dressing every day.

Patients whose limbs he had amputated he fitted with serviceable artificial ones, and for patients who were convalescent he ordered good food, good drink, and even music. Pare's innovation was far from being appreciated. He was even persecuted for his interfering with the rules of "regular medicine." He was compelled for his own safety to produce evidence from ancient authors to prove that they were not his innovations but those of the ancients.

Ambroise Pare, known as the "father of modern surgery" and the greatest surgeon of the Renaissance, was born about 1519 at Bourg-Hersent, near Laval in the province of Mann, France. His father was a barber and some of his relatives were physicians. His brother Jean was a barber surgeon at Vitre and his brother-in-law a master barber surgeon at Paris. His father was poor and was not able to give him any education, so he obtained for himself a position with a priest of the parish who needed a handyman to do odd jobs to cultivate his garden and groom his horses and in his leisure hours he was taught to read and write. Having received some elementary education he studied with his brother, Jean, and in 1532 he apprenticed himself for a period of three years to a barber surgeon, eager to acquire some additional knowledge in anatomy and surgery. He succeeded in obtaining a position as an orderly in the Hotel Dieu in Paris, then possibly the greatest hospital in the world. Realizing that the battlefield was the best surgical school, when he reached the age of nineteen, Pare enlisted as a regimental barber surgeon in the army at Piedmont during the campaign of Francis I and in the year 1536 he joined the forces of Marshal Monte-Jan as a regimental surgeon with the forces that crossed the Alps and laid siege to Turin. It was a new life for the young surgeon. He was, as he said, a novice not yet hardened to the cruelties of war. Here is a description of his experience:

"We thronged at the city and passed over the dead bodies and some that were not yet dead, hearing them cry under the feet of our horses, which made a great pity in my heart, and truly I repented that I had gone forth from Paris to see so pitiful a spectacle. Being in the city, I entered a stable, thinking to lodge my horse, where I found four dead soldiers and two others who were not yet dead propped against the wall, their faces wholly disfigured, and they neither saw, nor heard, nor spoke, and their clothes yet flamed with the gunpowder which had burnt them. Beholding them with pity, there came an old soldier who asked me if there was any means of curing them. I told him no. At once he approached them and cut their throats gently and without anger. Seeing the great cruelty, I said to him that he was an evil man. He answered me that he prayed God that when he should be in such a case, he might find some one who would do the same for him, to the end that he might not languish miserably." [2]

This was Pare's first taste of war. He watched next the retreat from Turin. The castle, Chateau de Villane, was attacked on the following day. A breach was made in the walls and all who manned them died to a man, but not before they had left Pare and his fellow-surgeons with more work than they could handle. Pare was inexperienced but he had been taught that wounds made by fire-arms were envenomed and poisoned by gunpowder. It was therefore necessary that they should be cauterized. Soldiers were brought to him by the men-at-arms and their wounds were lavishly and correctly treated with the boiling oil.

At last the oil was finished. He had to be satisfied with a simple mixture of yolk of eggs and oil of roses in turpentine, a substitute for boiling oils of elders. He was wondering what effect the poison from gunshot wounds which had not been cauterized by boiling oil would have on his patients. He had observed first the men who had had the benefit of boiling oil and found them, as usual, feverish and sleepless, tossing and turning, moaning from the pain in wounds which were swollen and reddened, and then he went to the "unfortunates" who were not healed by the burning oil to see how many remained alive. Most of them were asleep, but those who were awake were quiet and cheerful. They had no pain and their wounds were neither reddened, nor swollen, nor inflamed in any way. The inference was obvious, and from that moment onwards Pare discarded boiling oil and any other form of cautery in the treatment of gunshot wounds.[3]

Here was what Pare said of his experience in treating wounds: "Now I was at that time an untried soldier; I had not yet seen wounds made by gunshot at the first dressing. It is true that I had read in Jean di Vigo that wounds made by firearms were poisoned wounds, because of the powder, and for their cure he commands to cauterize them with oil of elder, scalding hot, in which should be mixed a little theriac; and in order not to err before using the oil, knowing that such a thing would bring great pain to the patient, I wished to know first, how the other surgeons did for the other dressing, which was to pour oil as hot as possible into the wounds, of whom I took courage to do as they did. At last my oil lacked and I was constrained to apply in its place a digestive made of the yolks of eggs, oil or roses, and turpentine. That night I could not sleep at my ease, fearing that by lack of cauterization I should find the wounded upon whom I had failed to put the oil dead or poisoned, which made me rise early to visit them, where beyond my hope I found those whom I had not put the oil feeling little pain, their wounds without inflammation or swelling, having rested fairly well throughout the night; the others, to whom I had applied the boiling oil, I found feverish, with great pain and swelling about their wounds. Then I resolved with myself never more to burn thus cruelly poor men wounded with gunshot."[4]

After the campaign was over, Pare returned to Paris and continued to study anatomy and surgery and in 1541 he was examined and passed the test for master barber-surgeon. Pare again returned to the army to practice military surgery from 1542-1545.

After he returned from the war his fame as surgeon spread all over France and he was appointed one of the twelve royal surgeons and was granted a fellowship at the College de St. Come against the opposition of the University professors who raised the objection against him that he did not understand Latin. He learned, however, enough Latin to translate into the French vernacular the *De Fabrica Humani Coporis* of Vesalius, thus making his master's work accessible and popular to those who did not know Latin. Vesalius and he had met in consultation at the death-bed of Henry II, who was mortally wounded while jousting with the Comte de Montgomery. He later became one of the leaders of the College.

Pare had been advanced to the position of surgeon to King Henry II, an office in which he was continued under Francis II (1544-1560) and later under Charles IX (1550). In 1573 appeared his *Deux Livres de Chirurgie* and in 1582 his *Discours de la Mumie des Venins de la licorne et de la Peste*.

As stated Pare quickly rose to fame in the army. His reputation was founded on his own courage, ability and common sense. The fees he was paid at different times speak eloquently enough of the services he rendered his patients and of the way they appreciated him. A cask of wine was his fee on one occasion, on another a diamond; a collection of half-crowns and crowns was presented to him by the soldiers of the French army; a nobleman gave him a horse and fifty double ducats; another diamond was from the finger of a duchess. The King himself gave Pare three hundred crowns, and promised that he would never let him want. According to Brantome and Sully, Pare was the only Protestant spared in the massacre of St. Bartholomew's Eve. The King made Pare stay in the royal apartment that night.[5]

Like Paracelsus, he wrote in the language of the people, but unlike the German medical iconoclast he was free from the encumbrance of mystical theories, which detracted from the merits of his fellow reformer in Germany.[6]

Here are some of Pare's maxims: "I dressed him and God healed him." "An approved remedy is much more valuable than one newly discovered." "He who becomes a surgeon for the sake of money, and not for the sake of knowledge, will accomplish nothing." "You will have to render an account not to the ancients, but to God for your humanity and skill."

Pare was responsible for many advances. He was the first surgeon habitually to employ trusses for support of ruptures. He introduced a form of massage, he linked up the symptom of pain in passing urine with the enlargement of the prostate gland which may cause it, and he was the first to suggest that syphilis might affect the walls of arteries and allow them to swell and dilate into aneurysms.

Pare invented numerous instruments including the feeding bottle for artificial nursing. He performed bronchotomy and employed ligatures in the treatment of fistula of the anus. He confined the use of the cautery for the treatment of cancer of the breast. He performed herniotomy in cases of strangulated hernia. He diagnosed fracture of the femur. He revived the operation of harelip repairing it with the figure-of-eight suture. He was the first surgeon to link up induration of the prostate gland with pain in urinating.

Pare introduced the implantation of teeth. The only dentist in Pare's time was the barber surgeon and his work consisted merely of pulling painful teeth. The extraction was performed with fierce looking instruments called pelicans or keys. The barber took a hold on the tooth as the plumber seizes a pipe with his wrench. In order to cover up missing teeth artificial teeth made of bone of ivory were made to fill in the empty place mostly for cosmetic purposes. Pare's method of implantation was to pull the aching tooth then insert into the wound of the jaw a sound tooth which was extracted from the mouth of some poor fellow who was willing to sell his tooth and insert it into the wound in the jaw. The tooth stuck in grew firmly into the bone and often lasted several years. He also revived the use of artificial eyes (of gold and silver) and introduced a method of staphyloplasty.

He died full of years and highly honored by his countrymen. His native town has erected a well merited monument in his honor.

GIOVANNI DE VIGO (1460-1525)

Among the well known surgeons in Italy was John of Vigo, of Genoa, author of *Practica Copiosa in Arte Chirurgica*, Rome (1514), a work that has passed through as many as four editions and was translated into English, French, Spanish, Italian and

German. His "Chirurgica" is divided into nine books. The first book describes the anatomy connected with surgical operations treated in his work. The other eight books are devoted to surgical operations and their treatment. Of particular interest is the direction how the large vessels were to be ligated, namely by inserting the needle beneath the vein and tightening the thread from above. It is the method described by Celsus but discontinued since. Vigo adhered to the Old Arabian doctrine: if disease is not curable by iron (knife) it is curable by fire. He favored the use of the cautery on wounds to counteract the poison which he believed gunshot wounds contained and he employed boiling oil in the treatment of wounds. He also believed in the use of plasters to promote healing of wounds. Vigo invented a number of surgical instruments. Vigo had a number of pupils, the most gifted one was Mariano Santo de Barletta.

MARIANO SANTO DE BARLETTA (1490-1550)

Barletta describes in his "De Lapide ex Vesica per Incisionem Extrabendo" Rome (1522), the "lateral incision" which gained the popularity of the French lithotomists. It is related that Germain Calot, a French physician, journeyed to Barletta to learn the method of Mariano Santo's secret operation for stones. Calot succeeded in winning the confidence of Mariano who permitted him to be present and even assist him in the operation. Returning to his native France with the secret, Calot experimented first on cadavers and then on patients with success. He then communicated the results to the medical faculty of Paris and to the court physician of Louis XI. He convinced the King that the operation must not be permitted to be performed by ignorant wandering stone cutters. With royal assent he operated on a prisoner sentenced to death, who suffered from a stone in the bladder. The man's sentence was commuted from death to lithotomy. The King himself and members of the court witnessed the operation which was successful. The prisoner was freed and Calot was acclaimed as a great lithotomist. Calot kept his method secret for several years and was called from one place to another to operate on distinguished patients who suffered from stones in the bladder. He refused the assistance of the local barber surgeon for fear he would learn his method. On one of his patients, Calot was assisted by Ambroise Pare.

THOMAS VICARY (d.1562)

The first surgical master of the English corporation of barber surgeons was Thomas Vicary, the royal chirurgeon. Thomas Vicary was also the first known surgeon of St. Bartholomew's Hospital. He was also the first to write a book on anatomy of the face *The Englishman's Treasure* or *The True Anatomy of Man's Body* (London 1548-1577), in which the author outlines the qualities with which "a surgeon should be imbued." "He should be learned, expert, ingenious and well mannered."

The anatomy of Vicary starts from the bones of the head to the lower extremities. Vicary died in 1562. He apparently was against Vesalius.

His successors in England were Thomas Gale (1507-1586), a contemporary of Pare, William Clowes (1575), and John Woodall (1526); the latter was surgeon general to the "East India Company," and William Herman of Salisbury, England (died in 1548), who according to Magnetus wrote an anatomy of the human body in two volumes.[7]

BARTOLOMEO MAGGI (1516-1552)

Pare's opposition to the use of hot oil and the cautery wounds inflicted by shotguns was seconded by Bartolomeo Maggi, professor of anatomy and surgery at Bologna and physician to Julius II. While Pare was investigating this problem on the battlefield, Maggi was approaching the subject experimentally. He fired from an old firearm (a harquebus) arrows tipped with wax. As the wax did not melt he concluded that the harquebus did not burn or envenom the tissue. He also tried the same experiment with sulphur and it did not ignite. The sulphur therefore could not have been too much heated.

He also suspended from a beam on the roof of his house a large bag full of gunpowder. Then he took up a harquebus, watched the friends and neighbors scuttling for cover, and fired a ball through the bulging bag. Nothing happened, and so Maggi dealt with John of Vigo's theory as Pare had done clinically on the battlefield. Even this did not convince many of the devotees of John of Vigo, and cudgels were taken up against him in England, by Thomas Gale and William Clowes.

THOMAS GALE (1507-1586)

Gale was a contemporary of Pare, becoming Master of the barber-surgeons (1561), two years after he published his *Certaine Works of Chirurgerie,* in four parts. The third part is entitled "An excellent treatise of wounds made with gunshot," in which is computed the gross errors of Jerome Brunshwig (1450-1533), John Wigo, Alfonse Ferri (born c. 1500) and others. . . . These three surgeons, as Gale would have it, were protagonists of the "envenomed" theory of gunshot wounds.

Gale was applying to wounds messy and complicated unguents and styptics and the like, which must have done more harm than good. He was not, however, as meddlesome as many of his contemporaries, for if a ball entered the body in such a way that there was a great difficulty in extracting it, he advised leaving it alone. He described the cases of eleven soldiers who had been shot in the body and whom he had treated in this wisely conservative manner and reported that "all did well."

The first part of his book contained "the sure grounds and principles of chirurgerie." He wrote bitterly of men who called themselves surgeons yet were "rude and unskillful . . . in an arte"; "and of carpenters, weavers, tinkers, cobblers, and women who were said to cure more patients than did the men engaged in surgery at the Royal Hospitals of St. Bartholomew and St.

Thomas." At these two hospitals Gale saw over three hundred patients, and estimated that at least one hundred and twenty of them would not recover without the loss of a limb or other gross deformity, if indeed they were fortunate enough to recover at all.

He laid down rules of conduct for surgeons. The surgeon was to be courteous and gentle and cause as little pain as possible; cure was to be effected as soon as might be, and treatment was never to be undertaken "for lucre or gayne's sake" only, though honest rewards could be rightly and properly claimed. The surgeon was never to promise a cure in cases of cancer or in cases of elephantiasis. The "sure grounds" on which surgery was to be based were that the student should be "lettered," "expert," "ingenious," "virtuous," and "well mannered."

This book includes the first mention of syphilis in English. It is referred to as the *morbus Gallicus* or the French pox. Thomas Gale did not help the education and character of the barber-surgeons. He waged polemics against quacks and pseudo-surgeons.[8]

WILLIAM CLOWES (1540-1604)

A junior contemporary of Thomas Gale was William Clowes, an experienced military surgeon and lecturer on surgery to barber apprentices. Clowes served for some period as physician to Queen Elizabeth and, according to Norman Moore, Clowes was the author of one of the best surgical treatises during the Elizabethan age. Of particular interest in his work *A proved Practice for All Young Chirurgians*[9] is the citation from Juan Almenar (a Spanish physician of the fifteenth century) as to the method of employing mercury in syphilis. In his treatise *De Morbo Gallico,* Clowes appears to have translated Almenar's treatment from Latin into English.

He was probably the greatest of the Elizabethan surgeons. Early in life he served in the Earl of Warwick's army at Le Havre, and later, as a naval surgeon he saw the defeat of the Armada. After long military and naval experience he was appointed surgeon on the staff of St. Bartholomew's Hospital. He came to the conclusion that an ordinary bullet could not possibly poison a wound, but on the other hand a bullet could be smeared with some poisonous liquid, and there was no reason why a poison introduced thus violently into someone's body should not prove as effective as if the poison had been swallowed. This conviction was supported by several eminent naval and military authorities.

Clowes appears to have had fairly good results, too, in the treatment of fractures. In cases of fracture of the thigh he would have two towels tied above and below the fracture so that his assistants by pulling upward and downward separated the fractured ends of the bone. He himself then manipulated the bones into correct position, and applied splints of willow and bandages soaked in egg-white and vinegar. Finally, the injured leg was laid in a bed of rushes. If, as sometimes happened in adults, the union was such that the affected leg was shorter than the uninjured one, then Clowes explained to the grumbling relatives that the results in adults were never quite as good as in children.[10]

Although his books bear a Latin name, Clowes wrote in the English vernacular of his period. In one of his works he quoted Sir Thomas Elyot in defence of "Vulgar Tongue." "The Greeks wrote in Greek, the Romans in Latin, and the great Arabians in Arabic, their own proper and maternal tongue. They had more charity than Christian physicians for they wrote in a language that could be understood." He wrote several works on syphilis. He expressed the belief that the "French disease" is equally prevailing in England as in the Latin countries. He ascribed syphilis to "licentious and beastly disorders of a great number of rogues and vagabonds, the filthy lives of many lewd and idle persons, men and women about the city of London." In St. Bartholomew's alone he had treated more than a thousand cases of syphilis in five years, chiefly by rubbing mercurial ointment on the skin.

In his essay on tuberculosis of the skin he showed himself to be a son of his period. He referred his patients for treatment by royal touch which was considered the best cure.

The revival of surgery may be said to have grown out of the change and method of carrying on war, which has always exercised great influence in promoting and retarding the course of civilization.

It is apparent that the few good surgeons were either in Italy or France and that they were self taught as a result of possessing extraordinary surgical ability.

In sixteenth century Germany, since the Pope had not yet issued an "indulgence" to practice the art, surgery was in a very low state. Generally speaking, in Germany surgery was in the hands of the itinerant herniotomists, eye cataract couchers, tooth pullers and bath house barbers whom Theophrastus von Hohenheim called "Arsch Kratzer." They carried their equipment in boxes from place to place proclaiming the kind of surgical work they were ready to do. There were a few Wundärzte also called Schneidärzte who studied in a school or trained under a master.

In Germany the high value of surgical practice was recognized by Paracelsus (1493-1541). His description of "hospital gangrene," for example, is perfectly true to nature; his numerous observations on syphilis are also sound and sensible. He was the first to point out the connection between cretinism of the offspring and goiter of the parents. He gives most prominence to the healing of wounds. His special surgical treatises are "Die kleine Chirurgie" (Minor Surgery) (1528) and "Die grosse Wundärznei" (Major Wound Treatment, 1536-1537); the latter being the best known of his works.

HANS VON GERSSDORFF (c. 1519)

A prominent German surgeon was Hans von Gerssdorff. His "Book of Treatment of Wounds" shows that he had performed from one to two hundred amputations, a greater number than were done by any of his contemporaries. To dull the pain of the operation, he administered opium and to check bleeding, he used the cautery. He covered the stump of the amputation with the bladder of a bull put on wet so that in drying it would contract and he applied an even pressure which would help to stop bleeding. Gerssdorff evidently had a good opinion of himself as a great surgeon. The legend which formed the illustration of his book reads:

> "To cure St. Anthony's fiery smart
> Removing arms has certain art
> Which is not in all men 'tis true
> So send your case to me to do.
> When I am stricken hip and thigh
> Or wounded grievously do lie
> I hope that God will bring to me
> Gerssdorff's artistic surgery." [11]

FELIX WURTZ (c. 1518-1574)

Another well known surgeon was Felix Wurtz of Zurich. His work "Practica der Wundartzney" is limited to the treatment of wounds, fractures and dislocations. He was a friend and admirer of Paracelsus whom he followed in the simple treatment of wounds and like the latter he wrote in the German vernacular which was characteristic of Paracelsus. His work shows that he was not interested in anatomy. He was among the first in Germany to combat the treatment of wounds by the cautery, ointments and plasters. He applied a clean dressing. His book went through thirty editions in the course of one century. It was first published in Basel in 1563.

FABRICIUS HILDANUS (1560-1624)

Perhaps the best known of the German surgeons of that period was Wilhelm Faby of Helden, near Düsseldorf, known as Fabricius Hildanus, referred to as the father of German surgery. He received his surgical training in Italy and France and practiced in Bern. His best known surgical work is the "Observationes Medico-Chirurgicae" (Basel, 1606). He is reported to be the first to advise amputation above the diseased part in case of gangrene.[12] He controlled hemorrhage with a tourniquet in amputation of the thigh. He, however, believed in the use of the cautery

CASPER STROMAYER

Casper Stromayer, author of the "Practica Copiosa" (1559) is another well known surgeon of Germany. His above mentioned work was hidden nearly four centuries in the municipal library of Lindau, Bodensee. The book revealed Stromayer's efforts to supplant market place charlatanism with practical therapeutics. It was edited by Walter von Brumm (Berlin, 1925) with its five colored drawings. The colored illustrations and the text offer an excellent survey of the state of surgery of his time. He emphasizes the importance of reliable instruments and demonstrates unusually high standards of technique and ethics.

CHAPTER XXXIX

THE ADVANCE OF OBSTETRICS

Great progress was also made in obstetrics. The old Roman law that stipulated that any woman dying in advance of pregnancy should be delivered of the fetus by Caesarian section, was endorsed. In 1608 the senate of Venice enforced the law that any medical practitioner who failed to perform the Caesarian operation on a pregnant woman who died, laid himself open to heavy punishment.

The practice of Caesarian section on the living mother was promoted, at least partially, during the Renaissance period when obstetrics became an independent profession.

The operation of "Caesarian section" nowadays is considered a usual surgical procedure, but in ancient and medieval times the operation was regarded with awe and was only resorted to upon the dead mother to save the child.[1] It was first mentioned by Numa Pompilius (700 B.C.,) who forbade the burial of a pregnant woman before the child was extracted from her uterus. (Incidentally this was one of the few operations permitted by the Church.)

The first caesarian section on a living woman was performed by a sow-gelder named Jacob Nufer of Siegershausen in Thurgau upon his own wife about the year 1500. After many midwives and lithotomists had tried in vain to relieve her, her husband received permission of the governor of Frauenfeld to operate. Nufer proved successful in his venture; both the mother and child survived and she lived to the age of 77 years, and after recovering from the operation, had several children including a pair of twins in a normal way.

According to Johann Weyer (Wierns) (1555-1588), a sow-gelder removed the ovaries of one of Nufer's daughters in consequence of her "lasciviousness". Thus it is seen that the most successful obstetricians and gynecologists were sow-gelders, even as the general surgeons were barbers.[2]

Caesarian section on living women seems in the course of the sixteenth century to have been practiced frequently in Italy. It was performed by Christof Bian (1540), in 1531 in Neusse and in 1559 by Paul Dirlewang on Marie of Vienna, and in France by Francois Rousset (about 1581) body physician of the Duke of Savoy. The latter in his writings describes various successful obstetrical operations. (Rousset planned his work carefully indicating the line of incision with ink and placing a cross mark on several points of guidance in attaining accurate approximation. He reports subsequent pregnancy without discomfort.)

In 1513 appeared Eucharius Rösslin's *Der Swangern Frawen und Hebammen Rosengarten*. This work is to all intents and purposes a survey of the works of the Greeks and Romans, which would have little value were it not for its twenty woodcuts and the fact that it is written in the German vernacular—a language used for the first time in obstetrics.

Rösslin was a German physician. His opus rendered in English *A Garden of Roses for Pregnant Women and Midwives* was the first printed work written for midwives. He first settled at Worms and afterward at Frankfort-on-Main. In 1493 he was an apothecary in Freiburg. In 1506 he was appointed physician to the city of Frankfort and two years later he entered the service of the Duchess of Brunswick and Luneberg to whom he dedicated his work.

According to G. Klein (1911) about one hundred editions of the *Rosengarten* are known to have been published. Rösslin's son issued a Latin translation. One Rosengarten edition was rendered into English by Jonas under the title of *The Berthey of Mankynde* (1520).

It was the first work dealing with the practice of obstetrics. It furnished for the first time printed figures of the birth chair, the lying chamber and the position of the fetus *in utero*. Some of the plates are of artistic merit. Rösslin took full advantage of the opportunity given him by the discovery of printing to publish his obstetrical work in German, so that it could be understood by midwives.

The history of Caesarean section may be said to extend over two periods, the first lasting from the earliest times in Alexandria, by Herophilus (335-280) and later by Soranus of Ephesus (c. 100 A.D.), to the beginning of the sixteenth century. During this period (as we have observed) the operation was occasionally tried after the death of the mother, in the hope of saving the child,[3] but it is improbable that it was practised upon the living woman. The second period extends from the year 1500 to 1876, when Eduardo Porro of Milan (1876) described his method of amputating the pregnant uterus.

Francois Rousset, a contemporary of Pare, wrote (as we have noted) a treatise upon the subject in 1581, in which he gave the histories of a number of Caesarean sections collected from various sources.[4] Several of them were probably apocryphal, while others, in all probability, were operations for advanced extra-uterine pregnancy. His article, however, had the merit of directing attention to the operation and the possibility of performing it upon the living woman. Pare, however, advised against this operation. The first authentic Caesarean section on a living woman by a doctor was probably done in 1610 by Dr. Jeremias Trautmann, of Wittenberg. His patient died three weeks after the operation. Following this, it was occasionally performed upon living women up to 1777, when it became temporarily eclipsed by sympheyseotomy, to be taken up again after the latter operation fell into disrepute.

In the operation of caesarean section the child is removed from the uterus through an incision in the abdominal and uterine walls. The origin of the term has given rise to a great deal of discussion. It has been generally asserted that Julius Caesar was brought into the world by this means and obtained his name from the manner in which he was delivered. This explanation, however, can hardly be correct, as his mother, Julia, lived many years after her son's birth; and, besides, Julius was not the first of his name, since there is mention of a priest named Caesar who lived several generations before. The following view, however, would at least appear to be more plausible. In the Roman law, as codified by Numa Pompilius, it was ordered that the operation should be performed upon women dying in the last few weeks of pregnancy. This "lex regia," as it was called at first, under the emperors, became converted into the "lex caesarea," and the procedure itself became known as the Caesarian operation.

Later Jeremias Trautmann of Wittenberg performed the operation of caesarian section on a woman who complained of a hernia of the gravid uterus which developed to be a living child, so it was necessary to do a laparotomy and opening of the uterus. The mother died twenty-five days after the operation, when the uterus had completely healed.

THE OBSTETRICAL FORCEPS

The obstetrical forceps was devised towards the later days of the Renaissance at the end of the 16th century by one of the Chamberlen family, who kept the instrument secret for three generations. It did not become known until the early part of the 18th century through a grandchild whose name was Hugh Chamberlen.

The forceps presents the following story: William Chamberlen who landed in South Hampton, England in 1569 fleeing from France as a Huguenot refugee had two sons, both were named Peter and both were students of medicine in London where they became successful practitioners devoting themselves to midwifery in which they became proficient. They gave instruction to midwives and claimed to be able to deliver patients when all other doctors failed. The younger Peter (died in 1626) was survived by several sons one of whom (born 1606) bore the name Hugh. He was well educated having studied in Cambridge, Heidelberg, and Padua. On his return to London he was elected a fellow of the Royal College of Physicians. He was most successful in his profession of midwifery and counted among his clients many of the Royal Family and nobility. He tried to monopolize the control of midwifery like his father and uncle but was hindered by the authorities.

The frequent attempt to take a hold on midwifery in London gave rise to a good deal of discussion among physicians. Many pamphlets were written questioning the morality of women who employ men. He left a large family and three of his sons Hugh, Paul and John, became physicians and paid special attention to obstetrics. The most important of his sons was Hugh (1630-1700), who possessed, like his father, certain ability and at the same time took a practical interest in politics. Some of his political views were not favorable and he was forced to leave England and while in Paris in 1673 attempted to sell the family secret to Francois Mauriceau (d. 1719) President of the College of St. Cerus for 10,000 livres claiming that by this means he could deliver the most difficult cases in a very short time. Mauriceau tried it on a rachitic dwarf whom he had been unable to deliver and Chamberlen after several strenuous efforts to deliver had to admit his inability to do so. Notwithstanding his failure he maintained friendly relations with Mauriceau so that upon his return to England he translated Mauriceau's book into English. In the preface he refers to forceps in the following words: "My father, brother, and myself (though no one else in Europe) I know have by God's blessing and our own industry obtained to a long-practiced way to deliver women in this case without prejudice to them or their infants." "I will now take leave to offer an apology for not publishing the secret I mentioned to extract children without hooks. . . . There being my father and two brothers living that practice this art I cannot esteem my own to dispose of nor publish it without injury to them and I think I have not been unserviceable to my own country although I do but inform them that the aforementioned three persons of our family and myself can serve them in these extremities with greater safety than others."

Some years later he went to Holland and sold his secret to

Roonhuysen (1663). Shortly afterwards the medico-pharmaceutical College of Amsterdam was given the sole privilege of licensing physicians to practice in Holland to each of whom, under pledge of secrecy was sold Chamberlen's invention for a large sum.

The practice continued for a number of years until Vischer and Van der Poll purchased the secret and made it public. Then it was found that the device consisted of only one blade of the forceps. Whether this was all that Chamberlen sold to Roonhuysen or whether the medico-pharmaceutical college had swindled the purchasers of the secret is not known.

The son of Hugh Chamberlen also named Hugh (1664-1725), was another successful practitioner and numbered among his clients the best in England. When he died, the Duke of Buckingham had a statue erected to him in Westminster Abbey. During the later years of his life he allowed the family secret to leak out.

In 1813 Kenbel, the housekeeper of a rich brewer who had purchased Dr. Peter Chamberlen's country house found in the garret a trunk containing numerous instruments and among them were four kinds of forceps.

Aveling, who has carefully investigated the matter believed that the three forceps were used by the three Peters and the not-so-good one was devised by the older Dr. William Peter. The forceps came into use in England during the life of Hugh Chamberlen. It was used by Mr. Drinkwater (1668-1728).

The secret mentioned by Dr. Chamberlen was the forceps now in use by the principal men in the profession. In 1747 and 1751 H. S. Levret (1703-1780) and Smellie (1697-1763) independently of each other added the pelvic curve and increased the length of the instrument. Levret's instrument was longer and possessed a more delicate curve. The instrument was used by Drinkwater, and was well known to Edmund Chapman and William Giffard (c. 1730). Chapman wrote in 1733 the secret mentioned by Dr. Chamberlen was the use of the forceps now well known by all the principal men of the profession both in town and country.

In breech presentation Pare recommended pedalic version or coming of the child so that it arrived head last as described before by Seronus of Ephesus. He stated that he had seen pedalic version practiced by Thiery de Hery (d. 1599) and Nicolo Lambert (1575) master barbers and surgeons in the town of Paris.

In Pare's *Generations of Man* we find illustrated the birth chair of Rösslin and Rueff. We find also in his writings, the recommendation of caesarean section on the living mother. It is through the practice of Pare that surgeons began to practice obstetrics and did not view its practice as undignified. Pare was a great obstetrician as well as a great surgeon, and was referred to by Smellie as "the famous restorer and improver of midwifery." Pare had the courage in case of severe bleeding from the womb during pregnancy to take the obvious course and stop the hemorrhage by artificially inducing labor.

William Harvey (1578-1657) of "circulation" fame later gave a stimulus to the study of obstetrics in England as Pare had done in France. William Harvey formulated in his work *De Generatione* the first scientific and original ideas on the subject of obstetrics to be published in England. He recommended the method of pedalic version suggested by Pare; version in difficult labor he stated was the only effective measure in the obstetric art. Harvey exhibits extensive personal experience in obstetrics. Much space is devoted in favor of careful watchfulness and patient assistance to the parturient woman. He warns against unnecessary interference.

Jacob Sylvius mentioned the operation of symphysiotomy theoretically. The employment of forceps, accouchement forcé and the artificial removal of the placenta are also innovations of the sixteenth century. Jacques Guillemeau opposes the removal of the placenta artificially but he recommends accouchement forcé in antepartum hemorrhage.[5]

The first known effort to extract the head by means of a vaginal speculum-shaped instrument was made in the sixteenth century by Pierre Franco (1560). He also removed the placenta artificially.[6]

SCIPIONE MERCURIO (1540-1616)

Another prominent physician was Scipione Mercurio who was born at Rome and studied medicine in Bologna and Padua. He traveled in France and Spain as physician to a German officer. After this he practiced medicine with great success in Padua and Milan. In Bologna he studied under Arantius whom he refers to as "the most learned anatomist of his kind, and my very kind preceptor." He states that this anatomist had performed many dissections of gravid women. He lived in Venice during the last fifteen years of his life.

Mercurio's work mentions pelvic contraction as an indication of Caesarean section. The author appears to have introduced the operation in Italy and published the first illustration of the operation in the position which Welcher described in 1889.[7] Bimanual version is also described by Mercurio, who furthermore provides an illustrated description of labor divided into three parts. The first deals with natural labor and the care of the woman and child. The second book takes up abnormal presentations and their mismanagement. The third section deals with various maladies which may occur in the parturient woman and the new born child. According to Fasender there were seventeen editions of this work published.

FRANCOIS MAURICEAU (1637-1709)

Since the time of Francois Mauriceau it has been believed that the uterus, when distended up to a certain point, must begin to contract and attempt to empty itself, just as happens in the case of any other hollow viscus. This presumption is supported by the frequency with which premature labor occurs in hydramnious or twin pregnancies. On the other hand, even an extreme distention does not necessarily give rise to labor, as is shown by the cases of prolonged pregnancy which are associated with large children.

Galen supposed that labor resulted from gradual dilatation of the cervix, which was brought about by the pressure of the presenting part, and the view has had numerous adherents ever since. That the condition of the cervix is not the sole factor is shown by the fact that in a certain number of instances, especially in twin pregnancies, considerable dilatation may exist for days or even weeks before the onset of labor.

As the mechanism of labor is essentially a process of accommodation between the foetus and the passage through which it must pass, it is apparent that obstetrics lacked a scientific foundation until the anatomy of the bony pelvis and of the soft parts connected with it was clearly understood.

We are indebted to Andreas Vesalius (1543) for the first accurate description of the pelvis. Prior to the publication of his observations, it had generally been believed that the child could not be effected until the pelvic cavity had become increased in size by the separation and gaping of the pelvic bones. Vesalius demonstrated the fallacy of this conception, and showed that the pelvis, for practical purposes, should be considered as an unyielding bony ring. His work was still further elaborated by his successor at the University of Padua, Realdus Columbus, who also demonstrated that each innominate bone was originally composed of three separate portions, the ilium, ischium, and pubis, which fused together just before the age of puberty. Julius Caesar Arantius, Professor of Anatomy in Bologna (1559), also made important contributions to the subject, and was the first to recognize the existence of contracted pelvis.

That the teachings of these three anatomists did not exert so great an influence as might have been expected, was largely due to the fact that no less an authority than Ambroise Pare still continued to adhere to the doctrine of the separation of the pubic bones during labor, and promulgated it in his obstetrical writings.

Inasmuch as Vesalius was the first to describe the normal pelvis correctly, it is clear that the conception of contracted pelvis could not have existed before his time. His pupil, J. C. Arantius

(1530-89), gave the first anatomical description of an abnormal pelvis.

During the next century knowledge of the subject advanced but slowly, and we find Mauriceau stating that in his very large experience he had observed only two instances of contracted pelvis. In one of these Chamberlen's forceps was applied, but failed to effect a delivery.

We consider a pelvis contracted when it is shortened to such an extent in one or more of its diameters as to affect materially the mechanism of labor, but without necessarily retarding the birth of the child. According to Litzmann (b. 1832) this is the case when the conjugata vera measures 9.5 centimeters or less in flat, and 10 centimeters or less in generally contracted pelvis.

MULTIPLE PREGNANCY

Vassalli has recorded the only credible instance of sextuplet pregnancy, but even his case has been subjected to considerable criticism. On the whole, it may be said that reports of the birth of more than six children at a single labor are to be regarded as apocryphal, although many such are to be found in the older literature, the most remarkable being the Rhine legend, according to which the Countess Hagenau was delivered of 365 embryos at a single labor—manifestly an hydatidiform mole. The Dionne quintuplets of whom all five were delivered alive in Canada are a famous exception.

CHAPTER XL

THE GROWTH OF OPHTHALMOLOGY

The advance made during the Renaissance Period in anatomy and surgery reflected in a great measure on the progress of ophthalmology. Andreas Vesalius himself made a number of discoveries some of which are that the color of the iris is derived from its pigmentation and is not due to a reflection from the aqueous humor as it was believed. He also made two other notes, one that when the crystalline lens is removed from the eye it acts as though a convex lens made of glass were removed, and the other that the aqueous humour is watery, not solid. He was in error however, in his belief that the crystalline lens is situated in the middle of the eye ball and that there is a retractor bulbi muscle in man as had been found in cattle in the time of Galen.

Fallopius (1532-1562) discovered the levator with the superior oblique muscles and its nerve. He also discovered the curvature of the cornea and stressed the difference in structure between the cornea and the schlera. He also gave a clearer view of the capsule of the lens and gave a description of the hyoline membrane. He differed from Vesalius in regarding the ciliary body as a membrane. He held it to be a ligament binding the lens to the choroid.

The location of the lens in the middle of the eye, however, did not tally with the optic measurement necessary to focus rays of light on the retina. This is supplied by Fabricius ab Aquapendente, student of Fallopius of Padua and teacher of Harvey. In his writings he presented a diagram indicating the correct position of the lens, posterior to the iris and not in the middle of the eye as accepted by tradition. Fabricius, however, did not realize the importance of his discovery.

The oculists before the sixteenth century were as a rule itinerant quacks and had no professional contact with the physician. Thanks to the careful observations of Leonardo da Vinci (1552-1619), and Franciscus Maurolycus (1494-1577), who demonstrated that the eyes work on the principle of an optical instrument, a new conception of the structure and function of the eye was obtained. Maurolycus was the first to disapprove the doctrine of Galen that the crystalline lens is the essential element of vision. He demonstrated that vision is accomplished by the retina and for the first time he explained the mechanism of far sight as due to a flat lens and near sight to the lens strongly curved.

FELIX PLATTER (1536-1614)

Felix Platter seconded the discovery of Maurolycus that the retina and not the crystalline lens was the receiving plate of the eye, but not until Johannes Kepler (1571-1630) demonstrated that the retina was the receiving plate and the cornea and lens are the refracting media was the significance of hyperopia and myopia and the rational use of glassses appreciated. He also denied the opinion of Leonardo da Vinci that the optic nerve is the receiver of the impressions of light.

AMBROISE PARE (1510-1590)

Pare, the greatest of the sixteenth century surgeons, was also interested in ophthalmology. He invented the speculum occuli. He recommended for strabismus the mask of Paul of Aegina and the use of horn spectacles with a hole on each disk. He mentions Trachoma (*aspiriduto*) without giving any details and he popularized the artificial glass eye which had been used for mummies but not for those who had lost an eye.

GIACOMO BERENGARIO DA CARPI (1470-1550)
(Berenger Berengarius)

Berengario described the conjunctiva and showed that the membrane is not a continuation of the cranial periosteum as had been believed since the time of Galen.

CHRISTOPHER SCHEINER (1575-1650)

The Jesuit Father Scheiner discovered that the pupil contracts during accommodation. This diminished the diffusion circles caused by the decreased size of the pupils and clarifies near vision. Scheiner was also responsible for measuring the indices of refraction of the components of the eye. He found that the refractive power of the aqueous humour is nearly the same as that of water and that of the crystalline lens resembles that of glasses and that the vitreous is between that of the aqueous and the lens. He measured the radius of curvature of the cornea by the simple expedient of placing glass spheres of known curvature alongside the cornea to find which sphere gave an image equal in size to that of the image of a window seen in the cornea. But apart from the accurate physical measurements that were being undertaken, the conception of the eye as an optical instrument precipitated the problem of accommodation. Obviously if the eye could register impressions of objects both near and far, it was a dynamic and not a static optical apparatus. Accommodation was thus recognized as a property of the healthy eye, and the problem of accommodation formulated by Kepler (1571-1630) was to baffle physiologists for well over two centuries.[1]

GEORGE BARTISCH (1535-1606)

The first who removed ophthalmology from the itinerant quacks and elevated it to the dignity of a medical specialty was George Bartisch of Königsbruk, near Dresden, Germany. He was a pupil of Meister Abraham Meyscheider. Bartisch like Pare, advanced himself from the position of unlettered barber surgeon to occupy the position of court oculist of the elector of Saxony. He was also an "ordinary" surgeon but he was independent in his practice. His *Augendienst* (Dresden, 1583), was widely read by physicians and students. He was among the first oculists to base his thesis on the science of anatomy, physiology and optics. His work contains a number of anatomical illustrations. He distinguished five different kinds of cataracts according to the color such as white, blue, gray, green and yellow. He describes the operations for pannus, ectropion, trichiasis symblepharon, fistula lachrymalis, ankyloblepharon, extirpatio bulli, tumors of the lids, ptosis, and for black cataract, etc. Diseases of the conjunctiva are well described. Trachoma is mentioned but not fully discussed. He limited the operation of enucliation to massive proptosis that render the eye hideous and could not be concealed. He insisted upon absolute technical dexterity.

Bartisch was a man of character inspired by a love of the medical profession and of humanity in general. He hated quacks and the like and was independent and rational in his practice. One is therefore surprised to find him in his books devoting chapters to sorcery and magic, and many astrological prescriptions for all diseases. However, as Baas remarks: "That this truly assiduous, upright and conscientious man should be free from the superstition and medical credulity of his time is not to be expected." Of great interest are the chapters dealing with the mouth, teeth, and skin and so forth as related to the eyes. He opposed wearing spectacles. "He could not conceive how an eye that does not already see well could see better with something in front of it."

He carefully specified the preparation for the operation on the part of both physician and patient. The operating room, he states, should be light, ventilated, and the bed well prepared. The physician should be well rested and avoid alcoholic drinks, and abstain entirely from conjugal duty with his wife for two days before the operation. He stressed also the use of proper instruments. The operation for cataract was that of depression through the sclerotic. The patient shall "fast" before the operation. He laid stress upon postoperative care.

It is to the credit of Franciscus Mauralycus (1494-1577), Leonardo da Vinci (1452-1519), Felix Platter (1536-1614), and Giovanni Battista della Porta (1538-1615), of Naples that the eyes were coming to be regarded as optic instruments.

GIOVANNI B. PORTA (1535-1615)

At the time when Maurolycus and Platter were advancing towards an understanding of the nature of vision, Porta threw much light upon the subject of the invention of the camera obscura (1590).[2]

According to his own story, when only fifteen years of age he observed that "if a small hole be made in the shutter of a window, all external objects will be visible, in their proper colors on the opposite wall," and further, "if a convex lens be fixed in the hole, the images in the focus of that lens will be rendered much more distinct; the images, however, becoming reversed." From his experiments with the camera, he became convinced that vision is performed by the "intermission of something into the eye and not by the visual rays proceeding from the eye." He made numerous observations concerning the reactions of the iris to light and darkness, and why weak sight is relieved by convex or concave glasses. He described, in 1590, the now well-known opera glass.[3]

Porta was the first botanist to group plants according to their geographic local (Phytognomonica, 1583). He was, however, a son of his period. He often went in for magic, and the academy he founded for this purpose was suppressed by Pope Paul III.

Popular books on the eye made their appearance in England in the sixteenth century. One is the *Brief Treatise Touching the Prevention of Injury to Eye Sight* partly in good order of diet and partly in the use of medicines. (Published anonymously in 1586, London?), by Walter Bayley of Portsham, professor of physics at Oxford and court physician to Queen Elizabeth. His knowledge of ophthalmology extended little beyond doubting the value of urine and wine for bathing the eye. He recommended ale to strengthen the sight. Another work by the same author was entitled *A Discourse of Three Kinds of Pepper in Common Use* (1588).

Of higher caliber was the work of Jacquesmeau *Maladies de L'Oeil* which was translated into English in 1586 and 1589. The sixteenth century closed with another English translation of Andreas Laurentius' *Discourse on the Preservation of Eye Sight*.

The sixteenth century saw the beginning of the use of concave glasses. Pope Leo X is depicted by Raphael holding concave lenses in hand. Thus at the end of the sixteenth century the principles of vision were fairly well understood. As Porta expressed himself: "Just as objects illuminated by the sun send their light through narrow holes in the window shutter upon a paper placed opposite, exactly so does light, passing through the hole of the pupil, produce an image upon the crystalline lens." There was no need of depending upon ambulant eye quacks as exemplified by Henry Blackbourn, one of the most famous itinerant mountebanks of the sixteenth century.

CHAPTER XLI

THEORIES AND STUDIES OF CONTAGION

While the Renaissance of surgery was primarily due to the unrelenting efforts of the barber surgeon the revival of medicine was accomplished by the independent spirits of the medical reformers. But the practice of the medical reformers did not blaze a new path of rational medicine. Their accomplishments were largely of a negative value, namely not to follow blindly Galen and the Arabian authorities. Astrology, demonology, uroscopy, herb-lore and numerous other types of quackery still played a prominent part in the medical systems.

There were some vague ideas that certain diseases are contracted from person to person and that it is safer to avoid the sick, especially during epidemics when many persons were suddenly stricken by the same illness in the same place. But there was no understanding as to the rationale of contagion.

PIETRO CURIALTI da TOSSIGNANO (c.1250)

At the close of the thirteenth century treatises on the cause of epidemic diseases appeared in Latin, Arabic and in Hebrew. The first distinguished writer who tried to explain the cause of contagion was Pietro Curialti da Tossignano or Petrus de Tossignano (near Imla, about 1250). His most important work entitled *Consilium pro Peste Evitante* which was dedicated to Giovanni Galeazzo Visconti, treats of the etiology of disease. The first part deals with astrologic causes of disease such as eclipses of the sun and moon, conjunction of planets, corrupt air, etc. The second part deals with regimen of a prophylactic nature. The third part describes disease and various preventives and the last part deals with therapeutic measures. But although Pietro discusses astrological causes of disease he recognized other methods of contagion such as contact with infected persons or places. Pietro states that he saw cases of infection by direct contact. Pietro appears to be more advanced than his contemporaries. He calls the home of plague-victims "contagious house" and warns doctors to be cautious when treating the impostums, since the discharge is highly infectious. He indicates clearly that the plague had entered Europe through the ports where ships arrived from the East and then spread from one country to another. He insists far more on preventive measures than on treatment. Pietro da Tossignano in a letter to Giovanni Galeazzo Visconi proposed a series of six remedies against the plague which were to be changed every day. He forbade marriage during the epidemic and advised strongly against political conversations. Pietro affirms that he saw cases of infection by direct contact. There was a widespread conviction that contagion could also be spread by cloth.

GIROLAMO FRACASTORIUS (1483-1553)

The first distinguished physician to advance a scientific understanding of contagion (syphilis) was the physicist, geologist, astronomer, poet and humanist, Fracastorius of Padua and Verona. His prose essay on *Contagion* (1546) is the first really comprehensive statement that syphilis may be transmitted by sexual contact. His earlier poem, *On the French Disease* (1530) which gave the name to the malady, was the most important contribution to our medical knowledge of this subject. The poem is divided into three books. The first deals with the origin of the disease which at that time he ascribes chiefly to atmospheric influences. The second with treatment, emphasizing the use of mercury. The third book discusses the new drug—guaiac—then coming into use. He links the discovery of guaiac with the story of the shepherd *Syphilus* from whose name Fracastorius was supposed to have derived his name Syphilis for the disease. This work remains one of the outstanding classics of Renaissance medicine.

The poem relates that the shepherd, Syphilus, who watched the flocks of King Alcithous, one day reproached Apollo for drying up the trees and ruining the springs in such a manner that his flock was dying because of want of shade and water. He swore that in the future he would sacrifice to his king and no longer to the sun. Apollo, enraged, thereupon loosed upon the land a shameful disease which attacked first of all Syphilus, and spread everywhere without sparing the king himself. "Syphilus had his body covered with shameful ulcers; it was he who gave his name to this disease, which was called syphilis from that time, on account of this circumstance."

The beauty of Fracastorius' poem is seen in his discussion of the etiology of the epidemic: "What causes after so many ages brought forth for us this unaccustomed disease? Was it borne by the Western Sea, and so came to our world at the same time when a chosen band set sail from the shores of Spain, and dared to attack the foam and the unknown waters of the wandering ocean and search out lands lying in a new world? For there, they say, that sickness held sway with everlasting ruin through all the cities, and wandered hither and thither by endless fault of heaven, sparing but few. Must we then think that by means of traffic this contagion was carried to reach us."[1] And again:

"Say, Goddess, to what Cause we shall last
Assign this plague, unknown to Ages past;
If from the Western Climes 'twas wafted o'er,
When daring Spaniards left their native shore;
Resolv'd beyond th' Atlantick to descry,
Conjectur'd Worlds, or in the search of dye."

Fracastorius distinguished three forms of contagion:[2] (1) by simple contact, as in scabies, phthisis and leprosy; (2) by indirect

704

contact, such as through clothing and bedclothes which can carry the seeds of contagion; and (3) by transmission from a distance, without direct or indirect contact, which may happen in plague, Egyptian ophthalmia, and smallpox. The seminaria spread themselves by selecting the humors for which they have an affinity, and by attraction, being drawn into the vessels. They can be absorbed by the breath and adhere to the humors which carry them to the heart. "There are diseases of plants which do not contaminate animals, and animal diseases which do not attack plants; there are other diseases limited to man or to certain animals, as cattle, horses and so on. Certain diseases have a special affinity for certain individuals or certain organs." [3]

Fracastorius discusses the problem as to whether infection is a kind of putrefaction: "Contagion which appears in fruit to be the most of that variety which is produced by contact alone, as from a grape to a grape and an apple to an apple for which reason it is asked what character of infection this may be: for that they are spoiled by contact first with one of them which became rotten is evident, but from what cause is not evident. But the first one from which all the infection passed to the others, became putrid, and it would be agreed that the second received a similar putrefaction if indeed contagion and infection are similar to each other. For putrefaction is a dissolution of this mixture by the evaporation of the innate heat and moisture, indeed the cause of this evaporation is always a strange heat, whether in the surrounding humidity; therefore although the cause of the putrefaction is one or the other, the cause of the contagion is identical, that is external heat.

"But this heat in the first place comes either from the air or from somewhere else and is not yet called infection; in the second place it comes from those insensible particles which evaporate from the first one and now there is contagion because the infection is similar in both cases. Moreover, the heat evaporating from the first could produce in the second, that which the air produced in the first, and in like manner cause putrefaction; in fruits, therefore, which contagion strikes, it is considered to be caused by this principle, and also in all other fruit too, which the putrefying fruit itself touches; if conditions be similar the same thing happens and it is right to consider it due to the same cause: moreover this principle consists of those small insensible particles which evaporate, indeed hot and acid but of a humid mixture which henceforth are called seeds of contagion. These seeds have the faculty of multiplying and propagating rapidly."[4]

Such statements, perhaps inspired by the atom theory of Lucretius (c. 400) show a good understanding of the specific nature of contagion, so that his concept is worthy of being accepted as one of the great precursors of the modern theory of infection and his name of being included among the greatest scientists of the Renaissance.

Girolamo Fracastorius was born at Verona in 1483. He studied at Padua, and became professor of philosophy there in 1502. He later was practicing physician in Verona. Fracastorius became eminently skilled, not only in medicine and belles-lettres, but in most arts and sciences. He was the author of many works, both poetical and medical, and was intimately acquainted with Cardinal Bembo to whom he dedicated his poem *Syphilidis, sive Morbi Gallici* (*libri tres,* Verona, 1530). Cardinal Bembo, writing to Fracastorius, said "You write with more charm than Lucretius . . . your lament of Marco Antonio and what follows make me think that the soul of Virgil has passed into you."

Fracastorius was the first scientist to refer to the magnetic poles of the earth and he gave one of the first good descriptions of typhus fever. He was the first to distinguish the three categories of infection; i.e., by contact, via fomites and at a distance.

He believed that the cause of contagion is to be found in *seminaria contagionis* (seeds of contagion) which he believed to be capable of reproduction in suitable media. He does not precisely refer to them as *contagia anima* (living contagious organisms) but the fact that he considered them to be capable of multiplication has led many historians to believe that Fracastorius had at least a premonition of the modern germ theory of disease.

It was said of him, "It was he who first opened man's eyes to the nature of contagion."

It is related that his mother was killed by lightning, while he, although in her arms at the moment, escaped unhurt. It is also reported that the lips of Fracastorius at birth adhered so closely together that a surgeon had to separate them with a scalpel. He died of apoplexy at Casi, near Verona, on the 8th day of August in the year 1553. In 1559 the town of Verona erected a statue in his honor.

Fracastorius recommended a large number of plants which he used in the form of infusions in treating syphilis and chief among these were moist hops, thyme and above all guaiac. He believed in the efficacy of diaphoresis: "When one perspires the rottenness leaves the body with the drops of sweat." Among other measures which he recommended for the treatment of syphilis was mercurial friction, inunction pushed to the point of salivation, purgation and bleeding.

Mercury was used as an inunction in the treatment of leprosy from the earliest times. The Arabs used such inunctions in treating infestations of lice and perhaps against bothor and asafati, which, as previously intimated, were probably syphilitic manifestations. The so-called "saracenic ointment" contained 9% of mercury. Physicians used weaker doses of mercury but the quacks administered massive doses. Although the first results with mercury were often encouraging, soon stomatitis, debility and other signs of mercurial poisoning often set in. The patient was often literally smeared from head to foot with the semi-fluid mercurial mixture. Those entrusted with the application of the ointment were called "greasers of pox." After the application, the patient was taken to a sweat bath and given cooling drinks with a base of wild cherry. It is said that the baths were so hot that some—particularly the poor were infrequently found dead in the chamber.

The object of this drastic treatment was to eliminate the syphilis poison via the salivation and the diaphoresis. Many of the patients became very debilitated either by the extreme sweating or by the absorption of the mercury into the system and died in the course of treatment. Those who appeared to be dying were made to drink the blood of a duck or gosling or eat the flesh of a freshly killed fowl.

FRANCISCO LOPEZ de VILLALOBOS (c. 1473-1549?)

Among the syphiliographers of the Renaissance may be mentioned Francisco Lopez de Villalobos. His *Tratado Sobre las Pestiferas Bubas* was the first book on syphilis in the Spanish language. It was written in the form of a poem of seventy-two stanzas each of ten lines. Some regard the poem as the equal in elegance of that of Fracastorius which appeared thirty-two years later.

Villalobos deals with the origin of syphilis and concludes that it is of recent origin. He gives his main reason that the Arabian writers do not refer to the primary lesion. The primary lesion of this disease was called "buba" or pimple. Thus the name of his book *Treatise on the Pestilentia Bubas*.

In stanza three of his tratado he describes the disease as exceedingly contagious.[5]

"It was a pestilence ne'er to be found at all
In verse or in prose, in science or in story,
So evil and perverse and cruel past control,
Exceedingly contagious, and in filth so prodigal,
So strong to hold its own, there is little got of glory;
And it makes one dark in feature and obscure in countenance,
Hunchback'd and indisposed, and seldom much at ease,
And it makes one pained and crippled in such sort as never was,
A scoundrel sort of thing, which also doth commence
In the rascalliest place that a man has."

In stanza thirty-seven he points out the fact that the small ulcer on the penis preceded by many days eruption of the disease elsewhere.[6]

"With this kind of ailment in the very first place,
The liver is distempered in the sense of dry and hot,
And gross and adust humors grow therein apace,
(but in the first beginning this is not so much the case)
And the strength to void it forth the liver will have got.
By all this noisome stuff diseased and much tormented,
Through its conduits forthwith some more or less it chases,
And this ere any portion in the veins is spread,
Thus 'tis that the passion on these members is presented
Many days before it yet hath appeared in other places."

In stanza sixty-three Villalobos speaks highly of the mercurial ointments.

"If something shall seem needed of a character more fine,
And stronger than the last, take both the arsenics
And bright yellow sulphur, with which you will combine
The black hellebore and the resin of pine,
All of these in the like proportion you mix;
With garlic ash rub, and after you will add
Some incense and myrrh, aloes and Negilla;
Hog's lard and kill'd quicksilver next should be had.
And oil, juice of lemon, or cider instead.
Make your ointment and lay it upon the pustilla."

He like his contemporary Fracastorius wrote his work on syphilis in verse. The syphiliographer Captain R. C. Holcomb, M.D. who has done so much to clear up the early history of syphilis writes: "I will say considering syphilis as a venereal disease, this poem gives a clearer description of its venereal etiology, its primary and its secondary symptoms than any other text produced up to the latter part of the fifteenth century. He lifts the veil to show many divergent opinions which had long been seething in medical groups, and which among other things would indicate to me that physicians were acquiring the courage to think for themselves and to break with a thralldom of centuries."

Francisco Lopez de Villalobos was born in the city of Toledo, Spain. His father and grandfather were physicians of the house of the Marquis of Astorga. He studied medicine in the University of Salamanca and, when still a student, composed his work *Treatise on the Pestilential Bubas.*

In 1514 he became court physician to King Ferdinand of Spain (1509-1516). He refers frequently in the letters to his dissatisfaction with court life. In 1515 he wrote that he "was often attending upon His Majesty." He expressed himself: "I intend, God willing, to quit it shortly."[7]

In 1518 he became physician to Emperor Charles and he did not retire until the age of seventy. He participated in the wars of the Emperor Charles V in Italy.

Villalobos stood in great favor because of his learning and wit. The exact date of his death is not known but he appears to have lived to a very old age. His work on syphilis was written in the Castilian dialect. As the author remarks in his preface: "The physicians in this domain being little familiar with Greek and Latin, the common tongue will popularize more easily the knowledge of scientific work."

ULRICH VON HUTTEN (1488-1523)

Ulrich von Hutten of Fulda, Germany, also made a great contribution to our knowledge of syphilis. His early training was in a Benedictine cloister. As a youth he was sickly and his father thought best to put him in a monastery where he could live quietly. However, the youth found the atmosphere in the monastery stifling and fled from the religious atmosphere. For nine years he wandered about aimlessly through Germany and Italy. Because of his poverty he entered the army of Emperor Maximilian. His poetic erudition finally brought him to the attention of the Bishop of Brandenberg through whom his long aspiration for literary attainments was realized.

His attacks on the Duke of Württemberg, who murdered his cousin, his criticism of the papal claims and his so-called exposure of the Lutheran cause brought the wrath of Albert of

Elector of Maynce down on his head and interrupted the fulfillment of his ambition.

Pope Leo X ordered his arrest and he fled to Basle for safety. From there he went to Zurich where he was kindly received by the reformer Zwingli. He died in Zurich at the age of thirty-five years, penniless and friendless.

Ulrich von Hutten's opus: *De Guaiaci Medicina et Morbo Gallico* (1519) dedicated to Cardinal Albert of Brandenberg, was translated into English by Thomas Paynell (b. 1563) in the year 1533 with the long title: "Of the Wood called Guiacum, that Healeth the Frenche-Pockes, and also Helpeth the Goute in the Feet, Stoone, the Palsey, Lepree, Dropsey, Fallynge Evill, and other Diseases."

In this work, von Hutten declares that he had suffered from the French disease since he was eight years old and that he presently had found a wonderful remedy in this Indian wood. The disease, he says, originated in Naples in 1493, which was before Charles VIII undertook his campaign, as he did not arrive in Naples until February 22, 1495. It appeared in the army of Charles VIII at Naples and in France at about the same time. The disease spread with terrorsome rapidity and reached this little eight year old boy in Hesse in 1496.

Not long after the disease appeared in Italy, he states, it made its appearance in Germany, where it prevailed more than in any other country in Europe. He ascribed this to national intemperance, explaining that the Germans were indulging both in excesses of eating and drinking, and as a consequence they suffered the most violent symptoms and worst course during the disease. He says that the German physicians avoided any contact with persons suffering from syphilis and that for two years after the epidemic broke out, the patients had to depend solely on the assistance of the blundering surgeons.

During the first seven or more years that the disease prevailed, cases occurred even among those who had no contact with the infected, but at the time of his book (1519), it was spread mostly by intercourse. The leutic ulcers, he declared, which at first had resembled acorns in size and shape, had become a little smaller, a little less prominent, and a little less hard, although sometimes the disease assumed a worse form and covered the skin with a dry, scaly, spreading scab.

At the time of the first appearance of the syphilis epidemic, he continues, philosophers generally agreed that lakes, rivers, springs, and even seas had been corrupted by some poisonous ferment in the air, which was thence communicated to the bodies of animals. This view was in thorough accord with the teachings of the learned Niccolo Leonicensus (1497) and Simon Pisor (1499) at Leipzig. It is also in accord with the account of Ruiz Diaz de Isla.

Von Hutten, himself, underwent long years of treatment for syphilis. He received inunctions with mercury until salivation ensued; he took alum, turpentine, and a long list of purges orally. All of these made the disease more tolerable without curing it. This task remained for guaiacum, which alone, according to his statement, accomplished the cure. "Its virtues were not increased by compounding it with any other drug; on the contrary, its efficiency was thus diminished." In the space of forty days, by the use of the decoction of guaiac, he was "cured" and his ulcers healed.

It seems sad to contemplate that with all his earnestness to contribute to the relief of mankind, von Hutten died prematurely, overwhelmed by the disease which he thought was cured, and beset by discouragement, poverty, and persecution.

The general view of physicians of that period concerning the origin of syphilis varies.

Paracelsus (1493-1541) in his *Chirurgia*, (1536) considers syphilis to be the result of a sort of combining of leprosy with venereal buboes. He states that gonorrhea is the first stage of syphilis and he calls gonorrhea "the French disease." According to Paracelsus: "Pox owes its origin to the impure intercourse (in 1478) of a French leper with a courtesan who had venereal buboes; the latter then infected all those who had to do with her. It is thus that the pox, proceeding from the leprosy and the venereal buboes—about in the way that the mule results from the coupling of a horse and an ass—spread by contagion throughout the universe." [8]

Andrea Cesalpino of Arezzo (1519-1603), physician of Pope Clement VII, relates an odd story, which he claims to have heard from various eye-witnesses, and notably from a soldier who had served in the Spanish army. This soldier related that the French besieged a city named Somma, near Mount Vesuvius, where numerous excellent vineyards producing "Greek wine" were cultivated. The Spaniards abandoned the place during the night and contaminated the wine which they left behind them with blood which they had drawn from patients of the hospital of St. Azarus (where lepers were treated). The French, having entered the city and gorged themselves with this wine, commenced to sicken and develop severe cases of *morbus Gallicus*.

A Musa Brassavole (1500-1555) of Ferrara tells the following tale: There was in the camp of the French, in 1495, a famous and beauteous courtesan who was affected with a foul ulcer of the vulva. The men who had commerce with her contracted a malignant affection, which ulcerated their sexual organs. . . . Many men were so infected and, as a result, a large number of women who had relations with these men acquired the disease. They, in turn, passed it on to other men.[9]

The Greek historian, John Maschus, relates the case of a Greek Church Father, Abbe Polychronus of the monastery of Pentucula, who lived in Pergamos, Asia Minor, toward the end of the sixth century under the reign of Maurice. This ecclesiastic, no longer able to resist his long-repressed sexual urge, went to Jericho to satiate this desire. When he returned to his monastery, he developed "leprosy." He then declared that God had chastised him in order to save his soul. Knowing that true leprosy is often not communicable even after long contact, one is forced to the conclusion that this Father of Pentucula really contracted syphilis.[10]

Le Monnier (1689) states that he found the explanation presented by several authors as to how a perfectly healthy woman might contract syphilis. Lues could be developed in her by the very fact that she had had intercourse with several men in a short space of time even though they were all perfectly healthy.[11] This calls to mind the explanation given as to why prostitutes have no children, "No grass grows in a path which is often trodden." [12] Gervais Ucay[13] (1699) says that syphilis has its origin in the eruption of several seeds in the same vagina: "It is well known that if a perfectly healthy girl and a virgin, if you will, . . . mingles with a dozen lads as healthy as she is, and debauches herself with each in turn . . . all together will finally acquire the pox by the repetition of the venereal acts."

The communication of pox, according to the historian Hume, (1711-1776) was believed to be also through odor and breath. Henry VIII, King of England, ordered Cardinal Wolsey to be beheaded in 1530. He declared that the Cardinal had infected him with the pox by his very breath when whispering in his ears. Royalty or persons of high rank often claimed that they had been infected in such a manner in order not to be suspected of immoral behavior.

In the beginning, patients in order to conceal their debauchery did not confess how they had come to contact this disease. This circumstance contributed to render more credible the opinion that the disease was of epidemic nature. A multitude of reasons were sought to explain its production. Every scientific man permitted himself to be drawn into the discussion. Torella (1500) appears to have been the one to suspect the true mode of propagation of the virus, for he says the disease comes about by transmission.

An early American account of syphilis, is given by Gov. John Winthrop.[14] He tells of a local sailor who, on returning from a voyage, infected his wife with syphilis. She gave birth to a child and during her lying-in period, developed a sore on the breast. Neighbors who thought that the milk was caked tried to relieve her breast condition by letting various of their children suck her breast and by "drawing her breast." In consequence of these breast manipulations, sixteen persons, including women and children, were infected. The magistrate examining the husband and wife could find "no dishonesty in either . . . so it was considered by some that the women were infected by the mixture of the spirits of man and woman as they drew their breath."

JEAN ASTRUC (c.1545-1605)

Astruc, physician to Louis XIV of France and famous Biblical commentator, was first to definitely recognize syphilis as an infectious malady. Among other things, he said: "And therefore it is by no means strange that many of the Neapolitans should be infected with the same distemper since they served under the same colors and had to do with the same women who followed the camp . . . the same towns were taken and reconquered by both parties; 'tis plain that the French must also have had communication with the same women who had lain with the Spaniards and the Neapolitans and thus the siege of the venereal disease must have naturally passed from one to the other." Astruc makes repeated reference to the presence of the disease in Europe in 1494. In fact he says the Spaniards took the disease to Naples the same year.

Jean Astruc, was born at Sauve, in Languedoc. He received his medical degree in 1572 from Montpellier and he was appointed to the chair of anatomy at Toulouse, which position he retained until he became professor of medicine at Montpellier.

Of his numerous works, his fame rests principally on the six-book treatise entitled, *De Morbis Veneris,* published in 1736.

Syphilis for a time played an important role even in politics. Many political opponents, including kings, dukes, and ambassadors, were effectively cut down more on medical than on moral grounds, presenting them with beautiful girls who were infected with syphilis. It is said that Wenzeslaus XI of Bohemia, and Ladislaus of Naples, were among those infected in this way.

According to Fallopius, Charles VII lost the war with Italy in 1495 because of the violent outbreak of syphilis. His army, occupying Naples was infected with the disease by the charming ladies of this city, who thus performed a patriotic duty in preventing the French and German armies from conquering their country.

In the Mohammedan countries, where lues was said to have been introduced by the Crusaders, it was treated with a prayer from the Koran, which reads: "By these words I am begging Allah to protect us from the irate acts of revenge, from all the adverse influences that may be inflicted upon the faithful servants by the wrathful demons."

A true perspective as to syphilis was lost because the facts were obscured by secrecy and distorted by religion and moralizing. There were many laymen who well understood the manner of transmission of this disease as the following incident shows: Francis I was infatuated with la belle Ferronniere. Her outraged husband got revenge on the King by voluntarily contracting the disease and transmitting it to his wife who promptly infected the King. The King, in spite of his great royal powers, died from this infection. A chronicler composed the following epitaph:

> "Twas in the month of June, the seventh
> In 1447 at Ramboullet with pox as cause
> The King went up to heaven." [15]

The discovery of the infectious nature of syphilis at first did not debase a gentleman's reputation since so many men were affected with this disease. Indeed, some went so far as to assume that a man who had not had the disease at least once was no gentleman. There was little attention paid to the thesis that syphilis was transmitted sexually. The disease was often assumed to be contracted through the air and therefore a person who had inhaled the "bad air" was advised to press his mouth against that of a child in order to inhale the child's pure breath, and exhale his own infected breath into the child's mouth. Prophylactic measures against syphilis included "purifying" the air by burning all sorts of material in the public highways and streets and covering the face with crude masks. Physicians encouraged their patients to travel to neighboring cities in order to escape the infected air of their own community. From time to time suspicion arose that syphilis is caused by contagion from animals. Thus, to avert the disease, horses were padded with heavy blankets so that the rider could not come into close contact with the animal and people were generally wary of touching domestic animals.

When at last the true cause of syphilis became known, men tried to unload it on young girls, who were bought or kidnapped and raped. It was believed that the purity of young children would suffice to accept and destroy the disease. Infected women paid heavy sums to the parents of adolescent boys for the same purpose. When the demand for young persons exceeded the available supply, man turned to domestic animals and mules, horses, and cows were employed to unload the disease.

Many a marriage was performed on condition that both bride and groom spend the first night with other partners to be sure of getting rid of luetic infection before the first conjugal act. For a long time bathhouses were recommended for syphilis, where women called "poison girls" were employed for "therapeutic" purposes.

Gian Francesco Poggio Bracciolini, a fifteenth century Italian scholar and lay secteratry in the Papal curi, had this to say about bath cures: "Every lover, every suitor, in fact everyone whose chief concern is amorous alliance, flocks to the baths that they may enjoy the object of their desire. Many feign bodily illness, although their only troubles are those of the mind."

Bath-houses in Germanic countries not only offered the attraction of mixed nude bathing in a common tank, but also engaged in lively competition for patrons with such additional lures as especially attractive bath maids, music, food, and drink. The impudence of certain bath-keepers in professing to cure the malady so frequently acquired on their own premises was a strong factor in hastening the interest of medical men in the problem of syphilis. In the last years of the fifteenth century, so fertile a focal point of infection as the baths, could not escape the attention of medical authorities who were frantically seeking to arrest the spread of syphilis. Public baths at Nuremberg and elsewhere in Germany were closed in 1496 by decree of the government more on medical than on moral grounds.

The gravity of lues was fully recognized in the early part of the sixteenth century: The Italian artist Benvenuto Cellini (1500-1571) wrote to a friend: ". . . The French Disease remained in me more than four months dormant . . . then it broke out over my whole body at one instant . . . I went on treating myself according to (my physician's) methods, but derived no benefit. At last I resolved to take the wood (an infusion of guaiacum) against the advice of the . . . physicians . . . and I took it with most scrupulous discipline . . . (so) that at the end of fifty days I was cured and as sound as a fish in the water."

There is no disease in medical literature that was known by so many names as syphilis. The reason for the frequent change of names rested on the fact that lues is so easily confounded with many other diseases bearing similar symptoms. The dictum, "To know syphilis and its differential diagnosis is to know medicine," is an established fact. Lues was often diagnosed as a form of leprosy. It was mistaken for smallpox because in the third stage it is characterized by a pox-like eruption. It was believed to be an aggravated form of gonorrhea because of the presence of buboes, and for the same reason it was mistaken for bubonic plague. When its venereal origin finally became unmistakably established, no nation wanted to believe that it had developed in their native country. Each country put the blame upon its neighbor for its etiology. The Spaniards claimed that until the French army under Charles III came to Naples in 1494-1495, they had never even heard of such a disease. In the fifteenth and sixteenth centuries it was known among the Italian physicians as Morbo Gallico and many of the Italian works on syphilis were entitled *De Morbo Gallico* (Concerning the French Disease).

The French physicians objecting to this name retaliated by calling lues The Disease of Naples. From that time on it became customary for the peoples of the Old World to attribute the disease to their enemies. The name French Disease or Morbo Gallico, however, became generally used by most writers. By order of Emperor Maximilian (1495), it was named Mala de Franzas. Later the Germans called it Französische Krankheit. The English termed it French Pox to differentiate the tertiary stage from smallpox. To the Arabs and the Turks and to the people of the Mediterranean shore, it became known as the Christian Disease or the Disease of the Franks. The Poles blamed it on the Germans and named it the German Disease. The Russians called it "Polish Disease." To the Iranians it became known as the Disease of the Turks. The Africans and Moors who were unfriendly to Spain termed it the Spanish Disease. The same name was applied by the Dutch and Portuguese. The Spanish, who apparently did not feel quite comfortable in blaming the disease on their neighbors, attributed its origin to the native Americans.

Syphilis was also named after various saints. These included St. Job, St. Roch, St. Rein, St. Marcella and St. Anthony. It was also aptly described as "Hell fire."

It was also known as "sacred disease." While all diseases were looked upon as punishment for religious transgressions, syphilis was one disease readily identifiable as representing punishment for sexual transgressions. "Lues venerea," a term which was applied by Fernel, is still frequently employed. Leoniceno introduced the term "Morbus Gallicus" which was used for two hundred years. The terms "clap" and "pox" were used indiscriminately.

In addition to the dozens of names for syphilis representing various countries, there are about three hundred other designations for it. In a decree of the Parliament of Paris (1496) the expression "grosse verole" (big pox) was used to represent lues. By decree of James IV of Scotland, the term "grand gor" was applied.

The term "syphilis," although introduced by Fracastorius in 1530, did not receive general recognition for a long time. During the whole of the seventeenth and eighteenth centuries only about a half dozen writers used it.

No mention of Columbus (1446-1506) in connection with the origin of syphilis was made for more than a third of a century after the discovery of America and such an association appears to have been first inferred nearly a decade after the introduction of guaiacum (the holy wood) in Europe, as a specific for the cure of *Morbus Gallicus,* as syphilis was called. Guaiacum and its use in syphilis was associated with the deeply rooted superstition that disease develops as a punishment for sin, which doctrine is so frequently encountered in the Scriptures.

The concept of "signature," i. e. that Divine Providence mercifully provides the antidote or remedy for a disease so inflicted, at the place where the disease originates, or among the people who are thus afflicted, also predominated. As this remedy was discovered in the newly found land, it was taken as a corollary that the disease which it "cured" surely originated there. This superstition, which was encouraged by the venders of guaiacum, found support among physicians and laymen who lauded the marvelous properties of this holy wood.

Guaiacum was an original American Indian remedy. In Spain guaiacum was called *"palo santo"* ("holy wood"). In Italy it was called *"legno santo"* (also "holy wood"). The Latin writers called it *"lignum sanctum," "lignum indicum"* or *"lignum vitae."* In Germany it was known as "Franzosenbaum" or "Pockenholzbaum" after the disease for which it was supposed to be specific.

The fame of guaiacum spread into Germany, and Emperor Maximilian dispatched a commission, one of the most important members of which was Cardinal Matthew Lang, Bishop of Gurk, for the purpose of securing information concerning its use for German sufferers.

In 1517, *The Cure of Morbus Gallicus by the Wood Guaiacum* (*De Cura Morbi Gallici per lignum Guayanum, libellus*) dated 1517 was written by Nicholas Pol or Poll (1470-1527). This short work consisting of nine chapters set forth a regimen of treatment with the wood which was consistently followed thereafter. It announced that some 3,000 Spaniards had recently been cured of *morbus gallicus* by means of guaiacum after many of them had tried a great number of remedies without benefit.

The method of preparing the wood was by making a decoction. The wood, being hard, heavier than water and incapable of being broken down by ordinary means, had to be attacked with hammers, chisels, and other tools.

The Spaniards, according to Dr. Pol, were mostly cured by the decoction in fifteen days although some patients required forty days, and a few as long as sixty days. In short, anyone who had been affected with the disease, even though he had suffered with it for over a decade and had extensive and deep ulcerations, might expect an early cure with the decoction and regimen as outlined. It was essential, however, that the decoction be freshly prepared and not kept for longer than two or three days. Dr. Pol states that guaiacum operates by increasing the sweat, the urine, the stool and promoting the production of vomitus.

A Spanish account of the virtues of the "holy wood" appeared in the *Summaria* of another layman, Gonsalvo Gernandez Oviedo Valdez (1478-1507) who states that some persons call guaiac "hebaeno." Other later writers identified it with the *ebenus* of Pliny and Dioscorides.

The *Summaria,* The Natural History of the Indies was published in 1526. This work contains a chapter entitled *The Holy Wood,* which the Indians call "Guaiacum." The *Summaria* was translated into English by Richard Eden, and this version was published in 1555. Christopher Columbus (c. 1446-1506) has been charged with the importation of the disease for which guaiac was considered a specific.

Oviedo, who was fifteen years of age when Columbus returned from his first voyage, is credited with making a first-hand investigation into the disease.

Oviedo asserts that the disease was common among the American Indians, but not so violent or dangerous among them as in Spain and other countries not in the tropics. The Indians were easily "cured" of the disease with guaiac. "This guaiac cures the *bubas* (the Spanish name for syphilis) more perfectly than any other medicine." "Divine clemency is so great," declares Oviedo, "that wherever it allows us to suffer for our sins, it grants that there should be found likewise the remedies for this suffering." [16]

Peter Martyr, a member of the Council in the Indies makes no mention of the virtues of the wood in an earlier work, *De Rebus Oceanicis et Novo Orbe*. He mentions a remarkable trained hunting fish which the Indians called Guaiacanum, and this is the nearest approach to the name. The only "wood" he includes is a hard polished wood which was converted into various utensils by the Indians. He writes that John Baptiste Elisius, physician to Charles V, identified this wood with hebene. He says nothing of its medicinal properties.

This book appeared in France shortly therafter and the French version is often called "the first French book on syphilis."

At the end of the fifteenth century syphilis was recognized as a morbid condition and was described together with its different symptoms under the name of morbus Gallicus. At all events from this time on there is no possible discussion regarding the nature of the disease so we can be permitted to follow its history from the works which have come down to us.

Dr. William Allen Pusey (1915), in his *History and Epidemology of Syphilis* admires the achievements of the period following the epidemic of Naples. In the three hundred years between 1500 and 1800 all the facts concerning syphilis that could then be ascertained were worked out. But while it is true that many advances were made in the description of the various forms of the disease and better understanding was gained of its descriptive pathology, yet the underlying principle of the causative factor which alone could lead to practical methods of treatment of course remained obscure.

The discovery of the spirochete of syphilis ("spirocheta pallida") was finally attained by Fritz Schaudinn (1871-1906) and Erich Hoffman (b. 1863——) in the year 1905.

Paul Ehrlich (1854-1915) laid the foundations of chemo-therapy with his attempted "therapia magna sterilisans" for syphilis (i.e., killing off the infecting organism with one big dose). His aim was to experiment with new chemical drugs until he found those best suited to destroy the causative agents of various diseases. Ehrlich experimented with innumerable arsenic compounds, attempting to deprive them of their toxicity for the host while retaining their lethal effect on the parasite. Finally in 1910, he announced that his 606th arsenical synthesis, salvarsan, was a specific destroyer of the Spirocheta pallida, the causative organism of syphilis. While it failed to attain his hoped for "therapia magna sterilisans" level, it nevertheless proved most valuable in the treatment of the disease and pointed the way to the whole modern chemotherapeutic drug science.

CHAPTER XLII

DISEASES RECOGNIZED DURING THE
RENAISSANCE

As the sixteenth century advanced and the secret of contagion was slowly disclosed, more attention was paid to hygienic and sanitary conditions and stricter measures were taken by the communities to protect themselves against diseases. The plague, during the whole sixteenth century, prevailed more generally, and in places more fatally, than ever before. This was true, too, in spite of a great number of "Plague ordinances," issued in the form of books, reports and pamphlets by the authorities, as measures of public sanitation. Still the plague ravaged all places. The plague was declared contagious and portable, and accordingly measures of isolation and disinfection were put in force against it, though without proving in any degree effectual. Horn, gunpowder, arsenic with sulphur or straw moistened with wine, etc., were burned in the streets as disinfectants without avail. The administration of preventive doses of disinfectants was also customary at that period. The "Pestmedici" anointed the uncovered portions of their bodies with oil, etc., or wore special "plague-dresses" and "plague-masks," "plague-gloves," etc. The plague-dresses were red or black: the masks were made of leather, had openings filled with glass for the eyes and a beak-like prolongation for the reception of disinfecting substances. Similar clothing has been considered a means of protection down even to the present day.

Leprosy, one of the oldest diseases known, disappeared earliest from Italy, so that while at the beginning of the sixteenth century a few cases were still observed, at the close of this century it no longer appeared there. In France, likewise, it lost its epidemic character but did not entirely disappear until the following century.

England in the course of the sixteenth century rid itself completely of leprosy, while Scotland, the Netherlands and Germany were forced to suffer from its ravages into the seventeenth century.

Syphilis laid aside its malignant, epidemic character only to extend more widely its milder sway. In spite of the introduction in the sixteenth century of the external and internal employment of mercury and the administration of guaiac, sarsaparilla, sassafras and China smilax, it still exists in endemic form among civilized and uncivilized people.

A destructive disease which attacked the Italians in the year 1492 and 1493 was typhus fever which is said to have been introduced by fugitive Jews who had been expelled from Spain, but it appears the disease broke out fifteen years before (1477). In a Parmese notebook published in Muratori, there is a description of a fever with a high mortality which plagued Milan. This epidemic of severe and acute fever attacked many people and appears to have been typhus fever.

Of course, it is possible that some of the alleged epidemics of typhus have been confused with other destructive febrile diseases, such as, for example, bubonic plague, malarial fever, and typhoid fever. But whether typhus was recognized or not, all the predisposing causes of typhus fever existed in great measure during the renaissance.

JEROME CARDAN (1501-1576)

The first physician scientifically to identify typhus was Jerome Cardan (Girolamo Cardano). He called it *Morbus pulicaris* and gave the first detailed description of this disease in 1536.

"Morbus pulicaris," he says, "differs from measles.... Measles are elevated above the skin, from their own nature healing, they affect all men; just as small-pox, as Averroes says, is seen on different years, and most rarely attacks a man more than once, seldom has mild symptoms, except in boys, and is seen in certain adolescents, is not associated with bubonic plague.

"Morbus pulicaris is wholly without elevations, and only spots on the skin are present; in its nature deadly, neither attacking half of the human race: it rages at certain times not during single years, in a vigorous manner; frequently, moreover, malignant, it attacks the same person twice or thrice and four times with the most severe symptoms, infecting all ages, even to extreme old age, with the familiar buboes of the plague and rarely these are lacking... Now also you should consider me to have separated blacciae from measles, and especially, as one who has been able to escape from the bad accounts which have been written.

"Therefore, in the disease, when it is pestilential and not only epidemic, it has been preferable to administer the treatment if necessary for plague, applying with this purpose only, whatever may increase in the thinned blood, soothing in nature so the skin, which is the sole refuge to such, it produces sweating the true crisis of this disease. Also do not fail with adjuvants, nor let up with restraints, give aid to the heart and few treated from the beginning will be in peril. Moreover, it is clear from this that those who desire water, no other remedy should have as much of this drink as healthful, if other things agree."[1]

Jerome Cardan was born in Pavia in the year 1501. He was the illegitimate son of Fazio Cardano, prominent physician, jurist and mathematician. His early education was probably received from his father. At the age of nineteen he was admitted to the University of Pavia, where he followed the subjects of mathematics, astrology and other sciences. At the age of twenty-five he received the degree of Doctor of Medicine from the University of Pavia.

After his graduation he practiced his profession for a period of three years in Sacco, a small town near Padua, where he wrote treatises on syphilis, plague and sputum. He then removed to Milan. There he sought admission to the College of Physicians, but owing to his illegitimate birth, his application for membership was refused. This evidently depressed him very much for he immediately left Milan and led the life of a vagabond traveling from town to town. When he finally returned with his wife and son to Milan, he was so destitute that he was obliged to find shelter in the city poorhouse.

At that time the head friar was troubled with a skin infection for whom none of Milan's physicians could find any relief and of which young Cardan cured him. In appreciation, the head friar appointed Cardan Physician of the Monastery of the Augustine Friars. The medical skill of young Cardan soon became known all over Milan and his ill fortunes abruptly changed. He built up a large medical practice and in the year 1536, published his first medical work entitled, *De Malo Recentiorum Medicorum Mendendi Usu* (The Bad Practice of Healing among Modern Doctors), which was a criticism of his fellow physicians. Cardan was probably motivated in writing this book by his deeply rooted desire to get even with those who had rejected him as a member of the College of Physicians.

This book (which was said to have been written in fifteen days) had a large sale. Its publication was ill advised for it naturally enough received most severe criticism from the medical profession of Milan. Cardan himself was eventually sorry for this publication. He is said to have remarked: "Where I had looked for honor, I reaped nothing but shame."

The condemnation of Cardan's work was largely of a personal character and not from a medical point of view, for this work contains much of scientific value and includes the account of typhus, as described above, which he called *morbus pulicaris* or flea-bite disease.

In 1543, Cardan was appointed to a professorship at the University of Pavia, and this appointment brought him fame throughout Europe. He refused many lucrative offers, including the post of physician to Pope Paul III and that of court physician to the King of Denmark.

He did not refuse, however, the post of medical adviser to Archbishop Hamilton of St. Andrews of Edinburgh, in which capacity he served for a period of three years. When he returned to Milan, he continued to prosper professionally for some time, but soon charges were trumped up against him which caused him to be banished from the city (1562). The following year he was appointed professor at the University of Bologna and the freedom of the city was conferred upon him.

It seems that even in his old age (70) he could not hide his free and rebellious temperament for he was suddenly cast into prison on a charge of impiety and, although he was finally liberated, he was prohibited from lecturing or publishing books. He finally moved to Rome where a pension was granted by Pope Pius V. Cardano left ten large volumes containing important information on many subjects. Among them was *De Varietate Rerum* published in the year 1557 and *De Subtitate Rerum* published in the year 1551.

Cardano was one of the fathers of medicine next to Paracelsus and Michael Nostrodamus (1503-1566) physician and graduate of Montpellier. He died in Rome in the year 1576.[2]

The merit of having even more accurately described typhus fever goes to Fracastoro in his classic poem, *De Morbis Contagiosis* published in 1546. He gives a clear account of typhus which up to that time had been confused with bubonic plague and other diseases. Fracastoro clearly emphasized the importance of the rash and connected the influence of war and famine on epidemic typhus.[3]

During the Dark Ages, epidemics of typhus usually followed military campaigns, unsanitary living conditions, overcrowdedness particularly among persons confined in jails or trenches, famines and other destructive influences that lowered the living standards and vitality of the people. The great Castillian army at the siege of Granada in 1487 was decimated by typhus which the Spaniards called "the cloak" or "tabordillo." During the Thirty Years War which began in 1618, Central Europe was ravaged by typhus.

A severe epidemic of typhus ravaged Italy during the years 1505 and 1528 which had been brought over from Cyprus and adjacent islands.

It has been calculated that more than 30,000 French soldiers died of the disease in Prague in 1741. A similar condition prevailed during the Napoleonic War against Italy. During the Crimean War (1853-1856), the casualties from typhus fever among the French and the English were very heavy. During and following the Balkan wars, the mortality from typhus has been estimated at over one million persons. The Turkish Russian War in 1876 was accompanied by an outbreak of typhus in both countries.

In the severe typhus epidemic in Ireland during the 1840's, one-fifth of the doctors on the island died of typhus. Typhus was the fever that was brought over to America from Ireland in 1846 and was spread by Irish immigration to many parts of America. Typhus has also taken a steady toll in Mexico and Central America.

The high mortality of typhus following the First World War in Eastern and Central Europe was staggering. It certainly did not spare the attending physicians and the mortality among the medical men and their attendants in those epidemics was particularly high. Many prominent physicians, including Maezukowski, Cornet, Husk, Jochmann, McGruder, Bacot, Prowazek, Ricketts, Weil and Schussler, made the supreme sacrifice.

The exciting cause of typhus fever has been demonstrated by Matthews C.S. (1828) to be due to the presence of fleas, lice and other vermin. Fleas and lice are considered the carriers of the infection. Every case examined in the Aberdeen Hospital by Dr. Matthews was flea bitten and those of the medical staff who had been flea bitten or had come in contact with vermin became prey to the epidemic. The disease did not spread in healthy surroundings or in clean homes even when there were known cases suffering from the contagion.

During the sixteenth century, epidemics of typhus occurred in Italy, Hungary and England and three "black assizes" occurred in England: one each in Cambridge, Oxford and Exeter. The London "black assizes" occurred in the eighteenth century (1750). To the last, medicine is indebted for a better knowledge of the etiology of typhus fever. This last episode affected such men of standing in London as the Lord Mayor, two judges and other prominent personages, and led to a careful search for the cause of the disease and for measures of prevention.[4]

The event in question happened in a Court of Justice in the year 1750, when a prisoner named Clark was ushered from the Newgate prison into the Old Bailey Courthouse. The presiding judge, Sir Thomas Abney, in his wig and robe, had near him the Lord Mayor of London and two other judges, for the case was one that attracted much attention. The courtroom was very crowded. With every new spectator the crowd was pushed closer to the prisoner's dock, and as the prisoner passed through the aisles of the court that lead to the dock, the whole courtroom was filled with such a foul odor that all close to the prisoner drew back.

The trial ended with the usual regularity and nothing was thought about the prisoner until a week after the conclusion of of the trial when the three judges, the Lord Mayor, eight members of the jury and forty clerks and spectators took very sick and died of fever. It was noted that those who succumbed to the pestilence were the ones who sat at the left side of the courtroom where the prisoner was placed during the trial. It was also observed that none of the relatives that lived in the same houses with the fatally attacked persons had become infected.

The idea that the prisoner infected the fifty men with the disease soon occurred to the physicians who attended to those men, and for want of a better name typhus became known as "jail fever." The general opinion prevailed that the bad air and fetid odor of the prisoner were the cause of the infection for there was no famine nor war at the time to breed this disease.

It was due to these "black assizes" which did not spare the higher classes of London, that the sanitary conditions of the jails and the slums were improved. The crowded and dirty cells in the prisons were gradually cleaned up and more air and light were permitted to enter the cell blocks. Gradually typhus fever disappeared from the scene, and if it did appear, it was in a mild and infrequent form.

Thanks to the efforts of the United States Army Medical Corps which kept away vermin and "cooties" as the fleas were called, from the trenches, that cause of the terrible typhus epidemics was averted in recent wars. Delousing stations were established and the hems of the soldiers' uniforms and clothes, where lice usually find their hiding places, were disinfected in hot, dry air.

The credit for differentiating typhus fever from typhoid fever goes to a Philadelphia physician William Wood Gerhard. Typhoid fever is an infectious disease entering the body through the digestive tract and caused by a specific bacillus of typhoid that attacks the walls of the small intestine. It is acquired by eating and drinking foods contaminated by the typhoid bacillus. The incidence of typhoid is in direct proportion to the sanitary conditions of a city, its sewage disposal, the purity of its water and food supply. On the other hand, typhus depends upon personal cleanliness. It is not transmitted by food, water, filth *per se* or by contact with the sick. It is transmitted by an insect, most often by the body louse.

Typhus fever has been known by various names depending upon the author's idea of the etiology and pathology of the disease. Among these names are spotted fever, petechial fever, jail fever, ship fever, camp fever, enthematique fever, fleck fieber (in Germany), tarbardillo, assizes fever, Hungarian disease, putrid fever, pestilane and morbus pulicaris.

The truth of the maxim, *salus populi suprema lex* (the health of the people is the supreme duty) was adequately demonstrated long before the germ theory of typhus was advanced. The connection of typhus with unsanitary conditions was realized early. It was long known that the flea, the body louse, the bed bug, the house fly, the mosquito and the tic have been carriers of this disease, and in many countries steps were taken to exterminate these insects. The scourge of typhus was wiped out in some countries within a period of twenty-five years. The cause was discovered early in the present century by Ricketts and Prowazek. Hence, the name of the infectious germ, Rickettsia prowazeki.

CHAPTER XLIII

SWEATING SICKNESS DURING THE RENAISSANCE

An epidemic disease which first made its appearance in England in the year 1485, was the so-called "sweating sickness" (miliary fever or Anglicus Sudor). It appears to have been brought to the coast of Wales, England, by the returning mercenary soldiers of Henry VII of France after the Battle of Bosworth and it soon spread to the capital where it caused a great mortality. Henry VIII left London frequently with the dissolution of court because of this epidemic.

The symptoms of sweating sickness caused it to be readily differentiated from the plague, typhus fever and other previously known epidemics, not only because of the sweating it produced, but also because of its extremely rapid and fatal course.

There were six major epidemics of this sickness and these epidemics reached their heights during the summers of 1485, 1506, 1518, 1528, 1529 and 1551. The severity of the outbreak in 1518 was of such magnitude that few who were attacked survived beyond the third day. It carried off a large proportion of the nobility and in many towns half of the population fell victim to the disease. This epidemic was especially fatal in Oxford and Cambridge where half the populations perished. There is evidence that this epidemic prevailed also in Calais and Antwerp, but with these exceptions it was confined to England.

In 1528, the disease recurred for the fourth time, and with great severity. It first showed itself in London at the end of May, and speedily spread over the whole of England, skipping only Scotland and Ireland. Victims of this epidemic for the most part died in the course of six hours.

"Sweating sickness" as described by Caius and other contemporaries, began very suddenly with a sense of apprehension, followed by cold shivers (sometimes very violent), giddiness, headache and severe pains in the neck, shoulders and limbs, accompanied by prostration. The cold state, which usually lasted from one-half hour to three hours, was followed by the stage of heat and sweating. The characteristic sweat broke out suddenly and with it came a sense of heat, an unendurable headache, delirium, rapid pulse and intense thirst. Palpitation and pain in the heart were frequent symptoms. In the later stages there was either general prostration and collapse or an irresistible tendency to sleep, which was considered fatal if the patient could not successfully fight it. A miliary eruption usually developed. The disease caused death most frequently within the first twenty-four hours. If, however, death did not ensue, a change for the better usually set in speedily and complete recovery followed in from eight to fourteen days.[1]

The first epidemic (1485) extended essentially over England only (Calais and Antwerp were the only mainland cities involved) as did the second epidemic (1506); the third, however, extended also over northern France (1518); the fourth and fifth (1528 and 1529) spread over Germany, the Netherlands, Sweden, Russia, France and Switzerland; the last (1551) again affected only England proper, excluding Ireland and Scotland. In 1551, its last appearance in England occasioned many deaths within the first twenty-four hours. It was most destructive in the county of Salop where the celebrated physician, Doctor Caius was practicing and it was he who graphically decribed the symptoms of the disease.

The mortality occasioned by the early epidemics was enormous. In Hamburg in 1529 when the epidemic had already become milder, over 1,000 persons died in twenty-two days. In Augsburg, of 15,000 afflicted, 800 died in the first five days after the appearance of the epidemic, while later, of 3,000 attacked,

600 died. In Germany the sudorific treatment originally practiced was responsible for a large share of the high mortality, which diminished as better physicians, after the English method, advocated only gentle sweating and for a brief period.[2]

The sweating stage, from which the name of the disease is derived, was merely a symptom, or rather the crisis of the complaint. Unlike other epidemics, children and aged persons appear to have been most immune to "sweating sickness" and the poor were less affected than the wealthier classes.

Physicians at first hesitated as to the plan of treatment to be adopted. They recommended total abstinence from meat throughout the course of the disease and from drink during the first six hours. Ascribing the complaint to an interruption of perspiration, they ultimately directed all their efforts to the restoration of this discharge. On this account the patient was closely confined to bed. When such conservative efforts appeared unable to attain proper perspiration, medicines, wines and warm coverings were employed to accomplish this objective. The severity of the attack abated, in general, after a continuance of about fifteen hours; however, the period of danger did not terminate before the twenty-fourth hour. In some cases, it was necessary to renew the diaphoresis a second time; and, in a few robust constitutions, even up to twelve times. The worst complication ensued when the patient left his bed too soon.

The malady was remarkably rapid in its course, being sometimes fatal even in two or three hours, and some patients died in less than that time. More commonly, the serious phase lasted for a period of twelve to twenty-four hours. Those who survived for twenty-four hours were considered to have a good prognosis.

The disease, unlike the plague, was not especially fatal to the poor, but rather, as Caius affirms, to the rich who were high livers "according to the custom of England in those days." "They which had this sweat sore with peril of death were either men of wealth, ease or welfare, or of the poorer sort, such as were idle persons, good ale drinkers and tavern haunters."

A most peculiar feature of "sweating sickness" was the fact

that, when abroad in England the Scotch uniformly escaped while the English suffered horribly and even foreigners residing in England were not subject to attack. This has been blamed on the fact that the English dietary regime was richer and the habits of the Englishmen grosser than those of the inhabitants of other countries.

In the epidemics of 1528 and 1529, the disease spread much the same way as did cholera, arriving at Switzerland in December, and also spreading northwards to Denmark, Sweden and Norway. It also spread eastwards to Lithuania, Poland and Russia, and westward to Flanders and Holland.

In each place, it prevailed for a short time only; generally not more than a fortnight. During each epidemic, by the end of the year it had entirely disappeared, except in eastern Switzerland, where it lingered until the next year.

The epidemic, which occurred simultaneously at Antwerp and Amsterdam on the morning of the 27th of September, 1528, apparently came directly from England. England was the last to suffer from an outbreak of this disease and this occurred in 1551. This epidemic did not affect females and this was attributed to their greater temperance. With regard to the last epidemic, we have the account of an eyewitness, the eminent physician, John Kaye or Caius.

The most remarkable fact about this epidemic is that it spread over the continent, suddenly appearing at Hamburg, and spreading so rapidly that in a few weeks more than a thousand persons died. For some unknown reason, France, Italy and the southern countries were spared.[3]

The following is a brief abstract from "The Book of John Caius, Against the Sweating Sickness:"[4]

"This disease is not a Sweat only (as it is thought and called), but a feuer, as I saied, in the spirites by putrefaction venemous, with a fight, trauaile, and laboure of nature againste the infection receyued in the spirites, whereupon by chaunce followeth a sweate.

"That it is a feuer, thus I have partly declared, and more wil streight by the notes of the disease, vnder one shewing also by the same notes, signes, and short tariance of the same, that it consisteth in the spirites. First by the peine in the backe, or shoulder, peine in the extreme partes, as arme, or legge, with a flushing, or wind, as it semeth to certaine of the pacientes, flien in the same. Secondly by the grief in the liuer and the nigh stomacke. Thirdely, by the peine in the head, and madness of the same. Fourthly by the passion of the hart. For the Flusshing or wynde comming in the utter and extreame partes, is nothing els but the spirites of those same gathered together, at the first entring of the euell aire, agaynste the infection thereof, and flyeng the same from place to place, for their owne sauegarde.

"Thus under one laboure shortelie haue declared—both what this disease is, wherein it consistath howe and with what accidents it grieueth and is differente from the Pestilence, and the propre signes, and tokens of the same, without the whiche, if any do sweate, I take theym not to Sweate by this Sicknesse, but rather by feare, heate of the yeare, many clothes, greate exercise, affection, excesses in diets, or at the worst, by a smal cause of ingection, and lesse disposition of the bodi to this sickness. So that, insomuche as the body was nat al voide of matter, sweate it did when infection came: but in that the mattere was not greate, the same cloude neyther be perilous nor paineful as in others in whom it was greater cause." [5]

The symptoms of the disease are described as follows by Osler:

"The onset is abrupt with or without prodromata, the cardinal symptoms being fever, excessive, continuous sweating, great anxiety and depression with rapid and often tumultuous heart action and respiratory distress. After three to four days a rash appears, and with this the fever subsides slowly and slow recovery follows. Death may occur in a few hours or in from three to four days after onset. There is little reason to doubt the essential identity of miliary fever with the 'sudor Anglicus' or sweating sickness which swept over England between 1485 and 1551." [6]

In his textbook *The Principles and Practice of Medicine,* Osler states: "They (the epidemics) are usually of short duration, lasting only three or four weeks—sometimes not more than seven or eight days. As in influenza, a very large number of persons are attacked in rapid succession. In the mild cases there is only slight fever, with loss of appetite, an erythematous eruption, profuse perspiration, and an outbreak of miliary vesicles. The severe cases present the symptoms of intense infection— delirium, high fever, profound prostration, and hemorrhage. The death-rate at the outset of the disease is usually high, and, as is so graphically described in the account of some of the epidemics of the Middle Ages, death may follow in a few hours."[7]

Hirsch gives a chronological account of 194 epidemics of this disease between 1718 and 1887, many of which were limited to a single village or a few localities.

JOHN CAIUS (1510-1573)

John Caius, English physician was born at Norwich on the 6th day of October, 1510. He was admitted as a student at what was then Gonville Hall, Cambridge, where he seems to have studied mainly divinity. After graduating in 1533, he visited Italy, where he studied under the celebrated Montanus and Vesalius at Padua; and in 1541 he took his degree in physic at Padua. In 1543 he visited several parts of Italy, Germany and France; and returned to England. He practiced in London in 1547 where he was admitted as a fellow of the College of Physicians, of which he was for many years president. In 1557, being then physician to Queen Mary, he enlarged the foundation of his old college, changed the name from "Gonville Hall" to "Gonville and Caius College," and endowed it with several considerable estates, adding an entire new court at the expense of £1834. Of this college he accepted the mastership. He was physician to Edward VI, Queen Mary and Queen Elizabeth. He returned to Cambridge from London for a few days in June 1573, about a month before his death.

Dr. Caius was a learned, active and benevolent man. In 1557

he erected a monument in St. Paul's to the memory of Linacre. In 1564 he obtained a grant for Gonville and Caius College to take the bodies of two malefactors annually for dissection; he was thus an important pioneer in advancing the science of anatomy. He probably devised and certainly presented the silver caduceus now in the possession of Caius College as part of its insignia; he first gave it to the College of Physicians and afterwards presented it to the London College.

He published several medical works. The account of the sweating fever from his "A boke or counseile against the disease commonly called the sweate of sweatying sicknesse made by John Caius doctour in phisicke" published in 1552, is classic. Caius makes no reference to miliary vesicles, a characteristic finding in miliary fever.[8]

GUILLAUME DE BAILLOU (1538-1614)

One of the most distinguished doctors of the Renaissance was Guillaume de Baillou (Ballonius) of France. He was especially interested in epidemic diseases and was the first to describe the epidemic of whooping cough (1578) under the name of quinta or quintanta.[9] He also left a description of the plague of rheumatic fever and diphtheria. He was in favor of tracheotomy in cases of angina when it does not respond to other remedies. He, however, did not attempt to perform the operation. The credit for frequently opening the trachea for diphtheria goes to Marco Aurelio Severino (1610).

Here is a passage from his work *Epidemiorum et Ephemeridum libri duo*. It is with reference to a number of people suffering from a disease characterized by rapid and shallow respiration until death "which has the earmarks of diphtheria."

"They seemed to breathe as if dried up. Neither cough nor sputum. They were not able to hold their breath for a moment. The fever was not great, nor should it have made such breathing necessary. The physicians accused the lungs; others thought it to be a catarrh, others an inflammation or burning of the lungs,

though it was not likely since the fever had not been at all marked. Neither venesection nor purging was of avail. . . ."
"Another boy seven years old died of the same disease. Nothing was found of the origin of the illness and the cause of the difficult breathing. At this time, there raged a cough, commonly called Quinta. And since at intervals the cause of the Quinta cough was fleeting, the same certain cause produced it . . . This difficulty in breathing persisted until death. The son of Doctor le Noir died from this difficulty in breathing, hence he had this dog-like raucity and a little swelling of the pharynx. The right part of the lung was partly diseased. Gervais Honore my father-in-law died in the same manner almost suffocated. The surgeon said he sectioned the body of the boy with this difficult breathing, and with the disease (as I said) of unknown cause; sluggish resisting phlegm, was found which covered the trachea like a membrane and the entry and exit of air to the exterior was not free; thus sudden suffocation."[10]

Baillou also described as "Rubiola" a disease, occurring in 1574, with the characteristics of scarlatina, thus anticipating Sydenham's better known description.[11] Baillou's *Liber de Rheumatismo*, according to Major is the first to describe an affection under the name "rheumatism," recognizing both acute and chronic forms. The term used, to be sure, in a humoral sense, goes back at least to Galen, but not to Celsus or Hippocrates.[12]

Baillou was the son of a well known architect and mathematician of Paris where he was born and attended school. In the year 1570 he graduated from Paris University where he was a pupil of Jean Fernel. Ten years after his graduation he was selected dean of the medical faculty. At the same time he practiced medicine in Paris for a period of forty-six years where he was greatly honored not only as the most skillful physician but also as a most prominent citizen; thus when Henry Navarre became king of France Baillou was selected to welcome him to the city of Paris and present him the key of the city.

Baillou was among the first, if not the very first physician in France to rebel against the uncritical authority of Galen and the Arabian writers. He insisted upon the careful examination and study of the patient following closely the methods of Hippocrates.

FRANCISCO BRAVO (c. 1571)

A countryman of Villalobos in the sixteenth century was Francisco Bravo in whose work *Opera Medicinalia* is found a graphic description of diphtheria. It reads as follows:

"A fairly intense fever frequently attacks those affected by this malady, which lasts many days without any intermission; with the greatest fullness and distention of the veins, with the most intense severe lassitude of the entire body, and with pains, especially in the head, in which they suffer the most severe heaviness and pain, and most frequently with dizziness or symptoms of coma and delirium, with extreme redness of the face, with the mouth swollen and of a red color, with a large, forceful, fast and hard pulse, with uneasiness of the heart, with inexplicable thirst, and much dryness and harshness of the tongue, and blackness produced by the humors, and heaviness in the temples, and most intense heat of the entire body: so that they seem to be consumed: and it comes from these above mentioned troubles, and difficulty in breathing: in this disease all these vexing accidents happen, so that on the first day, or the second, or the third or the fifth, or the seventh, and so on the other days, there break out on the entire skin of the body, spots (pustulae) similar to fleabites, at first red or livid, or showing a black color when the intensity and severity of the complications are most severe." [13]

Bravo was born at Osuma, Spain, where he studied medicine but in later years he went to Mexico where he practiced medicine. He is the author of the work *Opera Medicinalia* in four volumes which was published in the city of Mexico in the year 1570 and it was perhaps the earliest medical publication in the New World. This disease was described by Frank Von Wird who also speaks of the ailment in 1517 as an epidemic by which the mouth and tongue were covered with something like moulds.

Diphtheria appeared six different times between the years 1583 and 1600 and was mentioned by the Spanish physician Juan de Villareal in 1600.

EURICIUS CORDUS (1534)

Scurvy is a disease described by Euricius Cordus in 1534. It appeared epidemically at sea and often also on land, especially on the coasts of the North Sea (Sweden, Norway, Finland, Denmark, Friesland, Prussia, the Netherlands and Lower Saxony). At this period, however, other diseases were included in the term "scorbutus" a condition in which worms accompanied with great pain are said to have developed in ulcers. This disease was described under the title *De Lopende Waren* by Hendrich Von Bra (died 1601) a prominent physician in West Friesland who prescribed for it maybugs while others ordered for it angleworms. In the period of the Crusades scurvy was distinguished from all other diseases. In the fifteenth century with more frequent and longer sea voyages it became still more distinctly diagnosed; e.g., in the case of Vasco Da Gama, 1498, when fifty-five sailors died of the disease.

When in the year 1535, the sailors of Jacques Cartier, on their exploration of the upper St. Lawrence River, were threatened with a severe epidemic of scurvy, they were saved by a decoction of tree bark and leaves, probably sassafras, prepared by the Indians. The benevolent effect of certain herbs in scurvy was also known to some Europeans. It is related that the Roman legion which attacked northern Holland was saved from annihilation of scurvy by the Frieslaenders, who knew of a certain antiscorbutic herb which had been employed in the Netherlands as a household remedy since the earliest times. The identity of the vital element inherent in certain herbs to combat scurvy known to ancients as well as to primitive people of modern times remained a secret until comparatively recent times.[14]

Other diseases recognized are epidemic and pandemic influenza. The first authetic pandemic occurred about 1580 commencing in the orient and spreading over North America and most of Europe. Thereafter epidemics of more or less widespread distribution and severity had occurred at approximately ten-year intervals.

It usually followed the wake of war and famine when it was attended by rapid dissemination. A second epidemic, beginning in 1557, was less widely extended. On the other hand, in 1580 and 1593 it became again pandemic, while in 1591 Germany alone was visited. It was estimated that the epidemic of influenza of 1918 and 1919 carried off half a million souls in America alone.

Erogotism also continued its epidemic visitations, down into the Modern Era, though in much milder form. Instead, however of the gangrenous form of the Middle Ages, the nervous form of the disease was characterized by itching, pains, rigidity, cramps, loss of consciousness, etc.

Small-pox is an ancient disease. The fathers of the church described the disease, and Marius in 570 A.D. was the first to use the term Variola. Rhazes (860-932) left a very remarkable description of the disease.

The pox was pandemic in Europe (1614) and occurred in the United States, especially in New England, reaching Pennsylvania in 1601. The term pox is derived from the Anglo-Saxon word "Pocca" and the prefix "Small" which served to exclude syphilis. Variolation, or the intentional transmission of the disease in mild form, had been practiced. The Chinese placed old powder crust into the nostrils. The Brahmans applied crust to the skin and the Persians ingested the prepared crusts. While in Europe clear fluid from a vesicle was transferred by a lancet. Small-pox was first observed or described in Germany in 1493. Measles, whose specific nature was still unknown to the physicians of the West, appeared in the sixteenth century. The following new epidemic diseases also appeared in the sixteenth century. Lead-poisoning, resulting from improperly stored cider or wine, broke out in the year 1572 in Southern France. Under the title of "The Hungarian disease" appeared (1566) a form of sickness intermediate between the plague and typhus fever.

Typhoid pleuro-pneumonia appeared epidemically in the sixteenth century, especially in Italy, France (1571) and in Switzerland. Typhoid fever was not differentiated from other pestilential scourges, notably the plague. Adequate descriptions of the symptomatology of typhoid fever are available from the beginning of the sixteenth century to differentiate it from other epidemic diseases.

During the sixteenth century epidemics occurred in Italy, Hungary and England. During the Thirty Years War disease ravaged central Europe, as usually follows in the wake of war with overcrowding and unsanitary conditions.

Malaria fever was known to Hippocrates who gave a clear description of quotidian, tertian, quartan and semi-tertian fevers. It was however impossible to distinguish it from other febrile conditions until the discovery of Cinchona bark and its specific actions upon febrile disease of malarial origins which was introduced by the Countess Cinchon in 1638 who was stricken by malaria and was advised by Don Lopez to use the Peruvian bark which resulted in her recovery, hence the name Cinchona.

Cholera had been endemic in the East from time to time; from there it spread to every part of the earth. Improved sanitation and health conditions are responsible for its disappearance. (The crema bacillus was discovered by Koch in 1883.) Finally whooping cough appeared in the sixteenth century on the list of epidemic diseases. Ballonius was first (1578) to describe it.

In the investigation of the diseases, the following prominent epidemiologists of the sixteenth century rendered valuable service: Fracastori, Victor de Bonagentibus (16th century), Giovanni Battista DaMonte (Montanus 1498-1552), Aloysia (or Luigi) Mondella, Professor of Padua, Giovanni Manardi (1462-1536), Johanna Weyer (Wierus 1515-1588), Nicolo Massa (1499-1569), Antonia Musa Brassalova (1500-1555), Amatus Lusitanus, Ercole Sassania (1510-1598), Albertino Bottoni (d. 1596), Johann Heurrnis (1543-1601), Batista Codronchi of Imola (15th century) and Fortunato Fetelle (1550-1630).

CHAPTER XLIV

THE LIBERATION OF MEDICINE

Up to the sixteenth century the universities, which possessed the sole power of authorizing physicians to practice medicine were in the hands of ecclesiastics. They decided upon the curriculum and upon the qualifications of the students.

Personal observation on the part of the teaching staff or practical experience on behalf of the student was taboo[1] and was punished by the supervising priests who insisted upon the use of the writings of Galen and Avicenna as interpreted by scholastic masters, as textbooks.

The efficiency of a certain remedy was not established by laboratory tests or by careful and repeated observation of its action upon a large number of patients, but by merely a chance trial on one case or by the testimony of one person and particularly if that person happened to be a King or a Prince, as was the case with antimony (referred to in the chapter on the renaissance of pharmacology, which was administered to Louis XIV who was ill with typhoid fever and recovered after taking the antimony). In consequence of this cure, antimony became a specific for all or many pathologic conditions for over a century; or as in the case of guaiac, which for a similar time was thought to be a specific for syphilis. The spirit of experimentation dawned in the Renaissance. The physician was no longer satisfied with the aphorism "post hoc, ergo propter hoc" ("after it, therefore because of it"). The fact that after taking a certain drug the pain stopped, was no proof of the efficiency of the drug; it might have stopped without it, and even if the drug caused the stoppage, there is no guarantee that it will act in the same way in another person. All pain does not arise from the same cause.

During the sixteenth century the higher schools of learning, one after the other gradually liberated themselves from ecclesiastic bondage. The Italian schools were first to shake off their dependence from the church. Next came the French universities and last, the Germans.

The senate of the Venetian Republic was the first to open the door of higher education to the public regardless of creed or nationality. Protestant and Jew enjoyed the same privileges as Catholic. When Pope Pius IV in 1565 decreed that the degree of doctor could be granted only to those who profess the Catholic faith, the Venetian Senate named a procurator with the power to grant degrees regardless of the faith of the candidate. A Jewish physician, Salomone Lotio, received a diploma from Count Sigismonde Capodilista (1589). The same Count conferred a degree on William Harvey in 1602. This example was soon followed by the senate of Padua and other Italian cities. They refused all church interference in academic matters. And the attempt of the Jesuits to establish a university of their own in Padua in 1591 did not materialize.

The most famous medical faculties were those of Bologna, Pisa and Padua, next to which ranked Paris and Montpellier and then Basel.

At a time when the rest of Europe was being destroyed by religious war, Italian universities enjoyed democratic rule. The students chose the rector and officers of the universities and even the teachers, and assisted in determining the curriculum of study. They also watched over the execution of the curriculum.

Impecunious students travelled from one school to another, united together into bands, supporting themselves by serenading, by begging and even stealing money, geese, hens, goats, fruits, etc. They prepared their food in the nearest lodging or even in the open fields. Yet many of these travelling scholars attained respectable positions.

Students at all times freely indulged in intoxicating drinks, for liquors were cheap and tippling was the order of the day.

Those students who were better situated financially usually tried to enter the famous universities of Italy or France. Among the celebrated physicians who studied in Italy during the Renaissance were the astronomer, Copernicus of Poland, Josephus Struthius (1510-78) from Hungary, Amatus Lusitanus of Portugal, Caius and Harvey, of England, Vesalius of Brussels and others.[2]

Excesses of various kinds were common in the Italian universities, especially during the Carnival. Jews were compelled to pay a certain sum of money into the students' carnival treasury.

The number of the students in the universities varied in accordance with the reputation of the school. Thus in the small university of Wittenberg in 1520 there were five hundred seventy-eight students while in Vienna the same year there were seven thousand. The largest enrollments were in the universities of Italy and France.

The cost of obtaining the doctorate generally amounted to 52 ducats—at that time a considerable sum of money. To this must be added the expense of presentation—gloves, of a special mass and banquets, besides presents to the professors.

As early as 1590 the privilege of practicing was granted to the students by resolution of the Faculty. The degrees of all universities were considered equivalent everywhere. The ceremony of graduation took place generally in church.

In Bologna the graduation fee was 40 ducats. This was considered high. In a few other European universities the cost was as low as six ducats. In many universities the newly graduated doctor had to take the following oath from the medical faculty: "I swear to you, the Dean of the Medical Faculty, and to both Professors, as well as to the other Doctors of the Faculty, obedience and reverence in everything honorable and allowable; that I will keep all the present and future statutes of this alma mater, and wherever I go I will keep in view her best interests. So may God and his Evangels be gracious to me."[3]

In Germany, the younger scholars, like the apprentices of the artisans, were obliged to perform the most menial duties for the upper classmen. They were compelled to beg, often to steal, and they enjoyed in return such protection as the fists of their stronger comrades could afford. A student might be received with humiliating ceremonies into the noble fraternity of scholars, and even be obliged, like slaves, to endure wild jokes and insults. Hazing as in the American colleges was practiced on younger students in the form of disgusting drinks, composed of phlegm, ink, stinking butter and candle—snuffs. Initiation by cuffs and kicks led to the honorable position of an academic citizen.[4]

In Bologna the number of teachers was fixed in 1579 at 166; in Rome in 1514 at 88, including fifteen teachers of medicine. The regular duration of lectures was at first two hours; subsequently it was reduced to one hour and a half, and then to only three quarters of an hour, as at present. Foundations and bequests in aid of poor students were not rare, and professors, particularly, distinguished themselves in this matter much more frequently than at present.

As a rule the members of the faculty were chosen for only one year and had to be reappointed for a further term of office. This arrangement kept the professors as well as the students who were more attached to them, in continual movement from one university to another.

Even Vesalius taught now in Padua, now in Pisa, now in Louvain and again in Basel, Augsburg and in Spain and Gunther von Andernach (1487-1574) taught in Louvain, Strassburg and in Paris. Consequently, the universities frequently changed their corps of professors. Teachers who were less known were obliged frequently to give a course of lectures on trial and free in order to secure a teaching position. Many of these itinerant scholars were so poor that they had to eke out a livelihood by begging, attending to odd jobs, and occasionally even stealing food while on the road, from one school to another.

The curriculum for the most part in the sixteenth century remained as that of the later Middle Ages. It consisted of discussion and elucidation of the "Aphorisms" of Hippocrates, the "Ars Parva" of Galen and the "Canon" of Avicenna. It took courage to introduce the new independent features for which the Renaissance was noted in medical schools. A century passed by the time they applied the experimental methods of their new science of medicine and before the universities assumed a modern form.

The renaissance of medicine began with anatomy. The old custom for the professor of reading anatomical texts from a high platform while an assistant was dissecting the body was gradually going out of fashion. Teachers of anatomy began to realize the importance of teaching anatomy not from books but from the cadaver. Practical anatomy was no longer viewed as a subject below the dignity of a professor. The cadaver was made "respectable" by reading before the dissection an official decree from the authorities to the effect that the procedure was in accordance with the law. The body was stamped on its chest with the seal of the university. After it was removed from the charge of the executor to the anatomic hall, the body was beheaded for opening the cranial cavity. However, the dissection even of criminals, was looked upon with aversion by the church.

Towards the end of the sixteenth century a number of anatomic amphitheaters sprang up. The first one, at Padua (1549), was constructed by Fabricius ab Aquapendente at his own expense. The second was in Montpellier (1551) and the third in Basel (1588).

In England, laws permitting dissection were passed in 1540 by authorizing the use of four executed criminals a year for teaching purposes. Because of the scarcity of cadavers it became necessary for the professor of anatomy to own a skeleton, the price of which was rather high. The price of a skeleton in Heidelberg in 1569 was equivalent to seventy-two dollars. At the end of the sixteenth century Bologna and Padua created special chairs for anatomy and surgery which were formerly combined and it made anatomy an essential part of the curriculum. They had previously been taught together because both were forbidden, and had to be taught more or less in secrecy. Old documents of Padua (1587) show that pathology also was made an essential branch of the school.

The rates of salary of teachers in the universities naturally varied. In general they were low; those of the German schools were the poorest. The professors at Heidelberg received an annual salary of only 85-105 florins; those in Wurtzburg, 219 marks with free board in the Julius Hospital. Melanchthon (1497-1560), one of the most famous physicians of his day received during his first eight years of practice a salary of 171 marks ($43.00) per annum, so that, during this period, he was unable to buy his wife a new dress; after 1526 his salary increased. Vesalius received 4,000 ($1,000). To this salary are, of course, to be added the fees for lectures and examinations (Baas, p. 444). They were compelled to make up the deficiency by pursuing other reputable occupations.

The Linacre foundation of Oxford and Cambridge provided for two professorships at $60 each per annum and one at $30. According to J. J. Walsh[5] the physicians' fees were about an eighth the amount of modern fees. The fees charged and the fees received by doctors from municipalities were also proportionally low, ranging from $4.25 to $43.00 per annum. Court physicians received from $35.00 to $939.00.

In Germany the treatment of the poor was gratis by law. A single visit in Germany was 1.65 marks or about 40¢; a night call 1.71 marks or 41¢; to a patient of moderate means, half that much. A consultation by letter 5 marks or $1.20; a simple advice by letter 1.50 marks or 36¢; a simple uroscopy 3¢; to foreigners a single visit 36¢, a second call 15¢.[6] For setting a fractured bone the charges were 10.50 marks.

On the other hand, specialists were well paid. Fernel received from Catherine Medici for each obstetric delivery 10,000 ecus. This may be multiplied by ten for she had ten children. It is not known how much Fernel left but Fabricius is said to have left 20,000 ducats not counting the great anatomic theater he built at his own expense. Berengario da Carpi left 50,000 ducats besides expensive furniture. Nicolo Massa (1499-1569) left a similar fortune. Most physicians of the Renaissance, however, died poor.

Syphilis and gonorrhea specialists have always done well even down to the days of Casanova (1725-1798). Thiery de Hery (d. 1599), the deputy barber-surgeon of the King, a syphilis expert, became immensely rich. The common people, in the sixteenth century, like in the medieval Arabian Period, were not quite advanced enough to go to a physician. They still stuck to the miraculous cures of relics of saints, or resorted to itinerant charlatans, sorceresses, vagabonds, drug-peddlers and similar quacks.

The Nuremburg ordinance permitted only sworn physicians to practice. "Empirics, like peddlers of theriaca, tooth-drawers, alchemists, distillers, ruined tradesmen, dealers in the black art, as well as old women who are accustomed to attend the sick and to boast that they possess the art of the doctors, and all such persons, are forbidden to treat the sick or to administer drugs to them, either publicly or secretly, without the permission of the council, under penalty of banishment if foreigners, or of a fine of twenty marks ($5.00), if residents of the city. Those who conceal or patronize them, shall suffer an equal punishment." The ordinance was likewise directed against the practice of uroscopy, because "nothing certain could be concluded therefrom." [7]

The physicians in the long velvet-trimmed, official doctors' robe, or in their fur pelisses, enjoyed great respect. Regularly educated physicians were for gentlemen and rich merchants.

The apothecaries fared even better if one may judge from a quarterly bill amounting to $216.00 sent to Queen Elizabeth for medicines. Pharmacists appear not to have been scrupulous in the conduct of the profession; they were carefully watched. Regular visits were made to supervise the quality of the drugs. In some places prices for drugs were stipulated by law.

That the average person was too poor to pay the expensive physicians may be inferred from the existence of books such as *An Apothecary for the Common Man, who cannot call the physicians* (1564).

Clinical instruction which was common in Rome, is seen from the bitter satire of Martial (150 A. D.), and later among the Arabians, that was discontinued in the Christian West for several centuries. It was revived at the University of Padua by

Albertino Bathoni (d. 1598) who discussed with students the possible diagnosis of the case at the bedside.

J. B. Montanus (1498-1552) is said to have been the first to give bedside clinical instructions to students. The first judicial post mortem was made by Ambroise Pare in 1562 after which the practice became more common. Post mortem examinations to verify diagnoses appear to have been practiced during the sixteenth century by certain professors. Emilio Campolongo (1589), professor of Padua, who was on the side of Brissot in the famous controversy over phlebotomy and who wrote on the subject of diagnosis is said to have carried away to his house the uterus of a woman patient for study. This appears to have caused a rumpus among women who finally succeeded in effecting the prohibition of such examinations for religious reasons.

In Bavaria professors were compelled by the church to take an oath not to mutilate dead bodies. The practice of clinical instruction (particularly on women) and pathological anatomical dissections in general had to be carried out with the utmost secrecy. According to some religious teaching, after the day of resurrection the absence of an organ may cause one to remain a cripple and particularly the absence of the uterus might deprive the woman of fecundity in the world of eternal life.[8]

Generally speaking, internal medicine during the Renaissance was not fortunate enough to produce men to measure up to Vesalius, Servetus and Pare; but lesser lights appeared. Germany brought forth a long list of eminent physicians who revolutionized the art of pharmacology and internal medicine.

Among the lesser lights who paved the way for the revival of medicine that followed the Renaissance was Amatus Lusitanus (1511-1568).

His descriptions and case histories show careful inquiry and observation. His *scholia* are often profound and interesting and cover a wide range of subjects. Anatomy is frequently touched upon. He writes: "A physician or a surgeon, who ventures to treat disease without an exact localizing diagnosis cannot but be regarded, like a carpenter with cataract, trying to cut the wood to build a chair."

Though he was a devoted follower of Galen, he was ready to deviate from his master when his own experience found Galen in error. Thus Amatus describes the optic nerve as not being hollow and the cavity of the human uterus as not being divided as Galen thought.[9] He demonstrated the structure of the mammary gland and showed that this explained why it is frequently necessary in suppuration of this organ to make multiple incisions.[10]

His description of an influenza epidemic is accurate and characteristic,[11] and he made a number of other interesting medical observations, such as the cachexia and the tumors of the spleen in quartan fevers. In treating dropsy he reduced the fluid intake and made use of hot sand baths. Although most of the seven hundred cases recorded by Amatus are medical, there are a large number of surgical interest.

Amatus stresses the duty of the physician to work with the surgeon, advising operations when surgery is indicated. In his early years he was at times obliged to operate, having had much surgical experience in Salamanca, but later he relinquished this practice. He introduced scarification to the surgeons of Belgium and Ferrara. In the use of leeches, he applied the method of cutting the full sucking leech in two, thus causing it to continue its activity for a much longer time.

In his medical practice, he laid great stress upon proper diet and general hygiene. He prescribed laxatives freely and explained that Hippocrates opposed them because the Greeks were unacquainted with those of mild action. He applied rectal feeding.[12] He was deeply interested, as we have seen, in the question of bloodletting, and laid stress upon various contraindications and restrictions in its use.

Amatus made the differential diagnosis in hydrocele by the use of transillumination with a candle. One of the most important contributions was the treatment of empyema. It was the custom to make the incision for drainage high up in the chest. On the basis of his anatomical studies he urged that the opening should be made in the lower intercostal spaces, so as to secure best drainage and yet do no damage to the diaphragm.[13]

Amatus devised a method of effecting nursing in retracted nipples by the use of small heated cups. A similar procedure was used by him to relieve the depression in the skull of the newborn. His method of closing a perforation in the palate with a gold plate and peg held in place with a sponge was perhaps the first model of an obturator.[14] Jos. F. Malgaigne (1806-1865) credits him with the invention of the trocar.

He popularized the use of the urethral bogie invented by Professor Aldarete of Salamanca (c. 1550). This instrument came into frequent use in consequence of the increasing frequency of syphilitic and gonorrheal strictures.

AMATUS LUSITANUS (1511-1568)

Amatus Lusitanus (Juan Ruderigo), was born in Castello Branco in Portugal, the son of a Marrano (a crypto-Jew, ostensibly baptized,) who had fled to safety from Spain to Portugal (1492).

Amatus entered the University of Salamanca, Spain, the most celebrated institution at that period ranking with Oxford with Bologna and Paris. The first two years at school he studied Greek logic, mathematics and music; then he spent an additional four years on philosophy (Aristotle), ethics, metaphysics, and medicine. Among his teachers in medicine were the royal court physician Pontanus Olivares and Alteretes (1550) both distinguished physicians of the time. Even before he graduated in medicine, Amatus was to take care of two local hospitals. After graduation in the year 1530 Amatus resided in Spain two years and about 1532 he returned to Lisbon. Soon hostilities broke out against the Crypto-Jews and Amatus had to leave Portugal. His new home was Antwerp (1533). Here Amatus resumed the practice of medicine for a period of seven years and he became known as a scholar and physician.

There he published the *Index Dioscoridites*, his first book on medical botany under his christian name "Joannes Rodericus Castelli Ab Lusitanus" (in the later works he assumed his Hebrew name, Amatus, the equivalent to the Hebrew Habib

'Beloved'). As his scholarly reputation spread he was invited to the University of Ferrara to lecture on Hippocrates and Galen. In Ferrara, Amatus felt very much at home. He enjoyed the friendship of famous scholars including A. M. Brassavola (1500-1555) who wrote on medical plants, G. Canano (1515-1579) the anatomist, and Wm. Falconer (c. 1781) the botanist whose herbal was said to have been the first of its kind. It is related that Canano performed dissections while Amatus read the portions of Galen pertaining to the part dissected. Amatus himself performed twelve dissections which was, considering the time, a good number. For some reason he resigned his professorship in Ferrara in 1547 and took up residence in Ancona. Perhaps there he also completed his commentary on Dioscorides. He was now thirty-eight years of age. In 1550 he was called to treat Pope Julius II in Rome whose sister he had previously treated. In the meantime he finished writing the second volume of his *Centuria* which he dedicated to Cardinal d'Este. The *Centuria* is the chief medical work of Amatus Lusitanus. It is divided into seven volumes. Each volume deals with one hundred case histories, notes and discussions and is elucidated with literary and personal references. In each case the anatomy, pathology and therapeutics are thoroughly discussed. Many of these discussions take the form of dialogue between him and his colleagues, a method popular in those days.

He returned to Ancona where he spent some time in peace but it was not for long. Pope Paul IV, the successor of Pope Julius, promulgated a decree forbidding the practice of medicine to Jews and Marranos alike. Many Marranos were arrested and punished severely. Amatus' home was broken into, all his valuables including manuscripts and books were taken from him. He saved himself by flight to Ragusa. The fifth volume of the *Centuria* was in manuscript and saved by friends, but his commentary on Dioscorides was lost. There he again worked up a big practice but he did not stay long. He left for Salonica where a large Jewish community exiled from Spain existed. There Amatus reverted to Judaism.

In Salonica he finished the seventh volume of his *Centuria*

(1561) and with this work his life story closed. It is believed that he died from the plague which was raging in that town. His epitaph reads as follows:

"He who so often halted the spirit fleeing from the dying body,
  now has been summoned to the waters of Lethe;
He who showed loving kindness equally to the people and to the
  great—here lies mortal Amatus embracing this earth.
Lusitania was his home: His lonely grave finds its place in the
  Macedonian earth, far from his fatherland,
For his great day, his day of death, came and the fatal hour and
  led him to the Stygian river; the way goes forward
  directly to the other world." [15]

GEROLAMO MERCURIALE (1530-1606)

Psychiatry was studied carefully by Gerolamo Mercuriale (1530-1606), who, already in the sixteenth century, maintained that the frequency of melancholia was occasioned by the life of pleasure and luxury to which people were giving way in ever-growing numbers. It is caused by disturbances of the several faculties. He identifies three classes of mania: sanguinous, bilious and melancholic. For the first he recommends phlebotomy, for the second he prescribes cholegoges and the third frequent purgation and the cautery.[16]

FELIX PLATTER

Felix Platter referred to in the chapter of anatomy made the first attempt to classify psychoses. He distinguished four types of mental disease: (1) "Mentis imbecilitas" (state of mental weakness); (2) mentis consternatio, cases where mental activities are temporarily suspended as in epilepsy, catalepsy, and apoplexy; (3) mentis alienatio (Mania), hydrophobia and phrenitis and (4) mentis defatigatio (hyperexcited state). He was among the first who came out against using force in mental cases.

ABRAHAM ZACUTUS (LUSITANUS, 1575-1642)

Zacutus was born in Lisbon, Portugal. He was of the fourth generation of physicians by that name. His great grandfather,

Abraham Zacutus of Spain was a celebrated astronomer, philosopher and physician who left books on various scientific subjects.[17]

Zacutus Lusitanus studied medicine at Coimbra and Salamanca receiving the degree of M.D. when he was twenty-one years of age (1596). He then returned to Lisbon where he was engaged in the practice of medicine for a period of thirty years. He was known for his profound scholarship, for his linguistic abilities, his judgements and above all his professional skill. A cruel edict by the King of Lusitania against Jews forced him to seek refuge at the age of fifty in Amsterdam, Holland. Here too, his scholarly and professional talents soon became known. In 1629 appeared his *De Medicorum Principum Historia*. Then in rapid succession, came volume after volume, to the year of his death in 1642. It is interesting to note that none of his books were published in Lisbon where he practiced for thirty years; all of them were published in the last twelve years of his life in Amsterdam.

Zacutus was an experienced pathologist. He missed no opportunity to make autopsies in cases where the cause of death was in doubt, such as heart affections, renal and vessical calculi, malignant tumors, etc. In each case he published his findings. As a clinician he was skillful. He employed all means at his disposal to reach an accurate diagnosis. He was particularly known for his investigation of plague, eruptive fevers, diphtheria, malignant growths, etc. According to Garrison he was the first to describe "black water." He made valuable contributions to our knowledge of syphilis and its treatment.

While Zacutus was a faithful follower of Galen it did not prevent him from showing his independence and devotion to progressive tendencies.

In his description of the human body he places the veins under the head of the liver and the arteries with the heart. The vena cava has the function of carrying the blood to the stomach and intestines. In the controversy over the circulation of the blood following the discovery of Harvey, Zacutus stood on the side of Galen but this did not prevent him from showering praise on Harvey for his careful studies.

His *Opera Omnia* published shortly after his demise shows that he possessed a phenomenal knowledge of the medicines of his predecessors. Volume one deals with the "history of great physicians" being the histories of internal disease which are found scattered in the works of foremost physicians most carefully arranged in proper order and supplied with explanatory notes and commentaries together with a review of questions and matters of doubt as gathered from records. He described the histories of four hundred and thirty-three physicians.

Sprengel (1766-1833) praises him for the well ordered and carefully explained collection of cases of older writers as well as his own observations and experiences in rare cases.

The second volume of his *Opera Omnia* deals with the practice of cases in which all diseases are explained according to the views of the leading physicians. The book contains a synopsis of precepts to be followed by physicians entering upon practice. There are eighty precepts with their commentaries. Next comes the pharmacopoeia of sixty-two pages. The practice of medicine is divided into five books (1) treatment of the head; (2) treatments of disease affecting the "vital" and "natural" parts, Morbus Gallicus, pneumonia, pleurisy, aphonia, empyemia, gastric disturbances, disease of the liver, diabetes, vesical and renal calculi, dropsy, etc.; (3) diseases of women; (4) fevers; (5) treatment of fever symptoms. The volume ends with gratitude for divine help. In discussing objectively medical problems, he states "the physician should be a faithful worshipper." However, he remarks "for me physics are not theologies."

The text of the first volume covers nine hundred and eighty-four pages of double columns, that of the second volume, eight hundred and three pages.

JEAN FERNEL (1497-1558)

Jean Fernel classified diseases into three kinds (1) of tissues (2) of organs (3) and those depending upon loss of cohesion. Even though he still adhered to the humoral theory of diseases, his *Universa Medicina* is a work well systematized. He divides it into physiology, pathology, and therapeutics. His pathological description was perhaps the first book in Europe that may be called a text book on this subject.

He was of the opinion that the seat of the soul was in the brain where the sensory nerves originated. The motor nerves came from the membrane and the blood originated in the liver. He assigns semen to women as well as to men and holds that the testicles in men do not escape through the openings in the peritoneum but follows this membrane as a prolongation. He follows Galen in his two former ideas and opposes him in the two latter ideas. He is the famous author of the *Universa Medicina* of the Renaissance. He was born near Amiens, France, and served as physician to Henry II.

Among other physicians may be mentioned Alessandro Masari (1510-1598). He published some writings on small pox and plague. He was a Galenist and he originated Maxims; e.g., "It is better to err with Galen than to maintain the right with the moderns."

JOHANN SCHENCK (1531-1598)

A famous physician of Strassburg and Freiburg is the author of *Observationum Medicorum Rerum*, published in 1597, in which he combines his own experience with many concise pathological reports from practically all important works since classical times with an index and in orderly manner. Among others may be cited his reference to Avenzoar's work in ventrical gastric cancer. Schenck insisted upon the value of post mortem examination in all doubtful cases.

NICOLO MASSA (died in 1569)

Massa was the best known syphilographer of his time. He used mercury and decoctions of sarsaparilla in syphilis. Many patients came to him for treatment from all parts of Europe.

He described cases where the contagion reached them by

fomites. He was the first writer to point out that syphilis is the cause of mental disease. He regarded it as contagious and the cause of articular pain. He is thought to have been the first to describe gummata (materia alba viscosae) in his book *De Morbo Gallico*. His birth place was Padua.

FORTUNATO FEDELES (1550-1630)

A great independent physician of Palermo was Fortunato Fedeles. He disputed all authority particularly on therapeutics; even Hippocrates. He was against specifics. No medicine in many cases is the best treatment. He was the first physician to develop the subject of state medicine or legal medicine. His book the *Relationes Medicorum* was published in Palermo in 1602. He pointed out the injurious effect of lead pipe in the conduction of drinking water.

ANDREW BORDE (died in prison 1549)

Andrew Borde graduated from Montpellier and became professor at Oxford. He wrote, *A Breviarie of Health* and *A Dietary of Health* published at Oxford in 1562. He was humorous, and in the habit of frequenting gay parties. Hence arose the expression "merry Andrew."

If the Renaissance did not achieve the aim medicine was striving for (for indeed the science of medicine is endless), it served as the means to rid the art and science of medicine from much of the rubbish that had accumulated throughout the ages. Most practitioners still were disposed toward faith cures, astrology, uroscopy, relics, amulets, incantations and other superstitions.

The celebrated physician of Germany, Menlanchthon, was a devoted astrologer, and eminent physicians like Jean Fernel (1497-1558), Caspar Peucer (1525-1602), and Anthon De Haen (1704-1776), were known to believe in demons and devils. With regard to the etiology of disease, Luther recognized the influence of Satan as most prominent. His son Paul (1533-1593), who was a physician, believed in alchemy. He was physician and alchemist to Joachim II of Brandenburg and to Elector Augustus of Saxony.

THOMAS BROWNE (1605-1682)

One of the most eminent physicians in England at the early part of the next century was Thomas Browne author of *Religio Medici* and *Vulgar Errors*. He still believed in astrology and in alchemy. Although he studied in universities where ideas were more advanced, Dr. Browne was aware that he was living in a double faced age, one looking back to the old world of mystery, wonder and belief, and the other looking forward to the time when men would clear up the mystery with experiments and would substitute knowledge for belief.

ROBERT BOYLE (1627-1691)

The prominent English natural philosopher Robert Boyle, still hoped to find the philosophers' stone. He believed in alchemy, in the transmutation of metals, and carried on experiments in the hope of achieving it.

The most enlightened physicians, however, acquired a scientific knowledge of medicine, developed an independent view of tradition, and freed themselves from metaphysics and dialectics. The celebrated physician was not satisfied with studying only his own art, he also was interested in classic literature, in the sciences and in the arts in general.

The doctor of the Renaissance as pictured by his contemporary artists possessed a dignified expression and a scholarly demeanor seldom seen in the vendor of the medicinal herbs or the dealer displaying his urine bottle.

The physician, as depicted by Hans Holbein the Younger (1538), in his wood-cut series *The Dance of Death*, is dressed in the garb of the contemporary scholar. While death, holding a urine bottle in one hand, leads a patient into the office, the doctor is seated on a cushioned bench at his table upon which may be seen a book and an hourglass. On the shelf attached to the wall above the bench, eight books are arranged, quite a considerable collection considering the period.

The physicians mentioned by Benvenuto Cellini (16th century) in his *Memoirs* convey a vivid idea of the dignified manner in which medicine was practiced during the latter part of the sixteenth century. The most valuable edition of books in the newly invented press, had the most beautiful illustrations of anatomic works of Leonardo, and Michelangelo.

During the period of the Renaissance, Jewish physicians of Spain, Portugal and Italy helped each other to transmit Arabic medicine in the West. By the fourteenth century the Provençal Jews had lost the knowledge of the Arabic language but had learned Latin and set about translating medical works from Latin into Hebrew. Some of the writings of Bernard Gordon were translated by John de Avignon (Moses Ben Samuel of Roccambra) under the name Perah ha-Refua (1359) and a second time under the title of Shashan ha-Refuah (1387) were translated by Bonsenhor Solomon (Jekutiel Ben Solomon of Narbonne).

DIONYSIUS BRUDUS (1478-1522)

Another prominent physician who fled from Portugal to escape persecution was Brudus. A native of Portugal, he was court physician to King Manuel and professor at the University of Paris. He is the author of a criticism of Pierre Bissot for his opinion on blood letting. His son was Manuel Brudus (16th cent.). His work on diet and fevers passed through several editions as did his *De Ratione Victus* (Venice, 1544). He, like Amatus, fled from Portugal to escape the Inquisition.

ANDRES A. LAGUNA (1499)

Andres A. Laguna (1499) was the son of Fernando of Laguna who studied at the University of Salamanca and was given a degree of doctor of medicine in Toledo (1530). He wrote a commentary of Galen and a treatise on anatomy and materia medica. He died in 1563.

CRISTOVAL D'ACOSTA (16th century)

Acosta was a royal physician to the hospital of Cochin and was the author of five books, chief of which is *Tractado de Las Drogas Midicinos las India*. (Burgas, 1575).

ELIAHU (ELIJAH) MONTALTO (PHILOTHEUS 1550-1616)

He belonged to a family of Marranos[18] and is the author of *Optica* and *Arcipathology* (Paris, 1614). He was born in Castelbranco. He received his medical education in Salamanca but because of his religion he fled to Italy. He became physician to Ferdinand of Florence in 1606 and in 1611 he became personal physician to Maria de Medici and King Ludvig. His *Arcipathology* which appeared in 1614 was frequently mentioned by Burton in his *Anatomy of Melancholy* and by Abraham Zacutus Lucitanus.

RODRIGO DE CASTRO (1560-1675)

Another prominent physician was Rodrigo de Castro (1560-1675). Castro settled in Hamburg where he distinguished himself during the plague epidemic of 1596. In 1603 he wrote an extensive work on obstetrics and gynecology. His fame was so great that the King of Denmark repeatedly consulted him. He also left a description of the plague of Hamburg (1596). His son Benedict de Castro graduated from Leyden and also settled in Hamburg where he earned much fame as a physician. He was appointed personal physician to Queen Christine of Sweden.

GARCIA DA ORTA (16th century)

Garcia was born in Portugal toward the end of the fifteenth century and he acquired his medical degree from Salamanca (1534) where he practiced medicine for a period of thirty years. There he published his *Coloquios* a study of medical plants of India (1563). In commemoration of his 400th anniversary Silva Carvalho author of *History of the Lisbon School of Medicine and Surgery,* published an account on his life, in which he states that Garcia was of Jewish descent, that his sister was burned at the stake and that Garcia's bones were exhumed and burned because he relapsed back to his ancestral faith.

DAVID DE POMIS (c. 1555)

David de Pomis studied medicine in Perugia where he received his degree in 1551. He settled in Magliano where he occupied the dual position of Rabbi and doctor. On account of the anti-Jewish edicts of Pope Paul IV (1555-1559) he fled to Venice where he was allowed to practice. A decree which prohibited the practice of Jewish physicians at Venice caused him to flee again. He wrote a splendid defense of Jewish physicians and was the author of many other works among them the Hebrew work *Zemach David.*

Another famous physician was Joseph Solomon Delmedige (1591-1655). He was born in Candia and received his education at the University of Padua where he studied under the great Galileo who acquainted him with Copernicus' astronomical system. His chief interests were mathematics and astronomy.

The account of the Renaissance of medicine comes to an end with the translation into English of *The Regimen Sanitatis Salernitatis,* by Sir John Harrington (1561-1612). Harrington, although not a physician, was esteemed by his contemporaries as a man of great culture and wit. He is the author of *Metamorphosis of Ajax* and various works that introduce the reader to the improved knowledge of sanitary engineering, among them the invention of the modern water closet.

The frontiers that lay uncharted in the sixteenth century have yielded their secrets but today's discoveries are no less significant for they will profoundly affect man's enjoyment of his stay on this earth.

In our atomic age, the spectacular explorers have been the physicists and mathematicians. Quietly, however, the biochemists are widening our knowledge of our physical selves as they prove the mysteries of cellular life by identifying uncountable physiological and pathological chemical compounds and chemical reactions. The relations of these to physical and mental diseases and such complex processes as antibody formation are only now beginning to come to light.

NOTES

CHAPTER I

1. Gibbon, Edward: *The Decline and Fall of the Roman Empire,* New York, Collier, 1899, vol. IV, pp. 311-313.
2. Gibbon, Edward: Opus cited, p. 312.
3. Singer, C.: *Medieval Contributions to Modern Civilization,* Harrap, London, 1921.
4. Singer, C.: *A Short History of Medicine,* Oxford, Oxford University Press, 1928, p. 62.
5. Cited by Coulton, G. G.: *Medieval Panorama,* Cambridge, Cambridge University Press, 1939, p. 744.
6. Reliable sources date it to the 18th century because a few medical writers of the 18th century, including Boerhaave (c. 1736), Anton Van Haen (1758), and James Currie (1797), refer to it as a useful implement for diagnostic purposes. The first to describe the modern clinical thermometer was C. R. A. Wunderlich who did so in the year 1868.
7. Arturo Castiglioni: *A History of Medicine,* New York, Knopf, 1941, pp. 262-264.
8. A collected edition of the works of Constantine was published in Basle in 1539.
9. A leading production of the School of Salerno was the *Breslau-Codex* most of which has been produced in the collection of De Renzi in 1853-6 and Giasca 1901.
10. Jabir, ibn Hayyan, The Arabic works, ed. by E. J. Holmyard, London, 1928. Bertholot believed that the knowledge of Jabir was much less than that of the Latin "Geber." Sarton stated that the other Arabic work still untranslated shows that Jabir was a much better alchemist. *Introduction to History of Science,* ed. by E. J. Holmyard, London, 1928, vol. I, p. 532.

CHAPTER II

1. Cited by Draper, J. W.: *History of the Intellectual Development of Europe,* New York, Harper, 1876, vol. 1, p. 254.
2. Gordon, B. L.: *Medicine Throughout Antiquity,* Phila., F. A. Davis, 1949, pp. 619-621.
3. Castiglioni, A.: *A History of Medicine,* New York, Knopf, 1941, p. 273. Coulton, G. G.: *Medieval Panorama,* Cambridge, Cambridge University Press, 1939, p. 455.
4. John 5:14.
5. I Corinthians 11:30-33.
6. Luke 5:13.
7. Mark 5:26.
8. James 5:14-15.
9. Acts 19:12.
10. Gibbon, E.: *The Decline and Fall of the Roman Empire,* Collier, vol. I, p. 55.
11. St. Jerome: *Lives of the Fathers,* E. F. Farrar, Edinburgh, 1889, vol. II.
12. Ecclesiasticus 38:1 (Vulgate).
13. Ecclesiasticus 38:4.
14. Isaiah 26:12.
15. Translation by Wright, F. A.: in "Select Letters of St. Jerome," London and New York, letter 52, p. 225. Nepotian, an ex-soldier and nephew of a bishop in Venetia, had asked St. Jerome for advice as to a young cleric's duties.
16. The last is a teaching of Plato.
17. Gregory. *Lives of the Fathers,* E. F. Farrar, Edinburgh, 1889, vol. II.
18. Tertullian: *Lives of the Fathers,* E. F. Farrar, Edinburgh, 1889, vol. II.
19. Neuburger, M.: *History of Medicine,* London, Henry Prowde, 1910, pp. 314-316.
20. Neuburger, M.: *History of Medicine,* Oxford, Oxford University Press, 1925, vol. II, part I, p. 8.
21. Deaber, P.: *Body and Soul,* p. 268.
22. White, A. D.: *History of the Warfare of Science and Theology,* vol. II, p. 201.
23. Fort, G. F.: *History of Medical Economy during the Middle Ages,* p. 201.
24. Translation by Wallis Budge, E. C.: *The Book of the Dead,* New York, Barnes and Noble, 1951, p. 676.
25. Palestinian Talmud: Rosh Hashana 56a.
26. Gordon, B. L.: Oculists and Occultists; Demonology and

the Eye, *Archives of Ophthalmology,* July 1939, vol. 22, pp. 21-23.

27. Moses, A. J.: *Pathological Aspects of Religion,* p. 133.

28. Gordon, B. L.: Oculists and Occultists; Astrology and the Eye, *Archives of Ophthalmology,* Jan. 1941, vol. 25, pp. 36-61.

29. Gordon, B. L.: *The Romance of Medicine,* Phila., F. A. Davis, 1944, p. 307.

30. Cutten, G. B.: *Three Thousand Years of Mental Healing,* New York, Scribner, 1911, p. 66.

31. Montgomery, J. A.: Aramaic Incantation Texts from Nippur, Phila., University of Pennsylvania Museum, 1913, p. 67.

32. Cutten, G. B.: *Three Thousand Years of Mental Healing,* New York, Scribner, 1911, p. 102.

CHAPTER III

1. Lecky, W.: *History of European Morals from Augustus to Charlemagne,* vol. II, London, 1869.
2. A six volume edition of his remaining work was published by Bussemaker and Daremberg. *Oeuvres d'Oribase,* Paris, vol. VI, 1856-1876.
3. Meyerhof, M., and Sobhy, G. P.: *The Abridged Version of the Book of Simple Drugs,* Cairo, 1932, p. 8.
4. Neuburger, M.: *History of Medicine,* trans. by Playfair, E.: London, Oxford Univ., Press, 1910, vol. I, pp. 301-303.
5. In this chapter some of the quotations are from Caelius "On Acute and on Chronic Diseases" as translated by I. E. Drabkin and published by the University of Chicago in 1950. Caelius was the means for the transmission of Greek medicine to the *Middle Ages.* He belonged to the methodist school.
6. Neuburger, M.: Ibid, 332.
7. This is a Hippocratic method.
8. Aetius, Tetrabiblos, translated by Shastid, T. H.: *The American Encyclopedia and Dictionary of Ophthalmology,* Chicago, Cleveland Press, 1917, pp. 8633-8688.
9. For a complete translation of Aetius' ophthalmology, see the Tetrabiblos, translated by Shastid, T. H.: in *The American Encyclopedia and Dictionary of Ophthalmology,* Chicago, Cleveland Press, 1917, pp. 8633-8688.
10. *Outline of the History of Medicine*: by John Herman Baas, translated by H. E. Handerson, and published by Wm. R. Jenkins Co., New York, p. 201.
11. Hamilton W.: *History of Medicine, Surgery and Anatomy,* 1831, vol. 1, pp. 176-187.
12. Friend, J.: *History of Physic from the Time of Galen to the Beginning of the 16th Century,* London, 1725-26, p. 169.
13. Friend regards him as second only to Hippocrates, p. 169.
14. Neuburger, M.: Opus cited, p. 334.
15. Cited by Neuburger, M.: ibid., p. 335.
16. Hamilton, W.: *History of Medicine, Surgery and Anatomy,* London, 1831, vol. 1, part 1, pp. 176-186.
17. Adams, F.: *The Seven Books of Paulus Aegineta,* London, Sydenham Society, 1844, vol. I, p. XV, editor's preface.
18. Garrison, F. H.: *History of Medicine,* Philadelphia and London, W. B. Saunders Co., first edition 1914, p. 84.
19. Adams, F.: Opus cited, p. XVIII.
20. The first classical description of the plague was made by Thucydides (460-339 B.C.). Another was made by the poet Ovid

(43 B.C.-19 A.D.). Still later Boccaccio left a description in 1026 A.D.

21. Adams, F.: Opus cited, pp. 277-278.

22. Paul of Aegina, *Opus de re medica. Liber tertius,* Venice, Arrivabenum, 1542, chapter XLIII, p. 120b; cited by Major, R. H.: *Classic Descriptions of Disease,* Springfield, C. C. Thomas, 1948, p. 313.

23. Adams, F.: Opus cited, p. 414.

24. Adams, F.: *The Seven Books of Paulus Aegineta,* London, Sydenham Society, 1844-1847, in three volumes.

25. De Urinis, chapter 20, cited by Baas, J. H.: *Grundriss der Geschichte der Medizin und des Heilenden Stands,* Stuttgart, 1876, translated by Henderson, H. E.: under the title: *Outlines of the History of Medicine and the Medical Profession,* New York, 1889, p. 234.

CHAPTER IV

See: Gordon, B. L.: Lay Medicine during the Early Middle Ages, *The Journal of the Michigan State Medical Society*, v. 57, July 1958, pp. 1001-1007 and 1034.

1. Castiglioni, A.: *A History of Medicine*, trans. by Krumbhaar, E. B., New York, Alfred A. Knopf, 1941, p. 290.
2. Neuburger, M.: *History of Medicine*, translated by Playfair, E.; London, Oxford University Press, 1925, vol. 2, part 1, p. 6.
3. The Alemanni were an ancient people of Southwestern Germany.
4. This translation was made by order of Ferdinand III, in 1241, and formed the basis of Spanish medieval law.
5. Two *solidi* was the price of an ox. Hence this fee for a private venesection is very high.
6. Baas, J. H.: *Grundriss der Geschichte der Medizin und des Heilenden Stands*, Stuttgart, 1876, translated by Handerson, H. E., under the title: *Outlines of the History of Medicine and Medical Profession*, New York, J. H. Vail, 1889, p. 240.
7. Laws of Sudermania; compiled 1327.
8. Neuburger, M.: *Geschichte der Medizin;* Stuttgart, 1911, vol. 2, part 1, p. 246.
9. Baas, J. H.: Opus cited, p. 234.
10. Ibid. p. 242.
11. Neuburger, M.: Opus cited, note 2, pp. 4-11.
12. Baas, J. H.: Opus cited, p. 242.
13. Refer to fine English translation of the first two parts of Theodoric's *Chirurgia* by Eldridge Campbell and James Colton published in 1955 by Appleton and Company, New York.

CHAPTER V

See: Gordon, B. L.: Medicine in the Koran, *The Journal of the Medical Society of New Jersey*, v. 52, Oct. 1955, pp. 513-523.

1. It will be shown that many medical tenets in the Koran are found in the Talmud.
2. Leviticus 32:4.
3. Koran 12:41.
4. Old Testament: Genesis 40:9.
5. Koran 16:80.
6. According to Dschellal Edden it should read, "against cold." See Ulmann: *Der Koran*, Crefeld, 1840, 16:80.
7. In preparing this chapter on medicine in the Koran, the writer has availed himself of the English text of Al-Haj Hofiz Ghulam Sarwar's Koran, Singapore, 1923-1928, translated from the original Arabic text with critical essays on the life of Mohammed. The text of George Sale's (1647-1736) translation of the Koran published in Oxford in 1734, has also been employed. Frequent reference has also been made to Opitz, K.: *Die Medizin im Koran*, Stuttgart, Von Ferdinand Enke, 1906.
8. Koran 20:84.
9. Koran 6:46.
10. "The eyes flinched and the beats of the heart reached the throat." Koran 23:10, 40:18.
11. Koran 69:46.
12. Koran 76:2.
13. Koran 23:13-14.
14. Koran 32:8-9.
15. A similar concept is found in the Midrash (a term applied to a series of works which explain the Pentateuch): Leviticus Rabba 14.
16. Koran 86:6-7.
17. Perlman, M.: *Midrash haRephuah*, Tel Aviv, 1926, vol. 3, p. 3.
18. Koran 77:20.
19. Dicta of the Fathers 3:1.
20. Koran 39:6.
21. Koran 19:16.
22. Compare with Talmud: Kethuboth 60.
23. Koran 2:233.
24. Koran 2:233.
25. Koran 2:233, 65:6.
26. Koran 28:12, 20:40.
27. Sotha 12:6.

28. Koran 4:23.
29. Koran 4:23.
30. Koran 4:24.
31. Koran 24:3, 4:24-25.
32. Koran 5:49, 6:152.
33. Koran 58:2-3.
34. Koran 4:34.
35. Koran 4:34.
36. Koran 36:56-57.
37. Koran 37:43-48.
38. Koran 4:3.
39. Herbetat, D.: *Bibliotheque Orientale,* Paris, 1904, p. 602.
40. Koran 2:226, 72:28.
41. Koran 2:28.
42. Koran 33:48.
43. Koran 65:4-7.
44. Koran 2:234.
45. Ulmann: *Der Koran,* Crefeld, 1840, p. 483.
46. Koran 2:222.
47. Koran 112-223.
48. Koran 2:103.
49. Koran 2:233.
50. Old Testament: Leviticus 12:1-6.
51. Cited by Frazer, J. G.: The Golden Bough; Taboo and the Perils of the Soul, New York, Macmillan, 1935, p. 155.
52. Gordon, B. L.: *The Romance of Medicine,* Philadelphia, F. A. Davis, 1944, pp. 20-22.
53. Koran 7:80-81.
54. Koran 4:20.
55. Koran 16:60-61.
56. Koran 6:152.
57. Sprengel, K. P.: *Versuch Einer Pragmatischen Geschichte der Arzneikunde,* Halle, 1792-1799, vol. II, p. 76.
58. Koran 4:33.
59. Koran 4:91, 8:12.
60. Koran 17:35.
61. Koran 17:35.
62. Koran 2:173.
63. Koran 5:4, 8:175.
64. Koran 38:41.
65. Koran 26:27.
66. Koran 3:25.
67. Koran 3:25.
68. Koran 113:5.

69. Koran 16:16.
70. Koran 37:88, Sale's Koran p. 368.
71. Babylonian Talmud: Baba Bathra 16b.
72. Koran 25:7.
73. Koran 113:4.
74. Koran 12:82.
75. Psalms 6:8.
76. Koran 35:8.
77. See Old Testament: Genesis 18:12.
78. Koran 40:28.
79. Koran 65:16.
80. Koran 9:35.
81. Koran 9:35.
82. Koran 22:20.
83. Koran 54:11.
84. Koran 7.77-78.
85. Koran 26:189.
86. Koran 105:1-4.
87. Sprengel, K. P.: Opus cited, vol. I, p. 461.
88. Gottfried, G: *A History of Epidemology,* Halle, 1776.
89. Old Testament: Genesis 19:24.
90. Koran 19:24-25.
91. Koran 69:67.
92. Koran 69:8.
93. Koran 46:24-25.
94. Puschmann, T.: *Handbuch der Geschichte der Medizin,* Jena, Fischer, 1902, vol. I, p. 98.
95. Koran 2:49.
96. Koran 5:110.
97. Koran 7:108, 26:23.
98. Koran 20:22.
99. Sprengler: *Das Leben und die Lehre des Muhammed,* Berlin, 1869.
100. Moheprem Bey: War Muhammed Epileptiker? *Psychiatrisch-neurologische Wochenschrift,* 1902, pp. 355-367; see also Sprengler: Opus cited, p. 201.
101. Old Testament: Numbers 24:4.
102. Referring to Moses; Koran: 25:1.
103. Koran 26:80.
104. Bruzon: *La Médicine et les Religions,* Paris, 1901, p. 59.
105. Koran 38:42.
106. Koran 12:84.
107. Koran 12:96.
108. Koran 37:146.

109. Old Testament: Numbers 19:9.
110. Old Testament: Leviticus 19:8-9, 22:46.
111. Ibid., 15:5-10.
112. Old Testament: Ezekiel 26:25.
113. New Testament: Revelations 21:6.
114. Koran 47:1-5.
115. Koran 2:25.
116. Koran 47:16.
117. Koran 6:70.
118. Koran 76:5.
119. Koran 2:216, 5:90-91.
120. Koran 16:69.
121. Koran 67:17, 83:27.
122. Koran 4:43.
123. Koran 2:116, 48:27.
124. Koran 24:61.
125. Koran 2:183-184.
126. Koran 73:20.
127. Koran 2:55-61.
128. Koran 16:72.
129. Koran 52:22.
130. Koran 55:22.
131. Koran 49:12.
132. Koran 6:144-145.
133. Koran 6:146.
134. Koran 5:1.
135. Koran 6:140.
136. Koran 6:146.
137. Koran 6:147.
138. Koran 56:21.
139. Koran 56:21.
140. Koran 16:68-69.
141. Koran 44:43-45.
142. Old Testament: Genesis 40:16; Koran 12:36.
143. Koran 16:69.
144. Koran 16:48.
145. Koran 16:68.
146. Avicenna: Cannon, vol. 2, fen. 12, tractate 1, chap. 1.
147. Koran 16:38.
148. Old Testament: Genesis 17:10-11.
149. Koran 18:8-25.
150. Koran 18:17.

CHAPTER VI

See: Gordon, B. L.: Arabian Medicine in the Post-Koranic Period, *The Journal of the Michigan State Medical Society*, v. 55, Sept. 1956, pp. 1109-1116.
   1. Baas, J. H.: *Grundriss der Geschichte der Medizin und des Heilenden Stands*, Stuttgart, 1876, translated by Handerson, H. E., under the title: *Outlines of the History of Medicine and the Medical Profession*, New York, J. H. Vail, 1889, p. 220.
   2. Neuburger, M.: *History of Medicine*, translated by Playfair, E.; London, Oxford University Press, 1910, vol. 1, p. 363.
   3. The most complete English translation is that of Sir Richard Burton in 25 volumes which contains more than 200 stories, many of which include other stories making a total of almost 400 stories. The present writer has availed himself of the following edition: Burton, R. F.: *The Book of the Thousand Nights and a Night*, printed by the Burton Club for private subscribers only, 1885, vol. V, pp. 218-227.
   4. A number of Talmudic academies flourished at that period in Mesopotamia, namely: Nisibis, Nehardea, Pumpeditha and Sura. The last was still in existence at the end of the seventh century.
   5. Burton, R. F.: Opus cited, vol. V, p. 218.
   6. Ibid. p. 218.
   7. Ibid.; cf. Midrash:Tadshei 6.
   8. The chemical composition of four elements was the teaching of the ancient Greeks which was still in vogue at the time of Galen, and for centuries after.
   9. Burton, R. F.: Opus cited; cf. Targum:Jonathan ben Uziel; Old Testament:Genesis 3:77.
   10. Mishna:Oholot 1:8.
   11. Cf. Midrash:Genesis Rabba 3; Kohelet Rabba 7.
   12. Cf. Midrash:Genesis 2:2.
   13. Cf. Babylonian Talmud; Berochot 19; Hulin 45.
   14. This teaching is entirely modern. It is to be noted that these faculties were believed by all ancients including the Scripture and the Koran to be located in the heart.
   15. Cf. Mishna:Oholot 1:8.
   16. It is believed among the Hebrews that the body will be built from that bone on resurrection day. It was known as "luz" or "nut"; cf. Midrash:Leviticus Rabba 18; Kohelet Rabba 12:5.
   17. Cf. Mishna:Oholot 1:8.
   18. Zohar: vol. 3, pp. 221, 225 and 232.
   19. Koran 7:39.
   20. Educated Arabs can quote many a verse bearing upon

domestic medicine and reminding us of the thoughts bequeathed to Europe by the School of Salerno.

21. Personal cleanliness was a feature of the Arab world as the lack of it was characteristic of contemporary Europe. The scrupulous cleansing doubtless arose from the frequent ablution required by Moslem prayer and other rules of life.

22. Crumbled bread and hashed meat in broth; or bread, milk and meat. The Saridah of Ghassan, cooked with eggs and marrow, was held to be a dainty dish: hence, the Prophet's dictum.

23. Koran 2:216.

24. Liberal Moslems observe that the Koranic prohibition is not absolute and there is no threat of Hell for infraction. Yet Mohammed doubtlessly forbade all inebriatives and the occasion of his so doing is well known.

25. Many of these regulations are found in Talmudic literature.

26. According to the text, Tawaddud hesitated to answer this question and hung her head in shame and confusion before the Caliph's majesty. Thereupon the Caliph insisted that she answer.

27. This notion is of great antiquity.

28. The Hebrew Korah. Old Testament:Numbers 16. This follows a Talmudic tradition that Korah was immensely wealthy.

29. All the aforementioned text is taken from Burton, R. F.: Opus cited, vol. V, pp. 218-27.

30. Burton, R. F.: Opus cited.

31. Cf. Pickthall, M.: *The Cultural Side of Islam*, The Committee of "Madras Lectures" on Islam, 1927.

CHAPTER VII

1. Jonisabur or Gundê-Shāpūr was founded by the Sasanian Jundī-Sābūr (Arabic) or Gundê-Shāpūr. Campbell, D.: *Arabian Medicine and Its Influence on the Middle Ages*, London, Kegan Paul, Trench, Trubner, 1926, vol. 1, p. 46.
Shapur I, after he defeated Emperor Valerian and sacked Antioch, he named it Veh-az-Andevi-i-Shāpūr, which means "Shāpūr is better than Antioch." This in time became contracted into Jondisabur.

2. Bass, J. H.: *Grundriss der Geschichte der Medizin und des Heilenden Stands*, Stuttgart, 1876, translated by Handerson, H. E., under the title: *Outlines of the History of Medicine and the Medical Profession*, New York, J. H. Vail, 1889, p. 218.

3. Browne, E. G.: *Arabian Medicine*, Cambridge, Cambridge University Press, 1921, p. 23. Sarton, G.: *Introduction to History*, vol. 1, p. 435.

4. Wustenfeld, F.: *Geschichte der Arabischen Aerzte und Naturforscher*, Gottingen, 1840, p. 4-5.

5. Ibid., p. 5.

6. Translated by Meyerhof, M.: The abridged version of the *Book of Simple Drugs of Ahmad ibn Muhammad al Ghafiki*, Cairo, G. P. Sobhy, 1932.

7. In Arabic the proper name, *"abu"* or *"ebu"* signifies father and *"ben," "ebn"* or *"ibn"* denotes son or descendant; *"al," "el,"* or *"il"* is the article, and the name following represents the native country, city of birth, or father's occupation, etc. The Arabic sounds are not so sharply defined to our ears that variations in the mode of writing cannot arise. In the West, Arabic proper names often undergo such changes that the original and correct orthography is no longer recognizable. As examples of this process we may include the following names: Georgius, Averroes, Avicebron, Abimeron, Avicenna, Avenzoar, etc.

8. Derived from the Syriac or Hebrew *"keneseth"* meaning "collection."

9. Freind, J.: *The History of Physick*, London, 1750, part 2, p. 9.

10. Von Wolff: *Phil. Geschichte der Arabischen Aerzte und Naturforscher*, Stuttgart, 1837, vol. 2; cited by Wustenfeld, F.: Opus cited.

11. Pruefer, C. & Meyerhof, M.: *Die Augenheilkunde das Juhanna ibn Masawaih der Islam, Isis*, vol. 6, pp. 217-268; vol. 7, p. 108; vol. 8, p. 717.

12. Guilaume, A.: *Philosophy and Theology*; cited by Kertram Thomas: *The Arabs*, New York, Doubleday Doran, 1937, p. 187.

13. See Campbell, D., Opus cited, p. 64.
14. Meyerhof, M.: Introduction to "The Ten Treatises on the Eye," Cairo, 1928.
15. Steinschneider, M.: *Die Europaischen Übersetzungen aus dem Arabischen*, Vienna, 1904-1905, p. 18.
16. Campbell, D.: Opus cited, p. 62.
17. Meyerhof, M.: New Light on Hunain, *Isis*, 1926, vol. 8, p. 708.

CHAPTER VIII

1. Freind, J.: *The History of Physick*, London, 1750, p. 49.
2. Ibid., p. 41.
3. Campbell, D.: *Arabian Medicine and its Influence on the Middle Ages*, London, Kegan Paul, Trench, Trubner, 1926, vol. 1, pp. 72-73.
4. Wustenfeld, F.: *Geschichte der Arabischen Aertze und Naturforscher*, Gottingen, 1840, pp. 54-55; Brockelmann, C.: *Geschichte der Arabischen Litteratur*, Weimar, 1898, vol. 1, p. 231. According to Sarton, the first translation of the "Almagest" into Arabic was made by Ali al Tabari. Sarton, G.: *Introduction to the History of Science*, vol. 1, p. 565.
5. Wustenfeld, F.: Opus cited, p. 36.
6. The edition of 1486 weighs seventeen pounds. Haller believes it to be the best Arabic treatise ever published.
7. This is, incidentally, the only manuscript extant in the Egyptian National Library in Cairo.
8. According to the "Pandect" of Rhazes.
9. See Gordon, B. L.: *Medicine Throughout Antiquity*, Phila., F. A. Davis, 1949, pp. 676-677.
10. Abu Bekr Muhammad ibn Zakariya al Razi: *A Treatise on the Smallpox and Measles*; English translation by the Sydenham Society, 1848, p. 32.
11. Ibid., p. 32.
12. Al Razi: "A Treatise on Smallpox and Measles," cited by Major, R. H.: *Classic Descriptions of Disease*, third edition, Springfield, C. C. Thomas, 1948, pp. 196-197.
13. See Gordon, B. L.: Opus cited, pp. 708-719.
14. Meyerhof, M. and Sobhy, G. P.: *The Abridged Version of the Book of Simple Drugs of Ahmad ibn Muhammad al Ghafiki*, Cairo, 1932, p. 26.
15. Baas, J. H.: *Grundriss der Geschichte der Medizin und des Heilenden Stands*, Stuttgart, 1876, translated by Handerson, H. E., under the title: *Outlines of the History of Medicine and the Medical Profession*, New York, J. H. Vail, 1889, pp. 220-221.
16. Neuburger, M.: *History of Medicine*; translated by Playfair, E.: London, Oxford University Press, vol. 1.
17. Baas, J. H.: Opus cited, p. 221.
18. Major, R. H.: Opus cited, pp. 196-197.
19. The "Hawi" was posthumous, the work having been compiled from unfinished notes by Rhazes' pupils. Neuburger, M.: Opus cited, vol. 1, p. 361.
20. Leyden, 1903.
21. Campbell, D.: Opus cited, vol. 1, pp. 74-75.

22. The exact date of his birth is not clear but these dates are given by most of the Arabic authorities.

23. Ishak Israeli should not be confused with Ishak ibn Amran al Baghdadi, a Moslem physician of Bagdad who emigrated to North Africa and entered the service of Ziyadath Allah ibn al Aghlab, ruler of Kairawan, now Tunisia, who reigned 816-837 A.D.

24. Wustenfeld, F.: Opus cited, p. 32.

25. Hirsch, A.: *Biographisches Lexikon der Hervorragenden Aerzte alter Zeiten und Voelker,* Vienna and Leipzig, 1884, pp. 287-289.

26. Seligsohn, M.: *The Jewish Encyclopedia,* New York & London, Funk & Wagnalls, 1904, vol. 6, pp. 670-671.

27. Singer, C.: *Medieval Contributions to Modern Civilization,* London, Harrap, 1921, p. 144.

28. Campbell, D.: Opus cited, vol. 1, p. 74.

29. Wustenfeld, F.: Opus cited, pp. 51-52.

30. Neuburger, M.: Opus cited, vol. 1, p. 360.

31. Wustenfeld, F.: Opus cited, p. 51; also Sprenger, A.: *Geschichte der Aerzneikunde,* vol. 7, p. 270; also Seligsohn, M.: Opus cited, article on "Israeli, Isaac"; published in *The Jewish Encyclopedia,* New York & London, Funk and Wagnalls, 1904, vol. 6, pp. 670-671; also Husik, I.: *A History of Mediaeval Jewish Philosophy,* New York, Macmillan, 1916, pp. 1-16.

32. Dawson, B.: *The History of Medicine,* New York, Macmillan, 1932, pp. 66-76.

33. Garrison, F. H.: *History of Medicine,* Philadelphia & London, W. B. Saunders, first edition, 1914, p. 80.

34. Campbell, D.: Opus cited, vol. 1, p. 79.

35. Garrison, F. H.: Opus cited, p. 88.

36. Wallace, W., in an article on "Avicenna" in The Encyclopedia Britannica, 11th edition, Cambridge, 1910, vol. 3, pp. 62-63.

37. Wustenfeld, F.: Opus cited p. 13.

38. Steinschneider, M.: *Die Europäischen Übersetzungen aus dem Arabischen,* Vienna, 1904-5, vol. 1, pp. 39-40.

39. Neuburger, M.: Opus cited, vol. 1, p. 370.

40. Campbell, D.: Opus cited, vol. 1, p. 77.

41. Withington, E. T.: *Medical History from the Earliest Times,* London, 1894, p. 172.

CHAPTER IX

1. Arabic tradition ascribes the first grammar in the Arabic language to Abul Aswad Ud-Du-Ali (latter half of the seventh century). From early times the Arabians have been proud of their language and its systematic study was stimulated by their contact with the Persians and particularly because of their respect for the language of the Koran.
2. The ancient Tadmor in the Syrian desert; Old Testament: II Chronicles 8:4.
3. In northeastern Mesopotamia, the Biblical Accad; Old Testament: Genesis 10:10.
4. Browne, E. G.: *Arabian Medicine*, Cambridge, Cambridge University Press, 1921, p. 15.
5. Adams, F.: *The Seven Books of Paulus Aegineta*, London, Sydenham Society, 1844, vol. III, p. 17.
6. Gordon, B. L.: *Medicine Throughout Antiquity*, Philadelphia, F. A. Davis, 1949, p. 362.
7. Curiously enough, that which has appeared so utterly impossible, has become a reality in this Atomic Age. It has lately been demonstrated that base metals such as mercury can be converted into gold, but so far, the cost of this process is too prohibitive to make it remunerative.
8. Others hold that "chemia" is of Greek origin, meaning "pouring" or "infusion." They state that this word was first used in connection with the study of juices of plants and thence extended to cover chemical experiments in general.
9. All of these are Arabic terms, according to Garrison, F. H.: *History of Medicine*, Philadelphia and London, W. B. Saunders, first edition, 1914, pp. 86-96.
10. Meyerhof, M. and Sobhy, G. P.: *The Abridged Version of the Book of Simple Drugs*, Cairo, 1932, Introduction, p. 3.
11. Arabic "rabi al ghar" or "powder of the mine"; arsenic disulphide.
12. Campbell, D.: *Arabian Medicine and Its Influences on the Middle Ages*, London, Kegan Paul, Trench, Trubner, 1926, vol. I, pp. 54-55.
13. Jacobs, J.: *Jewish Contributions to Civilization*, N. Y., Jewish Publication Society, 1909, pp. 201-203.
14. Ibid., pp. 201-203.
15. Baas, J. H.: *Grundriss der Geschichte der Medizin und des Heilenden Stands*, Stuttgart, 1876, translated by Handerson, H. E., *Outlines of the History of Medicine and the Medical Profession*, N. Y., J. H. Vail, 1889, pp. 236-237.
16. Sherwood, F.: *The Founders of Modern Chemistry*, New York, 1949.

CHAPTER X

1. Gibbon, E.: *The Decline and Fall of the Roman Empire,* N. Y., P. F. Collier, 1899, vol. 3, p. 90.
2. Neuburger, M.: *History of Medicine,* translated by Playfair, E.; London, Oxford University Press, 1910, vol. 1, p. 353.
3. Abulkasim: *Chirurgia,* section 30.
4. Neuburger, M.: Opus cited, p. 366; also, Baas, J. H.: *Grundriss der Geschichte der Medizin und des Heilenden Standes,* Stuttgart, 1876, translated by Henderson, H. E., under the title: *Outlines of the History of Medicine and the Medical Profession,* N. Y., J. H. Vail, 1889, p. 231
5. Spink, M.: *Proceedings of the Royal Society of Medicine, 1936-1937,* 30, part 1, pp. 653-670.
6. Hamilton, W.: *History of Medicine, Surgery and Anatomy,* London, 1831, vol. I, pp. 280-288.
7. Neuburger, M.: Opus cited, vol. I, p. 379.
8. Friend, J.: *History of Physic,* London, 1750, part 2, p. 125.
9. Hamilton, W.: Opus cited, vol. I, p. 250.
10. Neuburger, M.: Opus cited, vol. I, p. 391.
11. Baas, J. H.: Opus cited, p. 231.
12. Campbell, D.: *Arabian Medicine and its Influence on the Middle Ages,* London, Kegan Paul, Trench, Trubner, 1926, vol. I, p. 91.
13. *Encyclopedia Britannica,* 11th edition, Cambridge, 1910, vol. 3, p. 54.
14. Wustenfeld, F.: *Geschichte der Arabischen Aerzte und Naturforscher,* Gottingen, 1840, pp. 88-91.
15. Garrison, F. H.: *History of Medicine,* Phila. and London, W. B. Saunders, first edition, 1914, p. 90; also Baas, J. H.: Opus cited, p. 231.
16. Steinschneider, M.: *Die Hebraischen Übersetzungen des Mittelalters,* Berlin, 1893, p. 65.
17. Wustenfeld, F.: Opus cited, pp. 88-91.
18. This was an ancient belief. It was based on the supposition that the male only possesses the fertilizing germ and that the female part in procreation is that of an incubator. This theory is also found in the Babylonian Talmud: Haaigah 16.
19. Garrison, F. H.: Cited by Campbell, D.: *Arabian Medicine and its Influence on the Middle Ages,* London, 1926, vol. I, p. 94.
20. The present writer is particularly prompted to enlarge upon the medical history of the literary giant because of the lack of proper appraisal of his greatness on the part of many historians.

21. Meyerhof, M.: In *Essays on Maimonides* (edited by Baron, S. W.), New York, Columbia University Press, 1941, p. 266.

22. This letter to Japhet, written eight years after the death of his brother David, is published in Graetz, H.: *History of the Jews,* Phila., Jewish Publication Society, vol. 4, p. 338, 1894.

23. Richard I, the Lion Hearted, of England. See article by Broyde, I.: *The Jewish Encyclopedia,* N. Y. and London, Funk & Wagnalls, 1905, vol. 9, p. 74.

24. Gordon, B. L.: *New Judea,* Philadelphia, Greenstone, 1909, pp. 12-13.

25. Meyerhof, M.: Opus cited, p. 270.

26. Broyde, I.: *Jewish Encyclopedia,* N. Y. and London, Funk & Wagnalls, 1905, vol. 9, p. 74.

27. Maimonides: Iggereth Temon, 2.5.

28. The passages in the Babylonian Talmud Berachath 10b and Pessahim 56a to the effect that King Hezekiah destroyed the medical books which had been approved by the sages is explained by Maimonides on the premise that the books contained magical, idolatrous and superstitious methods of treating the people which lured them into idolatry.

29. Morei Nebuchim, 3:29:37.

30. Sarton, G.: Introduction to the History of Science, Carnegie Institute, 1931, vol. 2, p. 371.

31. Meyerhof, M.: Opus cited, p. 274.

32. Steinschneider, M.: Opus cited, p. 763.

33. Meyerhof, M.: Opus cited, p. 265.

34. Ibid.

35. Meyerhof, M.: Opus cited, p. 282.

36. Responsa of Maimonides. Cited by Yellin, D. And Abraham, I.: *Maimonides,* 1913, pp. 140-146.

37. Adler, E.: Epistle, etc., Miscellany of Hebrew Literature, London, 1872, p. 219. Also see Marx, A.: *Moses Maimonides,* New York, 1935, Centennial Series, vol. II, p. 271.

38. Yellin, D. and Abraham, I.: Opus cited, pp. 155-156.

39. Dambary, J.: *Neubauer's Medical Jewish Chronicle,* p. 117.

40. Maimonides, M.: The Guide for the Perplexed, 2:4.

41. Ibid.

CHAPTER XI

1. As a matter of fact, it is difficult to say in the case of Arabic culture where the Jew ends and the Arab begins, so important and essential were its Jewish factors. (Wells, H. G.: *The Outline of History*, 1921, pp. 600-601.)
2. Cited by Jacobs, J.: *Jewish Contributions to Civilization*, Philadelphia, 1919, p. 194.
3. Cited by Steinschneider, M.: *Zeitschrift der Deutschen Morgenländischen Gesellschaft*, vol. 24, pp. 253-354.
4. Cited by Jacobs, J.: Cantor's Geschichte der Mathemitik, Leipzig, 1880, 1:612, p. 149.
5. Cited by Jacobs, J.: Opus cited, p. 151.
6. Sarton, G.:*Introduction to the History of Science*, 1927, vol. I, p. 479.
7. Meyerhof, M.: *The Book of Simple Drugs*, Cairo, 1932, p. 10; Wüstenfeld, F.: *Geschichte der arabischen Aerzte und Naturforscher*, Gottingen, 1840, pp. 79; Puschmann, T.: Gesch. der Medizin, 1:557, Vienna, 1902.
8. Aloy: *Dictionary of History of Medicine,* listed under *Isaac ben Imran.*
9. Wüstenfeld, F.: *Geschichte der arabischen Aerzte und Naturforscher,* Göttingen, 1840, p. 86.
10. *Jewish Encyclopedia,* vol. 8, pp. 414-415.
11. This abridged list of translators is based upon Steinschneider's "Hebraeische Uebersetzungen," pp. 770, 764, 769, 694, 704, 711, 780, 730; Sarton's "Introduction" II, 719-764.
12. The writer has availed himself of the privilege to draw upon the scholarly article on Jewish physicians of the Middle Ages by Dr. Fredrick T. Hanemann, *Jewish Encyclopedia*, 2nd edition, 1904, vol. 8, pp. 414-417, and Harry Friedenwald: *The Jews in Medicine,* vol. 2, pp. 551-700, Johns Hopkins Press, Baltimore, 1944.
13. Mémoires à l'Histoire de la Faculté de Médecine de Montpellier, Paris, 1767, pp. 8-15.
14. Ibid., pp. 6-18.
15. Ibid., p. 168.
16. Garrison, F. H.: *An Introduction to the History of Medicine,* Phila. and London, W. B. Saunders, first edition, 1914, p. 102.
17. The diploma was awarded by the "Sanctum Collegium" presided over by the local bishop as Chancellor of the University.
18. Sarton, G.: Opus cited, p. 614.
19. Venetianer, L.: *Deutsche Litterature Zeitung,* 1917, pp. 30,

388; Asaf Judeaus, der aelteste Medezinische Schriften in Hebraische Sprache, Präger, Budapest, 1915-16, p. 140.

20. Munter, S.: On the Age of Asaph the Physician, Harephuah, 1948, vol. 33, pp. 10-12.

21. Talmud, Oholoth 1:8.

22. The Talmud gives the number of blood vessels of the human body as 365: Makoth 23b.

23. A Talmudic concept.

24. Talmud Niddah 30, Mid. Terumah 3.

25. Talmud Niddah 38.

26. Talmud Niddah 31.

27. Talmud Niddah 30.

28. Munich Manuscript, folio 7, Venetianer, Asaph Judaeus, Budapest, 1916, p. 117, Sarton, G.: Opus cited, vol. I, p. 614; *Jewish Encyclopedia* vol. II, pp. 162-3.

29. Steinschneider, M.: *Sefer Hayakar,* Berlin, 1867, p. 1.

30. Sarton, G.: Opus cited, vol. I, p. 682.

31. Introduction to Sefer ha Yakar.

32. Steinschneider, M.: Donnolo, Fragment des aeltesten Medizinischen Werkes in hebräischer Sprache, Berlin, 1867, Introduction I.

33. Steinschneider, M.: Donnolo 38:71, cited by Gordon, B. L.: Curiosities of Jewish Medicine, *Bulletin of History of Medicine,* vol. 20: no. 2, July, 1946.

34. Another copy of this "Book on Pharmaceutical Products" was discovered by Professor Alexander Marks, and this is almost identical with Steinschneider's copy. The Marks manuscript was in the possession of the late Dr. Harry Friedenwald of Baltimore until willed to the University of Jerusalem.

35. See the scholarly thesis of Sigmund Muntner, Harofe Haivri, vol. 2:86-97, 1946.

36. Singer, C.: *Medieval Contributions to Modern Civilization,* Harrap, London, 1921, p. 120.

37. Bartholiny: *Revue des Etudes Juives,* vol. 46, cited by Friedenwald, opus cited, vol. I, p. 127.

38. Friedenwald, opus cited, vol. I, p. 287.

39. Ibid., vol. I, p. 218.

40. Ibid., vol. I, p. 218.

41. Ibid., vol. I, p. 219.

42. Ibid., vol. I, pp. 217-218.

43. Schleiden, M. J.: *Principles of Scientific Botany,* Berlin, 1942-43.

44. Address on Morgagni delivered in 1894 before the International Medical Congress in Rome.

45. Garrison, F. H.: Opus cited, p. 94.

CHAPTER XII

1. Isis N. 64, 1935, p. 543.
2. This is the person famous for his amour with Heloise (1105-1164) which finally occasioned his castration by his inhuman enemies.
3. Patterson, A. S.: *The Philosophical Radicals*, London, 1891, cited by *Encyclopedia Britannica*, 11th edition, vol. 19, p. 735.
4. Immense labor and intellectual enthusiasm were often vainly spent. The Royal Society itself is said to have devoted itself *ad nauseum* to the discussion of Charles II's malicious question: "Why does a living fish weigh more than a dead one?"
5. Neuburger, M.: *History of Medicine*, trans. Playfair, E.: London, 1910, Henry Frowde, Oxford University Press, 2 volumes, vol. II, p. 55.
6. Sarton G.: *Introduction to the History of Science*, Carnegie Institute of Washington, 1931, vol. II.
7. *Essays on the History of Medicine*, Oxford, 1924, p. 139.
8. Riesman, D.: *Medicine in the Middle Ages*, Paul B. Hoeber, New York, 1935, pp. 79-81.
9. Sarton, G.: Opus cited, 1931, vol. II, pp. 952-967.
10. Neuburger, M.: Opus cited, pp. 56-57.
11. The original Greek version of the Old Testament was begun about 270 B.C.
12. This very important translation was at first wrongly ascribed to William of Moerbeke.
13. Sarton, G.: Opus cited, vol. II, pp. 583-4.
14. This name seems odd as there were nineteen popes named John before him.
15. Thorndike, L.: *History of Magic and Experimental Science*, Macmillan, 1923, vol. 2, p. 490.
16. Corner: *Annals of Medical History*, January, 1931, New Series, 3:9.
17. Storches, T. D. von: *Annals of Medical History*, 1930, 2:614.
18. Diepgen, P.: *Des Meisters Arnold von Villanova*, Parabeln der Heilkunst, Leipzig, 1922.
19. Sarton enumerates 80 volumes by Arnold. Opus cited, vol. II, pp. 873-890.
20. Englernig, Gertrude:*Bulletin of the History of Medicine*, June, 1940, vol. 8, No. 8, pp. 770-784.
21. Le Mayen: *Medical Age*, Paris 1888, p. 24.
22. *Epistle*, 307.

23. Handerson: *Gilbertus Anglicus*, Cleveland, 1918.
24. Neuberger, M.: Opus cited, vol. II, p. 63.
25. Reisman, D.: Opus cited, pp. 87-89.
26. Baas, J. H.: *Seventeen Lectures*, 1886, p. 90, 422-23.

CHAPTER XIII

See: Gordon, B. L.: A Short History of Spectacles; *The Journal of the Medical Society of New Jersey*; January 1951, vol. 48, pp. 3-8.

1. Dampier, W. C.: *History of Science*, Cambridge University Press, p. 54, 1943.
2. George Sarton considers this work the most remarkable experimental research in history. "Introduction to the History of Science," vol. 1, p. 274, 1927.
3. Psalms 6:8.
4. Talmud:Yoma 76 B.
5. *Historia Naturalis*, Book 37, chap. 5.
6. Sarton, G.: Opus cited, vol. 2, pp. 1024-25.
7. Kitab al Manzir: "The Optical Thesaurus of Alhazen," translated from the Hebrew into Latin by Gerard of Cremona.
8. *Opus Majus*: Bridges' translation, 2:72, London.
9. On the testimony of Jardeno di Rivalto the discovery occurred sometime after 1285. See Sarton, vol. 2, p. 1025.
10. Thompson, C. J. S.: *The Origin and Development of Spectacles*, Turin, 1942, p. 8.
11. According to a letter sent by Dr. Andrea Corsini of Florence there is no such epitaph, but the Chapel of the Virgin in Santa Maria Maggiore contains a marble head said to represent Salvino and a marble tablet bearing the inscription quoted above. However, Salvino is not buried here. Sarton, vol. 2, p. 1025.
12. Thompson, C. J. S.: Opus cited, p. 8.
13. Donders, F. C.: *Hints on the Use and Selection of Spectacles* (Arch. of Ophth., 4:301, 1858); See also: *Astigmatismus und Cylindrische Glaser*, Berlin, 1862.
14. Littell: *Manual of Diseases of the Eye*, Philadelphia, 1836, p. 255.
15. Friedenwald, H.: *The First Medical Refraction*, Arch. of Ophth., January, 1934, vol. 11, pp. 67-80.
16. According to Sir Duke Elder the first to consider the question of astigmatism was Sir Isaac Newton; *Practice of Refraction*, P. Blakiston Sons & Company, 1928, p. 119. See also Gordon, B. L.: *The Problem of the Crystalline Lens*; Arch. of Opthth., May, 1936, vol. 15, pp. 859-889.
17. Posey, W. C.: *Wills Hospital of Philadelphia*, J. B. Lippincott Co., 1931, p. 5.

CHAPTER XIV

1. Baas considered the universities to be "the greatest element in the emancipation of the human spirit." Baas, J. H.: *Grundriss der Geschichte der Medizin*, Stuttgart, 1886. Translated by Handerson, H. E.: *Outlines of the History of Medicine*, New York, 1910.
2. Baas, J. H.: Ibid. p. 223.
3. Singer, C.: *Evolution of Anatomy*, London, 1921, p. 65.
4. Gurlt's classical *Geschichte der Chirurgie*, Berlin, 1898, vol. 1, p. 673.
5. Rashdall, H.: *Medieval Universities*, Oxford, 1895, vol. I, pp. 126-127.
6. Castiglioni, A.: *A History of Medicine*; translated by Krumbhaar, E. B.; New York, 1941, p. 327.
7. Rashdall, H.: Opus cited, vol. I, p. 126.
8. *Universities of Europe in the Middle Ages*, vol. I, opposite the introduction.
9. Rarely one of the books mentioned below is substituted. No examination or practice was apparently required for an M.A. to become an M.D. By a statute of Henry V, (Rot. Parl. iv, 130) the Council is empowered to make regulations for preventing non-graduates from practicing anywhere in England. However, the dearth of doctors in England rendered any such regulations quite futile.
10. Rashdall, H.: Opus cited, vol. III, p. 156.
11. Rashdall, H.: Ibid. vol. I, p. 245.
12. Baas, J. H.: Opus cited, p. 326.
13. Stampers, M.: cited by Puschmann, T.: *History of Medical Education from the Most Remote to the Most Recent Times*, trans. and edited by E. H. Hare, London, 1891, pp. 240-241.
14. Rashdall, H.: Opus cited; Coulton, G.: *The Medieval Panorama*, Cambridge University Press, 1939, pp. 431-432.
15. Perhaps the most exhaustive work is that of Rashdall referred to above.
16. Rashdall, H.: Opus cited, vol. I, p. 128.
17. Garrison, F. H.: *History of Medicine*, Philadelphia and London, W. B. Saunders, first edition, 1914, p. 117.
18. Rashdall, H.: Opus cited, vol. I, p. 128.

CHAPTER XV

1. The "heel and toe" of the Italian peninsula remained Greek in spirit and language throughout its domination by Rome except perhaps the southern part. After the decline of Rome's power it escaped much of the fury of barbaric invasion, so that some scholarship was still possible.
2. See Chapter 10.
3. Haeser, H.: *Lehrbuch der Geschichte der Medizin*, Jena, 1875-82, vol. 2:62.
4. Elinus was followed by Hillel ben Samuel of Verona (1220-95), who translated Bruno's work on surgery entitled "Chirurgia Bruni" into Hebrew.
5. Baas, J. H.: *Outlines of the History of Medicine and the Medical Profession*, translated by Handerson, H. E.: J. H. Vail & Co., New York, 1889, p. 261.
6. Garrison, F. H.: *History of Medicine*, Philadelphia and London, W. B. Saunders, first edition, 1914.
6a. Packard, Francis R.: *The School of Salerno*, Paul B. Hoeber, New York, N. Y., 1920, p. 30.
7. Graham, H.: *The Story of Surgery*, New York, pp. 896-897.
8. "Anatomia Porci" dedicated to Robert, eldest son of William the Conqueror.
9. Riesman, D.: *The Story of Medicine in the Middle Ages*, New York, 1935, p. 37.
10. Garrison, F. H.: Ibid., pp. 70-71.
11. Garrison, F. H.: Opus cited, pp. 100-101.
12. Osler, W.: *The Evolution of Modern Medicine*, Yale University Press, 1921, pp. 115-117.
13. Ashby, T.: *Encyclopedia Britannica*, 11th edition, vol. 4, pp. 178-179.
14. Franchini: *The Origin of the University of Bologna*, Annals of Medical History, 4:18, March, 1932.
15. Riesman, D.: Opus cited, pp. 133-136.
16. Osler, Sir William: Opus cited, 1921, p. 105.
17. Withington, who reports these cases, regards this last fee as the highest on record.
18. Cited by Cliford Allbut, *Historical Relations of Medicine and Surgery*, book 2, chapter 27.
19. Garrison, F. H.: Opus cited, pp. 115-117.
20. Baker, F.: *Johns Hopkins Hospital Bulletin*, Baltimore, 1909, XX, footnote to p. 331; quoted by Garrison p. 108.
21. *Ciba Symposia*, 1948, p. 960.

22. Ashby, T.: *Encyclopedia Britannica*, 11th edition, 1910-1911, vol. I p. 7.

23. "One must not forget," says Castiglioni, "none of those who had been influenced by Arabian thought could be hostile to the great commentator (Averroes) and to Maimonides who prepared the way for him." Castiglioni, A.: *History of Medicine,* New York, Knopf, 1941, p. 331

24. Castiglioni, A.: *Ciba Symposia, 1948,* pp. 959-960.

25. Riesman, D.: Opus cited, p. 130.

CHAPTER XVI

1. Laignel, M.: (Lavastine) *French Medicine*, Paul B. Hoeber, 1934, p. 15.
2. *Life in the Middle Ages*, II, p. 7.
3. Garrison, F. H.: *History of Medicine*, Philadephia and London, W. B. Saunders, first edition, 1914.
4. The similar inferiority of surgeons in England explains why they were, and still are, to some extent, addressed as "Mister."
5. Castiglioni, A.: *A History of Medicine*, New York, 1941, p. 338.
6. Benjamin of Tudela, A.D. 1160, *Early Traveler in Palestine*, edited by Thomas Wright, London, 1848, p. 65.
7. Castiglioni, A.: Opus cited, p. 388.
8. Astruc, J.: *Memoires*, translated by Steinschneider, M.: 166-168, p. 217, H. U. 795.
9. Friedenwald, H.: *The Jews and Medicine*, 1944, vol. 1, pp. 242-243.
10. *Jewish Encyclopedia*, under the title "Medicine," states that the name "Sasportos" originally Seisportas was later mispronounced Saportas, Saporta and Sforta.
11. Riesman, D.: *The Story of Medicine in the Middle Ages*, New York, 1935, pp. 148-59.
12. Garrison, F. H.: Opus cited, p. 105.
13. Withington, E. T.: *Medical History from the Earliest Times*, London, 1894, p. 217.

CHAPTER XVII

See: Gordon, B. L.: Medieval Medicine in England, *The Journal of the Medical Society of New Jersey*, v. 55, Aug. 1958, pp. 440-453.
 1. Hellsane, P.: *Dreck-Apotheke*, Stuttgart, 1847.
 2. Gibbon, E.: *History of the Decline and Fall of the Roman Empire*, London, 1854.
 3. Bede's Ecclesiastic History, Book 4, chapter 2.
 4. Ibid., pp. 386-394, Book 5:36, trans. by Rev. L. Gedley.
 5. Cited by Payne, J. F.: Biographical libraries, Anglo-Saxon Period, 1842, p. 70, Oxford, 1904, p. 15.
 6. Baas, J. H.: *Outlines of the History of Medicine and the Medical Profession*, trans. by Handerson, H. E.: J. H. Vail & Co., New York, 1889, p. 325.
 7. Payne, J. F.: *English Medicine in the Anglo-Saxon Times*, Oxford at the Clarendon Press, 1904, p. 35.
 8. Famen, low-Latin oratio, verbum.
 9. Cited by Dayne, J. F.: *English Medicine of the Anglo-Saxon Times*, Oxford, 1904, pp. 40-41.
 10. Smallpox was identified in France as early as 527 A.D. and in Arabia by 572 A.D.
 11. Uroscopy was highly regarded by the Greek physicians as an aid to diagnosis.
 12. Rashdall, H.: *The Universities of Europe in the Middle Ages*, Clarendon Press, Oxford, 1936, vol. III, pp. 12-13, 29.
 13. Rashdall, H.: Ibid., pp. 13-14.
 14. Rashdall, H.: Ibid., p. 29.
 15. Rashdall, H.: Ibid., pp. 328-329.
 16. Lyte, H. C. M.: *A History of the University of Oxford from the Earliest Times to 1530*, London, 1886, cited by Puschmann, T.: *A History of Medical Education*, trans. by Evan H. Hare, London, 1890, p. 233.
 17. Parker: *The Early History of Surgery in Great Britain*, London, 1920.
 18. Cited by Riesman, H.: Ibid., p. 169.
 19. Gilbert is covered in the chapter on Scholasticism.
 20. See "Signature and Other Healing Concepts" by Gordon, B. L.: *Romance of Medicine*, F. A. Davis Co., 1949, 2nd edition, p. 67. This practice is still common in the foreign settlements of our large cities. The writer had come across similar cases in his early practice.
 21. Graham, H.: *The Story of Surgery*, New York, 1942, pp. 116-117.

22. Cited by Collins: Medicine in Chaucer's Time, Charaka Club, Wm. Wood & Co., 1916, vol. IV, p. 141.
23. Cited by Coulton, G. G.: *Medieval Panorama,* Cambridge, Cambridge University Press, 1939, pp. 450-453.
24. Graham, H.: *The Story of Surgery,* New York, 1942, pp. 125-26.

CHAPTER XVIII

1. Among the ancient Germans Eir was the goddess of physicians. Baas, J. H.: *Outlines of the History of Medicine and the Medical Profession*, trans. by Handerson, J. E., J. H. Vail & Co., New York 1889, pp. 242-249.
2. It should be recalled that even Galen was accused of fleeing Rome when an epidemic broke out.
3. Rashdall, H.: *The Universities of Europe in the Middle Ages*, Clarendon Press, Oxford, 1895, vol. II, p. 213.
4. Rashdall, H.: Opus cited, p. 213.
5. Tomerk, W.: Gesch. der Prague University, Prague, 1849, Puschmann, T.: *History of Medical Education from the Most Remote to the Most Recent Times*, trans. and edited by E. H. Hare, London, 1891, p. 234.
6. Isschbach Gesch. der wiena Univ. Wien, 1605, s. 326.
7. Puschmann, T.: Ibid., pp. 237-41.
8. Haberling, W.: *German Medicine*, trans. by Freind, J., Paul B. Hoeber, New York, 1934, pp. 1-14.
9. This date coincides with age modern children enter first grade.
10. Neuburger, M.: *History of Medicine*, trans. by Playfair, E., London, 1910, vol. 2, p. 133.
11. Neuburger, M.: Opus cited, p. 147.

CHAPTER XIX

See: Gordon, B. L.: Roots of Russian Medicine, *The Journal of of the Medical Society of New Jersey*, v. 54, Feb. 1957, pp. 79-85.
 1. Hastings, J.: *Encyclopedia of Religion and Ethics*, New York, 1928, vol. III, pp. 465-466.
 2. Ramband, A.: *Russia*, New York, 1900, vol. I, p. 23, translated by L. B. Lang, Collier and Son.
 3. Ramband, A.: Ibid., p. 222.
 4. Ramband, A.: Opus cited, pp. 58-59.
 5. Ravitch, M. L.: *Romance of Russian Medicine*, New York, 1937, Liveright Publishing Co., p. 36.
 6. Garrison, F. H.: *History of Medicine*, Phila. and London, W. B. Saunders, first edition, 1914.
 7. Winter, A. C.: Russische Volksbräuche bei Seuchen, Globus, lxxix.
 8. Kohl, J. G.: *Die Deutsch-Russischen Ostsee Provinzen*, Dresden and Leipzig, 1841, 11, 278; Folk-lore Journal, vii, 1889, p. 174; cited by Frazer, J. G.: *The Golden Bough* (The Scapegoat), pp. 172-173.
 9. Buch, M.: *Die Wotjaken*, Stuttgart, 1882, pp. 153.
 10. Krauss, F. S.: *Kroatien, Slavonien*, Vienna, 1889, p. 108.
 11. Mannhardt, W.: *Baumkultus*, p. 257; cited by Frazer, J. G.: *The Golden Bough*, pp. 172-173.
 12. Ravitch, M. L.: Opus cited, p. 25.
 13. Kostomarov, Sketch of the Domestic Life and Customs of the Great Russians in the Sixteenth and Seventeenth Centuries, in *Sovremennik*, vol. XXXIII: cited by O. Schrader, J. Hastings, *Encyclopedia of Religion and Ethics*, vol. IV, Chas. Scribner & Sons, New York, 1928, pp. 814-16.
 14. Chapter 20.
 15. Note 13, page 816.
 16. Fletcher, G.: *Of the Russe Common Wealth*, (London, 1591): Hakluyt Society, London, 1856, p. 118 f; cited by Hastings, J.: *Encyc. of Religion and Ethics*, New York, 1928, Chas. Scribner & Sons, vol IV, pp. 815-816.
 17. Mackenzie, D.; Wallace: *Russia*, London, 1905, vol. I, p. 41.
 18. Ravitch, M. A.: Opus cited, p. 32.
 19. Ravitch, M. A.: Ibid., p. 33.
 20. Hastings J.: *Encyclopedia of Religion and Ethics*, New York, 1928, Chas. Scribner and Sons, p. 125.
 21. An alcoholic liquor of the Middle Ages made of honey, water and spices, and fermented by yeast.
 22. Ravitch, M. L.: Opus cited, 1937, pp. 34-38.

CHAPTER XX

1. Midrash: Lev. Rabba 15, Ecc. Rabba 127.
2. Hist. Nat. 7, 2.
3. Talmud: Nidda 27b, 28a.
4. Castiglioni, A.: Cleo Medicine Series, Italian Medicine, Hoeber, p. 28.
5. *The Guide of Physicians and Pharmacists,* Florence, 1927.
6. Singer C.: *A Short History of Medicine,* Oxford at the Clarendon Press, 1928, pp. 156-159.
7. Castiglioni, A.: *A History of Medicine,* Knopf, 1941, pp. 341-344.
8. Parsons, F. G.: Ency. Britannica, 11th edition, Vol. 1, pp. 921-928.
9. Singer: *A Short History of Medicine,* Oxford, The Clarendon Press, 1928, p. 76.

CHAPTER XXI

1. In his translation and commentary of Paulus, ii, 247.
2. See chapter 3, Byzantine Medicine.
3. See chapter 5, Medicine in the Koran.
4. Matthew 19:12.
5. Genesis 47:29.
5a. The incident of David who brought 200 prepuces to Saul was part of him proving himself worthy to be a man.
6. This practice which still persists in Southern Europe is performed by middle-aged matrons.
7. D'Arey, Sir P.: The History of Amputation of the Breast, 1904.
8. Genesis 3:16.
9. See chapter 15, Medieval Medicine in Italy.
10. See chapter 16, Medieval Medicine in France.
11. See Pilcher, P. E.: *Chauliac and Mondeville*, Philadelphia, 1895.
12. Cited by Garrison, F. H.: *History of Medicine*, Phila. and London, W. B. Saunders, first edition, 1914, p. 102, book 2, chapter 27.
13. Baas, J. H.: *Outlines of the History of Medicine and the Medical Profession*, trans. by Handerson, H.E.: J. H. Vail & Company, New York, 1889, pp. 330-337.
14. Cited by Streeter, E. C.: Education of the Barber Surgeon, The Proc. of Characa Club, Paul Hoeber, vol. 7, p. 87.
15. Ibid. p. 88.
16. The writer is pleased to acknowledge his sincere indebtedness to Dr. Edward. C. Streeter, Education of the Barber-Surgeons in France, pp. 82-95, The Charaka Club, New York, Paul B. Hoeber, 1931, vol. VII.

CHAPTER XXII

1. Adams, F.: *Seven Books of Paulus Aegineta,* London, Sydenham Society, 1844, vol. I.
2. Meyerhof, M.: *The Legacy of Islam,* Carro, p. 341; see also Sarton, G.: *Introduction to the History of Science,* 1927, vol. III, part I, p. 896.
3. Varron, A. G.: *Hygiene,* Ciba Symposia, October, 1939, pp. 227-278.
4. See Noah Webster, *History of Epidemic Diseases,* London, 1800, 2 volumes; a work which makes no pretension to medical learning, but exhibits the history of epidemics in connection with physical disaster, as earthquakes, famines, etc.
5. Gibbon, E.: *The Decline and Fall of the Roman Empire,* vol. 4, p. 312.
6. According to Surgeon-General Francis "hemorrhage is not an ordinary accompaniment" of Indian plague; when seen it is in the form of hemoptysis.
7. Baas, J. H.: *Outlines of the History of Medicine and the Medical Profession,* trans. by Handerson, H. E.: J. H. Vail & Company, New York, 1889, pp. 314-315.
8. Extract from "The Model of Mirth, Wit, Eloquence and Conversation," 1026; see also the English translation by Edward Hutton, 1909.
9. Hippocrates advised this to purify the pestiferous air.
10. Octavius Horatianus describes a similar disease which seems to generally fit erysipelas. See Adams, F.: *Commentary on Paulus Aegineta,* London, Sydenham Soc., 1844, vol. I, p. 253.
11. Cited by Reisman, D.: *Medicine in the Middle Ages,* New York, 1938, pp. 244-245.
12. Adams, F.: Opus cited, vol. I, p. 253.
13. Irish Lib. Hymn 1:206——:243.
14. Gaelic names of Disease, pp. 10, 23.

CHAPTER XXIII

1. Adams, F.: *The Genuine Works of Hippocrates,* English translation, New York, William Wood & Company, Aphorisms 5:9, 13:15, pp. 135-136.
2. Adams, F.: Opus cited, p 114.
3. Gordon, B. L.: *Medicine Throughout Antiquity,* Philadelphia, F. A. Davis Co., 1949, pp. 685-686.
4. Luke 5:12-13.
5. *Historia Naturalis*: 7.2.
6. Lecky, W. E. H.: *History of European Morals,* vol I, pp. 347-48. One version has it that Serapion revealed to invalids that they could be cured by the emperor. Tacitus says that Vespasian did not believe in his own power and it was only after much persuasion that he was induced to try the experiment.

CHAPTER XXIV

1. Adams, F.: *The Seven Books of Paulus Aegineta,* London, Sydenham Society, 1844, vol. 1, p. 330.
2. McLintock: Encyclopedia, vol. III, p. 312b.
3. Marston, A. W.: *The Great Closed Land* (Tibet), p. 41.
4. Noldeke: *Gesch. der Persen aus Tabari,* Leyden, 1879, p. 218.
5. Rhazes: *Liber di Pestilentia,* published in Villas Nacephoria Logica collection, Venice, 1498.
6. It seems that the early writers thought measles to be an early stage of smallpox.
7. Rhazes: Opus cited, Chapter 2.
8. Adams, F.: Opus cited, vol. I, p. 331.
9. Adams, F.: Opus cited, iii, 3, 4.
10. Avenzoar Theor. viii, 14.
11. Adams, Opus cited, vol. I, pp. 331-335.
12. Rhazes: *Liber di Pestilentia* in Villas Nacephoria Logica collection, Venice, 1498, chapter 10.
13. Haggard, H. W.: *The Lame, the Halt and the Blind,* New York, 1932, p. 219.

CHAPTER XXV

1. Evan Bloch believed it was psoriasis.
2. Leviticus 13:37-49.
3. Virchow, R.: *Zur Geschichte der Aussätze und der Spitäler, Arch. of Pathol. Anatomy,* etc., Berlin, 1860, 18:273, 19:43, 1861:20.
4. Numbers 12:10.
5. II Kings 5:27.
6. II Chronicles 26:21.
7. Riesman, D.: *The Story of Medicine in the Middle Ages,* New York, 1935, p. 238.
8. Sarton, G.: *Introduction to the History of Science,* 1947, vol. II, pp. 586-88; see also Riesman, D.: Ibid. pp. 223-240.

CHAPTER XXVI

1. Adams, F.: *Genuine Works of Hippocrates,* London, 1856, vol. 1, p. 210.
2. *De Causis et Signis Morbiarum,* translated and edited by Frances Adams, Sydenham Society, London, chap. 10, p. 253.
3. Major, R. H.: *Classic Descriptions of Disease,* Thomas, 1948, pp. 137-137.
4. Talmud Taanit 27b; Sata 35a.
5. Talmud Sofnim 17, 5.
6. Ibid. 35a.
7. Talmud Sabbath 33a.
8. Leviticus Rabba 18:4.
9. Talmud Brochoth 8a.
10. Talmud Megillah 17.
11. Preuss, J.: *Biblish-Talmudische Medizin,* Berlin, 1911, pp. 178-181
12. Pliny.: *Historia Naturalis,* 22:70.
13. Caelius Aurelianus: *On Acute and Chronic Diseases,* Trans. I. E. Drabkin, University of Chicago, pp. 301-303.
14. Castiglioni, A.: *A History of Medicine,* Knopf, 1941, p. 562.
15. Arch. Gen. de Med., 1826.

CHAPTER XXVII

1. Adams, F.: *Genuine Works of Hippocrates*, vol. I, p. 273.
2. Adams, F.: Opus cited, p. 273.
3. *Methodus Medendi*, Book V, f. 74b, Linacre, 1526 ed. Cited by: Castiglioni, A.: *A History of Medicine*, Knopf, 1941, p. 223.
4. Adams, F.: Opus cited, p. 273.
5. Gordon, B.: *Lilium* 14:1.
6. Sarton, G.: *Introduction to the History of Science*, Baltimore, 1947, III, p. 1669.
7. Translated by the American Philosophical Society, Philadelphia, 1770, vol I.
8. Adams, F.: Opus cited, pp. 166-167, 229 and in the chapter "On Regimen," vol. 1, p. 270.
9. Ibid., vol. II, p. 223.
10. Babylonian Talmud Nedarim 37b; Sabb. 12a.
11. Ibid. 41b.
12. Caelius Aurelianus: *On Acute and Chronic Diseases*, trans. by I. E. Drabkin, 1950, University of Chicago, pp. 869-871.
13. Cited by Kottelmann, L. W.: *Die Ophthalmologie bei den alten Hebräern*, Leipzig, 1910, p. 156.
14. Talmud: Kethuboth 77b.
15. Feigenbaum is convinced that trachoma in the Talmudic days was known by this name, Haayin, 1927, Tel-Aviv, p. 63.
16. Talmud Bekhoroth 43b.
17. Jastrow, M.: *Dictionary of the Targunim and Talmudim*, p. 1281.
18. Talmud Kethuboth 77b.
19. Adams, F.: *Seven Books of Paulus Aegineta*, London, Sydenham Society, 1844, vol. I, p. 428.
20. Dr. Feigenbaum, who has a large experience with cases of trachoma in Palestine and Egypt, found in many cases a profuse discharge from the nose spreading through the lacrimal canal. In such cases, he observed that the treatment of the disease is more difficult.
21. Cited by Hirschberg, J.: *Codex Arabicus, Centralbl. f. pract. Augenh.* 29:63, Feb. 1905.
22. Cited by Feigenbaum: *Haayin*, Jerusalem, 1927, p. 63.
23. Gordon, B. L.: *New Judea*, Philadelphia, Julius H. Greenberg, 1919, p. 90.

CHAPTER XXVIII

1. Leviticus 26:16; Deut. 28:22.
2. English translation by B.B. Rogers, G. P. Putnam's Son, 1924, New York, vol. I, p. 507.
3. Adams, F.: *The Genuine Works of Hippocrates*, vol. I, pp. 297-298.
4. Adams, F.: Ibid. 147-184.
5. McLintock: Encyclopedia, vol. IV, p. 154.
6. Garrison, F. H.: *History of Medicine*, Philadelphia & London, W. B. Saunders, first edition, 1914, p. 50.
7. Allen, T. H.: *Science and History of the Universe*, The Current Literature Publishing Company, 1914, New York, vol. 7, p. 134.
8. Celsus, A. C.: "De Re Medica" in eight books, translated by James Greive, London, Wilson and Durham, 1756, p. 114.
9. 1.5:6.
10. Martial: *Epigrams*, translated by Walter Kerr, New York, G. P. Putnam, 1920.
11. Babylonian Talmud Gittin 67b, shabbath 665.
12. Ibid.
13. Preuss, J.: *Biblish Talmudische Medizin*, Berlin, 1911, pp. 183-184.
14. Babylonian Talmud Pes. 112a.

CHAPTER XXIX

1. Bloch, E.: *Der Ursprung der Syphilis*, Jena, 1901, pp. 237; 297-308.
2. I Samuel 5:9.
3. Deuteronomy 28:27.
4. Preuss, J.: *Biblisch-Talmudische Medizin,* Berlin, 1911, pp. 176, 587.
5. Preuss, J.: Ibid. p. 557.
6. Williams identifies in the effigy pottery ("huacos") of Peru the possibility of leprosy, lupus, syphilis, verruca peruviana, and yaws.
7. Bull. de la Soc. D'Anthrop., 1876.
8. *Ciba Symposia*, vol. 2, No. 2, May 1940, pp. 442-443.
9. Ibid. pp. 548-60.
10. Ibid. vol. I, No. I, April 1939, p. 14.
11. Cited by Riesman, D.: *The Story of Medicine in the Middle Ages,* New York, 1935, Paul Hoeber & Co., pp. 285-6, *Die Welt,* 905, June 30, 1931.
12. Buret, F.: *Syphilis in the Middle Ages & Modern Times,* trans. by Ohmann-Dumesnil, A. H.: F. A. Davis Co., 1895, vol. II, p. 6.
13. Ibid. p. 7.
14. Lib. I, Cap. 48.
15. Buret, F.: Opus cited, p. 21.
16. La Cap. 2, Milan, 1290.
17. Ibid. 22-23.
18. Book vii, cap. 2, Montpellier, 1305.
19. The Antiquity of Congenital Syphilis, *Bull. of the Inst. of the Hist. of Med.,* vol. 10, July, 1941, pp. 148-167; Paris, 1088, p. 24.
20. Montpellier, c. 1400.
21. Buret, F.: Opus cited, pp. 27-28.
22. Major, R. H.: *Classic Descriptions of Disease,* Thomas, 1948, pp. 15-16.
23. Ann. Medical Hist., N. S. 3:465, Sept. 1931.

CHAPTER XXX

1. Aurelianus, C.: *On Acute Diseases and on Chronic Diseases,* translated by Drabkin, I. E.: University of Chicago Press, Chicago, 1950, p. 777.
2. Kleen, E.: *Diabetes Mellitus,* P. Blackstone Sons & Company, Phila., 1900, p. 10.
3. Aurelianus, C.: Opus cited, p. 777.
4. Adams, F.: *The Seven Books of Paulus Aegineta,* Sydenham Society, London, 1844, vol. I, p. 547.
5. Rhazes often quotes Sarud as an authority on Susruta and his ophthalmological operations, *Archives of Ophthalmology,* Oct. 1939, p. 552.
6. Adams, F.: *The Extant Works of Aretaeus the Cappadocian,* The Sydenham Society, 1856, p. 338.
7. Adams, F.: Ibid., p. 338.
8. Willis, T.: *Pharmaceutice Rationalis* or *An Excerptation of the Operations of Medicine in Human Bodies,* London, 1679, p. 79.

CHAPTER XXXI

1. The term "mania" has its origin in the Greek myth that the person suffering from a psychic disorder is dominated by the goddess Mania.
2. Caelius Aurelianus: *On Acute Diseases and on Chronic Diseases*, trans. by Drabkin, I. E.; The University of Chicago Press, Chicago, 1950, p. 539.
3. Freud, S.: *Hysteria and the Psychoneuroses*, translated by Brill, A.; 1909.
4. Numbers 24. 4.
5. Genesis 20, 6; 25, 12; 37, 5.
6. Samuel 16. 15.
7. Kohelet 4. 16.
8. A collection of documents of about 600 B. C., which constituted a written presentation of the efforts of the Hindus to construe the world as a rational whole.
9. Burges. Bohn Vol. VI, p. 160. Timaeus XIX, XLIV: Davis, Bohn Vol. II, pp. 349 and 380.
10. Kata Upanishad 3.10 and 11—Ref. 5, p. 352.
11. Davis, Bohn Vol. II, p. 260.
12. Translated by J. I. Beare, Oxford 1908.
13. Maretts, E. R.: *The Concept of the Unconscious in the History of Medical Psychology*. The Psychiatric Quarterly, January, 1953.
14. The others are: bubonic plague, tuberculosis, scabies, erysipelas, anthrax, trachoma and leprosy.
15. Numbers 24:4.
16. Caelius Aurelianus: Opus cited, p. 479.
17. Cited by Cutten, G. B.: *3000 years of Mental Healing*, Charles Scribner's Sons, New York, 1911, p. 196.
18. Von Storch, T. C.: *Essay on the History of Epilepsy; Annals of Medical History*, new series, 2:614, 1930.
19. Von Storch, T. C.: *Annals of Medical History*, new series, 10:251, 1938.
20. Von Storch, T. C.: *Essay on the History of Epilepsy; Annals of Medical History*, new series, 2:614, 1930.
21. Riesman, D.: *The Story of Medicine in the Middle Ages*, Paul B. Hoeber, Inc., New York, 1935, p. 249.
22. Frazer, J. G.: *The Golden Bough*, vol. VI: *The Scape Goat*; The Macmillan Co., New York, 1935, p. 330.
23. Gordon, B. L.: *The Romance of Medicine*, F. A. Davis Co., Philadelphia 2nd. ed., 1949, pp. 411-412.

24. Lyman, G.: *Witchcraft,* pp. 460-461.
25. Haggard, H. W.: *The Lame, the Halt, and the Blind,* Paul B. Hoeber, New York, 1932, p. 152.
26. Riddel, W. R.: *Medical Journal and Record,* 1930, pp. 131-217, 269.

CHAPTER XXXII

1. II Samuel 6:16.
2. Hecker, J. F. C.: *Epidemics of the Middle Ages*, London, 1844.
3. Hecker: Ibid.
4. Sarton, G.: Introduction to the History of Science, Baltimore, 1947, vol. III, p. 1666.
5. Carus, C. G.: *Geistes-Epidemien der Menscheit*, Leipzig, 1852, p. 23.
6. Carus, C. G.: Opus cited, p. 18.
7. Sarton, G.: Opus cited, vol. III, pt. 2, pp. 1666-1667.
8. *Opera Omnia Medico-Practica et Anatomica*, 9th edition, pp. 599-640.
9. Caelius Aurelianus, *On Acute Diseases and On Chronic Diseases*, edited and translated by I. E. Drabkin, University of Chicago Press, 1950, p. 22.
10. Caelius Aurelianus, Opus cited, pp. 919-21.
11. Soranus of Ephesus, *Chronic Diseases*, Caelius Aurelianus, pp. 2-40, 61.
12. Herodotus Euterpe, 11.42.
13. W. Mannhardt, Mythol. Forsch. Strassburg, 1884, p. 72.
14. Augustine, ep. 159 ad Marcellus.
14a. Jewish Court of Justice; See Mafteach, to the *Responsa of the Geonim*, p. 1922.
15. Hecker, J. F. C.: *Epidemics of the Middle Ages*, London, 1844; trans. by B. G. Babington, London, 1853, p. 82.
16. Cooper, W. M.: *Flagellation and the Flagellants*, London, 1908.
17. Rufus M. Jones, *Hastings Encyclopedia of Religion and Ethics*, vol. 6, p. 51, Chas. Scribner & Son, 1928.
18. Paul Daniel Alphandery, *Encyc. Britannica*, p. 463-66, vol. 10, 11th edition.
19. The badge worn by them was the sign of the cross; crusade is the Portuguese form of cross.
20. The writer is indebted for much of the information with reference to the returning crusaders to Baas, J. H.: *Outlines of the History of Medicine and the Medical Profession*, trans. by Handerson, H. E.: J. H. Vail and Co., N. Y., 1889, pp. 333-341.
21. The quarter assigned to prostitutes in Paris acquired the not inappropriate designation of "Clapier"; the term "Clap" for gonorrhea, probably is derived from this designation.

CHAPTER XXXIII

1. See *Dictionnaire Philosophique,* and C. Waddington, *Ramus,* Paris, 1855, p. 256.
2. Garrison, F. H.: p. 131.
3. Copernicus studied medicine in Padua. He was a classmate of Giralamo Frascatora and a pupil of Achilini.
4. *De Avaritia,* vol. 2.
5. Symond, J. A.: *A Short History of the Renaissance in Italy,* by Lieut. Colonel A. Pearson, Henry Holt & Co., New York, 1926, pp. 188-195.
6. "De Sanitate Trienda" (Paris, 1517), "Methodus Medendi" (Paris, 1519), "De Temperamentis" (Cambridge, 1521), "De Naturabilus Facultatibus" (London, 1523), "Symptomatum Differentiis," et Causes (London, 1524), "De Pulsum Usu" (London, without date).

CHAPTER XXXIV

1. Friedenwald, H.: *The Jews and Medicine,* Johns Hopkins Press, Baltimore, vol. II, pp. 460-461.
2. Baas, J. H.: *The History of Medicine,* translated by H. E. Handerson, New York, 1910, pp. 375-376.
3. Major, R. H.: *Classic Descriptions of Diseases,* Charles C. Thomas, 1948, p. 648.
4. Sudhoff, ed. vol XI, p. 196, Strunz, p. 135.
5. Ed. Huser, vol. V, p. 180, ed. Sudhoff, vol. X, p. 227.
6. C. D. Leake, Isis. No. 21, 1925, p. 22.
7. Garrison, F. H.: *Introduction to the History of Medicine,* W. B. Saunders Co., 1914, pp. 141-142.
8. Paracelsus was the first to prescribe mercury for syphilis and skin diseases.
9. *Grosse Chirurgie* III, p. 259, quoted by Dr. Iago Galdston.
10. This seems to be an old notion also found in the Talmud.
11. Volumen Paramirum, ed. Leidecker, p. 16.
12. Ibid. p. 14.
13. Baas, Opus cited, pp. 379-389.
14. Payne, J. F.: *Encyc. Brit.,* 11th ed., vol. 18, p. 48.
15. The system of signature still persists among certain classes of people. The writer recalls that during his early practice, when summoned to treat cases of icterus neonatorum (jaundice of the newborn) he occasionally noticed a yellow coin on the umbilicus or a yellow ribbon from the neck of the newborn baby.
16. Gordon, B. L.: *Romance of Medicine,* F. A. Davis & Co., 1944, pp. 367-370.
17. Albrecht Burckhardt, "Nochmals der Doktortitel von Paracelsus," *Correspondenz-Blatt für Schweizer Aerzte,* vol. 44, 1914, pp. 884-887.
18. According to Burkhardt, Paracelsus received an M.D. degree at Ferrara.
19. The complete text of the letter will be found in Chapter 14.
20. *Four Treatises of Theophrastus von Hohenheim,* p. 12, by Temkin, etc.
21. S. Grunder, Baas, p. 381.
22. Walter Artelt, "Paracelsus im Urteil der Medizinhistorik," *Fortschritte der Medizin,* 1932, vol. 51, no. 22.
23. Tranlated by C. L. Temkin, Gregory Zilboerg, George Rosen, and H. E. Sigerist, Johns Hopkins Press, 1941.
24. Castiglioni, A.: *A History of Medicine,* Alfred A. Knopf, New York, 1941, 539-40.

25. An alternative date for his birth is 1579 and for his death 1635, see Bull. Roy. Acad. Belg., 1907, 7, p. 732.

26. For his chief writings, see *Encyc. Brit.*, 11th edition, vol. 20, pp. 149-150, 1911.

27. Uroscopy in the sixteenth century was considered an honorable occupation of the physician.

28. *Epistolarium Medicinalium*, Basel, 554, p. 488.

29. In this chapter the present author is indebted to Henry M. Pachter for his work *Paracelsus*, Henry Schuman, New York, 1951.

CHAPTER XXXV

1. D. Riesman: *The Story of the Middle Ages,* p. 173, p. 113-18.
2. Parson, F. G.: *Encyc. Brit.,* 11th ed., vol. 2, pp. 996-997.
3. Dampier, Sir W. C.: *A History of Science and Its Relations with Philosophy and Religion,* Cambridge, Cambridge University Press, 3rd edition, 1942, pp. 117-118.
4. Akerknecht, E. M.: *Ciba Symposia,* vol. 3, p. 1816.
5. Taylor, R. A.: *Leonardo The Florentine,* New York, 1928, p. 268.
6. It is regrettable that Leonardo did not publish his researches. It is only recently that his notebook has become fully accessible.
7. Castiglioni, A.: *A History of Medicine,* Knopf, N. Y., 1941, p. 437.
8. The physiologist, P. Flourens, investigated the various parts of the brain.
9. Neuburger actually attributes the progress of anatomy in Italy to its union with the fine arts.
10. "How far his method was progressing, may be gathered" said Garrison, (*History of Medicine,* p. 150), "from the title page picture of the 'Mellerstadt's Mudidno' (1493) in which the scholastic instructor, in long robe and beretta, wand in hand, gravely expounds Galen by the book from his pulpit chair, while below the long haired barber surgeon makes a desperate show."
11. F. H. Garrison, *History of Medicine,* first ed., W. B. Saunders Co., p. 150, Phila., 1914.
12. *History of Medicine,* F. H. Garrison, 1914, p. 152.
13. Singer, Chas.: *A Short History of Medicine,* Oxford, 1928, p. 88.
14. *Encyc. Brit.,* 11th ed., p. 684-685.
15. Castiglioni, Opus cited, p. 436.
16. Fredrich Gymier Parsons, *Encyc. Brit.,* 11th ed., vol. I, p. 934.
17. *History of Anatomy,* Puschmann's Handbook.
18. Castiglioni, Opus cited, p. 427.
19. F. G. Parsons, *The Encyc. Brit.,* 11th ed., 1910, vol. I, p. 930, Cambridge University Press, Cambridge.
20. Centuria 1, Curat, 52.

CHAPTER XXXVI

1. Gordon, Benj., L.: *The Romance of Medicine,* F. A. Davis Co.
2. Marcellus Malpighi, 1628-1694.
3. Robinson, *Story of Medicine,* Vol. I.
4. Singer, S.: *A Short History of Medicine,* p. 108, Oxford, 1928.
5. Singer, C.: *History of Medicine,* pp. 105-106, Oxford, 1926.
6. Faster, Sir Michael: *History of Physiology during the 16th, 17th and 18th centuries,* 1901.
7. Giovanni da Gesuau, Carlo, Rome, 1680.
8. *Encyc. Brit.,* 11th ed., vol. XIII, pp. 42-43.

CHAPTER XXXVII

1. Friedenwald, H.: *The Jews and Medicine*, The Johns Hopkins Press, 1944, vol. 1, p. 352.
2. Baas, J. H.: Outlines of the History of Medicine and the Medical Profession; translated by Handerson, H. E.; William R. Jenkins Co., N. Y., 1910, pp. 435-437.
3. In his later works, Pare condemns as a gross fraud the medicinal use of "mumia" (allegedly derived from Egyptian mummies) and unicorn's horn (from the entirely mythical animal).
4. Baas, J. H.: Opus cited, p. 401.
5. Robinson, V.: *The Story of Medicine*, Tudor Publishing Co., N. Y., 1936, pp. 167-168.
6. Haggard, H. W.: *The Doctor in History*, Yale University Press, New Haven, 1934, pp. 231-232.

CHAPTER XXXVIII

1. Baas, p. 429.
2. Haggard, H. W.: *The Doctor in History,* Yale University Press, New Haven, Conn., 1934, p. 223.
3. Graham, H.: *The Story of Surgery,* Doubleday, Doran & Co., Inc., Garden City, N. Y., 1942, pp. 141-142.
4. Haggard, H. W.: *The Doctor in History,* Yale University Press, New Haven, Conn., 1934, pp. 224-225.
5. Pare's religion has been disputed. While he conformed externally to the Catholic faith, at heart he was a Huguenot.
6. It is only in his book on monsters, written towards the end of his career, that he shows himself to have been by no means free from superstition.
7. Baas, 429.
8. Graham, H.: Opus cited, pp. 148-150.
9. London, 1588.
10. Graham, H.: Opus cited, pp. 151-152.
11. Graham, H.: Ibid., p. 147.
12. De Gangraena et Spahacelo (Cologne, 1593).

CHAPTER XXXIX

1. The Jews appear to have known the operation of Caesarian section in the 12th century. The commentary *tosephot* on the Babylonian Talmud *avoda zarah*, p. 20, connects this operation with Julius Caesar.

2. Johan Weyer was a great reformer. In his work *De Proestigiis Daemonum* he maintains that witchcraft is a manifestation of anguish and apprehension and may lead to insanity and that the confessions extracted from the accused should not frighten anyone as they have no bearing on the magic art. He examined many confessions and showed that they were either obtained after a loss of control of the accused's emotions when the mind became distorted or by outright torture.

3. Rabbi Nachman, quotes Samuel, that when a women dies during childbirth the abdomen must immediately be opened and the child removed. Babylonian Talmud: *Erubin*, p. 14.

4. Rousset planned his work carefully indicating the line of incision with ink and placing a cross mark of several points of guidance in later attaining accurate approximation. He reports subsequent pregnancy without discomfort.

5. Jacques Guillemeau (1550-1590) performed the operation in the presence of Ambroise Pare in the year 1590.

6. Authorities are inclined to believe that Caesarean section performed among the natives of Uganda renders it possible that this procedure may have been employed upon living women at an early period by certain primitive races.

7. This so-called "Welcher's position" goes back to Renaissance times.

CHAPTER XL

1. Sorsby, A.: *A Short History of Ophthalmology*, p. 29, John Bale Sons and Danielson, London, 1933.
2. He was the forerunner of Lavater in appraising human character by the facial features in his work *De Humana Physiognomia*, Sorento, 1586.
3. Chance, B.: Clio Medica, *Ophthalmology*, p. 42, Paul B. Hoeber, Inc., New York, 1939.

CHAPTER XLI

1. Girolamo Fracastoro, *Syphilis*, 1530, pp. 32-37.
2. *De Contagione et Condogasis Morbis,* Venice 1546.
3. Book 1, Chapter 7.
4. Major, R. H.: *Classic Description of Disease,* Springfield, Charles C. Thomas, 1948, pp. 8-9.
5. *Tratado Sobre Las Pestiferas Bubas* (Salamanca); Translated by *Major*, opus cited, pp. 17-19.
6. Fabie furnishes proof that Villalobos was of Jewish descent and that he suffered at the hands of the Inquisition.
7. Baas: *History of Medicine,* opus cited, p. 383.
8. A Mussa Varrslova De Morbo gallico, Ferrara, 1551.
9. Moschus, J.: *Paterology,* Paris, p. 137.
10. Ohman Dumesinil, translated by F. Buret; *Syphilis in the Middle Ages,* p. 150.
11. Theophilus Parvin, *Treatise on the Venereal Disease.*
12. *Traite et Pathologique et Therapeutique des Maladies Veneris*, Paris, 1834.
13. Winthrop was governor of Connecticut 1606-1616.
14. As translated into prose by Wynne-Finch. Astruc, *De Morbis Veneris,* libri novem, 2nd ed., Paris 1740. In this work, he gives a bibliography of syphilis.
15. Holcomb, R. C.: *Christopher Columbus and the American Origin of Syphilis,* U.S. Naval Med. Bull., vol XXXII, October, 1934, No. 4, pp. 403-30.
16. Ibid. pp. 401-430.

CHAPTER XLII

1. Major, R.: *Classic Descriptions of Disease,* Charles C. Thomas, Springfield, Illinois, 1948, p. 103.
2. Richard Garnett, *Encyclopedia Britannica,* 11th edition, vol. V, pp. 314-315.
3. Castiglioni, Arturo: *History of Medicine,* 1941, opus cited, p. 467.

CHAPTER XLIII

1. Morley, H.: *Life of Girolamo Cardano of Milan*, Physician, London, 1898.
2. Baas, J. H.: *Outlines of the History of Medicine and the Medical Profession*, trans. Handerson, H. E.: J. H. Vail & Co., New York, 1889, pp. 317-319.
3. John Caius, a Book or Conseille against the disease commonly called the sweate or sweating sickness, *Encyclopedia Britannica*, London, 1552, 11th edition, vol. 26, pp. 186-187.
4. Major, R. H.: *Classic Description of Disease*, Springfield, Ill., 1948, p. 202.
5. Ibid.
6. Reisman, D.: *The Story of Medicine in the Middle Ages*, New York, 1935, p. 241.
7. New York, 1897, p. 290.
8. Major, R. H.: Opus cited, p. 204.
9. Baillou, G.: *Epidemiorum et Ephemeridum*, Lib. II, p. 237, 1640.
10. Baillou, G.: *Epidemiorum et Ephemeridum libri duo*, Opera Omnia, Venice, 1934, p. 130.
11. Ibid, Bk. 1, p. 55.
12. Major, R. H.: Opus cited, second edition, p. 220.
13. Ibid.
14. Gordon, Benjamin L.: *The Romance of Medicine*, p. 388.

CHAPTER XLIV

1. A Huguenot scholar of Paris, Petrus Ramus (1515-1572), who opposed Aristotle's doctrine, was shot, dragged, decapitated and thrown in the water.
2. This group included the greatest Renaissance luminaries.
3. This regulation is indicative of the difficulties encountered in keeping dissenting students and graduates in line.
4. Compare with the hazing practices I encountered in my student days at Jefferson Medical College. Gordon, B. L.: *Between Two Worlds*, Bookman Associates, 1952, pp. 162-165.
5. Walsh, J. J.: *Physicians' Fees down through the Ages*, International Clinics, Philadelphia.
6. Baas, J. H.: *Outline of the History of Medicine and the Medical Profession*, translated by Handerson, H. E.; William R. Jenkins Co., N. Y., 1910, p. 452.
7. "Uroscopy" is the pseudoscience of ascertaining a diagnosis by merely inspecting the urine.
8. Baas, J. H.: Opus cited, pp. 437-447.
9. Amatus Lusitanus: Centuria I, Curat 27.
10. Ibid I, 47.
11. Ibid IV, 1.
12. Ibid I, 100.
13. Friedenwald, H.: *The Jews and Medicine*, Johns Hopkins Press, 1944, vol. 1, pp. 353-357.
14. Malgaigne, J. F.: *Manuel de Medicine Operations*, I, 401.
15. Friedenwald, H.: Opus cited, vol. I, p. 345.
16. Geralamo is the author of several books, *De Morbus Puerorum* (Venice, 1583), a treatise on medical gymnastics *De Gymnastica* (Venice, 1569), and *De Morbus Cutanea* (Venice, 1572).
17. I am indebted to the late Dr. Harry Friedewald for much of the information pertaining to Zacutus.
18. "Marrano," derived from the New Testament phrase "Marran athat" ("Our Lord hath come"), denotes in Spanish "accused" or "damned" and is applied to Spanish Jews who through compulsion became converted to Christianity.

INDEX

A

Aahad Al Daula, 164
Aaron, 37, 214
Aaron Harun, 241
Aaron the Presbyter, 482-483
Ab Aquapendente, Fabricius, 625, 637-638, 643, 653, 669, 748
Abbas, Haly, 140, 322
Abbela, 316
Abd Ar Rahim Ali Al Baysani, 229
Abderrahman I, 129
Abderrahman III, 194, 199, 201, 243-244
Abd Ul Arab Ibn-Muisha, 220
Abd Ul Latif, 182-183, 224, 420
Abdullah Ibn Sawada, 151
Abelard, 76, 265, 348
Able, 634
Abner, 490
Abney, Sir Thomas, 730
Abon, Rabbi, 247
Abraham, 55, 89, 101
Abraham Bar Hiyya, 240
Abraham Ben Hasdai, 170
Abraham Ben Moses Ben Maimon, 225, 235, 244
Abraham De Balmes, 248
Abraham De Saint Gilles, 258
Abraham Ibn Daud or John of Seville, 240
Abraham Ibn Ezrah, 239, 245
Abraham Ibn Zarkali, 240
Abraham Maimonides II, 238
Abu Al Bayzan Al Undawwar, 243
Abu Al-Hakim of Turin, 247
Abu Al Hasan, 235
Abu Al Husn, 116, 124
Abu Al Maali, 243
Abu Al Muna Al Kuhim, 235
Abu Al Walid Merwan Ibn Gasmah, 244
Abu Baks, 129, 133
Abu Beks Muhammed Ben Abd Al Malik Ibn Zuhr, 208, 213, 222
Abu Gurraig, 154
Abu Haza Yazid, 240
Abu Hanifa, 89, 100
Abu Koreish Isa, 154
Abul Aina Al Misri, 214
Abul Allah Zuhr Ben Abu Mervan Abd Ul Malik, 213
Abul Casim, 8, 64, 190, 201-207, 211, 226, 242, 319, 427, 437, 513, 530
Abul Faradsh Bar Hebraeus, 79
Abul Faradsh, Physician, 79
Abufeda, 112
Abulfeda, 433
Abu Mansur, 190, 243
Abu Merwan Ibn Zuhr, 244
Abul Qasim Al Zahrawi, 245-246
Abu Yafar Ali Abdaulah, 172
Abu Yafar Ibn Al Yazzar, 165
Abu Yakub Ibn Ishaq, 141, 147
Abu Yusuf, 222
Achilles, 127
Achillini, Alessandro, 425, 619-620
Adachi, 528
Adam, 92, 117, 266, 274, 418
Adams, Francis, 61, 65, 427, 515
Adhad Ed-Dalla Ben Buweih, 136
Adolph of Nassau, 583
Adrian V, Pope, 277
Aesculapius, 19, 32, 37, 223, 364, 466, 567
Aetius of Amida, 10, 45, 50-57, 59, 64, 150, 159, 201, 307, 338, 489, 506, 510-512, 520, 541, 554

825

Agapit, Holy, 404
Agatha, Saint, 35, 434
Aharun Al Quis, 141, 154, 164
Aignan, Saint, 35
Airy, Sir J. B., 297
Aknin, Joseph, 224-225, 236
Al Afdal, 230, 232
Al Amin, 135
Albert of Mayence and Brandenburg, 711-712
Albertus Magnus, 24, 190, 266, 268, 272-275, 350
Albrecht, Emperor, 75
Al Candurs, 258
Alcithous, 704
Alcuin, 11, 30, 261, 358
Aldarete or Alterete, 753
Alderotti, Thaddeus, 325-328, 421-422
Aldhelm, Saint, 357, 359
Aldus, 50, 4, 581, 583
Alexander Ab Alexandro, 566
Alexander of Hales, 262
Alexander of Tralles, 10, 45, 56, 59, 69, 140, 150, 154, 285, 307, 316, 350, 361-362, 501, 505, 553
Alexei Mikhailovich, Tsar, 415
Alexius, Byzantine emperor, 575
Alfonso X, of Castile, 240
Alfonso XI, of Castile, 245
Alfred the Great, 11, 79-80, 301
Al Ghafiqui, 147, 165, 189, 202, 223
Al Ghazzali, 200, 262-263
Al Hafiz, 243
Al Hakem II, 194, 199-200
Al Hakem III, 200
Al Harith Ben Kalada Al Thakefi, 89-90, 111, 133
Al Hazan or Ibn Al Haitam, 164, 179-180, 291-292
Ali, 123
Ali Al Tabari, 151-152, 154
Ali Ben Isa, 165-166
Ali Ibn Al Abbas, 164-165, 173
Ali Ibn Khatma Al Ansari, 457
Ali Ibn Sahl Ibn Rabban Al Tabari, 242
Ali Ibn Talif, 133
Ali Ibn Yusuf Ibn Tashwin, 222, 229
Ali of Seville, 245

Ali Usaybi, 225
Al Kadi Al Fadil Al Baisami, 222, 224, 229, 230
Al-Kahir, 151
Al Kifti or Ibn Al Quifti, 221-222, 224-225
Al Kindi or Al Kindus, 140-141, 144-145, 217
Al Mahdi, 154, 167
Al Mamun, 135-139, 144
Al Mansur, Caliph, 134, 136-137, 153, 163, 170
Al Mansur of Khorasan, 189
Al Menar, Juan, 681
Al Milik Al Hshraf, 243
Al Moctader or Al Muktadir, 136, 151-152
Al Munatirah, Lord of, 436
Al Mustamin, 139
Al Mutassim, 139, 143-144, 242
Al Mutawakkil, 139, 144, 151, 242
Al Nader Ben Harith Ben Kalad, 133
Al-Radi, 151
Al Said Ibn Sina, 234
Amalaswintha, 71
Aman, Saint, 35
Amathi, Nathan, 178
Ambrosius, 580
Ammar Ben Ali Al Mausuli, 245
Anglicus, Bartholimaeus, 493-494
Anna of Byzance, 401-402
Anne of England, 555
Anselm of Canterbury, 262, 264-265, 268, 345
Anthemius, 56
Anthimus, 72-73, 77
Anthony, Saint, 34-35, 284, 469-472, 524-525, 684, 719
Anthony the German, 400
Antyllus, 45, 55, 159, 427
Aonio, Paleario, 581
Apion, 528
Apollonair, 339
Apollonia, Saint, 35
Apollonius of Memphis, 539
Apuleius, 661
Apulus Platonici, 380
Ara Gon, Cardinal of, 617
Aquinas, Saint Thomas, 24, 190, 263

Aranzio, Julius Caesar, 638, 693-694
Arcadius, 16
Archigens of Afanna, 45, 54, 58, 140, 427, 541
Archimatteus, 318-319
Arculanus, Johannes, 308
Aretaeus, 57-58, 456, 476, 495, 498, 501, 539-541, 552
Aretino, Guido, 318
Argelata, Petrus Ab, 426
Ariosto, Lodovico, 581
Aristophanes, 228, 508
Aristotle, 24-26, 58, 92, 130, 139, 144, 169-171, 179, 191, 215, 217-219, 222, 245, 262, 265-266, 268, 273-274, 276, 285, 311, 318, 334-335, 348, 391, 393, 493, 550, 587-588, 593, 605, 638, 649
Arlt, C. F., 297
Armati, Salvino, 284, 293-294, 296, 418
Arnold of Villanova, 173, 190, 268, 277-281, 317, 320, 345, 381, 393, 554-555
Arnollet, Balthasar, 634
Asaf Judaeus or Samuel Yarhinas or Judam Ha-Jerichoni, 250-256, 631
Astorga, Marquis of, 710
Astruc, Jean, 247, 345, 715
Atalaric, 71
Augustine, Saint, 263-264, 417
Augustus of Saxony, 760
Austrichides, Queen of the Franks, 384
Avempac, 245
Avenzoar or Ibn Zuhr, 6, 163, 173, 190, 201, 208-215, 220, 223, 226, 231, 242, 245, 321, 394, 428, 485, 530, 667
Averroes or Ibn Rushd, 172, 209, 214-220, 227, 242, 245, 263, 269, 273, 285, 334, 336, 365, 371, 428, 530, 726
Avertin, Saint, 35, 558
Avicenna or Ibn Sina, 6, 8, 27, 83, 111, 140, 164-165, 170-179, 189-190, 207, 217, 226-227, 229, 243, 245-246, 263, 268, 285, 307-309, 321, 328, 330, 334, 336, 349-350, 365, 371, 302, 391, 394, 423, 427-428, 453, 458, 484, 502, 506, 520, 530-531, 537, 540-541, 589, 592, 598, 606-608, 615, 630-631, 744, 747
Azzo D'este, Marquis, 334
Azzolino, 422

B

Baas, 133, 699
Bacon, Roger, 2, 180, 191, 263, 268, 272, 276, 288, 292-294, 350, 370, 533, 538, 566, 581
Bacot, 729
Baglivi, Giorgio, 566, 650, 653
Bailly De Troyes, 445
Bakhtishua, 134
Bailaam, 551
Bald, 11, 360-362, 461, 473, 482, 520
Baldwin, King of Flanders, 340
Baldwin, the Monk, 367
Balescan De Tarante, 345
Baliol, John, 371
Ballonius or De Baillov Guillaume 738-740, 743
Balsham, Hugh, 372
Balthazar, 555
Balthazzar De Tusca, 388
Banacasa of Padua, 215-216
Banting, 544
Barbara, the Physician, 259
Barbarus, Hermelaus, 587
Barbeyrac, 345
Bard, Samuel, 503
Barthelemy, 345
Barthez, 345
Bartholomeus Da Varignana, 328
Bartholomew, Saint, 36, 380-381, 581
Bartisch 592, 698-700
Basil, Emperor of Byzance, 401
Basil, Saint, 27
Bathoni, Albertino, 751
Battista, Giovanni, 595
Baudouin, 339
Bauhin, 345
Bayley, Walter, 700
Bechus, Saint, 35
Bede, Venerable, 3, 11, 356, 358-360, 365, 460, 478
Bedford, Duke of, 383
Bellan, 248

Bellini, Corenzo, 652
Bembo, Cardinal, 706
Benedetti, Alexander, 620
Benedict XIII, Pope, 246
Benedict, Saint, 19, 26-30, 36, 313, 315
Benesch De Wartinnel, 388
Benignus, Saint, 339
Benivieni, Antonio, 620
Berengar of Tours, 265, 346
Berenger Berengarius, 638, 698, 749
Beowulf, 357
Bergmann, Ernst Von, 431, 433
Bernabo, Duke of Milan, 467
Bernard, Claude, 544
Bernard De Gordon, 268, 283-295, 345, 365, 371, 381, 439, 456, 502, 531-533, 554, 761
Bertharius, 29
Bertuccio Lombardo, 331, 426
Best, 544
Bian, Christoph, 687
Bidpai, 142
Biondo, Michael Angelo or Blondus 625
Blackbourn, Henry, 701
Blasius (Blaise), Saint, 35-36, 56
Bloch, Ivan, 524-525
Blumentrost, Lavrenti, 415
Boccaccio, Giovanni, 463-467, 582
Boccaccio, Jacopo, 466
Bocke, Jerome, 659-660
Boerhave, 51
Boethius, 11, 71, 285
Bonacosa, Jacob, 242
Bonapart, Pietro, 296
Boniface VIII, Pope, 278, 421-422
Boniface, Saint, 357
Borde, Andrew, 759-760
Borde, Paul, 759
Borelli, Giovanni Alfonso, 180, 650
Borgognoni, Theodoric, 330-331, 442
Boso of Parma, 426
Botticelli, Sandro, 619
Bottoni, Albertino, 743
Boyle, Robert, 760
Brantome, 676
Brassavole, Amuza, 658, 713, 743, 754
Brown, P., 165
Browne, Thomas, 760

Brudus, Dionysus, 761
Brudus, Manuel, 761
Brunfels Otto, 657-660
Bruno De Carbo, 329
Bruno, Giordano, 581
Brunschwig, Hieronymus, 396, 680
Buckingham, Duke of, 691
Budaeus, 591
Buddha, 89
Burkart, F., 528
Burzwei Ibn Adesher, 141-142
Bravo, Francisco, 740-741
Brettoneau, Pierre, 495, 499
Brissot, Pierre, 594-595, 657, 663, 751
Broca, Paul, 527
Browley, William, 487

C

Caelius Aurelianus, 10, 28, 45-50, 78, 498, 504-505, 539-540, 545, 546, 552
Caesar, Julius, 13, 106, 519, 557, 686-689, 693
Caius, John or Kaye, 589, 734-738, 746
Cajetanus, Cardinal, 567
Calcar, Stephan, 627
Caliazzo De Sophia, 388
Calimet, Don, 546
Calot, Germain, 177, 678-679
Calvin, John, 629, 634-635
Cambyses, 106, 557
Campalogo, Emilio, 595, 751
Campanella, Tomaso, 581
Campbell, 166, 173
Canano, Giovanni Battista, 621-622, 640, 755
Canappe, Jean, 454-455
Capho, 247
Capilius Pector, 337
Capodilista, Count Sigismonde, 745
Carabelli, 528
Carbonari, Gregory, 415
Cardan, Fazio, 726
Cardan, Jerome, 595, 725-728
Cardona, 543
Carnarius, 51
Cartier, Jacques, 741
Carus, 519-520

828

Casanova, 749
Casserius, Julius, 654
Cassiodorus, Archius, 11, 28, 71, 77-79, 313
Castiglioni, 334, 336
Catherine II, of Russia, 411
Catherine De Medici, 596, 749
Cato, 518
Celli, 518
Cellini, Benvenuto, 38, 717, 761
Celsus, 38, 206, 353, 446, 469, 505, 508-509, 517, 527, 539, 552, 580-581, 605, 678, 739
Cesalpinus, Andrea, 622-625, 638, 643, 647, 654, 713
Chabas, 114
Chalmley, H. P., 376
Chamberlen, Hugh, I, 689-690
Chamberlen, Hugh II, 689, 691
Chamberlen, John, 690
Chamberlen, Paul, 690
Chamberlen, Peter I, 689, 691
Chamberlen, Peter II, 689, 691
Chamberlen, Peter III, 691
Chamberlen, William, 689
Chancellor, Richard, 415
Champier, 453
Chapman, Edward, 691
Charaka, 517
Charcot, 242
Charlemagne, 30, 79, 197, 261, 301, 339, 384-385, 491
Charles IV, Emperor, 323, 387, 392
Charles V, Emperor, 627-629, 633, 710, 722
Charles of Anjou, 242, 247, 322
Charles I of England, 477, 654
Charles II of England, 478, 480
Charles III of France, 718
Charles V of France, 449, 595
Charles IX of France, 668-669, 676
Charles VII of Portugal, 715
Charles VIII of France, 345, 525, 536
Charles the Bald, King, 339
Chasdai Ben Isaac Ibn Shaprut, 170, 223, 242-244, 257
Chaucer, Geoffrey, 364, 371, 584
Chiari, Johann, 639
Chilperic, King, 339

Chinchon, Countess of, 743
Christ, Jesus, 19-20, 32, 39, 89, 105, 130, 362, 480, 555, 587, 634
Christina of Sweden, 652, 762
Ciasca, 332, 421
Cicero, 25, 585
Cild, 360, 362
Clair, Saint, 35
Claudius, Emperor, 534
Clement III, Pope, 623
Clement IV, Pope, 269
Clement V, Pope, 398
Clement VI, Pope, 354, 572
Clement VII, Pope, 713
Clement of Alexandria, 20
Cleomedes, 290
Clesius, Bernardus, 659
Clovis, King, 338, 480
Clowes, William, 450, 592, 679, 681-683
Cockayne, Rev. Oswald, 360
Codronchi, Batista, 743
Cole, William, 650
Colet, John, 518, 589
Colinaeus, 583
Collins, Samuel, 415
Columbus, Christopher, 526, 537, 719, 721
Columbus, Realdar, 627, 635, 636, 638, 643, 654, 658, 694
Confucius, 89
Constantine Africanus, 7, 38, 164, 167-169, 285, 310, 318, 321-322, 365, 371, 394
Constantine the Great, 41-42
Cooper, 570
Copernicus, 310, 583-584, 631-632, 647, 746
Copho, 316-317
Copin, 248
Corbolensis, Aegidius, 310, 316, 391
Cordus, Euricius, 741
Cordus, Valerius, 590, 599, 659-661
Cornet, 729
Cosmas, Saint, 22, 38, 438
Crawford, 555
Culpepper, Nicholas, 605
Cunel, Jacob, 248
Curialti Da Tossignauo, 702-703
Curtius, Matthew, 453

Cuvier, 661
Cynewulf, 537
Cynfrid, 359
Cyriacus, Saint, 36

D

Da Cappi, Girolamo, 622
Da Carpi, Jacopo Berengario, 425, 621, 625
D'acosta, Cristoval, 762
Da Gama, Vasco, 741
Damian, Saint, 22, 38, 438
Da Monte, 595
Dante, 106, 557, 581
D'ascali, Cecco, 310
David, 37, 104, 561
David Ben Abraham Ben Mosses Ben Maimon, 235
David Ben Maimon, 221, 224, 244
David Ben Solomon, 243
David of Bourgneuf, 258
Da Vinci, Catarina, 618
Da Vinci, Leonardo, 581, 615-619, 621, 697, 700, 761
Da Vinci, Ser Piero, 618
De Blaise, Armengaud, 230
De Castel, Pierre, 591
De Castro, Benedict, 762
De Castro, Rodrigo, 762
Defoe, Daniel, 463
De Frigeis, Lazarus, 630
De Gradibve, Matthew, 620
De Haen, Anton, 759
De Hery, Thiery, 692, 749
Delator, George, 414
Della Porta, Giovanni Battista, 700-701
Della Spina, Alessandro, 293-294
Della Torre, Marcantonio, 611
Delmedige, Joseph Solomon, 763
Delmedigo, Elijah, 249
Demetrius of Apameh, 540
Democritus, 184, 265
Demosthenes, 55
Deninger, 527
De Pomis, David, 763
Derenberg, 322
De Renzi, 315, 320, 473

De Sandris, Giacomo, 652
Descarts, Joachim, 650
Descartes, Rene 648-651, 655-656
D'este, Cardinal, 754
De Vigo, Giovanni, 674, 677-678, 680
De Zerbis, Gabriello, 620
Diaz De Isla, Ruiz, 712
Di Azzolino, Pietro, 331
Di Credi, Lorenzo, 619
Diniz of Portugal 246
Dinus De Garbo, 308, 329, 334
Diocletian, 38, 438
Dioscorides, 11, 28, 44, 78, 134, 145, 189, 223, 250, 257, 307, 313, 349-350, 364, 371, 460, 587, 657-660, 754
Diocorus, 56
Dirlewang, Paul, 687
D'israeli, Isaac, 417
Dolan, 248
Dolet, Etienne, 581
Dominic, Saint, 5
Donders, 296
Donnolo or Abraham Ben Joseph, 250, 256-258, 315, 631
Drinkwater, 691
Dryander, Johann, 247, 425
Du Chesne, Joseph, 610
Du Crevis, 650
Dun, 360
Dunash Ibn Tumin, 166, 170
Dupony, 284
Dymphna, Saint, 35
Dyonisius, 454

E

Ebers, 507, 509, 539
Ebn Bahbul, 150
Eckard, 386
Eden, Richard, 721
Edward I of England, 371, 477, 575
Edward II of England, 374
Edward III of England, 461, 492
Edward IV of England, 448, 450, 670
Edward VI of England, 737
Edward the Confessor, King of England, 367, 477, 479, 555
Ehrlich, Paul, 722-723

Elias of Arles, 248
Eliezer Ben Jose, Rabbi, 497
Elinus, 316
Elisha, 490
Elisius, Jean Baptiste, 722
Elizabeth, Saint, 490
Elizabeth, Empress of Russia, 411
Elizabeth I of England, 667, 681, 701, 737, 750
El Malik El Mansur Jacub Ben Jusuf, 213
El Milik Al Mansur Gilavun, 196
Elzevir, 583
Elyot, Sir Thomas, 682
Endicott, Governor, 667
Engelhardt, Andrew, 415
Ennodius, 71
Erasmus of Rotterdam, 581, 586-588
Erasmus, Saint, 35
Erastus, Thomas, 595
Erhard, Saint, 75
Erigena, 218, 261, 263
Ernst, Archbishop of Salzburg, 609
Es Jaffiah, 239
Euclid, 144, 289
Eudoxia, 15
Eustacchius, Bartolomeo, 636, 638
Eustathius, 46, 61
Eve, 266, 274
Evelyn, John, 478
Ezekiel, 108
Ezzeglin, 333

F

Fabricius, H., 654
Falco or Falcon, John, 452, 454
Falconer, William, 755
Falconieri, 295
Fallopius, 592, 622, 630, 635-638, 696, 715
Faraguth or Faragrius, 316, 339
Faraj Ben Salim, 247
Fasender, 693
Fayard of Perigueux, 455
Fedeles, Fortunato, 759
Felder, Hilarin, 5
Feliban, Michel, 470

Felix IV, Pope, 38
Ferdinand I of Portugal, 246
Ferdinand III of Castile, 245
Ferdinand of Florence, 762
Ferdinand the Catholic, 710
Fermicus III, 186
Fernel, John, 524, 596-597, 633, 739, 749, 757-759
Ferrari, 324
Ferrarius, 317-318
Ferri, Alfonse, 680
Ferronliere, La Belle, 716
Fetelle, Fortunato, 743
Fiacre, Saint, 35
Fileffo, Francesco, 505
Floridus, Macer, 381
Flourens, P., 623
Fouquet, 528
Fracastoro, Gerolamo, 525, 703-708, 728, 743
Francis, Saint, 5, 35, 429
Francis I of France, 581, 671, 673, 716
Francis II of France, 676
Franco, Piere, 692
Franklin, Benjamin, 297
Frazer, 555
Fredrick I, Emperor, 325
Frederick II, Emperor, 82-83 320, 340, 390, 420, 438
Frederick III, Emperor, 589
Freind, Doctor, 7, 56, 150
Frerichs. F. T., Von, 522
Freud, Sigmund, 547-548, 554
Friedlander, M., 236
Friedrich, Isaac, 397
Froben, 583
Frobinus, 608
Fuchs, Leonard, 658-660
Fulcher, 575

G

Gabriele Mussi, 461
Galeazzi, Giovanni, 323
Gale, Thomas, 679-681
Galen, 3, 5-7, 11, 18, 24-28, 44-48, 51, 53-54, 58-61, 65, 68, 78, 80, 83, 115-118, 140, 145-146, 149-150, 152-154, 157-159, 164-165, 170, 173-175, 179, 202,

831

207, 209-213, 217, 222-223, 227-228, 231, 241, 243, 246, 251-252, 268, 273, 277, 279, 285, 303, 305-309, 313, 316, 322, 328-330, 332, 335, 338-339, 349, 365, 370-371, 382, 391, 393-394, 416-417, 419-420, 423, 425, 440, 442, 446, 451, 454, 456-457, 460, 466, 472, 477, 488, 495, 499, 504, 510, 520, 527, 535-536, 539, 541, 583, 588-589, 591-592, 594-595, 598, 600, 602, 606-609, 614-617, 622, 625, 630, 632, 636, 638, 641-642, 655, 663-664, 697-698, 702, 739, 744, 747, 752, 754, 756
Galilei, Galileo, 295, 581, 584, 610, 645-648, 651, 763
Galile, Vincenzo, 647
Gall, Saint, 38
Gallioi, Johann, 388
Garcia Da Orta, 762-763
Garipontus, 316-317
Garrison, Colonel F. H., 61, 173, 260, 756
Gaspard, 555
Gastfreund, J., 102
Gedaliah Ibn Yahia the Elder, 246
Gedaliah Ibn Yahia the Younger, 246
Genseric, 15
Gentile Da Foligno, 334, 457
George, Saint, 39
Gerard of Cremona, 145, 150, 167, 178, 201, 537
Gerbert, Later Pope Sylvester II, 31, 261, 339
Gerhard, William Wood, 731
German, Saint, 36
Gernandez Oviedo Valdez Gonsalvo, 721-722
Gersdorff, 592
Gervasius, Saint, 35
Gesner, Conrad, 658-661
Gete, Saint, 35
Ghazi, 490
Gibbon, Edward, 3, 20, 199, 357
Giffard, William, 691
Gilbertus Anglicus, 285-287, 345, 350, 365, 371, 373, 486
Gilbertyn, 365
Giles, Saint, 35, 524

Gillies, 472
Giovanni Da Ravenna, 586
Giovanni De Vigo, 453
Girling, Mrs, 568
Givnti, 583
Glavcon, 78
Godfrey of Bovillon, 577
Godin, Nicholas, 453
Godunof, Boris, 400, 409
Goethals, Heinrich, 294
Gohory, Jacques, 610
Golgi, 522
Goliath, 105
Gonsalez De Velasgo, Pedro, **635**
Gothard, Saint, 34, 38
Gottschalk, 575
Graciano, Zerahiah, 631
Gram, 77
Grangier, 667
Grapheus or Grassus, 316
Grasset, 345
Gregory of Nazianzus, 24
Gregory of Nissa, 22-24
Gregory of Tours, 29, 33, **482**
Gregory IX, Pope, 82
Gregory X, Pope, 277, **537**
Gregory, Saint, 4, 11, 69
Grimani, Cardinal, 248
Grimbald, 339
Griphis, 452, 454
Grocyn, William, 581, 589
Gryphius, Sebastian, 591
Guarino Da Verona, 586
Guglielmini, Domenico, 653
Guibert De Nogent, 340
Guidi, Guido, 595, 629
Guillemeau, Jacques, 692
Guinterius Von Andernach, Johannes, 64
Guise, Duke of, 453
Gunther, Johann, 633
Gunther Von Andernach, 595, 625, 747
Guntram, King of Burgundy, 340
Gutenberg, John, 582, 661
Gutleben, 397
Guy, Saint, 34
Guy De Chauliac, 226, 227, 295, 331, 345, 350, 352-355, 383, 392, 421, 426, 438-439, 442, 451-454, 461, 672

H

Hadrian, Emperor, 418
Haeser, 308, 395
Hagenau, Countess, 695
Hakim Imad-El Mahmud Ibn Mascud Ibn Mahmud, 537
Hall, John, 587
Halle, John, 450
Haller, 354
Haly, Count, 209
Haly Ibn Al Abbas, 319-321, 365, 371, 427, 456-457, 471, 484-485, 501-502, 506, 541, 553
Hamilton, Archbishop of St. Andrews, 727
Hammond, 429
Hamza, 112, 433
Hananeel of Amalfi, 246
Hansen, 494
Harrington, Sir John, 763
Harun Al Rashid, 9, 116, 134-135, 137, 139, 143, 328
Harvey, Eliab, 655
Harvey, Thomas, 656
Harvey, Sir William, 24, 337, 623, 629, 635, 637-638, 643-644, 654-656, 692, 696, 745-746, 756
Hays, Dr. Isaac, 298
Heckr, A. F., 462
Hecker, J. F. C., 561-562, 570
Heinrich Von Pfolspeundt, 395-396
Heliodorus, 45, 430
Hellin, 595
Helmholtz, 54
Heloise, 76
Henri De Mondeville, 226, 328, 345, 350, 352-353, 355, 438-440
Heurrnis, Johann, 743
Henry II of England, 368-369, 575, 578
Henry III of England, 370
Henry VII of England, 477
Henry VIII of England, 450, 578, 589, 714, 732
Henry I of France, 414
Henry II of France, 676, 758
Henry IV of France, 651
Heraclius, 59
Herbert, Saint, 35

Herbst or Oporinus, 583, 631
Hercules, 106, 551
Herman, William, 679
Herman Von Treysa, 388
Herod of Judea, 526
Herodotus, 113, 569
Heron, 144
Herophilus, 24, 688
Hierax, 509
Hildanus, Fabricius or Wilhelm Faby, 684-685
Hildebert, 281
Hildebrandt, Philippe, 529
Hildegard of Bingen, Saint, 38, 281-283, 385
Hippocrates, 5-7, 11, 27-28, 48, 51, 53, 64-65, 68, 78, 80, 83, 89, 117, 130, 134, 140, 145-147, 152-154, 158-159, 164, 166, 170, 174-175, 222-223, 228, 231, 242, 245, 251-252, 267, 273, 277, 285-286, 303, 305-309 313, 317, 322, 328, 330, 339, 343-344, 348-350, 365, 370, 382, 391, 393-394, 419, 446, 453, 465-457, 466, 474-477, 495, 498, 500, 503-504, 509, 515-516, 520, 522, 526, 534-536, 551-553, 581, 583, 588-589, 591-592, 594-595, 607, 614-615, 641, 653, 657, 739-740, 743, 747, 752, 754, 759
Hirsch, 165, 738
Hirschfeld, H., 102
Hitler, Adolf, 642
Hoffmann, Erich, 722
Hohenheim, Wilhelm Von, 605
Holbein, 490, 760
Holcomb, R. C., 532-533, 709
Holmes, Oliver Wendell, 75, 667
Homer, 137, 567, 585
Honorius, 16, 240
Honorius III, Pope, 326
Honorius IV, Pope, 334
Honorius XII, Pope, 328
Horace, 314, 585
Hubaish Ibn Al-Hasan, 141, 147, 154, 167
Hugh of Lucca, 307, 330
Hugo, 308
Huham, John, 503
Hume, David, 714

833

Hunain Ibn Ishaq, 8, 47, 132, 139, 141, 145-148, 154, 164, 223, 226, 328
Huntington, 564
Husk, 729
Huygens, Constantine, 647
Hygeia, 37
Hyrtle, Joseph, 426

Isa, Ibn Yahia, 47, 141, 147-148
Ishaq Ibn Amran Al Baghdadi, 165
Ishaq Ibn Imran the Younger, 241
Ishmael, 112, 239, 433
Isidore of Sevilla, 11, 28-29, 38, 81
Israel Ben Joseph, 630
Ivan III of Russia, 400, 413
Ivanchenco, 407

I

Iarospolk, 402
Ibn Abi Usabia, 146, 234, 242
Ibn Al Baiter, 241
Ibn Al Baxthor, 142
Ibn Al Haitham, 140, 271, 276
Ibn Al Maulim, 222
Ibn Hanbal, 138
Ibn Hayan, Abu Musa Jabir, 10
Ibn Janah, 223
Ibn Julful Al Tamimi, 223
Ibn Khordadhbeh, 238
Ibn Masawaih, 132, 137, 141, 143-145, 146, 154
Ibn Tufail or Abubacer, 215
Ibn Wafid, 223, 229
Idris, Imam, 241
Ifa Ibn Shalahta, 134
Imram Al Isra Ali, 325
Ingrassias, Julius Caesar, 638
Innocent III, Pope, 428
Innocent IV, Pope, 299
Innocent VI, Pope, 325
Innocent VIII, Pope, 589
Irnerius, 323
Isaac, 55
Isaac, Rabbi, 248
Isaac, Ben Obadiah Maimonides, 235
Isaac Ben Shaprut, 243
Issac Ben Shealtiel, 227, 229
Isaac Ben Shem Tob, 246-247
Isaac Ibn Sid, 240
Isaac Israeli, 165-170, 238, 240, 242-243, 308
Isaac Judaeus, 8, 274, 285, 303, 322, 520, 530
Isa Ben Ali or Jesus Haly, 141, 145-146
Isaiah, 22, 513
Ishaq Ibn Amram, 240

J

Jabir or Geber, 8, 185-186, 188-190
Jabril (Gabriel) Ben Baktishua, 134-135, 143, 328
Jabril Ben Obeidullah, 136
Jacob, 39, 55, 102, 107, 432
Jacob Ben Ishaq, 235
Jacob Ben Obadiah Maimonides, 235
Jacob Ibn Machir, 343
Jacob of Forli, 308
Jacob, the Jewish Physician, 212
Jacobs, Joseph, 194
Jacque, 308
Jacquesmeau, 701
Jaeger, 297
Jahja (Johannes) Ben Bakhtishua, 135
Jamerius Bruno De Longoburgo, 421
James I of England, 477, 654
James IV of Scotland, 719
James, Saint, 20, 36
Japhet of Acco, Rabbi, 221
Jardeno Di Rivalto, 293
Jefferson, Thomas, 488
Jehuda Ben Samuel Ben Abbas, 243
Jenner, Edward, 487.
Jensen, 526
Jenson, Nicholas, 207
Jerome, Saint, 21-22
Jhel-Al-Eddin, 97
Joab, 490
Joachim II of Brandenburg 760
Job, 101, 106
Job, Saint, 719
Jocelyn, 445
Jochmann, 729
Johanan of Zavda, 254, 256
Johannes Actuarius, 10, 45, 65-68, 489, 541

Johannes Platearius, 316-318
Johannitus, 305, 307, 349
John, King of Bohemia, 340
John II of Aragon, 246
John, King of Naples, 422
John I of Portugal, 246
John II of Portugal, 246
John I of Wurzburg, 397
John II of Wurzburg, 258-259, 397
John of Arderne, 373, 376-380
John of Avignon or Moses Ben Samuel, 761
John of Beverley, 359
John De Calabria, Sir, 324
John of Capua, 231, 246
John of Damascus or Yahia Ibn Serabi, 24, 143, 150, 165, 365, 371
John of Gaddesden, 345, 365, 370, 373-376, 381, 467, 533
John of Gaunt, 383
John of Milan, 317
John of Mirfield, 5, 284, 380-383
John of St. Amand, 80
John of Salisbury, 306, 345, 368
John of Tervisa, 494
John of Toledo, 318
John, Saint, 35, 39, 555
Jonah, 56, 107
Jonas, 687
Jordshis or Georgeus, 134, 141
Joseph, 90, 102, 107, 432
Joseph Ben Isaac Kimhi, 246
Joseph Ben Yehuda, 225
Joseph Ibn Vives Al-Lorqui or Hieronymus De Santa Fe, 246
Joseph, King of the Chazars, 244
Joseph of Salerno, 315
Josephus, 526
Joshua Ben Chananyah, Rabbi, 418
Joshua Ben Jacob Maimonides, 235
Joshua Ben Nun, 137, 240
Joshua of Salerno, 315
Jossel, Doctor, 397
Judah Ben Asher, Rabbi, 259
Judah Ben Bathrai, 183
Judah Ben Joseph Ibn Al Fakhkhar, 245
Judah Ha-Levi, 245
Judah Ibn Shoshan, 220

Judah Ibn Tibbon, 246
Julianus Apostata, 45-46
Julius II, Pope, 679, 754
Justinian, 3, 51, 57, 87, 460, 471-472
Jusuf, Prince, 215
Juvenal, 429-430

K

Karakech, Tartar Prince, 413
Karun, 124
Kenbel, 691
Kepler, 180, 697-698
Kerler, 34
Khalid Ibn Yazid Ibn Muswiya, 141, 143, 186
Kimhi, David, 170
Kircher, Athanasius, 565
Klebs, Edward, 499, 522
Klein G., 396, 687
Kobad of Persia, 240
Koch, Robert, 503, 743
Kohl, 404
Kolman, 472
Kosta Ibn Luka, 141, 148
Krogman, 528
Kroner, Doctor, 232
Kuechler, 297
Kunrat Von Ammenhausen, 258
Kunrat Von Megenberg, 75, 393

L

Laban, 98
Lactan Tius Firmianus, 24-25, 538
Ladislaus of Naples, 715
Lafargue, 113
Laguna, Andres A., 761
Lancisi, 636
Lane-Poole, Stanley, 9
Lanfranc, 262, 284, 346, 350-352, 376-377, 381, 392, 421, 437-438, 451, 531, 533
Lang, Matthew, Bishop of Gurk, 720
Lange, Johannes, 614-615
Langerhans, 544
Largus, Scribonius, 526

835

Lartet, 528
Latimer, William, 589
Laurentius, Andreas, 701
Laveran, Charles Louis Alphonse, 522
Layard, Sir John, 289
Lazzarus, Saint, 35, 55, 576
Lazzi, Solomon, 337
Le Baron, 527
Lecky, 42
Leclerc, 61
Leibnitz, 656
Lemery, Nicolas, 668
Le Monnier, 713
Leo X, Pope, 701, 711
Leo XIII, Pope, 432
Leo Africanus, 181, 209, 220, 533
Leon the Armenian, Emperor, 139
Leon the Jew, 423
Leonicenus, Nicolo, 534-536, 538, 588-589, 614-615, 712
Leonides, 51, 53-54
Leopold I, Emperor, 415
Leopold, Duke of Austria, 444
Levret, 691
Lignanime, J. P., 661
Linacre, Thomas, 588-589, 623, 738, 749
Littell, Doctor, 297
Litzmann, 695
Livingstone, 112
Locartus, 509
Locke, John, 655-656
Loeffler, 499
Loesch, 507
Lombroso, Cesare, 557
Long, Crawford Williamson, 446
Lopez De Villalobos, Francisco, 708-710
Lopez, Don, 743
Lorci, Joshua, 631
Lorenz of Bibra, 397
Lorenzo De Medici, 581
Lot, 100
Lotio, Saldmone, 745
Louis of Bavaria, 571, 581
Louis X of France, 437, 439
Louis XI of France, 303, 678
Louis XII of France, 452, 581
Louis XIII of France 762
Louis XIV of France, 715, 744
Louis the Bald, 397

Lucretius, 99, 518, 706
Lucy, Saint, 35-36
Luke, Saint, 22, 36, 39
Lullius, Raymondus, 190
Lusitanus, Abraham Zacutus, 755-757
Lusitanus, Amatus, 246, 595, 622, 639-640, 657-659, 663, 743, 746, 751-755, 761
Lusitanus, Dionysius, 595
Luther, Martin, 584, 587, 595, 597, 610, 759
Luyev of Lubek, Nicolo, 414
Lydgate, 296

M

Macbeth, 479
Macchiavelli, Niccolo, 581
Macquer, P. J., 668
Maezukowski, 729
Magdalen, 577
Maggi, Bartolomeo, 679
Magitot, 527
Magnetus, 679
Magnus, 68
Maimonides or Moses Ben Maimon, 6, 8, 141, 201, 219-236, 242-243, 245-246, 263, 520
Main, Saint, 35
Malgaigne, Jos. F., 753
Malpighi, Marcello, 644-645, 651
Manardi, Giovanni, 591, 658, 743
Manfred, King of Naples, 33
Maninot, Gilbert, 339
Mantino, Jacob, 249
Manu, 89
Manuel, Eunuch, 431
Manuel I of Portugal, 761
Manzoni, Allessandro, 463
Marcella, Saint, 719
Marcellus, Saint, 524
Marcellus Empiricus, 338, 501, 529
Marcus Aurelius, 450
Margaret, Saint, 35, 39
Maria de Medici, 762
Marianos, 143
Marianus, 69
Maribif, 339

Marie of Vienna, 687
Marinus, 289
Marius, Bishop of Avenchia, 481, 742
Mar, Joseph, 251
Mar Mor, 251
Mar Samuel, 251-152, 520
Mark Anthony, 706
Mark, Saint, 296
Maron, 519
Marsh, Adam, 269
Marsilius, 390
Martial, 519, 750
Martin IV, Pope, 294
Martin V, Pope, 348, 397
Martin, Saint, 27, 33, 35
Martyr, Peter, 721
Mary I of England, 737
Mary the Jewess, 184
Mary, Virgin, 39, 93, 130, 470
Masari, Alessandro, 758
Masarjawaihi, 141- 142, 154, 241
Masawaih Al Marindi, 180
Maschus, John, 713
Masona, 81
Massa, Nicolo, 743, 749, 758-759
Mathurin, Saint, 35
Mattheolus or Mattioli, Pietro Andrea, 590, 657-659, 663
Matthew, Saint, 296, 429
Matthews, C. S., 729
Matthias, King of Hungary, 340
Maur, Saint, 35
Maurice, Emperor of Byzance, 713
Maurice of Orange, 651
Mauriceau, François, 690, 693
Maurolicus, Franciscus, 697, 700
Maximilian I, Emperor, 413, 536, 538, 710, 719
Maximus, 519
Macia, Doctor, 510
McGruder, 729
Mead, William, 337
Meckel, J. F., 522
Mehring, 544
Melanchthon, Philip, 614, 749
Melchior, 555
Mendel, Gregory, 31
Mercuriale, Gerolamo, 755
Mercurio, Scipione, 693

Merianus, 186
Mersenne, 651
Meryon, Edward, 375
Meshullam Ben Avigdor, 248
Mesue, 8, 530, 606-607
Mesue Junior, 181
Metlinger, Bartholomaeus, 394-395
Metrodorus, 56
Meyerhof, 159
Meyscheider, Abraham, 699
Michael, 135
Michael De Capella, 165
Michael, Saint, 477
Michelangelo, 12, 277, 581, 615, 647, 761
Middeldorpf, 395
Mikhail Fiodorovich, Tsar, 415
Mill, David, 101
Milo of Crotona, 20
Minkowski, 544
Miriam, 93, 490
Modestus, Saint, 35
Mohammed, 61, 86-89, 91, 93-96, 101-103, 105-112, 114, 121-112, 128, 132-133, 136, 145, 556
Moliere, 106
Mondella, Aloysia or Luigi, 743
Mondino Da Luzzi, 306-307, 325, 328, 331-333, 421-426, 615, 619, 621, 625, 638
Montagu, Lady Mary Wortley, 487
Montalto, Eliahu or Philoteus, 762
Montanus or Da Monte, 737, 743, 751
Montejan, 673
Montgomery, 37
Montgomery, Comte De, 676
Moore, Norman, 681
More Thomas, 581
Mortier, 557
Morton, William, Thomas Green, 446
Moses, 37, 39, 89, 93-94, 105, 290, 490, 520, 526
Moses Ben Abraham Maimonides, 235
Moses Ben Solomo Faraj, 242
Moses Ben Samuel Ibn Tibbon, 229, 231, 245
Moses Ibn Al Jazzar, 245
Moses Solomon, 246
Moses, the Physician, 248
Mosley, Benjamin, 487

837

Mourat, 489
Muawiyyah I, Caliph, 241
Mohammad Ibn Abdullah of Granada, 128
Muhammad Ibn Zuhr Al Ijadi, 213
Muller, Johann, 586
Munk, S., 236
Muntner, 250
Murat, 112
Muratori, 725
Musa Ben Abraham Al Hodaith, 150
Mydorge, Claude, 651

N

Nacht, A., 297
Napoleon, 106, 322, 557
Nathan Ha-Meati, 227-228, 245-246
Nathan, Rabbi, 504
Nathaniel Israeli, 243
Nemchin, Anton, 413
Nemesius, 24-25, 638
Nepotian, 21
Nerino, 422
Nero, 290
Nestor of Russia, 400-402
Nestorius, 28, 70, 81, 129-132, 137, 145, 184
Neuberger, Max, 81, 161
Newbold, 272
Newton, Sir Isaac, 295, 647
Nicholas, 244
Nicholas, the Child Crusader, 575
Nicholas IV, Pope, 343
Nicholas V, Pope, 580
Nicholas Davydovich, Prince of Chernigov, 414
Nicholas of Cusa, 270
Nicholas of Salerno, 303, 305, 316-318, 331
Nicolaus De Gevicka, 388
Nilus, Saint, 256
Nola, F., 499
Noldecke, Theodor, 482
Nostradamus, Michael, 728
Nufer, Jacob, 686
Numa Pompilius, 686, 689
Nur Ad Din, Sultan, 224, 229

Nushirwan the Just or Chosroes or Kisra, 133, 142

O

Obadiah Ben Abraham Ben Moses Ben Maimon, 235
Obadiah Ben Isaac Maimonides, 235
Obadiah of Bertinoro, Rabbi, 513
Obeidallah Ben Jabril Ben Baktishua, 136
Occam, William, 2, 266, 581
Odoacer, 16
Oleg, 402
Olivares, Pontanus, 753
Olympus, 56
Omar, Caliph, 61, 198, 240
Oribasius, 10, 45-47, 50-51, 57, 61-62, 140, 154, 164, 201, 460, 489
Origen, 429
Osenburg, Ivan, 415
Osler, Sir William, 324, 522, 736-737
Ovid, 17, 155, 463
Oxa, 360

P

Paback, 38
Palasiano, Coluccio, 590
Paleolog, Andrei, 413
Pales, L., 527
Palevy, 413
Panacea, 37
Panis, Nicolas, 452
Paracelsus, Theophrastus von Hohenheim, 99, 550, 592, 597-614, 662, 668, 676, 683-684, 712-713, 728
Paravicius, 212
Pare, Ambroise, 455, 592, 595, 665-668, 671-677, 679-680, 688, 692, 695, 697, 699, 751
Pare, Jean, 673
Parrot, 527
Parsons, F. G., 424
Pasquale, the Physician, 258
Patin, Guy, 445
Patrick, Saint, 80

Paul III, Pope, 249, 700, 727
Paul IV, Pope, 755, 763
Paul of Aegina, 10, 45, 60-64, 140, 142, 150, 154, 159, 164, 186, 201-202, 205-207, 307, 316, 350, 361-362, 427, 437, 456, 489, 501, 506-507, 512-513, 529, 535, 540, 554, 697
Paul, Saint, 19-20, 296
Paulmier, Pierre, 634
Paynell, Thomas, 711
Pellarino, Jacob, 415
Pengestus, Bubalya, 339
Pernel, Saint, 34
Perugino, Pietro, 619
Peter, Saint, 73, 561
Peter Damiane, 569
Peter De Abano, 268, 270, 333-337
Peter of Merida, 81
Peter of Pisa, 261
Peter the Hermit, 574-576
Petrarch, 580, 582
Petrocellus or Petronius, 316-318
Petronius Maximus, 15
Petrus Hispanus or John XXI, Pope, 80, 268, 273, 276-277, 285, 345, 530
Petrus Lombardus, 266, 274, 347
Petrus Physicus, 392
Pevcer, Casper, 614, 759
Philagrius, 154
Philip II of Macedon, 41
Philip II of France, 368, 577
Philip IV of France, 278, 351-352, 439
Philip V of France, 493
Philip II of Spain, 630
Philip of Arlois, 248
Philiston, 568
Philomenus, 51-52
Philo Judaeus, 262
Pinel, Philippe, 559
Pisor, Simon, 712
Pitard, Jean, 341, 437, 439
Pitcairne, Archibald, 650
Pius IV, Pope, 745
Pius V, Pope, 728
Plantin, 583
Plato, 3, 58, 117, 114, 217, 262, 265, 285, 418, 517, 549-550
Plato of Tripoli 240
Platter, Felix, 638-639, 697, 700, 755

Platter, Thomas, 638
Pletsch, Solmomon, 397
Pliny, 11-12, 38, 44, 99, 189, 288, 290, 419, 432, 498, 519, 589-590, 657 661
Plutarch, 569
Pococke, 112
Pocockі, Doctor, 182
Poggio, Bracciolini, Gian Francesco, 717
Poll or Pol, Nicholas, 720-721
Polo, Marco, 290
Polychronus, 713
Pomet, 665
Pompey, 444
Porro, Eduardo, 688
Pose, W. C., 298
Poseidonius, 25, 444
Potiphar, 102
Poupart, 637
Prevost, Nicolo, 452
Priestley, Joseph, 446
Proclus, 289
Procopius, 460
Prowazek, 729, 731
Prujean, Francis, 655
Psammetich, 113
Pseudo, Apuleius, 661
Ptolemy, 139, 144, 241, 289, 584, 586
Puccineotti, 336
Pusey, William Allen, 525, 722
Puschmann, 51
Pyrrhus, 419, 480
Pythagoras, 25, 113, 285, 567

Q

Quaritch, 383
Qulhuman, 154

R

Rabelais, François, 345, 590-592
Rachael, 98
Rameses II, 114
Ramus, Petrus, 581
Raphael, 581, 615, 701

839

Rashdall, 302, 304, 368-369, 387
Rashi, 290
Redi, Francesco, 295
Rein, Saint, 719
Reovalis, 73, 339
Rhabanus Maurus, 385
Rhazes or Al Razi, Abu Bakr, 4, 6, 8, 115, 140, 142-143, 145, 149, 163, 168, 172, 190, 202-203, 207-208, 223, 226, 229, 241-243, 245-246, 285, 303, 307-309, 316, 321, 324, 328, 338, 349, 361-362, 365, 382, 391, 423, 427-428, 473, 482-484, 486, 489, 499, 502, 520, 530, 536, 540, 543, 550, 589, 606-607, 742
Richard Coeur De Lion, 224, 577
Richard, Master, 420
Richard of Wendover, 531, 537
Ricketts, 729-731
Ricord, Philip, 525
Robert, Duke of Normandy, 577
Robert De Grosseteste, 268-269, 275-276
Robert Guiscard, 7
Robert, King of Naples, 422
Robert of Lincoln, 271, 370
Robinson, Victor, 528
Robmonatz, J. M., 230
Roch, Saint, 35, 718
Rodriquez, 246
Roger II, of Sicily, 82
Roger Frugardi of Palermo, 318-320, 331, 381, 421, 439, 441-442, 672
Rogneda, 402
Rogvaled, 402
Roland of Parma, 318, 331, 421, 434, 442, 672
Rollo, John, 544
Romulus Augustulus, 1, 16
Roonhuysen, 691
Roscellinus, 264-266, 268, 345
Roslin, 258
Rösslin, Eucharius, 687-688, 692
Rousset, François, 687-688
Rudolph of Worms, 251
Rueff, 692
Ruelius, 658
Rufus of Ephesus, 47, 51, 53, 62-63, 140, 154, 285, 365, 371, 460
Rupert, Elector, 389

S

Saadyah Ben Yusuf, 8, 238
Sack of Mainz, 583
Sadili of Cairo, 513
Sahl Al Tabari, 151, 241-242
Said Ben Ahmad Ben Said, 165
Saladin, 222, 229, 242, 577
Saliceto, William of, 284, 328-330, 350, 353, 392, 421, 437, 439, 451-452, 530-531, 533
Salimbene, 340, 572
Salvet De Bourgnef, 258
Samberg, 525
Sam Tob Falaquere, 243
Samuel, 526
Samuel, Rabbi, 504
Samuel Abu Al Nasr Ibn Abbas, 235
Samuel Ibn Tibbon, 232-233, 236, 343
Samuel Ibn Wakar, 245
Samuel, the Physician, 248, 251
Santo De Barletta, Mariano, 678-679
Santro, Santrio, 645-646, 648, 651
Saporta, Antoine, 345
Saparto, Jean, 345
Saporta, Louis the Elder, 345
Saporta, Louis the Younger, 345
Sarah, 102
Sarah De Saint Gilles, 258
Sarah La Mirgesse, 258
Sarah of Wurzburg, 258-259
Sarton, George, 241, 250, 255, 315
Sassania, Ercole, 743
Saul, 104, 548
Schaudinn, Fritz, 507, 722
Scheiner, Christopher, 689
Schickele, 526
Schleiden, Matthias Jacob, 259-260
Schoeffer, Peter, 661
Schussler, 729
Scotus, Duns, 2, 263, 268, 581
Sebastian, Saint, 35, 38
Sedicus, 339
Seleme, Jean, 527
Seligman, 397
Sement, Saint, 35
Seneca, Lucius Annaeus, 290
Serapion, 365, 371, 502
Sergius, Saint, 135

Seronus, 692
Servetus, Michael, 629, 632-635, 638, 643-644, 654, 751
Setheldryth, Abbess, 359
Setzer, John, 633
Severino, Marco Aurelio, 499, 738
Severus, 55
Shakespeare, William, 479
Shammakh, 241
Shams Abdullah, 171
Shepps, Philip, 533
Sibelist, Doctor 415
Siegfried, 127
Sigerist, 396
Sigismund, Emperor, 81
Sigismundus Albicus, 392
Silva, Carvalho, 762
Silvaticus, G. B., 537
Simear, John, 403
Simon Bar Zeman Duran, 246
Simon De Cordo, 80
Sinan Ibn Thabit, 151
Singer, 3, 526
Sirianin, Peter, 414
Sixtus, Pope, 430
Skorokhodov, 406
Smellie, 691-692
Smith, 528
Snegirov, 410
Snellen, 297
Socrates, 265
Solomon Ben Joseph, 243
Solomon Ben Joseph Ben Ayyub, 246-247
Solomon Ben Nathan, 246
Solomon, Bonsenhor, 761
Solomon Ibn Gabirol or Avicebron, 9, 201, 245
Sophocles, 561
Soranus, 47-49, 51, 53, 55, 64, 350, 567, 688
Spencer, Herbert, 567
Spink, Martin, 204
Spinoza, 218, 296
Sprengel, Kurt, 65, 767
Steinschneider, 250, 257, 316
Steno or Stensen, Nicolas, 620, 650
Stephanus, Printer, 583
Stephanus of Tralles, 56

Stephen of Antioch, 165
Sternberg, 522
Stokeley, Thomas, 442
Stromayer, Casper, 685
Struthius, Josephus, 746
Stubbs, George, 287
Sudhoff, Karl, 525-528, 555
Suleiman the Magnificent, 615
Suleiman Ibn Al Musallim, 245
Sully, 676
Susruta the Hindu, 154, 517, 539-540, 543
Svatopolk Yaroslavich, Prince, 414
Sviatoslav, 402
Swift, 106, 637
Swinburne, 106, 557
Sydenham, Thomas, 345, 564, 566, 655
Sylvius, Jacques Dubois, 345, 625, 627, 629, 633, 637, 658, 668-669, 692
Syphilus, 704

T

Tacitus, 15, 385
Tagaultius, 479
Tahir Ben Hasin, 135
Tamasi-Crudeli, 522
Tancred, 577
Tarewta, 56
Tawaddud, 116-118, 124
Tertullian, 24
Thabet Ibn Corra, 126, 141, 145-146 154
Thabit, 436
Thabit Ibn Senan, 196
Thaddeus of Florence, 306
Theodoceus, 154
Theodore of Tarsus, 358
Theodore Severus, 508
Theodoric, King of the Franks, 72-73
Theodoric the Great, 28, 71-72, 301 313
Theodoric, the Physician of Bologna, 353, 355, 439
Theodoric of Cervia, 84, 533, 537
Theodorus Priscianus, 316
Theodosius the Great, 16, 240, 338, 529
Theodosious of Russia, Saint, 407

841

Theophilus, 10, 68, 198-199, 285, 512
Theophilus Protospatharius, 45, 59-60
Thomas, Saint, 36
Thomas A Becket, Saint, 368, 467
Thomas Da Sarzana, 580
Thomas of Cantimbre, 393
Thorndike, 277
Thucydides, 155, 460, 463, 477
Tilly, William of Selling, 588
Tingewick, Nicholas, 371
Titus, Emperor, 200
Tizian, Vecelli, 581, 631
Tongilius, 519
Torella, 714
Torrigiano, 308
Trajan, 86, 460
Traube. L., 544
Trautmann, Jeremias, 688-689
Trechsel, 633
Trincavella, Vittore, 595
Trotula, 316-317
Turgenev, 407
Turquet of Mayerne, Theodore, 663-664

U

Ubaid Allah Al Mahdi Al Karawani 241
Ucay, Gervais, 714
Urban IV, Pope, 389
Ursula, Saint, 39
Usamah Ibn Munquidh, 436
Uziah, 490

V

Valens, 46
Valentine, Saint, 35
Valentine, Basil, 599, 664
Valentinus I, 46
Valentinus III, 15
Valescus of Tarentum, 533
Valla, Giorgio, 587
Van Der Linden, 61
Van Der Poll, 691
Van Helmont, Jean Baptista, 611-614
Varignana, Guilelmo, 421
Van Leuwenhoeck, Anton, 296, 644

Varo, 25
Varro, Marcus Terentius, 518
Vassalli, 695
Venceslaus XI of Bohemia, 715
Venetianer, 250
Vesalius, Andreas, 337, 417-418, 426, 592, 595, 621-623, 625-633, 636-637, 639, 643, 657-658, 663, 668, 671, 675-676, 679, 694, 696, 737, 746, 751
Vicary, Thomas, 450, 679
Vicente, 494
Vierordt, 65
Villanueva, Hernando, 633
Villareal, Juan De, 741
Villemore, 595
Vincent, 189
Vindician, 528, 529
Virchow, Rudolf, 260, 490, 522
Virgil, 585, 706
Virgil, Polydore, 479
Vischer, 691
Visconti, Gian Galeazzo, 702-703
Vital Ben Isaac, 248
Vitelo, 180
Vitruvious, 519
Vittorino Da Feltre, 586
Vitus, Saint, 34-35, 551, 564-565
Vives, Juan Luis, 550-551
Vizisch, Joseph, 246
Vladimir, Emperor of Russia, 400-404, 411-412
Voltaire, 432
Von Bra, Hendrich, 741
Von Brumm, 685
Von Calcar, Johann, 631
Von Gersdorff, Hans, 683-684
Von Graffenberg, Johann Schenck, 758
Von Hutten, Ulrich, 662, 710-712
Von Lichtenfels, Cornelius, 509
Von Muschebroeck, Peter, 294, 418
Von Storchs, 280, 554
Von Wird, Frank, 740
Von Wochenberg, Johann, Tollat, 664

W

Waghabota, 517
Waite, 190

Walafried Strabo, 38, 385
Walcher, 204
Wallaston, Dr. William H., 297
Walmann, 51
Walsh, J. J., 749
Walter De Merton, 369
Walter the Penniless, 575
Walther the Physician, 388
Ward 193
Warton, Thomas, 620
Wartt, Doctor, 435
Warwick, Earl of, 681
Washington, George, 488
Washington, Martha, 488
Wate, Physician, 385
Waterhouse, Benjamin, 488
Weil, 729
Wei-Powei-Yang, 186
Welch, 522
Welchner, 693
Weyer, Johann, 687, 743
White, Joseph, 182
Wickersscheimer, 31
Widmann, Johannes, 536, 665
William the Conqueror, 339
William of Champeaux, 268, 346
William IV of Montpellier, 343
William VII of Montpellier, 248
William Christian of Orleans, 455
Williams, F. E., 527
Williams, H. V., 525
Willibrod, Saint, 561
Willis, Thomas, 543, 544
Willoughby, Percivall, 435
Winthrop, John, 667, 714
Wintraw, 29
Wiseman, Richard, 478
Wittington, 11, 198
Wolsey, Cardinal, 589, 714
Wood, Casey, 165
Woodall, John, 679
Wright, A. E., 525

Wurtz, Felix, 684
Wustenfeld, Ferdinand, 585
Wyclif, John, 371
Wyer, 583
Wynkyn De Worde, 583

X

Xenophon, 585

Y

Yakub Ibn Ishaq, 137
Yohanan, Rabbi, 498
Young, Thomas, 297
Yperman, Jean, 350, 438, 672
Yusuf Al Saliti, 235
Yusuf Ibn Abdallah Abul Maali, 227

Z

Zachary, Saint, 35
Zacutus, Abraham of Spain, 756
Zambaco, Doctor, 533
Zarach, 316
Zecharia, 474
Zedekiah, 397
Zeno, Emperor, 130
Zeno of Cyprus, 45
Zerahiah Ben Isaac Ben Shealtiel, 227, 229, 246
Zerlin, 397
Zimmermann, J. G., 610
Ziyadat Allah II, 167, 241
Ziyadat Allah III, 241
Zoilus, 454
Zoroaster, 86, 89, 164
Zosimos of Constantinople, 184
Zwingli, 711

DEC 0 8 2005